AF778932

AMERICAN ACADEMY OF
OTOLARYNGOLOGY–
HEAD AND NECK SURGERY
FOUNDATION

Thieme

Geriatric Otolaryngology

Robert T. Sataloff, MD, DMA
Professor and Chairman
Department of Otolaryngology–Head and Neck Surgery
Senior Associate Dean for Clinical Academic Specialties
Drexel University College of Medicine
Philadelphia, Pennsylvania

Michael M. Johns, MD
Associate Professor of Otolaryngology
Director, Emory Voice Center
Emory University
Atlanta, Georgia

Karen M. Kost, MD, FRCSC
Assistant Professor of Otolaryngology–Head and Neck Surgery
Montreal General Hospital
Montreal, Quebec, Canada

64 illustrations

Thieme
New York • Stuttgart • Delhi • Rio de Janeiro

Executive Editor: Timothy Hiscock
Managing Editor: J. Owen Zurhellen IV
Editorial Assistant: Kate Barron
Production Editor: Kenneth L. Chumbley
International Production Director: Andreas Schabert
Senior Vice President, Editorial and E-Product Development: Cornelia Schulze
International Marketing Director: Fiona Henderson
International Sales Director: Louisa Turrell
Director of Sales, North America: Mike Roseman
Senior Vice President and Chief Operating Officer: Sarah Vanderbilt
President: Brian D. Scanlan

Library of Congress Cataloging-in-Publication Data

Geriatric otolaryngology (Sataloff)
Geriatric otolaryngology / [edited by] Robert T. Sataloff, Michael M. Johns III, Karen M. Kost.
p. ; cm.
ISBN 978-1-62623-977-7 (alk. paper) — ISBN 978-1-62623-978-4 (eISBN)
I. Sataloff, Robert Thayer, editor. II. Johns, Michael M., editor. III. Kost, Karen M., editor. IV. Title.
[DNLM: 1. Otorhinolaryngologic Diseases. 2. Aged. WV 140]
RF47.A35
618.97'751—dc23
2014044051

© 2015 Thieme Medical Publishers, Inc., and American Academy of Otolaryngology–Head and Neck Surgery Foundation
Thieme Publishers New York
333 Seventh Avenue, New York, NY 10001 USA
+1 800 782 3488, customerservice@thieme.com

Thieme Publishers Stuttgart
Rüdigerstrasse 14, 70469 Stuttgart, Germany
+49 [0]711 8931 421, customerservice@thieme.de

Thieme Publishers Delhi
A-12, Second Floor, Sector-2, Noida-201301
Uttar Pradesh, India
+91 120 45 566 00, customerservice@thieme.in

Thieme Publishers Rio de Janeiro, Thieme Publicações Ltda.
Argentina Building 16th floor, Ala A, 228 Praia do Botafogo
Rio de Janeiro 22250-040 Brazil
+55 21 3736-3631

Cover design: Thieme Publishing Group
Typesetting by Prairie Papers

Printed in India by Replika Press Pvt Ltd 5 4 3 2 1

ISBN 978-1-62623-977-7

Also available as an e-book:
eISBN 978-1-62623-978-4

Important note: Medicine is an ever-changing science undergoing continual development. Research and clinical experience are continually expanding our knowledge, in particular our knowledge of proper treatment and drug therapy. Insofar as this book mentions any dosage or application, readers may rest assured that the authors, editors, and publishers have made every effort to ensure that such references are in accordance with the state of knowledge at the time of production of the book.

Nevertheless, this does not involve, imply, or express any guarantee or responsibility on the part of the publishers in respect to any dosage instructions and forms of applications stated in the book. Every user is requested to examine carefully the manufacturers' leaflets accompanying each drug and to check, if necessary in consultation with a physician or specialist, whether the dosage schedules mentioned therein or the contraindications stated by the manufacturers differ from the statements made in the present book. Such examination is particularly important with drugs that are either rarely used or have been newly released on the market. Every dosage schedule or every form of application used is entirely at the user's own risk and responsibility. The authors and publishers request every user to report to the publishers any discrepancies or inaccuracies noticed. If errors in this work are found after publication, errata will be posted at www.thieme.com on the product description page.

Some of the product names, patents, and registered designs referred to in this book are in fact registered trademarks or proprietary names even though specific reference to this fact is not always made in the text. Therefore, the appearance of a name without designation as proprietary is not to be construed as a representation by the publisher that it is in the public domain.

MIX
Paper from responsible sources
FSC® C016779

This book, including all parts thereof, is legally protected by copyright. Any use, exploitation, or commercialization outside the narrow limits set by copyright legislation without the publisher's consent is illegal and liable to prosecution. This applies in particular to photostat reproduction, copying, mimeographing or duplication of any kind, translating, preparation of microfilms, and electronic data processing and storage.

To our families.

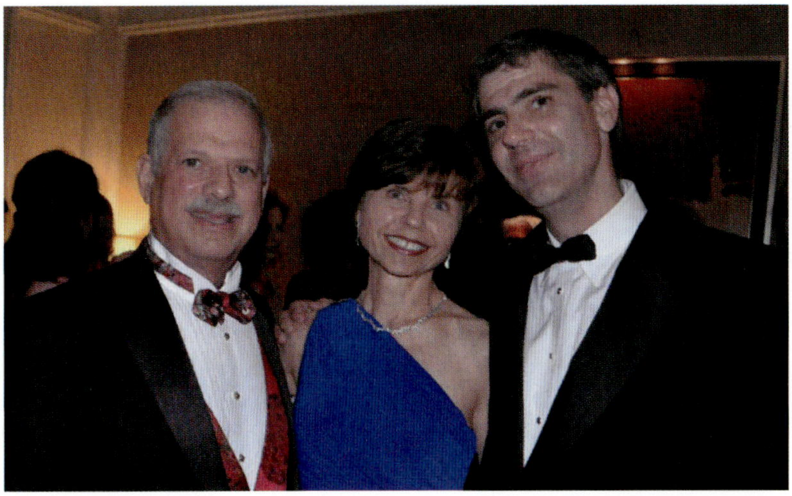

The editors (from left), Robert T. Sataloff, Karen M. Kost, and Michael M. Johns, at the 43rd Annual Voice Foundation Gala in Philadelphia, Pennsylvania, USA, May, 2014.

Contents

Foreword

Robert T. Sataloff, MD, DMA, FACS, has done it again, this time for the fiftieth time, and this time in collaboration with two expert colleagues Drs. Michael Johns and Karen Kost.

Geriatric Otolaryngology, published by Thieme and the American Academy of Otolaryngology–Head and Neck Surgery Foundation, represents the fiftieth book published by Dr. Sataloff. For this milestone book, he is joined by Dr. Michael Johns and Dr. Karen Kost. Bob is one of the most important and prolific writers in the field of otolaryngology and in Academic medicine. My relationship with Dr. Sataloff spans almost ten years, having had the privilege of recruiting him as professor and chair of the Department of Otolaryngology and Head and Neck Surgery and the senior associate dean for Clinical Academic Specialties at Drexel University College of Medicine, when I served as president and dean of the College of Medicine. During the search and recruitment process for the chairperson of the Department of Otolaryngology, I recall requesting that my executive assistant provide me the curriculum vitae of Dr. Sataloff for my review in preparation for my assessment of the candidates. At the time, it was customary for her to leave any important documents on my chair for my review upon returning to my office. Later that day, to my surprise, I saw a neatly stacked pile of documents, approximately three or four inches high, and I commented to my executive assistant that I did not need all of the curriculum vitae of all of the candidates, just that of Dr. Sataloff. She smiled and replied, "That is Dr. Sataloff's curriculum vitae, Dr. Homan."

Very few faculty members in academic medicine have been able to accomplish so much clinically and academically as Dr. Sataloff. He is the consummate physician, scholar, academician, and gentleman. He maintains an extremely busy practice and is world renowned in the fields of laryngology/voice disorders and neurotology. Nonetheless, in this edition of *Geriatric Otolaryngology,* Dr. Sataloff, with his coeditors Drs. Johns and Kost, has assembled a compendium which addresses the most common, acute, chronic, and disabling diseases and conditions which challenge every practitioner caring for the elderly in his field.

The demographics of our aging population continue to place extraordinary demands on clinicians, health care delivery systems, and payers. As a medical educator, primary care physician, and geriatrician, I recognize the urgent need to improve the skills of the healthcare workforce to address the needs of elderly patients across all specialties. Our role as physicians and health care professionals is to be best prepared to address conditions that are potentially treatable, while focusing on improvement of function to improve quality of life in the personalized context of the patient and family. *Geriatric Otolaryngology* will serve as an essential reference for those in the field of otolaryngology, as well as for many primary care physicians and other health-care professionals in need of improving their diagnostic and therapeutic expertise in a wide array of acute and chronic diseases afflicting the elderly. I congratulate Dr. Sataloff and his coeditors and contributors for publishing this important body of work.

Richard V. Homan, MD
Professor, Family and Community Medicine
CAQ, Geriatric Medicine
CAQ, Sports Medicine
President, Provost, and Dean
Eastern Virginia Medical School
Norfolk, Virginia

Foreword

The American Academy of Otolaryngology–Head and Neck Surgery is pleased to introduce *Geriatric Otolaryngology.* In keeping with its vision to empower otolaryngologist–head and neck surgeons to deliver the best patient care, this Foundation publication provides expert guidance and the most up-to-date information regarding the diagnosis and treatment of ear, nose, and throat disorders in the elderly.

As the population ages, education and training related to geriatric otolaryngology will become an important issue for healthcare providers of older adults. *Geriatric Otolaryngology* represents a complete and current textbook covering the entire field. Filling a major gap, this book provides the reader with increased knowledge of current research and advances in geriatric otolaryngology; greater competence in performing diagnostic and treatment measures to provide quality service to geriatric otolaryngology patients; and improved practice skills, abilities, and strategies for delivery of high-quality, evidence-based geriatric otolaryngology healthcare. This book is an essential resource for all physicians caring for the geriatric patient, from otolaryngologists to primary care physicians including residents, medical students, and allied health professionals.

Geriatric Otolaryngology is a welcome addition to the Foundation's vast collection of education programming. All of the Foundation's education initiatives support lifelong learning aimed at improving the quality of patient outcomes through knowledgeable, competent, and professional physicians. Thanks to a copublishing agreement with Thieme, the Foundation looks forward to continued production of high-quality and practical education opportunities for our members.

Drs. Sataloff, Kost, and Johns, along with the many contributors, are to be congratulated for their practical approach and comprehensive review. Their enthusiasm and passion for the specialty, and tireless dedication to the profession, are not only admirable but greatly appreciated.

Sonya Malekzadeh, MD
Coordinator, Education
AAO-HNSF

Preface

As the population ages, most otolaryngologists are seeing an increasing percentage of elderly patients. Just as pediatric otolaryngologists recognize that children are not small adults, otolaryngologists should understand that appropriate treatment of geriatric patients requires special knowledge and skills. This book was written to provide otolaryngologists with a comprehensive overview of the current principles of geriatric otolaryngology.

In the first chapter, Dr. Christian Sell and colleagues provide a succinct review of current concepts in the science of aging. This information is invaluable in helping otolaryngologists understand and advance clinical management. In Chapter 2, Dr. Karen Kost offers an overview of the practice of geriatric otolaryngology. Chapter 3 provides a summary of geriatric syndromes, as well as insight into the establishment of interdisciplinary teams for geriatric management. Dr. Kagan also offers information about resources to assist the otolaryngologist in providing optimal care for geriatric patients. In Chapter 4, Dr. David Eibling outlines the special aspects of outpatient clinical evaluation of older patients, and in Chapter 5, Drs. Justicz and Hatcher elucidate unique concerns for operative evaluation for the older patient. In Chapter 6, Drs. Parham, Lin, and Blakley discuss the latest concepts in presbycusis, one of the most common problems in otolaryngologic practice. Chapter 7 offers an elegant summary of research into regenerative treatments for sensorineural hearing loss, provided by Drs. Chow and Gubbels. In Chapter 8, Dr. Sataloff and colleagues outline the latest concepts in hearing aids, including new research suggesting that binaural amplification may not always be the best approach in elderly patients. Drs. Daniel Coelho and Brian McKinnon have contributed an excellent update on cochlear implantation in the elderly in Chapter 9. Tinnitus is an extremely common problem in older patients, and this subject is reviewed in detail by Drs. Shea and McKinnon in Chapter 10. Dizziness from aging and other causes is ubiquitous in elderly patients and may be life-threatening if it results in fall-related injury. Drs. Agrawal, Rubin, and Wetmore cover this topic in detail in Chapter 11. In Chapter 12, Dr. David Edelstein summarizes the state-of-the-art management of sinonasal disease in older patients, while in Chapter 13, Drs. Richard Doty and Hussam Tallab review the diagnosis and treatment of taste and smell disorders in older patients. In Chapter 14, Dr. Karen Calhoun provides insight into the special considerations in the clinical management of allergies and asthma in the geriatric population.

Diagnosis and treatment of voice disorders in the elderly are reviewed in depth by Drs. Sataloff and Kost in Chapter 15; and in Chapter 16, Dr. Ozlem Tulunay-Ugar summarizes the complex issues of managing swallowing disorders in older patients. Sleep disturbance is seen almost routinely in the geriatric population, and this complex subject is discussed in a clinically practical manner in Chapter 17 by Drs. Larsen and Gillespie. Facial plastic surgery is sought commonly by elderly patients who wish to look less elderly. Dr. J. Regan Thomas provides a superb review of this subject in Chapter 18. Disorders of the oral cavity are seen frequently in the geriatric population and are reviewed in elegant detail by Drs. Regenbogen and Trochesset in Chapter 19. Chapters 20 and 21 include comprehensive discussions of the management of cancer in older patients, and Drs. Malloy, Stucken, Patel, Chai, and Chalian stress important concepts that might make management different from that which would be offered to younger patients. In the final chapter, Drs. Swirsky-Sacchetti and Mosti have contributed a thorough discussion of the neuropsychological evaluation and treatment of geriatric patients. Cognitive assessment may be invaluable to the otolaryngologist in making decisions about treatment approaches and surgical management, including issues surrounding surgical consent.

Like all books on relatively new subjects, *Geriatric Otolaryngology* is not completely inclusive. Rather, it is intended to provide an introductory, comprehensive overview of selected topics. The discipline is evolving rapidly; we suspect that we will be well along in preparation of the second edition when the first edition is released. Nevertheless, we hope that our readers find this book informative, convenient, and clinically practical.

Contributors

Yuri Agrawal, MD
Assistant Professor
Department of Otolaryngology–Head and Neck Surgery
Johns Hopkins University School of Medicine
Baltimore, Maryland

Alessandro Bitto, PhD
Department of Pathology
University of Washington Medical Center
Seattle, Washington

Brian W. Blakley, MD, PhD, FRCSC
Professor
Department of Otolaryngology
University of Manitoba
Winnipeg, Manitoba, Canada

Karen H. Calhoun, MD, FACS, FAAOA
Professor
Department of Otolaryngology
The Ohio State University
Columbus, Ohio

Raymond Chai, MD
Assistant Professor
Department of Otolaryngology
Mount Sinai Beth Israel
New York, New York

Ara Chalian, MD
Professor
Member, Head and Neck Cancer Center
Reconstructive Surgery
Hospital of the University of Pennsylvania
Philadelphia, Pennsylvania

Cynthia L. Chow, BS
Department of Communication Sciences and Disorders
University of Wisconsin
Madison, Wisconsin

Daniel H. Coelho, MD, FACS
G. Douglas Hayden Associate Professor
Otologic and Neurotologic Surgery
Director, VCU Cochlear Implant Center
Department of Otolaryngology–Head and Neck Surgery
MCV/Virginian Commonwealth University School of Medicine
Richmond, Virginia

Richard L. Doty, PhD
Professor and Director
Smell and Taste Center
Perelman School of Medicine
University of Pennsylvania
Philadelphia, Pennsylvania

David R. Edelstein, MD, FACS
Chief, Otolaryngology–Head and Neck Surgery
Manhattan Eye, Ear, and Throat Hospital
Clinical Professor of Otorhinolaryngology–Head and Neck Surgery
Weill Medical College of Cornell University
Chairman-Elect, Board of Governors
American Academy of Otolaryngology–Head and Neck Surgery
New York, New York

David Eibling, MD, FACS
Department of Otolaryngology–Head and Neck Surgery
University of Pittsburgh
Pittsburgh, Pennsylvania

M. Boyd Gillespie, MD, MSc
Professor
Department of Otolaryngology–Head and Neck Surgery
Medical University of South Carolina
Charleston, South Carolina

Samuel P. Gubbels, MD, FACS
Assistant Professor and Waisman Center Investigator
Department of Surgery
University of Wisconsin School of Medicine and Public Health
Madison, Wisconsin

Jeanne Hatcher, MD
Assistant Professor
Department of Otolaryngology–Head and Neck Surgery
Emory University Hospital Midtown
Atlanta, Georgia

Mary Hawkshaw, BSN, RN, CORLN
Research Associate Professor
Department of Otolaryngology–Head and Neck Surgery
Drexel University College of Medicine
Philadelphia, Pennsylvania

Michael M. Johns, MD
Associate Professor of Otolaryngology
Director, Emory Voice Center
Emory University
Atlanta, Georgia

Natalie Justicz, BA
Emory University School of Medicine
Atlanta, Georgia

Sarah H. Kagan, PhD, RN
Lucy Walker Honorary Term Professor of Gerontological Nursing
School of Nursing
University of Pennsylvania
Philadelphia, Pennsylvania

Amanda Kantor, AuD, CCC–A
Instructor
Department of Otolaryngology–Head and Neck Surgery
Drexel University College of Medicine
Philadelphia, Pennsylvania

Karen M. Kost, MD, FRCSC
Assistant Professor of Otolaryngology–Head and Neck Surgery
Montreal General Hospital
Montreal, Quebec, Canada

Christopher G. Larsen, MD, FACS
Assistant Professor
General Otolaryngology
University of Kansas Medical Center
Kansas City, Kansas

Chad A. Lerner, PhD
Environmental Medicine
University of Rochester
Rochester, New York

Frank R. Lin, MD, PhD
Associate Professor of Otolaryngology-Head and Neck Surgery, Geriatric Medicine, Mental Health, and Epidemiology
Johns Hopkins University
Baltimore, Maryland

John Luckhurst, MS
Clinical Audiologist/Instructor
Department of Otolaryngology
Philadelphia Ear, Nose, and Throat Associates
Drexel University College of Medicine
Philadelphia, Pennsylvania

Kelly Michele Malloy, MD, FACS
Assistant Professor
Department of Otolaryngology–Head and Neck Surgery
Division of Head and Neck Surgical Oncology and Microvascular Reconstruction
University of Michigan School of Medicine
Ann Arbor, Michigan

Brian J. McKinnon, MD, FACS
Associate, Shea Ear Clinic
Clinical Associate Professor
Department of Otolaryngology–Head and Neck Surgery
University of Tennessee Health Sciences Center
Memphis, Tennessee

Erica Miele, BS
Advanced Audiology
Boran and Puzzi ENT Associates
Pottsville, Pennsylvania

Caterina B. Mosti, BS
Drexel University
Philadelphia, Pennsylvania

Kourosh Parham, MD, PhD, FACS
Associate Professor
Assistant Program Director
Director of Research
Department of SurgeryDivision of Otolaryngology–Head and Neck Surgery
University of Connecticut Health Center
Farmington, Connecticut

Mihir R. Patel, MD
Assistant Professor
Department of Otolaryngology–Head and Neck Surgery
Emory University
Atlanta, Georgia

Elliot Regenbogen, MD
Assistant Clinical Professor
Department of Surgery
Division of Otolaryngology–Head and Neck Surgery
Stony Brook University Medical Center
Stony Brook, New York

Allan Rubin, MD
Clinical Professor
Department of Surgery
Promedica Physician
Toledo, Ohio

Robert T. Sataloff, MD, DMA
Professor and Chairman
Department of Otolaryngology–Head and Neck Surgery
Senior Associate Dean for Clinical Academic Specialties
Drexel University College of Medicine
Philadelphia, Pennsylvania

Christian Sell, PhD
Department of Pathology and Laboratory Medicine
Drexel University College of Medicine
Philadelphia, Pennsylvania

Paul F. Shea, MD
Neurotologist
Shea Ear Clinic
Memphis, Tennessee

Chaz L. Stucken, MD
Clinical Assistant Professor
Department of Otolaryngology–Head and Neck Surgery
University of Michigan
Ann Arbor, Michigan

Thomas Swirsky-Sacchetti, PhD, ABPP-CN
Associate Professor
Psychiatry and Human Behavior
Jefferson Medical College
Philadelphia, Pennsylvania

Hussam F. Tallab, MD
Department of Otorhinolaryngology–Head and Neck Surgery
University of Pennsylvania School of Medicine
Philadelphia, Pennsylvania

J. Regan Thomas, MD
Mansueto Professor and Chairman
Department of Otolaryngology–Head and Neck Surgery
College of Medicine
University of Illinois at Chicago
Chicago, Illinois

Denise A. Trochesset, DDS
Associate Professor
Director of Oral Pathology
Department of Oral Biology and Pathology
School of Medicine
Stony Brook University
Stony Brook, New York

Ozlem E. Tulunay-Ugur, MD
Associate Professor
Director, Division of Laryngology
Department of Otolaryngology Head and Neck Surgery
University of Arkansas for Medical Sciences
Little Rock, Arkansas

Stephen J. Wetmore, MD
Romeo Yap Lim and Maria Corazon Wong Lim Chair
Department of Otolaryngology
West Virginia University School of Medicine
Morgantown, West Virginia

1 The Science of Aging

Alessandro Bitto, Chad A. Lerner, and Christian Sell

Introduction

The demographics of the developed world are shifting dramatically due to an increase in life expectancy and a decline in the fertility rate. By the year 2030, the U.S. Census Bureau projects that individuals aged > 65 years will make up almost 20% of the total population.[1,2] This represents an increase of 36 million in the > 65 age group, with an increase of 10 million among those aged > 80 years.[1] **Fig. 1.1** demonstrates the changing survival curve for the U.S. population based on data from the U.S. Social Security Administration projected out to 2100.[3] The survival curve becomes more "square" over time, indicating an increased time to first deaths, due largely to a decreased death rate in the first half of life. Mean lifespan increases dramatically, while the increase in maximum lifespan, represented by the final 10% of the population, is far from dramatic. The discrepancy between gains in mean and maximum lifespan can be understood if one considers that early life losses are primarily due to extrinsic factors, the impact of which were diminished over the past century through advances in sanitation and health care and the availability of antibiotics and vaccines.[4] The decrease in early life mortality produces the shifts in the survival curves seen in **Fig. 1.1**. The data for age-specific mortality broken down by 10-year intervals for the U.S. population in 1900, 1939, and 2000 (**Fig. 1.2**) indicate a reduction in mortality rates at all ages, with the most dramatic reduction in the first 15 years of life.[5] Interestingly, for all time periods examined, the lowest mortality rate occurs in the 5 to 14 year age group. The mortality rates increase

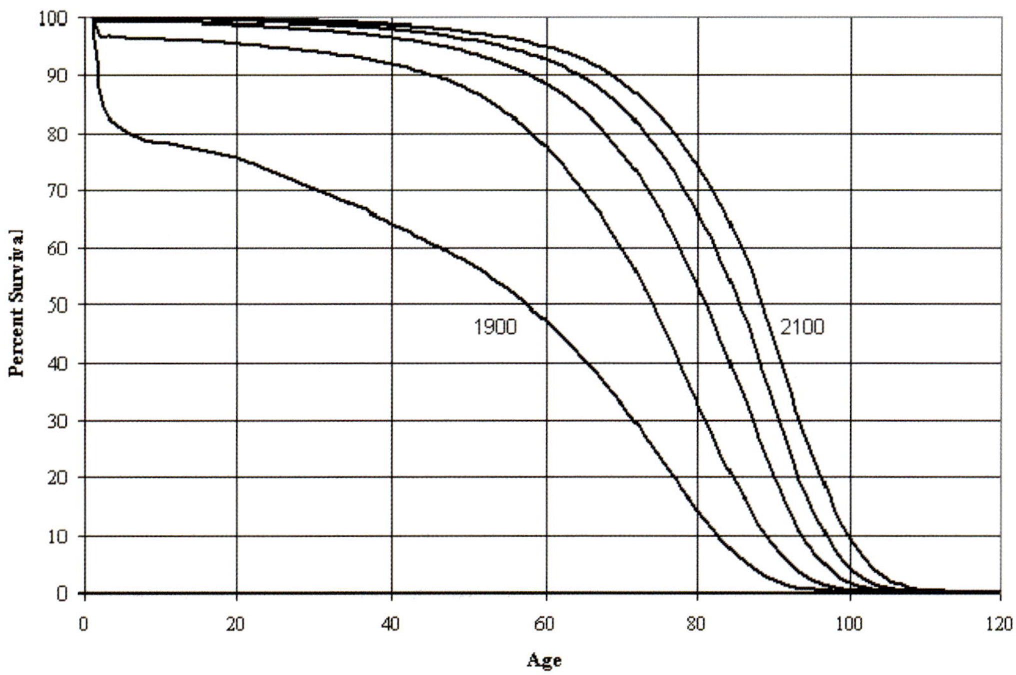

Fig. 1.1 Projected survival curves for the United States in the years 1900, 2000, 2025, 2050, and 2100. (From Bell FC, Miller ML. Life Tables for the United States Social Security Area 1900–2100. Actuarial Study No. 120. Social Security Administration; 2000. http://www.ssa.gov/oact/NOTES/as120/LifeTables_Body.html.)

with increasing age from this time on in all three populations. In contrast to mean lifespan, maximum lifespan exhibits only a modest increase, from 95 to 100 years, between 1900 and 2000. This reflects the fact that the intrinsic aging process has not been impacted to the same degree as the specific pathologies that underlie early life mortality.

Interestingly, the effects of the intrinsic aging process can be observed across species. For example, the mortality rate in mice, when examined as a percentage of lifespan completed, is very similar to that in humans (**Fig. 1.2**), despite a relatively abbreviated mouse lifespan, on the order of 2 to 3 years. Note that the shape of the polynomial trend line for the mouse mortality rate in **Fig. 1.3** exhibits a nadir early in life similar to that in humans (~ 10 years in **Fig. 1.2**). Similarly, a late-life rise in the mortality rate is evident in both species, beginning at ~ 50% of lifespan completed. In humans, this correlates with the 45 to 55 year age range. The similarity in mortality rate curves between the mouse and human suggests that the intrinsic rate of aging is similar in the two species, but it follows a very different trajectory in absolute terms. At the cellular level, the genomic stability of cells from these two species reflects this difference.

Cells from primary explants of tissues from multiple species have been tested for their growth properties.[6] Normal cells proliferate for a finite period and eventually undergo a growth arrest known as cellular senescence. The senescence growth arrest is a p53-mediated arrest that appears to serve multiple functions, including tumor suppression and immune activation.[7] Interestingly, cells from shorter-lived species such as the mouse demonstrate a greatly reduced genomic stability relative to cells from long-lived species such as humans. Mouse cells escape senescence and generate immortal transformed cell lines that have unstable genomes and exhibit multiple genetic rearrangements.[8] In contrast, human cells will transform spontaneously at a rate of less than 1×10^{-6}.[9] The difference in genomic stability between these species is thought to contribute to differences in the rates of both cancer and mortality.

Aging Is Characterized by an Increased Vulnerability to Disease

The most accurate definition of the aging process as it relates to an organism is that aging is characterized by an increasing inability to maintain homeostasis in multiple organ systems, giving rise to an increased vulnerability to disease. Data

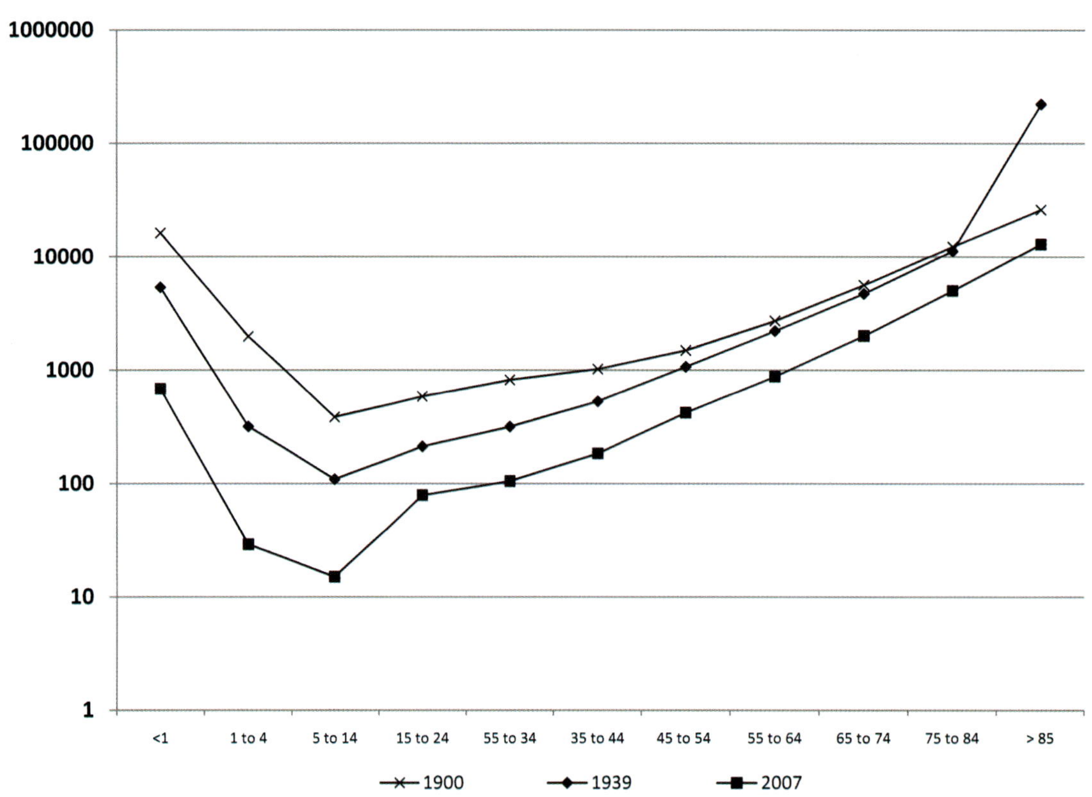

Fig. 1.2 Age-specific mortality rates for the United States in the years 1900, 1937, and 2000. (Calculated from Bell FC, Miller ML. Life Tables for the United States Social Security Area 1900–2100. Actuarial Study No. 120. Social Security Administration; 2000. http://www.ssa.gov/oact/NOTES/as120/LifeTables_Body.html.)

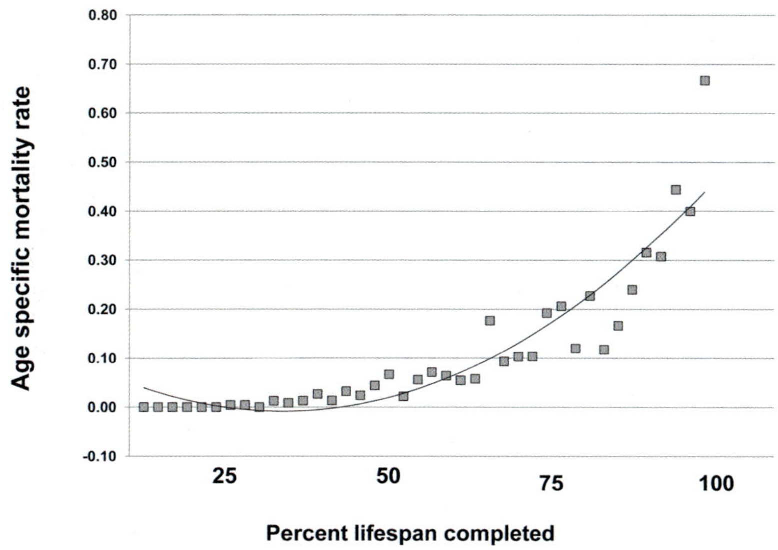

Fig. 1.3 Age-specific mortality rates in a laboratory mouse strain housed under pathogen-free conditions. (Data are recalculated from Lorenzini A, Salmon AB, Lerner C, et al. Mice producing reduced levels of insulin-like growth factor type 1 display an increase in maximum, but not mean, life span. J Gerontol A Biol Sci Med Sci 2014;69(4):410–419.)

from the Centers for Disease Control and Prevention support this definition. In **Fig. 1.4**, deaths per 100,000 population from cancer, heart disease, and cerebrovascular disease are shown as a function of age. Deaths from these diseases increase sharply in middle age and rise progressively thereafter, reflecting the greater vulnerability to multiple diseases in line with an intrinsic aging process. The inability to maintain homeostasis, which contributes to this vulnerability, is evident in the example

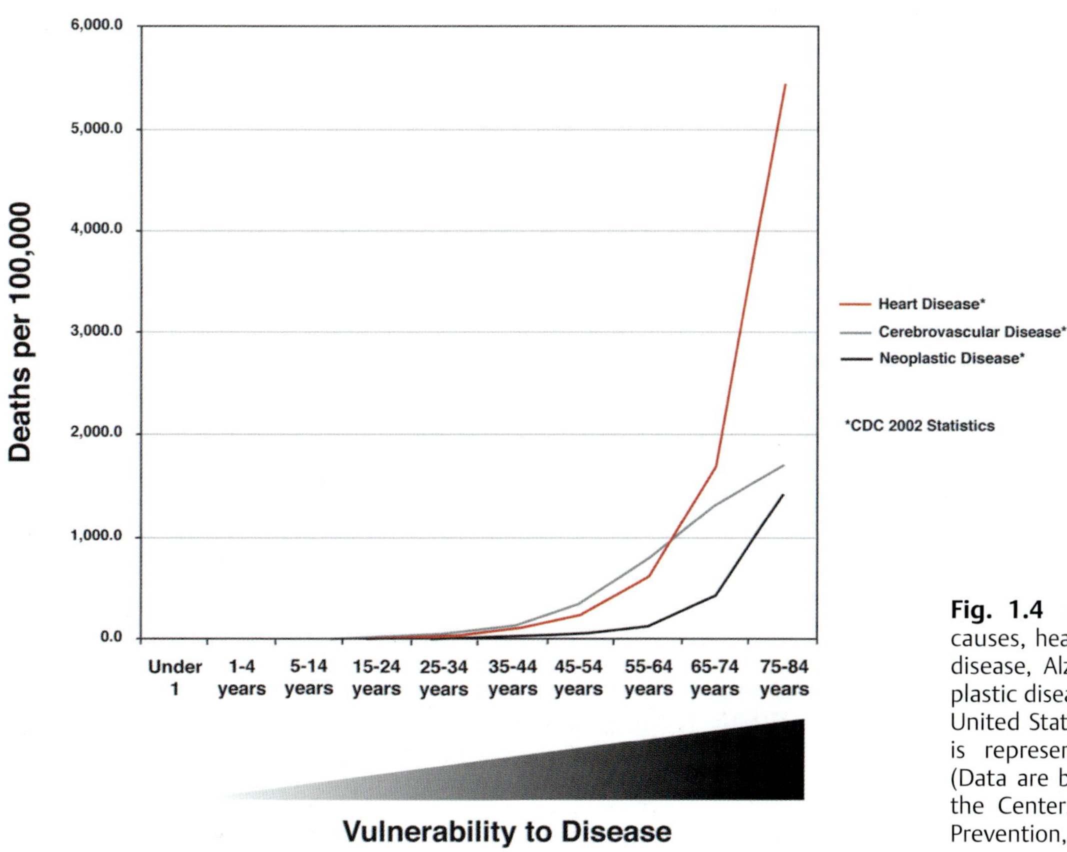

Fig. 1.4 Mortality rates due to all causes, heart disease, cerebrovascular disease, Alzheimer disease, and neoplastic disease in the year 2011 for the United States. Vulnerability to disease is represented beneath the graph. (Data are based on 2011 tables from the Centers for Disease Control and Prevention, Atlanta, GA.)

of age-related changes in lung function. Both forced expiratory volume and response to hypoxia are reduced with age, reflecting a progressive decline in lung function, whereas the loss of reserve capacity in the lungs is an excellent example of the reduced dynamic capacity that characterizes aged organisms.[10,11] Underlying the differences in functional parameters are changes in lung architecture due to intrinsic aging. These changes lead to reduced function that requires compensation to maintain normal physiology. Age-related changes and compensatory responses become more pronounced with increasing age, eventually producing the greater vulnerability to disease characterized by the curves in **Fig. 1.4**. Similar change occurs in all organ systems as a function of age, resulting in the eventual loss of dynamic range and lack of compensatory response typical of the aged organism.

Biological versus Chronological Age

Individual variation in the aging process suggests that chronological age may not be the best nor the most clinically relevant measure of the age of an individual. Efforts have therefore been undertaken to identify biomarkers of age that can be used to assess the true age of an individual. Although these efforts have not yet produced any marker or group of markers that can serve this purpose to the satisfaction of the scientific community, the National Institute on Aging continues to support efforts to define biomarkers of aging for their potential clinical impact.[12] In addition, systematic approaches to understand individual differences in the rate of aging involve large-scale genetic analyses of populations that enjoy exceptional longevity. The Einstein Ashkenazi Longevity Study in New York has enrolled more than 700 individuals. The New England Centenarian Study at Harvard likewise has also enrolled more than 700 individuals, whereas the Southern Italian Centenarian Study has enrolled more than 900 individuals. Thus far, these groups have identified polymorphisms associated with longevity in the ApoE, IGF receptor, and Lamin A genes.[13–15]

Theories of Aging

Multiple theories of aging have been proposed. Some suggest that specific types of damage, such as DNA damage or mitochondrial dysfunction, drive the aging process, whereas others examine aging from an evolutionary perspective. The most general question regarding aging asks why organisms age at all. In 1889, August Weismann made the observation that aging is a property of the somatic tissues and not the germline, which possesses an unlimited capacity for self-renewal. The concept Weismann developed stands on two principles: (1) that the germline is immortal, whereas the somatic cells are mortal; and (2) that aging allows for the removal of older individuals to make space for the next generation.[16] A synthesis of evolutionary theory and the aging process by Peter Medawar in 1952 led to the concept that aging is not under selective pressure, because reproduction occurs relatively early in life and few organisms in the wild live to advanced age. Thus, aging as a phenomenon is restricted to protected environments and is likely due to an inability to repair damage beyond the reproductive phase of life.[17] The concept that aging occurs in postreproductive organisms has led to the theory of antagonistic pleiotropy.[18] This theory states that mutations which benefit an organism early in life may have negative effects later in life. According to antagonistic pleiotropy, mutations that increase reproductive fitness may contribute to age-related declines in the same organism. For example, a rapid developmental rate may enhance reproductive fitness in a subset of organisms within a population, but this advantage may lead to increased cancer risk in these individuals as they age.

Building on the concept of a tradeoff between fitness and longevity inherent in the antagonistic pleiotropy theory and based on the idea that an organism must allocate limiting resources to either maintenance or longevity, Thomas Kirkwood developed the disposable soma theory of aging.[19] The disposable soma theory postulates that insufficient energy is available to the organism for the maintenance of both germline and soma, forcing an allocation of resources that leads to the eventual deterioration of the somatic tissues. The theory has traditionally centered on the allocation of energy in the form of adenosine triphosphate (ATP); however, we have developed the concept that time is the most likely limiting resource that constrains longevity.[20,21] In this iteration of the disposable soma theory, the time allotted for repair of genomic damage is limited due to evolutionary pressure, and it is time, rather than energy, that represents the limiting resource for an organism.

Recently, the possibility that aging may be subject to a level of regulation has been put forth. Trivial arguments have been made based on the fact that single gene mutations can influence longevity, but more rigorous arguments have been posed by population biologists.[22] These arguments propose that aging of individuals is an altruistic trait that may lead to enhanced overall fitness of the population.[23]

Several theories proposing the accumulation of specific types of damage as a primary cause of aging have gained widespread attention. These theories are properly placed under the umbrella of the disposable soma theory because they deal with potential mechanisms whereby the soma may become dysfunctional with age. One of the more prominent of these wear and tear theories is the free radical theory of aging championed by Denham Harman in the 1950s. At this time, the role of the oxygen free radical as a mediator of radiation damage was discovered, and it was postulated that the accumulation of free radical damage might underlie age-related functional decline.[24] Because mitochondria are believed to be the primary source of free radicals within the cell, the free radical theory has been intertwined with the mitochondrial theory of aging, which postulates that mitochondrial-generated free radicals are a major source of age-related damage.[25] However, free radicals can be generated by other cellular organelles such as peroxisomes,[26] and mutations inducing mitochondrial dysfunction have been found to increase lifespan in some cases, generating discussion as to the true role of mitochondrial dysfunction in aging.[27] Similarly, DNA damage has been put forth as the primary cause of aging.[28] There is evidence for an accumulation of DNA damage with age,[29] and mutations that decrease DNA repair capacity induce premature aging, but it has recently become clear that DNA damage *responses* are more important in aging than DNA damage per se.[30] Some arguments have implicated other types of damage, such as glycation end products (caused by nonenzymatic protein linkage of carbohydrates) as primary drivers of aging. But, rather than the absolute level of damage, it is likely that the balance between the accumulation of damage to macromolecules or organelles and the integrity of the complex repair and clearance mechanisms that exist to remove this damage is critical to the aging process.

Increased Longevity Resulting from Single Gene Mutations

A remarkable series of experiments has demonstrated that longevity can be influenced strongly by single gene mutations. The insulin-like signaling (ILS) pathway has emerged as a major mediator of longevity in multiple species. In mammals, the ILS pathway is mediated through the binding of insulin-like growth factor type 1 (IGF-1) to the IGF-1 receptor (IGF-1R) in the plasma membrane. Although IGF-1 is expressed in almost all tissues in an autocrine and paracrine fashion, the majority of circulating IGF-1 is released into the circulation by the liver. The regulation of IGF-1 expression is intimately linked to growth hormone (GH) signals emanating from the neuroendocrine system. GH is released into the blood by the pituitary gland in response to growth hormone releasing hormone (GHRH) produced in the hypothalamus. After IGF-1 is produced, it feeds back on the hypothalamus and suppresses GHRH, thereby completing part of a regulatory circuit known as the somatotropic axis. Six IGF-1 binding proteins (IGFBPs) are involved in regulating IGF-1 bioavailability. The major carrier for IGF-1 in the blood is IGFBP3, which combines with a protein known as the acid labile subunit to form the circulating IGF-1 complex. The remaining IGFBPs are expressed in a tissue-specific manner and are important for bioactivity in specific tissues and cells. The specific IGFBPs expressed can affect cell responses to IGF-1, including whether to adopt a proliferative or migratory phenotype, for example.[31]

IGF-1 is a major determinant of body size during prenatal growth and development. In mice, the IGF-1 knockout and IGF-1/IGF-1R double knockout are lethal to neonates, which show reductions of 60% and 45% in birth weight, respectively, compared with normal pups.[32] The influence of IGF-1 on growth in humans is similar. In one case report, a patient homozygous for IGF-1 deletions in exons 4 and 5 was 40% of normal weight at birth, with continued growth retardation at 15 years.[33] In Laron syndrome, a type of dwarfism, the GH receptor is mutated and unable to stimulate IGF-1 expression. Children born with this disorder exhibit reduced GH signaling and present with several growth-related defects, including small organ size, weakened hair and nail growth, and sarcopenia.[34] There are no reports indicating that patients with Laron syndrome experience increased lifespan; however, mice modeled after the Laron mutation, through ablation of the GH receptor, are dwarfs and exhibit a significant increase in lifespan (**Table 1.1**).

The deleterious effect that a severe loss of IGF-1 or its receptor confers on viability in mice is in remarkable contrast to low to moderate reductions in ILS. Kenyon et al first reported that a hypomorphic mutation in the *Caenorhabditis elegans* IR homologue Daf-2, increases lifespan. The worms harboring this mutation achieved a 300% increase in lifespan.[35] Studies in *Drosophila* expressing a hypomorphic IR showed an 85% increase in lifespan as well as decreased body size.[36] The IR homologues in worms and flies both respond to a variety of "insulin-like peptides" and are evolutionarily diverged from the IR and IGF-1R in vertebrates, which respond to distinct hormone ligands. Despite these differences, ILS is a highly conserved intracellular signaling pathway and transgenic mouse models that express reduced levels of IGF-1 or that are heterozygous for the IGF-1R achieve a range of small to modest increases in lifespan accompanied by dwarf phenotypes (**Table 1.1**). Mouse models such as the Ames dwarf that achieve a reduction in circulating IGF-1 through impaired GH production reach the longest lifespan, sparking debate as to whether GH signaling has an independent role in lifespan extension that enhances reduced ILS. Fibroblasts derived from the long-lived Ames and Snell dwarf mice, for example, exhibit resistance

Table 1.1 Lifespan extension in mice harboring mutations in the GH/IGF-1 axis

Mouse	Mutation	Mechanism	Key phenotype	Max lifespan % increase	Studies (see page 10)
Ames dwarf	Prop1	Pituitary defect	GH and IGF-1 deficiency	68	1
Snell dwarf	Pit1	Pituitary defect	GH and IGF-1 deficiency	42	2
Little	(lit/lit), $ghrhr^{-/-}$	Suppressed GH release	GH and IGF-1 deficiency	24	2,3
Laron	$GHR/BP^{-/-}$	Unresponsive to GH	IGF-1 deficiency	55	4,5
IGF-1R KO	$IGF\text{-}1R^{+/-}$	Heterozygous for IGF-1R	Reduced number of IGF-1 receptors	33	6
Midi	IGF-1 exon $3^{neo/neo}$	Hypomorphic for IGF-1	Reduced IGF-1 and increased GH	18	7
$p66^{sch}$ KO	$p66^{sch\ -/-}$	IGF-1 intracellular signaling molecule	No change in IGF-1	30	8
PAPP-A KO	$PAPPA^{-/-}$	Metalloproteinase	Reduced IGF-1 and GH	41	9
IRS1 KO	$IRS1^{-/-}$	IGF-1 intracellular signaling molecule	No change in IGF-1	32	10
IRS2 KO	$IRS2^{+/-}$	IGF-1 intracellular signaling molecule	No change in IGF-1	17, 18 in brain specific	11

Abbreviations: GH, growth hormone; GHR, growth hormone receptor; ghrhr, growth hormone releasing hormone receptor; IGF-1, insulin-like growth factor type 1; IRS, insulin receptor substrate; PAPPA, pregnancy-assisted plasma protein-A; Pit, POU domain, class 1, transcription factor 1; Prop, prophet of PIT-1.

to H_2O_2, paraquat, and ultraviolet (UV) light.[37] Cells from other long-lived mouse models have also been assessed and exhibit stress resistance to various toxins and oxidants as well.[38] Thus resistance to stress appears to be an important factor contributing to the increased lifespans in these mice.

Decreased Cellular Function during Aging

Aging tissues present increasing loss of function that is associated with structural damage and alteration. For example, the liver of aged mammals has reduced xenobiotic metabolism and hepatobiliary function, among other functional declines.[39] In skeletal muscle, loss of mass and reduced contractile capacity correlate with reduced plasticity and loss of neuromuscular junctions, causing atrophy of muscle fibers[40]; and in the heart, reduced function arises from increased fat deposits, fibrosis, and changes in conductivity.[41] As discussed previously, changes are also seen in the lungs, where reduced function is affected primarily by structural changes in the alveoli and capillaries.[11]

These age-related changes are often the consequence of loss of homeostasis at the cellular level, a process common to many species across the evolutionary spectrum. For example, *S. cerevisiae* accumulate extrachromosomal ribosomal-DNA circles and depolarized mitochondria with age,[42,43] whereas aging *C. elegans* accumulate lipofuscin,[44] an insoluble aggregate of oxidized proteins and lipids,[45] in their intestinal cells. In higher eukaryotes, damaged organelles and proteins accumulate in long-lived postmitotic tissues, such as skeletal muscle, heart, liver, and brain.[8,17,18,46,47] Cells in these organs exhibit higher levels of damaged and dysfunctional cellular components with age. Neurons, astrocytes, microglia, hepatocytes, and cardiomyocytes accumulate lipofuscin deposits and other protein aggregates[48–50]; rhabdomyocytes accumulate mitochondria with oxidized bases in their DNA and show increased production of reactive oxygen species and decreased activity[51]; whereas cardiac myocytes accumulate impaired mitochondria with increased fragmentation of mitochondrial DNA.[50,52] In regenerating tissues, cellular damage can impair the proliferative capacity by affecting stem cells and the stem cell niche, reducing the organism's ability to restore bone, intestine, skin, muscle, kidney, and blood. Compared with mesenchymal stem cells from younger donors, those from older donors have been shown to exhibit higher levels of oxidized proteins, lipofuscin aggregates, and advanced glycation end products, as well as reduced proliferation and differentiation potential.[53]

It is generally accepted that dysfunctional organelles, oxidized and aggregate-prone proteins, DNA damage, and other damaged macromolecules contribute to the loss of biological function seen in aged organisms.[29,30] In line with this idea, several models of accelerated aging are characterized by either increased accumulation or reduced turnover of dysfunctional organelles and/or proteins. "Mutator" mice, for example, rapidly accumulate dysfunctional mitochondria because of a mutation that impairs the proofreading activity of mitochondrial DNA polymerase γ. Increased levels of dysfunctional mitochondria reduce lifespan in these mice and increase the incidence of age-related conditions, including alopecia, anemia, kyphosis, osteoporosis, weight loss, and cardiac hypertrophy.[31,32] Importantly, mitochondrial DNA mutations also accumulate in aging humans and impair mitochondrial function in many tissues, including heart, skeletal muscle, brain, and colon.[30]

Cellular Senescence as a Contributor to Aging

Senescence is a cellular stress response to insults that include oxidative and genotoxic stress, telomere attrition, and dysregulated mitogenic signaling. In mammals, the response is mediated through two pathways, the $p53/p21^{CIP1/WAF1}$ and $p16^{INK4A/Rb}$ pathways, which appear to establish senescence with different kinetics.[7,54–56] The DNA damage response pathway generally mediates the initial response by increasing levels of $p21^{CIP1/WAF1}$; only at later times is senescence reinforced by expression of $p16^{INK4A/RB}$.[55,57] The p38 mitogen-activated protein kinase (p38 MAPK) pathway also may play a role in establishing senescence via signaling into the DNA damage response pathways.[7,58,59]

The senescent state is characterized by significant changes in cell morphology and activity. Senescent cells are increased in size,[60] and they exhibit increased activity of the lysosomal senescence-associated β-galactosidase,[61] persistent DNA-damage response signaling, DNA damage foci (DNA segments with chromatin alterations reinforcing senescence known as senescence-associated heterochromatin foci [SAHFs], and telomere-dysfunction-induced foci [TIFs]),[56,62,63] chromatin rearrangements and formation of SAHFs,[64] increased activation of p38 MAPK,[65,66] and loss of lamin B1 expression.[67] In addition, the expression of specific cytokines, growth factors, and proteases creates a senescence secretion profile that differs markedly from that of the presenescent cell.[68,69] Importantly, the clearing of senescent cells positive for $p16^{INK4A}$ has been shown to ameliorate the premature aging phenotype in at least one progeroid mouse model,[70] suggesting that the accumulation of senescent cells contributes to age-related pathologies. Moreover, senescent cells have been shown to promote the proliferation of preneoplastic cell lines in vivo.[71] The senescence-associated secretory phenotype, which contains proinflammatory cytokines, matrix metalloproteinases, and growth factors may contribute to cancer progression and metastasis, as well as neurodegenerative disorders, inflammatory disease, metabolic dysfunction, and other conditions that preferentially affect the elderly.[7,72] The expression of retinal pigmented epithelial differentiation factor, a key mediator of angiogenesis and stem cell survival, is also decreased in senescent mesenchymal cells.[73]

The immune system undergoes a series of changes during aging that result in a decreased response to new pathogens, termed immune senescence. Immune senescence is characterized by decreases in cell signaling, cytokine secretion, and proliferation that result in impaired effector B and T cell responses.[74,75] Shifts in CD4 and CD8 lymphocyte subsets and proliferative responses have been demonstrated in aged individuals and have been associated with increased mortality.[76] Thymic involution, due to the potential loss of newly emigrating naive CD4+ T cells, may contribute to loss of immune response during aging.[77] However, homeostatic proliferation in the periphery is sufficient to maintain the naive T cell population, making for a complex relationship between thymic involution and immune senescence. Reduced vaccine response in aged individuals limits the efficiency of vaccination and reflects immune senescence in the B cell lineage.[78] Interestingly, the loss of immune function during aging occurs in a situation in which generalized inflammation is increased. Increased levels of proinflammatory cytokines and acute-phase proteins are typical of advanced age in both humans and mice.[79] The concept that inflammation is a key component of decreased functionality in aged individuals has become central in biogerontology.[80,81]

Stem Cells and Aging

Functional attrition in stem cell compartments with age has been documented in mice in multiple tissues, including skeletal muscle, bone, and brain.[82–84] The idea of tissue stem cell exhaustion as a potential contributor to aging has become an attractive concept, given the reduced ability of multiple tissues to repair and regenerate in aged individuals. An intriguing series of experiments has shown that exposure of an aged stem cell compartment to circulating factors from younger animals via heterochronic parabiosis allows greater regeneration following injury[85]; the factor GDF11 has been implicated.[86] Supplementation with GDF11 in mice appears to improve several aspects of aging, including thymic involution and skeletal muscle repair. However, other studies suggest that intrinsic defects present in stem cells from aged skeletal muscle preclude simple restoration of circulating factors to restore these aged tissues.[87] Studies on bone marrow–derived stem cells indicate that the proliferation of these cells decreases with age and that the differentiation pathway becomes biased toward a myeloid lineage.[88,89] Further studies on a population of very small embryonic stem cells indicate that this interesting population of circulating stem cells also decreases with age. Notably, these cells are influenced by the GH/IGF-1 signaling pathway linked to lifespan modulation.[90] From this limited sampling of the literature, it appears likely that the potential for functional intervention during aging will develop as our understanding of adult stem cell compartments and biology increases.

Frailty and Aging

Frailty in the elderly is a major clinical concern, and measures of frailty are predictors of clinical outcomes in multiple settings.[91–93] A simple 6-minute walk test can provide an assessment of frailty, and a functional frailty score has been developed to objectively assess frailty in individuals and assist with clinical management of the elderly.[94] Interestingly, an accumulating body of evidence suggests that relatively simple interventions targeted toward increasing mobility and strength have a measurable impact on clinical outcomes.[95] Lifestyle changes are likely to have the most dramatic effect on functional outcomes in the elderly, particularly in developed countries where dietary changes and sedentary lifestyle have created an epidemic of obesity and type 2 diabetes.[96,97] Increasing physical activity in a meaningful way for a large portion of the population will be a challenge for health care in the United States and may require a broad public awareness campaign similar to that initiated to reduce smoking. These types of interventions, in combination with advanced therapies involving stem cells, cell targeting therapies, and targeted hormone therapies, are likely to provide a positive impact on the aging process.

References

1. International database, U.S.C. Bureau, Editor U.S. Census Bureau. International database: Table 094. Midyear population, by age and sex. http://www.census.gov/population/projections/.
2. Kinsella K, Velkoff V; U.S. Census Bureau. An Aging World: 2001. series P95/01–1. U.S. Government Printing Office; 2001
3. Bell FC, Miller ML. Life Tables for the United States Social Security Area 1900–2100. Actuarial Study No. 120. Social Security Administration; 2000. http://www.ssa.gov/oact/NOTES/as120/LifeTables_Body.html.
4. Olshansky SJ, Carnes BA, Cassel CK. The aging of the human species. Sci Am 1993;268(4):46–52
5. Center for Disease Control. Mortality rates: Public Health and Aging: Trends in Aging. United States and Worldwide; 2002
6. Lorenzini A, Tresini M, Austad SN, Cristofalo VJ. Cellular replicative capacity correlates primarily with species body mass not longevity. Mech Ageing Dev 2005;126(10):1130–1133
7. Campisi J. Aging, cellular senescence, and cancer. Annu Rev Physiol 2013;75:685–705
8. Todaro GJ, Wolman SR, Green H. Rapid Transformation of Human Fibroblasts with Low Growth Potential into Established Cell Lines by Sv40. J Cell Physiol 1963;62:257–265
9. Hayflick L, Moorhead PS. The serial cultivation of human diploid cell strains. Exp Cell Res 1961;25:585–621
10. Sharma G, Goodwin J. Effect of aging on respiratory system physiology and immunology. Clin Interv Aging 2006;1(3): 253–260
11. Lalley PM. The aging respiratory system—pulmonary structure, function and neural control. Respir Physiol Neurobiol 2013;187(3):199–210
12. The Quest for Biomarkers Takes Many Pathways, National Institute on Aging, 2013: http://www.nia.nih.gov/about/living-long-well-21st-century-strategic-directions-research-aging/quest-biomarkers-takes-many
13. Conneely KN, Capell BC, Erdos MR, et al. Human longevity and common variations in the LMNA gene: a meta-analysis. Aging Cell 2012;11(3):475–481
14. Rincon M, Rudin E, Barzilai N. The insulin/IGF-1 signaling in mammals and its relevance to human longevity. Exp Gerontol 2005;40(11):873–877
15. Verghese J, Holtzer R, Wang C, Katz MJ, Barzilai N, Lipton RB. Role of APOE genotype in gait decline and disability in aging. J Gerontol A Biol Sci Med Sci 2013;68(11):1395–1401
16. Weismann A. Essays upon heredity and kindred biological problems. In: Poulton E, ed. Translations of Foreign Biological Memoirs. Oxford, UK: Claredon Press; 1889
17. Medawar P. An Unsolved Problem of Biology. London, UK: HK Lewis; 1952
18. Williams G. Pleiotropy, natural selection and the evolution of senescence. Evolution 1957;11(4):398–411
19. Kirkwood TB. Evolution of ageing. Nature 1977;270(5635): 301–304
20. Lorenzini A, Johnson FB, Oliver A, et al. Significant correlation of species longevity with DNA double strand break recognition but not with telomere length. Mech Ageing Dev 2009; 130(11-12):784–792
21. Lorenzini A, Stamato T, Sell C. The disposable soma theory revisited: time as a resource in the theories of aging. Cell Cycle 2011;10(22):3853–3856
22. Wynne-Edwards V. Animal Dispersion in Relation to Social Behaviour. Can Med Assoc J 1963;88(25):1255–1256
23. Mitteldorf J, Wilson DS. Population viscosity and the evolution of altruism. J Theor Biol 2000;204(4):481–496
24. Harman D. Aging: a theory based on free radical and radiation chemistry. J Gerontol 1956;11(3):298–300
25. Loeb LA, Wallace DC, Martin GM. The mitochondrial theory of aging and its relationship to reactive oxygen species damage and somatic mtDNA mutations. Proc Natl Acad Sci USA 2005;102(52):18769–18770
26. Brown GC, Borutaite V. There is no evidence that mitochondria are the main source of reactive oxygen species in mammalian cells. Mitochondrion 2012;12(1):1–4
27. Pulliam DA, Bhattacharya A, Van Remmen H. Mitochondrial dysfunction in aging and longevity: a causal or protective role? Antioxid Redox Signal 2013;19(12):1373–1387

28. Li H, Mitchell JR, Hasty P. DNA double-strand breaks: a potential causative factor for mammalian aging? Mech Ageing Dev 2008;129(7-8):416–424
29. Wang J, Clauson CL, Robbins PD, Niedernhofer LJ, Wang Y. The oxidative DNA lesions 8,5′-cyclopurines accumulate with aging in a tissue-specific manner. Aging Cell 2012;11(4): 714–716
30. Maslov AY, Ganapathi S, Westerhof M, et al. DNA damage in normally and prematurely aged mice. Aging Cell 2013; 12(3):467–477
31. Duan C. Specifying the cellular responses to IGF signals: roles of IGF-binding proteins. J Endocrinol 2002;175(1):41–54
32. Liu JP, Baker J, Perkins AS, Robertson EJ, Efstratiadis A. Mice carrying null mutations of the genes encoding insulin-like growth factor I (Igf-1) and type 1 IGF receptor (Igf1r). Cell 1993; 75(1):59–72
33. Woods KA, Camacho-Hübner C, Savage MO, Clark AJ. Intrauterine growth retardation and postnatal growth failure associated with deletion of the insulin-like growth factor I gene. N Engl J Med 1996;335(18):1363–1367
34. Laron Z. Laron syndrome (primary growth hormone resistance or insensitivity): the personal experience 1958-2003. J Clin Endocrinol Metab 2004;89(3):1031–1044
35. Kenyon C, Chang J, Gensch E, Rudner A, Tabtiang R. A *C. elegans* mutant that lives twice as long as wild type. Nature 1993;366(6454):461–464
36. Tatar M, Kopelman A, Epstein D, Tu MP, Yin CM, Garofalo RS. A mutant Drosophila insulin receptor homolog that extends life-span and impairs neuroendocrine function. Science 2001;292(5514):107–110
37. Salmon AB, Murakami S, Bartke A, Kopchick J, Yasumura K, Miller RA. Fibroblast cell lines from young adult mice of long-lived mutant strains are resistant to multiple forms of stress. Am J Physiol Endocrinol Metab 2005;289(1):E23–E29
38. Murakami S. Stress resistance in long-lived mouse models. Exp Gerontol 2006;41(10):1014–1019
39. Schmucker DL. Age-related changes in liver structure and function: Implications for disease? Exp Gerontol 2005; 40(8-9):650–659
40. Jang YC, Van Remmen H. Age-associated alterations of the neuromuscular junction. Exp Gerontol 2011;46(2-3): 193–198
41. Kitzman DW, Edwards WD. Age-related changes in the anatomy of the normal human heart. J Gerontol 1990;45(2): M33–M39
42. Sinclair DA, Guarente L. Extrachromosomal rDNA circles—a cause of aging in yeast. Cell 1997;91(7):1033–1042
43. Hughes AL, Gottschling DE. An early age increase in vacuolar pH limits mitochondrial function and lifespan in yeast. Nature 2012;492(7428):261–265
44. Klass MR. Aging in the nematode Caenorhabditis elegans: major biological and environmental factors influencing life span. Mech Ageing Dev 1977;6(6):413–429
45. Toth SE. The origin of lipofuscin age pigments. Exp Gerontol 1968;3(1):19–30
46. Szweda PA, Camouse M, Lundberg KC, Oberley TD, Szweda LI. Aging, lipofuscin formation, and free radical-mediated inhibition of cellular proteolytic systems. Ageing Res Rev 2003; 2(4):383–405
47. Chaudhary KR, El-Sikhry H, Seubert JM. Mitochondria and the aging heart. J Geriatr Cardiol 2011;8(3):159–167
48. Landfield PW, Braun LD, Pitler TA, Lindsey JD, Lynch G. Hippocampal aging in rats: a morphometric study of multiple variables in semithin sections. Neurobiol Aging 1981; 2(4):265–275
49. Salminen A, Ojala J, Kaarniranta K, Haapasalo A, Hiltunen M, Soininen H. Astrocytes in the aging brain express characteristics of senescence-associated secretory phenotype. Eur J Neurosci 2011;34(1):3–11
50. Frenzel H, Feimann J. Age-dependent structural changes in the myocardium of rats. A quantitative light- and electron-microscopic study on the right and left chamber wall. Mech Ageing Dev 1984;27(1):29–41
51. Mansouri A, Muller FL, Liu Y, et al. Alterations in mitochondrial function, hydrogen peroxide release and oxidative damage in mouse hind-limb skeletal muscle during aging. Mech Ageing Dev 2006;127(3):298–306
52. Ozawa T. Mitochondrial DNA mutations and age. Ann N Y Acad Sci 1998;854:128–154
53. Stolzing A, Jones E, McGonagle D, Scutt A. Age-related changes in human bone marrow-derived mesenchymal stem cells: consequences for cell therapies. Mech Ageing Dev 2008; 129(3):163–173
54. Rodier F, Campisi J. Four faces of cellular senescence. J Cell Biol 2011;192(4):547–556
55. Stein GH, Drullinger LF, Soulard A, Dulić V. Differential roles for cyclin-dependent kinase inhibitors p21 and p16 in the mechanisms of senescence and differentiation in human fibroblasts. Mol Cell Biol 1999;19(3):2109–2117
56. Herbig U, Jobling WA, Chen BP, Chen DJ, Sedivy JM. Telomere shortening triggers senescence of human cells through a pathway involving ATM, p53, and p21(CIP1), but not p16(INK4a). Mol Cell 2004;14(4):501–513
57. Alcorta DA, Xiong Y, Phelps D, Hannon G, Beach D, Barrett JC. Involvement of the cyclin-dependent kinase inhibitor p16 (INK4a) in replicative senescence of normal human fibroblasts. Proc Natl Acad Sci U S A 1996;93(24):13742–13747
58. Naka K, Tachibana A, Ikeda K, Motoyama N. Stress-induced premature senescence in hTERT-expressing ataxia telangiectasia fibroblasts. J Biol Chem 2004;279(3):2030–2037
59. Freund A, Patil CK, Campisi J. p38MAPK is a novel DNA damage response-independent regulator of the senescence-associated secretory phenotype. EMBO J 2011;30(8):1536–1548
60. Hayflick L. The limited in vitro lifetime of human diploid strains. Exp Cell Res 1965;37:614–636
61. Dimri GP, Lee X, Basile G, et al. A biomarker that identifies senescent human cells in culture and in aging skin in vivo. Proc Natl Acad Sci USA 1995;92(20):9363–9367
62. d'Adda di Fagagna F, Reaper PM, Clay-Farrace L, et al. A DNA damage checkpoint response in telomere-initiated senescence. Nature 2003;426(6963):194–198
63. Rodier F, Muñoz DP, Teachenor R, et al. DNA-SCARS: distinct nuclear structures that sustain damage-induced senescence growth arrest and inflammatory cytokine secretion. J Cell Sci 2011;124(Pt 1):68–81
64. Adams PD. Remodeling of chromatin structure in senescent cells and its potential impact on tumor suppression and aging. Gene 2007;397(1-2):84–93
65. Iwasa H, Han J, Ishikawa F. Mitogen-activated protein kinase p38 defines the common senescence-signalling pathway. Genes Cells 2003;8(2):131–144
66. Wang W, Chen JX, Liao R, et al. Sequential activation of the MEK-extracellular signal-regulated kinase and MKK3/6-p38 mitogen-activated protein kinase pathways mediates oncogenic ras-induced premature senescence. Mol Cell Biol 2002;22(10):3389–3403
67. Freund A, Laberge RM, Demaria M, Campisi J. Lamin B1 loss is a senescence-associated biomarker. Mol Biol Cell 2012;23(11):2066–2075
68. Coppe JP, Boysen M, Sun CH, et al. A role for fibroblasts in mediating the effects of tobacco-induced epithelial cell growth and invasion. Mol Cancer Res 2008;6(7):1085–1098
69. Coppé JP, Patil CK, Rodier F, et al. Senescence-associated secretory phenotypes reveal cell-nonautonomous functions

of oncogenic RAS and the p53 tumor suppressor. PLoS Biol 2008;6(12):2853–2868

70. Baker DJ, Wijshake T, Tchkonia T, et al. Clearance of p16Ink4a-positive senescent cells delays ageing-associated disorders. Nature 2011;479(7372):232–236

71. Krtolica A, Parrinello S, Lockett S, Desprez PY, Campisi J. Senescent fibroblasts promote epithelial cell growth and tumorigenesis: a link between cancer and aging. Proc Natl Acad Sci USA 2001;98(21):12072–12077

72. Naylor RM, Baker DJ, van Deursen JM. Senescent cells: a novel therapeutic target for aging and age-related diseases. Clin Pharmacol Ther 2013;93(1):105–116

73. Pignolo RJ, Cristofalo VJ, Rotenberg MO. Senescent WI-38 cells fail to express EPC-1, a gene induced in young cells upon entry into the G0 state. J Biol Chem 1993;268(12):8949–8957

74. Nikolich-Zugich J. Ageing and life-long maintenance of T-cell subsets in the face of latent persistent infections. Nat Rev Immunol 2008;8(7):512–522

75. Akbar AN, Fletcher JM. Memory T cell homeostasis and senescence during aging. Curr Opin Immunol 2005;17(5): 480–485

76. Wikby A, Maxson P, Olsson J, Johansson B, Ferguson FG. Changes in CD8 and CD4 lymphocyte subsets, T cell proliferation responses and non-survival in the very old: the Swedish longitudinal OCTO-immune study. Mech Ageing Dev 1998;102(2-3):187–198

77. Kohler S, Thiel A. Life after the thymus: CD31+ and CD31- human naive CD4+ T-cell subsets. Blood 2009;113(4):769–774

78. Boraschi D, Aguado MT, Dutel C, et al. The gracefully aging immune system. Sci Transl Med 2013;5(185):ps8

79. Shaw AC, Goldstein DR, Montgomery RR. Age-dependent dysregulation of innate immunity. Nat Rev Immunol 2013; 13(12):875–887

80. Collerton J, Martin-Ruiz C, Davies K, et al. Frailty and the role of inflammation, immunosenescence and cellular ageing in the very old: cross-sectional findings from the Newcastle 85+ Study. Mech Ageing Dev 2012;133(6):456–466

81. López-Otín C, Blasco MA, Partridge L, Serrano M, Kroemer G. The hallmarks of aging. Cell 2013;153(6):1194–1217

82. Conboy IM, Rando TA. Heterochronic parabiosis for the study of the effects of aging on stem cells and their niches. Cell Cycle 2012;11(12):2260–2267

83. Gruber R, Koch H, Doll BA, Tegtmeier F, Einhorn TA, Hollinger JO. Fracture healing in the elderly patient. Exp Gerontol 2006;41(11):1080–1093

84. Molofsky AV, Slutsky SG, Joseph NM, et al. Increasing p16INK4a expression decreases forebrain progenitors and neurogenesis during ageing. Nature 2006;443(7110):448–452

85. Conboy IM, Conboy MJ, Wagers AJ, Girma ER, Weissman IL, Rando TA. Rejuvenation of aged progenitor cells by exposure to a young systemic environment. Nature 2005;433(7027): 760–764

86. Loffredo FS, Steinhauser ML, Jay SM, et al. Growth differentiation factor 11 is a circulating factor that reverses age-related cardiac hypertrophy. Cell 2013;153(4):828–839

87. Bernet JD, Doles JD, Hall JK, Kelly Tanaka K, Carter TA, Olwin BB. p38 MAPK signaling underlies a cell-autonomous loss of stem cell self-renewal in skeletal muscle of aged mice. Nat Med 2014;20(3):265–271

88. Gekas C, Graf T. CD41 expression marks myeloid-biased adult hematopoietic stem cells and increases with age. Blood 2013;121(22):4463–4472

89. Pang WW, Price EA, Sahoo D, et al. Human bone marrow hematopoietic stem cells are increased in frequency and myeloid-biased with age. Proc Natl Acad Sci USA 2011; 108(50):20012–20017

90. Kucia M, Masternak M, Liu R, et al. The negative effect of prolonged somatotrophic/insulin signaling on an adult bone marrow-residing population of pluripotent very small embryonic-like stem cells (VSELs). Age (Dordr) 2013;35(2):315–330

91. Ekerstad N, et al. Frailty is independently associated with 1-year mortality for elderly patients with non-ST-segment elevation myocardial infarction. Eur J Prev Cardiol, 2013.

92. Makary MA, Segev DL, Pronovost PJ, et al. Frailty as a predictor of surgical outcomes in older patients. J Am Coll Surg 2010;210(6):901–908

93. Partridge JS, Harari D, Dhesi JK. Frailty in the older surgical patient: a review. Age Ageing 2012;41(2):142–147

94. Fried LP, Tangen CM, Walston J, et al; Cardiovascular Health Study Collaborative Research Group. Frailty in older adults: evidence for a phenotype. J Gerontol A Biol Sci Med Sci 2001;56(3):M146–M156

95. Williams SC. Frailty research strengthens with biomarker and treatment leads. Nat Med 2013;19(5):517

96. Seidell JC. Obesity, insulin resistance and diabetes—a worldwide epidemic. Br J Nutr 2000;83(Suppl 1):S5–S8

97. Naser KA, Gruber A, Thomson GA. The emerging pandemic of obesity and diabetes: are we doing enough to prevent a disaster? Int J Clin Pract 2006;60(9):1093–1097

Studies for Table 1.1

1. Brown-Borg HM, Borg KE, Meliska CJ, Bartke A. Dwarf mice and the ageing process. Nature 1996;384(6604):33

2. Flurkey K, Papaconstantinou J, Miller RA, Harrison DE. Lifespan extension and delayed immune and collagen aging in mutant mice with defects in growth hormone production. Proc Natl Acad Sci USA 2001;98(12):6736–6741

3. Donahue LR, Beamer WG. Growth hormone deficiency in 'little' mice results in aberrant body composition, reduced insulin-like growth factor-I and insulin-like growth factor-binding protein-3 (IGFBP-3), but does not affect IGFBP-2, -1 or -4. J Endocrinol 1993;136(1):91–104

4. Coschigano KT, Clemmons D, Bellush LL, Kopchick JJ. Assessment of growth parameters and life span of GHR/BP gene-disrupted mice. Endocrinology 2000;141(7):2608–2613

5. Coschigano KT, Holland AN, Riders ME, List EO, Flyvbjerg A, Kopchick JJ. Deletion, but not antagonism, of the mouse growth hormone receptor results in severely decreased body weights, insulin, and insulin-like growth factor I levels and increased life span. Endocrinology 2003;144(9):3799–3810

6. Holzenberger M, Dupont J, Ducos B, et al. IGF-1 receptor regulates lifespan and resistance to oxidative stress in mice. Nature 2003;421(6919):182–187

7. Lorenzini A, Salmon AB, Lerner C, et al. Mice producing reduced levels of insulin-like growth factor type 1 display an increase in maximum, but not mean, life span. J Gerontol A Biol Sci Med Sci 2014;69(4):410–419

8. Migliaccio E, Giorgio M, Mele S, et al. The p66shc adaptor protein controls oxidative stress response and life span in mammals. Nature 1999;402(6759):309–313

9. Conover CA, Bale LK. Loss of pregnancy-associated plasma protein A extends lifespan in mice. Aging Cell 2007;6(5):727–729

10. Selman C, Lingard S, Choudhury AI, et al. Evidence for lifespan extension and delayed age-related biomarkers in insulin receptor substrate 1 null mice. FASEB J 2008;22(3):807–818

11. Taguchi A, Wartschow LM, White MF. Brain IRS2 signaling coordinates life span and nutrient homeostasis. Science 2007;317(5836):369–372

2 Geriatric Otolaryngology: An Overview

Karen M. Kost

Changing Demographics

Since the beginning of recorded human history, young children have outnumbered older people. In a shifting global trend, people over the age of 65 will soon outnumber children under the age of 5. As a result of declining birth rates and increasing life spans, the geriatric age group is the fastest-growing segment of our society.[1] In 2006, almost 500 million people worldwide were 65 and older, accounting for 8% of the world's population. By 2030, that total is projected to increase to 1 billion or more, amounting to one out of every eight, or 12.5% of the Earth's inhabitants. Of note, the most rapid increases in the 65 and older population are occurring in developing countries, which will witness a jump of 140% by the year 2030. In the United States alone, fully 20% of the population will be 65 or older by the year 2030. The median age of North Americans has seen a rise from 30 in 1960, to 34 in 1994, and is estimated to reach 41 by 2030.[1] An important, and sometimes overlooked, feature of population aging is the progressive aging of the older population itself.[2,3]

Over time, more older people are surviving to even more advanced ages. The "oldest old" are often defined as people age 85 and over. Because of chronic disease, the oldest old have the highest population levels of disability that require long-term care. Consequently, they also consume public resources disproportionately when compared with those in younger age groups. The health, economic, and social needs of this group differ significantly from those of patients aged 65 to 84. The oldest old currently account for 7% of the world's population aged 65 and over: this number rises to 10% in more developed countries and falls to 5% in less developed countries. In the United States, as the number of oldest old increases, it is estimated that they will account for 14% of the population by 2040. People of extreme old age, defined as 100 years of age or more, are referred to as centenarians. Although they currently constitute a small portion of the total population in most countries, their numbers are growing quite dramatically, having doubled each decade since 1950 in more developed countries.[2,3] These changes affect the traditional representation of populations as a pyramid. As the number of older people increases, and the number of younger people decreases, the pyramid takes on a square configuration, possibly eventually becoming inverted if current trends continue (**Fig. 2.1**).[4]

Global aging is a success story with people living longer and generally healthier lives, particularly in developed countries. Increased life expectancy reflects several health transitions occurring around the globe at different rates. Changes affecting life expectancy include the following:

- Shift from high to low fertility
- Increase in life expectancy at birth and at older ages
- Shift from infectious and parasitic diseases to noncommunicable diseases and chronic conditions
- Economic development
- Ongoing medical advances
- New drugs

Sustained growth of the world's older population, however, also creates important challenges.[5] Population aging affects economic growth, formal and informal social support systems, and the ability of states and communities to provide resources for older citizens. The "old-age dependency ratio" reflects the proportion of young individuals available to support the old in our society.[1] Currently, there are ~ 5 individuals supporting every elderly person, with a ratio of ~ 20. By 2050, it is estimated that there will only be 2.5 supporting individuals for every elderly person, with a ratio of ~ 40. Despite some recognized shortcomings of this ratio, it is nonetheless useful as a crude indicator of the level of economic and physical dependency of the geriatric population. Furthermore, the elderly consume a disproportionate amount of the total health care resources available. Attempting policy adjustments such as changes in retirement ages and medical benefits may be painful and unpopular. Nonetheless, it is incumbent upon

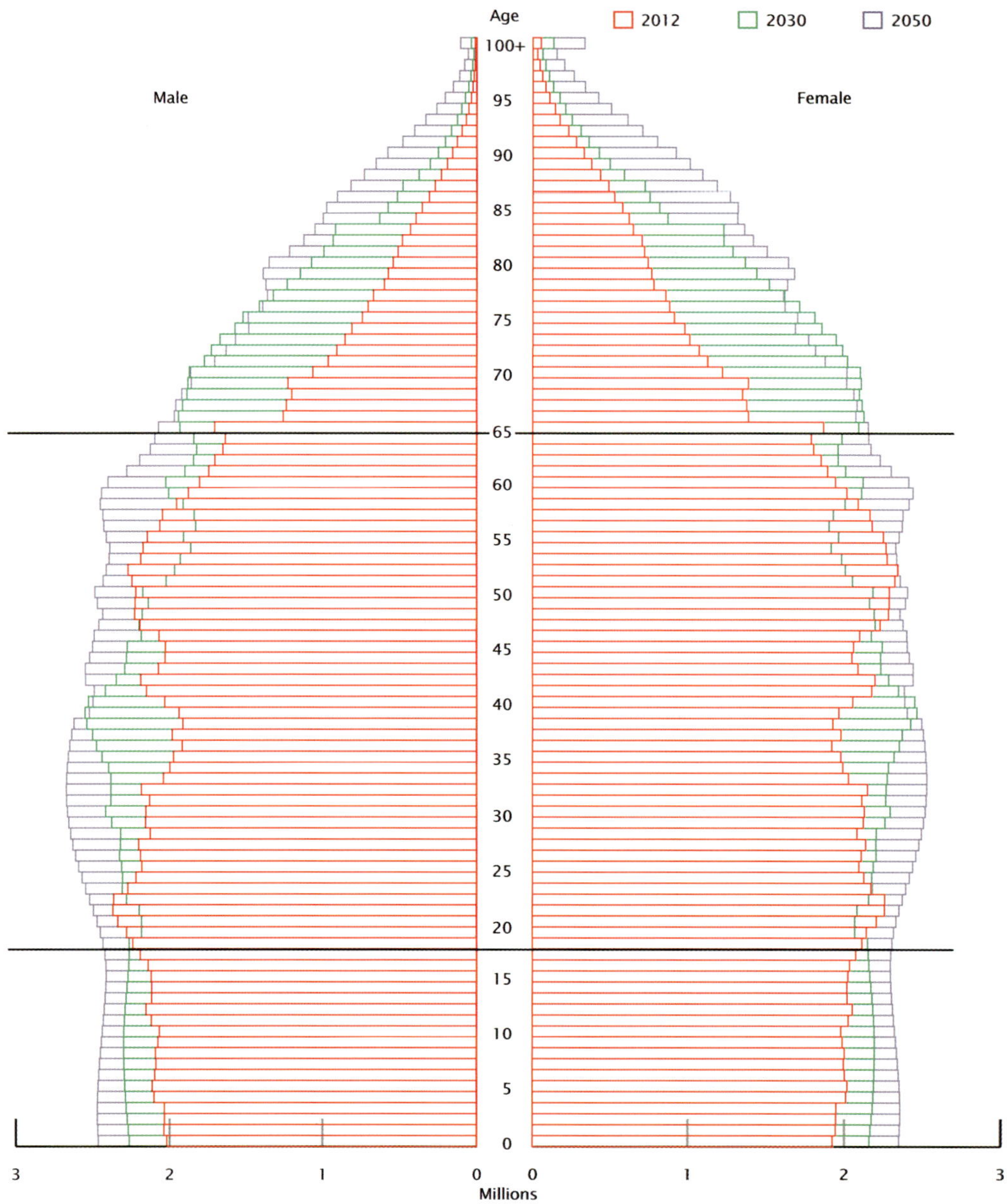

Fig. 2.1 Age and sex structure of the population for the United States for the years 2010, 2030, and 2050. (Courtesy of U.S. Census Bureau, 2012 Population Estimates and 2012 National Projections.)

nations to quickly recognize the scope of the new demographic reality and adjust current and future policies accordingly.[2,3]

■ General Concepts in Geriatrics

The *Canon of Medicine*, written by Avicenna in 1025, was the first book to offer instruction in the care of the elderly, foreshadowing modern gerontology and geriatrics. In a chapter entitled "Regimen of Old Age," Avicenna expressed concern with his observation that "old folk need plenty of sleep"; he suggested that their bodies should be anointed with oil and even recommended exercises such as walking or horseback riding. Thesis III of the *Canon* discussed a diet felt to be suitable for the elderly and dedicated several sections to the problem of constipation in geriatric patients. George Day published the *A Practical Treatise on the Domestic Management and Most Important Diseases of Advanced Life* in 1851, one of the first publications on the subject of geriatric medicine. The first modern geriatric hospital was founded in Belgrade, Serbia, in 1881 by doctor Laza Lazarević. In 1909, the term *geriatrics* was proposed by

Dr. Ignatz Leo Nascher from New York, who was subsequently recognized as a "father of geriatrics" in the United States. As with other areas of medicine, however, some traditional guiding ethical principles continue to apply. These include (1) beneficence, doing no harm, but only what will benefit the patient; (2) autonomy, or the right of the patient to decide what is best for him or her; and (3) justice, the rights of the patient considered in the context of what is best for society as a whole.[4]

Geriatric medicine differs from standard adult medicine because it focuses on the unique needs of the elderly person. This fundamental difference was formally recognized when, in July 2007, the Association of American Medical Colleges (AAMC) and the John A. Hartford Foundation[6] hosted a National Consensus Conference on Competencies in Geriatric Education. At this conference, a consensus was reached on minimum competencies, or learning outcomes, that were required of graduating medical students to assure that new residents could provide competent care for older patients. The American Geriatric Society (AGS), the American Medical Association (AMA), and the Association of Directors of Geriatric Academic Programs (ADGAP) established and endorsed 26 Minimum Geriatric Competencies in eight content domains. Each content domain specifies three or more observable, measurable competencies.

The eight domains are as follows:

- Cognitive and behavioral disorders
- Medication management
- Self-care capacity
- Falls, balance, gait disorders
- Atypical presentation of disease
- Palliative care
- Hospital care for elders
- Health care planning and promotion

The elderly are physiologically different from younger adults, with an expected but variable decline of almost all organ systems. In many cases these changes may be slowed or stopped with appropriate interventions. Indeed, there is evidence that age-specific medical care can reduce the rate of decline. With age, there is a relative loss of muscle mass (termed sarcopenia) and an increase in body fat. Exercise dramatically reduces, and to some degree, even reverses these changes. Similarly, although bone density decreases after age 30, exercise is a well-recognized and powerful means of slowing the process. In some cases, pharmacological intervention is also necessary. Common cardiovascular changes with age include a rise in systolic blood pressure and decreased cardiac output, both of which, again, may be mitigated by exercise. Visual acuity often declines with time and may be accelerated by macular degeneration or cataracts. Hearing loss is an extremely common complaint in the elderly and can most often be attributed to presbycusis. Other causes include noise-induced hearing loss, ototoxicity, and cerumen impaction. The vestibular system is affected by peripheral degenerative changes and slowing of central processing. Geriatricians distinguish between these effects of normal aging and disease. The extent to which older individuals are affected by symptoms and disease is often a reflection of lifestyle choices and the degree of available "functional reserve." The importance of this concept is recognized daily in health care centers. Healthy, high-functioning older individuals may present with a seemingly small medical problem, which, because of diminished functional reserves in multiple organ systems, leads to a cascade effect with multiorgan involvement and possibly critical illness. Several validated "barometers" currently exist with which to objectively determine functional reserve:

- Comprehensive geriatric assessment (CGA)
- Activities of daily living (ADL)
- Instrumental activities of daily living
- Exercise tolerance or gait speed
- Frailty (0–5)

Disease often presents very differently in the elderly, with a vague and nonspecific history that may include falls and confusion. Older individuals may minimize symptoms or delay seeking medical care. The multiple medications taken by many of these patients (polypharmacy) compound the difficulty of arriving at an accurate diagnosis because of possible drug interactions, dosing errors, and central nervous system side effects. In a geriatric patient, acute bacterial sinusitis may present with low-grade fever and confusion, in contradistinction to the higher fever, facial pressure/headache, and rhinorrhea described by younger patients.

Functional abilities, independence, and a high quality of life feature prominently in the top priorities of geriatric patients and the physicians caring for them. A multidisciplinary team knowledgeable in the complexities of geriatric care and dedicated to promoting and restoring autonomy and maximizing quality of life in this patient population is required to achieve these goals. In some cases this may mean enlisting the help of home care services or skilled nurses. Assisted living facilities may constitute a good option for some individuals, with long-term care or hospices reserved for those unable to achieve any independence, even with appropriate care and support.

Frailty is an important and relatively common issue in the elderly and alters the risk–benefit ratio of many treatment algorithms designed for younger patients. Accurate evaluations of treatment risks based on validated measures may assist geriatric patients in making reasoned and thoughtful choices about their available options. In some instances, for example, they may decline risky or toxic treatments if they are at higher risk of dying from other causes. The presence of frailty significantly increases the risk of postoperative complications, prolongs recovery times, and increases the probability of requiring extended care. Objective assessment of frailty in the elderly preoperatively allows for accurate predictions of recovery trajectories.[7] One frequently used, practical frailty scale uses five items:

- Unintentional weight loss
- Muscle weakness
- Exhaustion
- Low physical activity
- Slowed walking speed

Each item is assigned a score of 0 if absent, 1 if present. A healthy individual would then have the minimum score of 0, whereas a very frail person would have the maximum score of 5. Elderly individuals with intermediate frailty scores of 2 or 3 are twice as likely as healthy geriatric patients to have postoperative complications and spend 50% more time in the hospital, and they are three times as likely to be discharged to a skilled nursing facility instead of to their own home.[7] Very frail elderly patients with scores of 4 or 5 who were living at home before the surgery have even poorer outcomes, with the risk of being discharged to a nursing home rising to 20 times the rate for nonfrail elderly patients.

Polypharmacy refers to the concurrent use of several medications and is a particularly common problem in the elderly. It is defined either by the absolute number of medications taken (more than five), or by the use of excessive or unnecessary prescriptions. In addition, more than half of seniors take supplements in the form of vitamins, minerals, or herbal preparations. Polypharmacy is associated with an increased risk of adverse drug reactions, drug interactions, and patient noncompliance. This is the result of the number of medications taken as well as altered pharmacokinetics in the elderly, which include a change in the distribution, metabolism, and excretion of drugs. More specifically, a decrease in serum albumin, particularly in cases of malnutrition, may affect drug binding. Additionally, oxidative metabolism by the liver is diminished, and renal drug clearance is reduced.

Although the lists of geriatric syndromes vary, the following are frequently recognized: dementia, delirium, falls, hearing impairment, sarcopenia, malnutrition, frailty, incontinence, and visual impairment.

Geriatric Otolaryngology

The effect of the shifting demographics on medical and surgical subspecialties, including that of otolaryngology, has been noted for some time. Three major events contributed to the emergence of geriatric otolaryngology as a firmly established subspecialty.[8] The first was the Geriatric Otolaryngology Cherry Blossom Conference held in Washington, DC, in 1988. The meeting was attended by several farsighted physicians and was led by Jerome C. Goldstein, MD. It resulted in the publication of a monograph entitled *Clinical Geriatric Otolaryngology*. The second event was the Geriatrics for Specialists Initiative. Dr. Joseph LoCicero III, formerly the chairman of the interspecialty group formed by the American Geriatric Society (AGS), recognized the brewing crisis in elderly care. The AGS realized 20 years ago that it could not, by itself, handle the increasing volume of geriatric patients. It therefore reached out to several specialties, including otolaryngology, to embrace this focused subspecialty area, foster research and education, and ultimately better prepare otolaryngologists for the evolving needs of the ever-increasing population of older patients. Recognition of the scope of the new demographic reality led to the third event, the birth of the American Society of Geriatric Otolaryngology (ASGO) in 2007, a result of the foresight and leadership of its first president, Jerome C. Goldstein, MD.

Elderly patients account for a large and disproportionate number of outpatient visits. Similarly, it is reasonable to expect the number of geriatric otolaryngology patients to account for an increasing proportion of the practice of otolaryngologists. Indeed, in a review of geriatric patients in a general otolaryngology practice between 2004 and 2010, Creighton et al noted a statistically significant increase in the number of geriatric patients from 14.3% in 2004 to 17.9% in 2010.[9] That number is expected to dramatically increase to 30% by the year 2030. It appears that the cross section or profile of otolaryngological pathologies encountered during these outpatient visits lacks uniformity across various age groups. In the same study, Creighton et al demonstrated that as patients age, otologic complaints are increasingly common. The following, in order of frequency, were the most common diagnoses in patients over the age of 65[9]:

- Hearing loss
- Disorders of the external ear
- Other ear disorders, mainly tinnitus
- Nonsuppurative otitis media/eustachian tube disorders
- Vertiginous syndromes/vestibular disorders

Familiarity with the unique otolaryngological pathology profiles of elderly patients is important in providing optimal care to this increasing subset of the population. Going forward, awareness of these important demographic changes in otolaryngology practices should translate into appropriate representation in training programs.

References

1. Shapiro DP. Geriatric demographics and the practice of otolaryngology. Ear Nose Throat J 1999;78(6):418–421
2. Kost K. American Society of Geriatric Otolaryngology (ASGO)–AAO-HNS Bulletin. 2011; Vol 30(9)
3. National Institute on Aging, National Institutes of Health, U.S. Department of Health and Human Services, and the U.S. Department of State
4. Vincent KV, Velkoff VA. The next four decades: the older population in the United States: 2010 to 2050. U.S. Census Bureau; 2010
5. Lucente FE. Ethical challenges in geriatric care. Otolaryngol Head Neck Surg 2009;140(6):809–811
6. http://www.jhartfound.org/
7. Makary MA, Segev DL, Pronovost PJ, et al. Frailty as a predictor of surgical outcomes in older patients. J Am Coll Surg 2010;210(6):901–908
8. Chalian AA. Accomplishment and opportunity in geriatric otolaryngology. Ear Nose Throat J 2009;88(10):1156–1161
9. Creighton FX Jr, Poliashenko SM, Statham MM, Abramson P, Johns MM III. The growing geriatric otolaryngology patient population: a study of 131,700 new patient encounters. Laryngoscope 2013;123(1):97–102

3 Understanding Geriatric Syndromes, the Geriatric Interdisciplinary Team, and Resources to Optimize Care for Older Patients

Sarah H. Kagan

■ Introduction

Otolaryngologists, like all specialist physicians in any aging society, face important challenges in effectively caring for older adults. Effective care requires looking beyond the bounds of otolaryngology to develop an understanding of frailty, multimorbidity, and geriatric syndromes that intersect with otolaryngological conditions. This clinical knowledge provides the foundation for geriatric competence, affording a better capacity to collaborate with the geriatric interdisciplinary team (GIDT) as well as to target and access resources for older patients. As a result, geriatric patients and their family caregivers benefit from better integrated and coordinated care as well as from GIDT surveillance to reduce unmet needs and avoid complications.

Aging societies bear an increasing burden of health care need that emerges from the intertwined forces of elder dependency and compression of morbidity.[1–4] Elder dependency occurs as more people live longer while birth rates decline. This extension of life with reduction in births creates a larger proportion of dependent older people to younger people who provide the economic base as well as care for elders.[5] Dependent elders are those who, in demographic terms, no longer contribute economically to society. Underlying that dependency are implicit concerns of frailty and multimorbidity. However, compression of morbidity may mitigate dependency by moving time of greatest need closer to the point of death.[1,3] Consequently, the demographic of an aging society creates manifold and dynamic consequences for health and social care needs.[5] At the population level, frailty and multimorbidity contribute to both volume and complexity in care of older patients. Nonetheless, not all consequences in an aging society are easily and clearly projected.[1,6] Thus specialist physicians, as with all clinicians who are not specialists in the care of older people, benefit from preparation that supports competent practice in the rapidly evolving context of an aging society.

Geriatric competence describes the application of requisite knowledge for safe, effective, and quality care for older adults. The Institute of Medicine, along with authors from geriatric medicine and nursing, explicitly outlines that continued inattention to the unique characteristics and resultant needs of older adults in education and practice generates dire present and future consequences to health care and to society.[7–9] The Institute of Medicine amalgamated a vast collection of literature addressing the care of older adults, calling for a "retooling" of American clinical education, health care training, and care delivery.[7] This report established the current foundation for enacting geriatric competence as a requirement, and not an option, for all clinicians caring for older adults.

Geriatric competence broadly includes knowledge of aging as an integral biological, psychological, and social process; the functional consequences of aging along with diseases, conditions, and syndromes common to later life; and the means to recognize and mitigate the risks of adverse events in the care of older people. Specific competencies, which are particular to individual disciplines, are reliant on social contract and scope of practice. The Association of American Medical Colleges (AAMC) enacted a set of geriatric competencies for medical students, contemporaneously with the Institute of Medicine's *Retooling for an Aging America* report.[7,8] The AAMC requires that graduating medical students possess the following competencies: medication management; cognitive and behavioral disorders; self-care capacity; falls, balance, and gait disorders; health care planning and promotion; atypical presentation of disease; palliative care; and hospital care for elders.[8] Each of these competencies is detailed in the Appendix of this chapter.

Practice in an aging society requires otolaryngologists then to look beyond their own specialty care toward geriatric competence. As clinicians who do not specialize in aging, otolaryngologists must achieve competence through both knowledge and collaboration. The larger aim is to coordinate care and integrate resources to optimize care quality, safety, and patient and family satisfaction. This chapter describes the elements necessary to achieve that optimal level of care for older patients.

Three elements are necessary in order for otolaryngologists to optimize care for older adults. First, knowledge of important clinical phenomena that are common to older adults enables the otolaryngologist to identify the interface between these clinical conditions and otolaryngological diseases, conditions, and syndromes as well as to target areas for collaboration with the GIDT. Second, familiarity with roles and responsibilities with the geriatric interdisciplinary team as well as colleagues who can offer collaboration when a GIDT is not available enables the otolaryngologist to promote care coordination, ensure transitional care, and avoid fragmentation. Both knowledge of geriatric phenomena and collaboration with a GIDT or geriatric colleagues require routine continuing education and the savvy use of geriatric resources. Third, knowledge of and means to access local and national resources for continuing clinician education, for patient education and services, and for family support streamlines otolaryngological care for older adults as well as support for their family caregivers. The chapter concludes with a summary of implications for future geriatric otolaryngology practice, education, and research in the context of our aging world.

Frailty, Multimorbidity, and Geriatric Syndromes

Conditions and syndromes of very late life are characterized by intricate biological, physical, and psychological processes that intersect and commonly cascade, resulting in functional decline at all levels. As a result, clinicians face assessment and identification of subtle, complicated phenomena despite relatively straightforward presenting complaints among older adults. Frailty is increasingly understood as playing a critical role in this intersecting cascade that results in several etiologies converging in intersecting pathogenesis and leading to syndromes common to frail older adults.[10–12] These conditions emerge from cascading etiologies and are generally termed geriatric syndromes. There is no common definition for geriatric syndromes.[10] Geriatric syndromes, whereas they have multiple intersecting etiologies, have a complex manifestation with observable hallmarks like falls or pressure ulcers. Whether "frailty" is a geriatric syndrome as are "falls" and "incontinence" or whether it stands alone as a syndrome that contributes to others is not yet clear from extant evidence.[10,11] Nonetheless, the issues of complex and intersecting pathogenesis and presentation along with risks of disability and continuing care needs are well established.[10–13] Inouye and colleagues, in a classic work, demonstrate the complexity that characterizes geriatric syndromes in a widely known figure (**Fig. 3.1**).[10]

Frailty is ever better understood as an expression of aging processes that result in declining functional reserve. Clegg and colleagues vividly depict the distinction between fit and frail elders (**Fig. 3.2**). Declining reserves lead to vulnerability, which magnifies the effects of insults, resulting in deleterious events like a fall, disability, and escalating needs for care.[12] Although debate continues over whether frailty emerges from phenotypic flaws[13,14] or multiple deficits accumulated over time,[15,16] vast evidence points to the manifest impact on older individuals and on aging societies. Clegg and colleagues schematize the pathophysiology of frailty, clearly outlining the relationships from the cellular to the social levels in this epigenetic phenomenon from which geriatric syndromes and functional debility in late life emerge (**Fig. 3.3**).[11]

Classification of geriatric syndromes remains somewhat confusing. There is no universal and widely accepted definition or definitive list that might guide nonspecialist clinicians. Geriatric syndromes may be more easily understood if classified into antecedent and consequent syndromes. Specifically, some geriatric syndromes like frailty and sarcopenia seem to presage declining constitutional reserve.[11] In essence, these syndromes are characterized by declining reserve at the level of cells and tissues (e.g., muscle function in sarcopenia) that then contribute to clinically manifest syndromes like osteoporosis and potentiate normal aging changes like presbystasis. The result is consequent syndromes like falls. In this example, falls are obviously connected to sarcopenia, presbystasis, and osteoporosis. However, falls result from functional effects of sarcopenia, presbystasis, and sometimes osteoporosis, whereas osteoporosis also exacerbates risk of injury from falls. All of the syndromes implicated here converge in the clinical manifestation of the apparently simple syndrome of falls in older adults. Moreover, a fall event also results in risk for other syndromes like delirium and pressure ulcers and engenders the need for an array of health and social care services in the frail older adult.[12] In general, consensus regarding geriatric syndromes suggests that, at minimum, falls, fear of falling, incontinence, pressure ulcers, sleep disorders, and anorexia with failure to thrive are included in the classification.

Importantly, frail older adults experiencing geriatric syndromes are likely to be multimorbid, a term describing the state of sustained, multiple comorbid conditions. Older adults are widely acknowledged, both in epidemiological studies and in clinical wis-

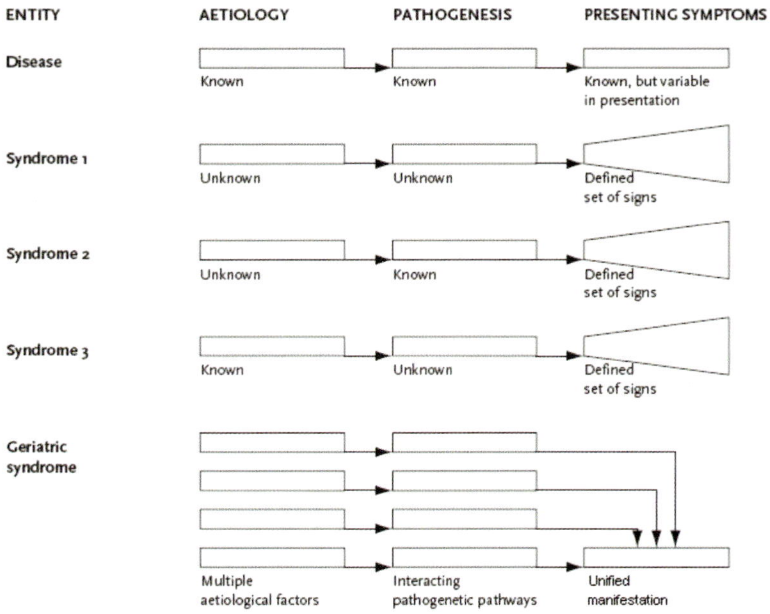

Fig. 3.1 Schematic conceptual representation of clinical conditions defined by the terms *disease*, *syndrome*, and *geriatric syndrome*, illustrating differences in numbers and complexity of relevant factors, including etiological risk factors, pathophysiological mechanisms, and presenting symptoms. (Used with permission from Inouye SK, Studenski S, Tinetti ME, Kuchel GA. Geriatric syndromes: clinical, research, and policy implications of a core geriatric concept. J Am Geriatr Soc 2007;55(5):780–791.)

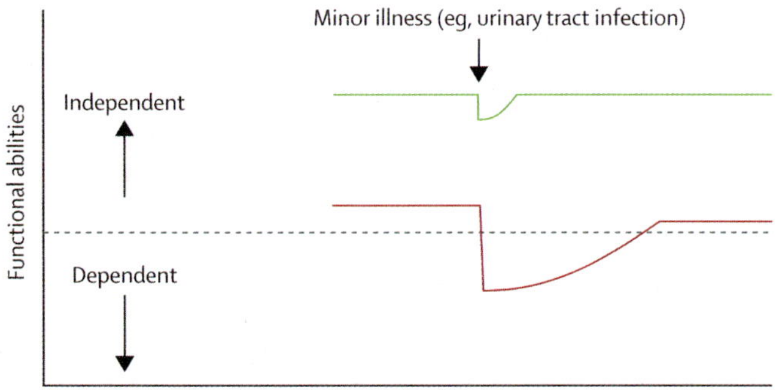

Fig. 3.2 Vulnerability of frail elderly people to a sudden change in health status after a minor illness. The green line represents a fit elderly individual who, after a minor stressor event such as an infection, has a small deterioration in function and then returns to homoeostasis. The red line represents a frail elderly individual who, after a similar stressor event, undergoes a larger deterioration, which may manifest as functional dependency, and who does not return to baseline homeostasis. The horizontal dashed line represents the cutoff between a dependent and an independent functional status. (Used with permission from Clegg A. The frailty syndrome. Clin Med 2011;11(1):72–75.)

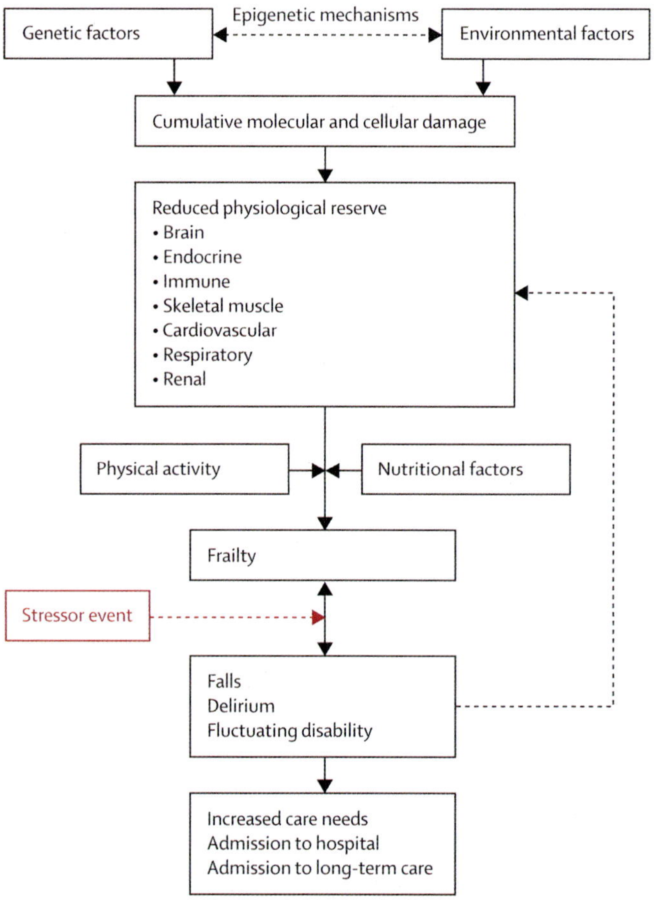

Fig. 3.3 Schematic representation of the pathophysiology of frailty. (Used with permission from Clegg A. The frailty syndrome. Clin Med 2011;11(1):72–75.)

dom, as often presenting with a constellation of chronic, noncommunicable diseases and conditions that coexist. These coexistent diseases and conditions complicate presentation, assessment, treatment, and outcomes.[17,18] Nonetheless, the presence of comorbid conditions as the phenomenon now termed multimorbidity is incompletely studied.[17] Physiological connections between frailty and multimorbidity are poorly elucidated as are the contributions of social determinants of health. Social determinants of health obviously influence development of chronic noncommunicable disease, which accounts for the major burden of health care globally.[17,19] Social determinants of health may also aggravate the antecedents and consequences of frailty and geriatric syndromes.[12] However, definitive investigation of the interrelationships of frailty, multimorbidity, and geriatric syndromes is as yet unreported in the world literature on aging. As a result, erudite clinicians must remain aware of the risks and consequences of this aging triad, pursuing developing evidence with the goal of optimizing clinical care.

The exemplar geriatric syndrome used here, falls, illustrates critical aspects of the intersections of frailty, multimorbidity, and geriatric syndromes for otolaryngological practice. In this case, the otolaryngologist possesses the expertise necessary to address presbystasis[20] as a major factor resulting in fall risk and actual falls for any given older patient. This exemplar further underscores the interdisciplinary and collaborative nature of optimal geriatric care. In this case, best practice warrants fall risk assessment, fall event grading, and investigation of fear of falling syndrome, depending on the individual presentation.[21,22] Likewise, evidence-based and best practices suggest an interdisciplinary plan for treatment that includes consideration of sarcopenia and osteoporosis in both pharmacological and behavioral therapies. Specific interventions easily incorporated into such an interdisciplinary plan encompass strength and balance exercises; home survey for trip and other safety hazards; home safety adaptations, including grab bars and the like; and patient and caregiver education to promote activity, reduce anxiety, and limit behavioral falls risk. Thus the role of the otolaryngologist in improving care for an older person experiencing fall risk and falls is clear. Needs for a team approach to promote astute identification and use of clinical, community, and social resources and for collaboration between the geriatric team and the otolaryngologist are equally clear. The case of falls as a geriatric syndrome provides a template for analyzing the interrelationships between and among frailty, multimorbidity, and geriatric syndromes and understanding the value of geriatric competence and collaboration with the GIDT in geriatric otolaryngology.

The Geriatric Interdisciplinary Team

Geriatric medicine possesses a fascinating 150-year history, tied initially to developments in pathology and expanding understandings of the aging process.[23] Geriatrics benefited—as do most major innovations—from the contributions of luminary advocates and leaders in the young science of aging and practice of geriatrics. Morley points up, however, that modern geriatrics arose in the middle of the 20th century, a time of many major advances in American medicine.[23] In the decades since geriatrics entered modern medicine and health care, its practitioners have cultivated values of interdisciplinary collaboration and presumption of benefit in the team approach to patients and clinicians. In the late 1970s and early 1980s, many investigations of the presupposed value of interdisciplinary geriatric teams were conducted and reported, attempting to establish differential value in the outcomes of care and supporting the belief among clinicians on those teams that care of the elderly improves with this approach.[24–26]

Interest in the contributions of GIDTs to safe, high-quality care for older patients continues through the present day.[27] However, issues of logistics, cost, and reimbursement commonly temper both capacity and enthusiasm. GIDTs present the obstacles of limited evidence on comparative and cost-effectiveness.[27–30] However, if the primary function of GIDTs is to complete comprehensive geriatric assessment and ensure that high-risk aspects of care are not neglected, then evidence supports their use.[26,28,31] A recent meta-analysis of the effectiveness of comprehensive geriatric assessment completed by a roving interdisciplinary team or in a dedicated hospital ward revealed increased likelihood of recipient patients being alive and in their own homes after nonelective hospital admission.[28] Nonetheless, the conceptual, methodological, and pragmatic challenges of showing improved care processes and outcomes for frail older patients are long-standing and unlikely to be overcome within clinical trials.[32]

Some academic medical centers maintain complete consultative GIDTs—often as part of a larger program that may include dedicated inpatient teams and wards.[30] In academic medical centers with geriatric programs, GIDTs are generally led, or jointly facilitated, by a geriatrician, a geriatric advanced practice nurse (G-APN), or both. Together, these clinicians offer a variety of specialist services that move beyond the capacity of geriatric-competent generalists. The team they lead is ideally comprehensive and holistic in both approach and composition. Disciplines commonly represented within GIDTs, in addition to medicine and nursing, include physical therapy, social work, and psychology or geropsychiatric nursing, or possibly geriatric psychiatry. Well-developed teams, taking a lesson from rehabilitation, may also include occupational therapy and speech language pathology. Team composition varies, as may availability of specific team members who may hold other positions or have commitments to other departments in addition to the GIDT. Most GIDTs are now consultative in nature, a feature that may have emerged out of research that explores consultation as a means to distribute geriatric expertise as a scarce resource in many institutions.[33,34] Some community-based institutions and academic medical centers often rely on consultation provided by one or two geriatric specialists rather than a complete GIDT. These specialists are often geriatricians or G-APNs who offer consultation, make recommendations, and help coordinate care resources.

In many community hospitals and many ambulatory settings, financial constraints and limited personnel commonly mean limited or no dedicated interdisciplinary geriatric resources exist. Some institutions invest in capacity to offer these resources by relying on a G-APN who is either a nurse practitioner or a clinical nurse specialist, who possesses many of the skills used in consultation by geriatricians combined with an ability to educate nurses and other direct care providers in best practices and individualized care for particular patients. Other institutions may endorse systematic advancement of care for older adults by pursuing certification through an international best practices program, Nurses Improving Care for Health System Elders (NICHE), which is dedicated to achieving geriatric competence among all levels of nurses and supporting it within the generalist interdisciplinary team.[33,35] Both the consultation and systemwide options offer valuable resources to improve the processes and outcomes of care for older patients. They can also be successfully combined. Nonetheless, many specialist physicians, including otolaryngologists, may prefer the convenience of being able to call a G-APN to request specialist geriatric consultation in institutions where dedicated geriatric resources are scarce.

Some institutions are without dedicated geriatric specialists; thus clinicians without training in the field wishing to provide optimal care to older people find themselves in a conundrum. The question of what to do in the absence of geriatric specialist colleagues to offer safe, high-quality care requires a detailed appraisal of institutional colleagues who may contribute important expertise to the care of older adults and support to their family members. Most notably, physical therapists and social workers are present in most settings and offer invaluable knowledge, insight, and skills relevant to the care of frail older people. Physical therapists commonly anchor plans of care in which the cross-cutting intervention of exercise addresses frailty and the downward spiral in which it is often apparent. The value of physical therapy links back to the possible association among sarcopenia, frailty, and consequent geriatric syndromes like falls.[11] Likewise, social workers provide essential education and support to geriatric patients by helping them locate and access community-based resources, thereby reducing the ill effects of diminished social support. These resources, when successfully managed, mitigate the risk of institutional long-term care and unexpected hospitalization.

Finally, otolaryngologists and their clinical teams may attain a level of geriatric competence and care coordination for older patients even in the absence of specific geriatric resources and colleagues. The otolaryngology team can develop competence by seeking out continuing education and networking with community and regional resources to essentially become their own geriatric consultants.[36] The otolaryngologist often bears much of the responsibility in increasing geriatric competence in the practice. However, a registered nurse within the team, or one hired to focus on care for older adults, may also share or assume this role with equal effect. More practically, many otolaryngology practices may benefit from having a nurse, medical assistant, or even medical secretary to locate, network with, and recommend local, regional, and national resources to enhance the care of individual older patients.

Geriatric Resources

Achieving geriatric competence as a clinician and delivering coordinated care to older adults are inextricably linked aspects of a larger process of understanding the dimensions of health care in an aging society. The Institute of Medicine's landmark report calling for retooling is emblematic of the inescapable fact that health care in an aging society must be constructed very differently to achieve safe, quality care for older adults.[7] Simultaneous education and improvements are necessary to meet the needs of patients today, because the crisis referred to in *Retooling for an Aging America* is upon us, though it remains unrecognized or misidentified by many.[7] Fortunately, a wide array of resources exists to support geriatric competence and care coordination and referrals alike. However, it is difficult to classify resources that support geriatric education and care because many are local or even institutionally specific, and a single organization or other entity often serves many resource functions.

Local and institutional resources are best identified by understanding some basic categories and then searching for those in the neighboring community.

Surveying local resources best begins with identifying the nearest academic geriatric and gerontological programs along with the services they offer. Actively seeking programs outside of medicine ensures that robust programs provided in schools of nursing, social work, or gerontology are not overlooked. Specific institutional resources, especially those focused on student and clinician education and training, may be supported by and thus searchable with the source of funding in mind. Two leading foundations support institutional centers of excellence and exceptional national resources. The John A. Hartford Foundation (http://www.jhartfound.org/) is a major source of support for discipline-specific and interdisciplinary educational programs and centers in aging and geriatric care across the United States. The Hartford Foundation supports, among other programs, the Hartford Institute for Geriatric Nursing, run by the New York University College of Nursing. The Institute is home to a variety of national programs, including the NICHE Program (http://www.hartfordign.org/). The Donald W. Reynolds Foundation is similarly influential, focusing exclusively on physician education (http://www.dwreynolds.org/Programs/National/Aging/Aging.htm). The Reynolds Foundation supports the Portal of Geriatrics Online Education, more popularly known by its acronym POGOe, and administered by the Icahn School of Medicine at Mount Sinai, Department of Geriatrics and Palliative Medicine on behalf of the Association of Directors of Geriatric Academic Programs (http://www.pogoe.org/). POGOe is an indispensable source of continuing education for otolaryngologists and other physicians aiming to become competent in geriatrics. Many academic medical centers may house programs supported by the Hartford or the Reynolds foundations, providing a repository of information and expertise for those in the larger health care community. Finally, the John T. and Catherine D. MacArthur Foundation (http://www.macfound.org/) also maintains a considered interest in aging, focusing largely on the societal level of knowledge and action.

Regional resources are largely designed to offer services that assist older adults and their families. Counties throughout the United States provide a service, largely funded by lottery proceeds, called Area Agencies on Aging. Native American Aging Programs are similarly present in regions of the United States that include native communities. These local programs and agencies can be located through the National Association of Area Agencies Web site (http://www.n4a.org/index.cfm). These programs provide a broad array of services that generally require both functional and financial eligibility. Most state governments have a department of aging or similar unit that offers a range of state specific resources. Some larger metropolitan population centers, such as New York City, maintain similar departments (http://www.nyc.gov/html/dfta/html/home/home.shtml). As America's population continues to age, more municipalities are likely to launch departments of aging and similar units strategically positioned to address the needs of older communities.

National resources are more varied than those at local and regional levels. Important national organizations and coalitions provide information for clinicians and the public alike. The Administration on Aging (AOA) is the section of the Department of Health and Human Services dedicated to aging and older Americans (http://www.aoa.gov/). Clinicians will find statistics on aging valuable, whereas older adults and their families may find the Eldercare Locator useful (http://eldercare.gov/Eldercare.NET/Public/Index.aspx). Like the AOA, the Centers for Disease Control and Prevention (CDC) provides easy access to U.S. aging statistics and several other topics on its Healthy Aging page (http://www.cdc.gov/aging/index.htm). The Centers for Medicare and Medicaid Services (http:// www.cms.gov) offer vast amounts of information about Medicare and Medicaid. Among the most important sites for both clinicians and family members of frail older adults is Nursing Home Compare, the resource for comparative state- and institution-level data assessing nursing home quality (http://www.medicare.gov/nursinghomecompare/).

Clinicians seeking learning and networking opportunities value the remarkable choice of organizations dedicated to professionals working in aging. The American Geriatrics Society is focused on health care (http://www.americangeriatrics.org/) with a large physician membership, whereas the Gerontological Society of America is explicitly interdisciplinary, offering discourse valuable to colleagues in biological, psychological, and social gerontology as well as those in clinical care (http://www.geron.org/). Disease- and condition-specific associations are appreciated by patients, family members, and even clinicians who seek current information and access to programs like clinical trials. Good examples of these resources include the Alzheimer's Association (http://www.alz.org/) and the National Parkinson Foundation (http://www.parkinson.org/). Private charities and advocacy groups such as the Michael J. Fox Foundation for Parkinson's Research are often equally if not more useful sources of information for diseases common in aging (https://www.michaeljfox.org/).

■ The Future

The contribution of otolaryngology to an aging society is distinct and important, given the otolaryngological nature of complaints common among older patients and the demographics of our aging society and rapidly aging world.[4,5,7,37] Otolaryngologists, with their current and ever expanding contribution to American health care and indeed to health care in all aging societies around the globe, must invest evermore in geriatric competence and wise use of geriatric resources, including the interdisciplinary team. Geriatric competence is predicated in large part on knowledge of the ramifications of aging among individuals and populations. Understanding frailty, multimorbidity, and geriatric syndromes is requisite to effective clinical care of older patients and to fully using geriatric interdisciplinary teams or their analogues to collaboratively deliver safe, quality care for older adults and their families. Understanding foundational knowledge in geriatrics enables the otolaryngologist to avoid the false security of believing standard of care for adults is sufficient and instead to incorporate geriatric considerations and best practices into evidence-based, goal-directed assessment, intervention, and evaluation of process and outcomes. The projected need for geriatric competence in otolaryngology as well as for specialist geriatric otolaryngology care mandates a long view of the future and investment in career-long continuing education and practice improvement as well as in geriatric research and education.

References

1. Bayer A. Clinical issues in old age—the challenges of geriatric medicine. Quality in Ageing and Older Adults 2011; 12(1):44–49
2. Fries JF. The compression of morbidity. Milbank Mem Fund Q Health Soc 1983;61(3):397–419
3. Cai L, Lubitz J. Was there compression of disability for older Americans from 1992 to 2003? Demography 2007;44(3): 479–495
4. United Nations Population Division. World Population Aging: 1950–2050. United Nations Publications; 2001. http://www.un.org/esa/population/publications/worldageing19502050/
5. Olshansky SJ, Goldman DP, Zheng Y, Rowe JW. Aging in America in the twenty-first century: demographic forecasts from the MacArthur Foundation Research Network on an Aging Society. Milbank Q 2009;87(4):842–862
6. Lunney JR, Lynn J, Foley DJ, Lipson S, Guralnik JM. Patterns of functional decline at the end of life. JAMA 2003;289(18): 2387–2392
7. Institute of Medicine. Retooling for an Aging America: Building the Health Care Workforce. Washington, DC: National Academies Press; 2008
8. Leipzig RM, Granville L, Simpson D, Anderson MB, Sauvigné K, Soriano RP. Keeping granny safe on July 1: a consensus on minimum geriatrics competencies for graduating medical students. Acad Med 2009;84(5):604–610
9. Kagan SH. The plateau of recognition in specialty acute care. Geriatr Nurs 2009;30(2):130–131
10. Inouye SK, Studenski S, Tinetti ME, Kuchel GA. Geriatric syndromes: clinical, research, and policy implications of a core geriatric concept. J Am Geriatr Soc 2007;55(5):780–791
11. Clegg A, Young J. The frailty syndrome. Clin Med 2011; 11(1):72–75
12. Clegg A, Young J, Iliffe S, Rikkert MO, Rockwood K. Frailty in elderly people. Lancet 2013;381(9868):752–762
13. Fried LP, Ferrucci L, Darer J, Williamson JD, Anderson G. Untangling the concepts of disability, frailty, and comorbidity: implications for improved targeting and care. J Gerontol A Biol Sci Med Sci 2004;59(3):255–263
14. Fried LP, Hadley EC, Walston JD, et al. From bedside to bench: research agenda for frailty. Sci SAGE KE 2005; 2005(31):pe24
15. Rockwood K, Mitnitski A. Frailty in relation to the accumulation of deficits. J Gerontol A Biol Sci Med Sci 2007;62(7): 722–727
16. Rockwood K, Song X, MacKnight C, et al. A global clinical measure of fitness and frailty in elderly people. CMAJ 2005;173(5):489–495
17. Barnett K, Mercer SW, Norbury M, Watt G, Wyke S, Guthrie B. Epidemiology of multimorbidity and implications for health care, research, and medical education: a cross-sectional study. Lancet 2012;380(9836):37–43
18. Marengoni A, Angleman S, Melis R, et al. Aging with multimorbidity: a systematic review of the literature. Ageing Res Rev 2011;10(4):430–439
19. United Nations General Assembly. Political Declaration of the High-level Meeting of the General Assembly on the Prevention and Control of Non-communicable Diseases. 2011. http://www.who.int/nmh/events/un_ncd_summit2011/political_declaration_en.pdf
20. Agrawal Y, Carey JP, Della Santina CC, Schubert MC, Minor LB. Disorders of balance and vestibular function in US adults: data from the National Health and Nutrition Examination Survey, 2001-2004. Arch Intern Med 2009;169(10):938–944
21. Hadjistavropoulos T, Delbaere K, Fitzgerald TD. Reconceptualizing the role of fear of falling and balance confidence in fall risk. J Aging Health 2011;23(1):3–23
22. Davalos-Bichara M, Lin FR, Carey JP, et al. Development and validation of a falls-grading scale. J Geriatr Phys Ther 2013;36(2):63–67
23. Morley JE. A brief history of geriatrics. J Gerontol A Biol Sci Med Sci 2004;59(11):1132–1152
24. Blumenfield S, Morris J, Sherman FT. The geriatric team in the acute care hospital: an educational and consultation modality. J Am Geriatr Soc 1982;30(10):660–664
25. Steel K, Hays A. A consultation service in geriatric medicine at a university hospital. JAMA 1981;245(14):1410–1411
26. Allen CM, Becker PM, McVey LJ, Saltz C, Feussner JR, Cohen HJ. A randomized, controlled clinical trial of a geriatric consultation team. Compliance with recommendations. JAMA 1986;255(19):2617–2621
27. Yoo JW, Kim S, Seol H, et al. Effects of an internal medicine floor interdisciplinary team on hospital and clinical outcomes of seniors with acute medical illness. Geriatr Gerontol Int 2013;13(4):942–948
28. Ellis G, Whitehead MA, Robinson D, O'Neill D, Langhorne P. Comprehensive geriatric assessment for older adults admitted to hospital: meta-analysis of randomised controlled trials. BMJ 2011;343:d6553 doi: 10.1136/bmj.d6553

29. Cohen HJ, Feussner JR, Weinberger M, et al. A controlled trial of inpatient and outpatient geriatric evaluation and management. N Engl J Med 2002;346(12):905–912

30. Landefeld CS, Palmer RM, Kresevic DM, Fortinsky RH, Kowal J. A randomized trial of care in a hospital medical unit especially designed to improve the functional outcomes of acutely ill older patients. N Engl J Med 1995;332(20):1338–1344

31. Stuck AE, Siu AL, Wieland GD, Adams J, Rubenstein LZ. Comprehensive geriatric assessment: a meta-analysis of controlled trials. Lancet 1993;342(8878):1032–1036

32. Schmitt MH, Farrell MP, Heinemann GD. Conceptual and methodological problems in studying the effects of interdisciplinary geriatric teams. Gerontologist 1988;28(6):753–764

33. Fletcher K, Hawkes P, Williams-Rosenthal S, Mariscal CS, Cox BA. Using nurse practitioners to implement best practice care for the elderly during hospitalization: the NICHE journey at the University of Virginia Medical Center. Crit Care Nurs Clin North Am 2007;19(3):321–337, vii

34. Fallon WFJ Jr, Rader E, Zyzanski S, et al. Geriatric outcomes are improved by a geriatric trauma consultation service. J Trauma 2006;61(5):1040–1046

35. Pfaff J. The Geriatric Resource Nurse Model: a culture change. Geriatr Nurs 2002;23(3):140–144

36. van Vuuren PAC, Kagan SH, Chalian AA. Geriatric otolaryngology toolbox: what you and your nurse can do to improve outcomes for older adults. Ear Nose Throat J 2009; 88(10):1162–1168

37. Creighton FX Jr, Poliashenko SM, Statham MM, Abramson P, Johns MM III. The growing geriatric otolaryngology patient population: a study of 131,700 new patient encounters. Laryngoscope 2013;123(1):97–102

Appendix: Geriatric Competencies for Medical Students

1. Medication management
   - Explain impact of age-related changes on drug selection and dose based on knowledge of age-related changes in renal and hepatic function, body composition, and central nervous system sensitivity.
   - Identify medications, including anticholinergic, psychoactive, anticoagulant, analgesic, hypoglycemic, and cardiovascular drugs that should be avoided or used with caution in older adults and explain the potential problems associated with each.
   - Document a patient's complete medication list, including prescribed, herbal, and over-the-counter medications, and for each medication provide the dose, frequency, indication, benefit, side effects, and an assessment of adherence.
2. Cognitive and behavioral disorders
   - Compare and contrast among the clinical presentations of delirium, dementia, and depression.
   - Formulate a differential diagnosis and implement initial evaluation in a patient who exhibits delirium, dementia, or depression.
   - In an older patient with delirium, urgently initiate a diagnostic workup to determine the root cause (etiology of the delirium).
   - Perform and interpret a cognitive assessment in older patients for whom there are concerns regarding memory or function.
   - Develop an evaluation and nonpharmacological management plan for agitated demented or delirious patients.
3. Self-care capacity
   - Assess and describe baseline and current functional abilities in an older patient by collecting historical data from multiple sources, making sure to include instrumental activities of daily living and activities of daily living, and performing a confirmatory hearing and vision examination.
   - Develop a preliminary management plan for patients presenting with functional deficits, including adaptive interventions and involvement of interdisciplinary team members from appropriate disciplines, such as social work, nursing, rehabilitation, nutrition, and pharmacy.
   - Identify and assess safety risks in the home environment, and make recommendations to mitigate these.
4. Falls, balance, and gait disorders
   - Ask all patients older than 65 years of age, or their caregivers, about falls in the last year, watch the patient rise from a chair and walk (or transfer), then record and interpret the findings.
   - In a patient who has fallen, construct a differential diagnosis and evaluation plan that addresses the multiple etiologies identified by history, physical examination, and functional assessment.
5. Health care planning and promotion
   - Define and differentiate among types of code status, health care proxies, and advance directives in the state where one is training.
   - Accurately identify clinical situations where life expectancy, functional status, patient preference, or goals of care should override standard recommendations for screening tests in older adults.

- Accurately identify clinical situations where life expectancy, functional status, patient preference, or goals of care should override standard recommendations for treatment in older adults.

6. Atypical presentation of disease
   - Identify at least three physiological changes of aging for each organ system and their impact on the patient, including their contribution to homeostenosis (the age-related narrowing of homeostatic reserve mechanisms).
   - Generate a differential diagnosis based on recognition of the unique presentations of common conditions in older adults, including acute coronary syndrome, dehydration, urinary tract infection, acute abdomen, and pneumonia.
7. Palliative care
   - Assess and provide initial management of pain and key nonpain symptoms based on the patient's goals of care.
   - Identify the psychological, social, and spiritual needs of patients with advanced illness and their family members, and link these identified needs with the appropriate interdisciplinary team members.
   - Present palliative care (including hospice) as a positive, active treatment option for a patient with advanced disease.
8. Hospital care for elders
   - Identify potential hazards of hospitalization for all older adult patients (including immobility, delirium, medication side effects, malnutrition, pressure ulcers, procedures, peri- and postoperative periods, transient urinary incontinence, and hospital-acquired infections) and identify potential prevention strategies.
   - Explain the risks, indications, alternatives, and contraindications for indwelling (Foley) catheter use in the older adult patient.
   - Explain the risks, indications, alternatives, and contraindications for physical and pharmacological restraint use.
   - Communicate the key components of a safe discharge plan (e.g., accurate medication list, plan for follow-up), including comparing/contrasting potential sites for discharge.
   - Conduct a surveillance examination of areas of the skin at high risk for pressure ulcers and describe existing ulcers.

Adapted from Leipzig RM, Granville L, Simpson D, Anderson MB, Sauvigné K, Soriano RP. Keeping Granny safe on July 1: a consensus on minimum geriatrics competencies for graduating medical students. Acad Med 2009;84(5):604–610 doi: 10.1097/ACM.0b013e31819fab70; and from The Portal of Online Geriatrics Education. AAMC Geriatric Competencies for Medical Students 2009. http://www.pogoe.org/Minimum_Geriatric_Competencies. Accessed March 17, 2014.

4 Evaluation of the Outpatient Geriatric Patient

David Eibling

Introduction

Older adults differ from younger adults in many ways that can affect evaluation strategies and, ultimately, treatment decision making. This chapter reviews the most salient of these characteristics and offers guidance to otolaryngologists with geriatric patients.

Population demographics mean that ever-increasing numbers of older adults will seek otolaryngology care in the coming decades.[1] The impact of these changes will be ubiquitous, affecting the entire discipline with the exception of pediatric specialties and practices. Otolaryngologists readily understand that outpatient evaluation of a child differs from that of an adult, but many physicians do not recognize that the evaluation of an elderly adult also requires modification. Some of the differences between older adults and younger or middle-aged adults may not be readily apparent. Moreover, older adults vary dramatically within specific age ranges, with far more heterogeneity than children or even young adults. It is not uncommon to encounter patients in their 90s who appear to have lower disease burden than many in their 50s and 60s. The potential reasons for these disparities are numerous and collectively drive the need to comprehensively evaluate older patients who present for otolaryngological care.

The unique characteristics of older adults that impact outpatient evaluation in the typical otolaryngology practice include, but are not limited to, the following:

- Reduced functional reserve (frailty)
- Multiple comorbidities
- Polypharmacy
- Multiple physicians
- Sensory impairment (vision, hearing loss, olfaction)
- Reduced mobility
- Impaired balance with increased risk of falls
- Dysphagia, eating disorders
- Cognitive decline
- Inadequate social support
- Goals and expectations differ from those of younger adults

Comprehensive Geriatric Assessment (CGA)

The standard benchmark for geriatric evaluation is the comprehensive geriatric assessment (CGA), which is a standard assessment performed by geriatricians.[2] The CGA is intended to serve as a baseline for the geriatrician in directing a patient's medical care. As its name implies, it is comprehensive, requires hours to complete, and is usually unnecessary for the purposes of decision making in an otolaryngological office. Performance of a CGA should therefore be delegated to geriatricians. However, there are multiple evaluation components that should be performed by otolaryngologists, particularly those regarding surgical candidacy for older adults. These are discussed in this chapter in roughly descending order of importance. A useful tool is the Vulnerable Elderly Survey 13 (VES-13), which assesses physical well-being and strength as well as the subject's ability to perform common activities of daily living (ADLs) without assistance.[3]

Reduced Functional Reserve

Increased risk of frailty is the most critical defining characteristic of the elderly of which otolaryngologists must be aware. Frailty, a measure of reduced functional reserve, places the older adult at risk for a plethora of adverse and unanticipated consequences from seemingly minor interventions, including increased likelihood of surgical complications as well as ultimate hospital discharge to a setting other than home.[4,5] Younger adults have substantial functional reserves in all organ systems in that they routinely use only a percentage of the total capacity of the organ system. Older adults may appear to be just as resilient as younger adults at first glance, but when stressed they may quickly exhaust their resources and suffer multiple-system organ failure. Therefore, assessment of frailty must be considered a fundamental part of any evaluation of older adults when surgical intervention is a consideration. Like Justice Potter's famous statement regarding pornography, most people would state they are unable to define frailty, although they "recognize it when (they) see it." However, as practitioners of the science as well as the art of medicine physicians are obligated to be more rigorous in their assessments than merely relying on subjective impression. Evaluation of frailty falls into this paradigm because objective measures of frailty exist and are used by some practitioners. These measures have been validated by several longitudinal studies, including studies that demonstrate a strong correlation with surgical outcomes.[4–6] Measures may be demonstrated either on examination or via biochemical assessment. Several biochemical measures, such as circulating levels of D dimer (D-dimer assay) and interleukin-6 (IL-6) have been reported to correlate with other measures of frailty.[6] For the purposes of outpatient evaluation there are several easily performed tests that all otolaryngologists can incorporate into their clinical practice. The reader will note that these can be divided roughly into subjective (exhaustion; reduced anxiety level) and objective (unintentional weight loss > 10 lb; get-up-and-go test; grip strength) criteria.[4]

The get-up-and-go test is performed by arising from a sitting position, walking 8 feet, and returning and sitting. Scoring is 1 through 3, with loss of a point for (1) using arms to get up, (2) uncertain gait, and (3) taking longer than 10 seconds.[7] Another test often used is measurement of walking speed (15 feet in 6 seconds or less).[8]

Grip strength is measured with a dynamometer, a low-cost device in common use. Normal men should produce more than 29 kg (median 39 kg), women somewhat less.[9] Both of these measures correlate with both short-term and long-term survival and are considered valid measures of frailty.

Comorbidities and Polypharmacy

As patients age, they commonly collect new diagnoses as well as accumulate an ever-increasing list of medications to manage these illnesses. This characteristic is not unique to older adults, and otolaryngologists frequently encounter younger patients with more extensive comorbidities and longer medication lists than some of their elderly patients. Nonetheless, evaluation of geriatric patients requires diligent review of comorbid conditions with particular attention to medication lists. "Medication reconciliation" is recognized as a key component of high-quality health care and is particularly critical—and challenging—in the elderly. As the number of medications increases, the opportunity for unanticipated or unrecognized adverse effects increases as well. Elderly patients are at much higher risk for several reasons, including alterations in drug metabolism as well as pharmacokinetics. Diseases and conditions managed by otolaryngologists, particularly balance and swallowing disorders, are frequently impacted by medications being administered for other disorders. Well-established guidelines such as the Beers criteria list of potentially inappropriate medications[10] and the American Geriatrics Society clinical practice guideline on fall prevention[11] emphasize the significance of prescribed medications in increasing morbidity. Often the otolaryngologist is the first provider to note a relationship between balance or swallowing complaints and the patient's medication list. Common offenders are psychoactive medications, including selective serotonin reuptake inhibitors (SSRIs), and anticholinergics, although other medication classes are often implicated as well. As such, it is incumbent on the otolaryngologist to review medication lists carefully, verify them with the patient (or the patient's caregiver), and review possible interactions and untoward effects. This task is daunting because even the newer electronic health records (EHRs) typically fail to capture all medications that the patient is taking. The author of this chapter has himself been "victimized" by failure of the EHR (in this case the Veterans Health Administration Computerized Patient Record System [VHA CPRS]) to capture accurately all the medications being taken by elderly or cognitively impaired patients. In the absence of a truly interoperable health information exchange system in the United States, it falls to the provider and office staff to seek and update carefully and compulsively lists of all medications being taken by patients in the practice.

Cognitive Decline

Older adults are often quite adept at compensating for cognitive changes until late in disease progression. As such, casual conversation may fail to identify those with short-term memory loss or other information-processing defects. Standardized tests are available, of which the Mini-mental State Examination (MMSE) is the best known. This examination is copyrighted by Folstein[12] but has been excerpted by many groups and organizations.[13] Carefully scripted questioning by the otolaryngologist may provide valuable clues that cognitive decline is becoming potentially significant and should be investigated further. Inquiries regarding recent activities, family issues, other medical problems, schedules, and so forth, may yield enlightening results, particularly if the answers are associated with obvious confusion or confabulation. The following MMSE sample questions are excerpted from http://www.health.gov.bc.ca/pharmacare/adti/clinician/pdf/ADTI%20SMMSE-GDS%20Reference%20Card.pdf:

- Questions: What day of the week is this? What is tomorrow's date? What country are we in? What city are we in?
- Say: "I am going to name three objects. When I am done, I will want you to repeat them. Remember them because I am going to ask you to repeat them later."
- Spell the word *world*. Now spell it backward.
- "Now, what were the three objects I asked you to remember?"
- Show pencil, wristwatch. "What is this called?"

Recent evidence linking cognitive decline to unaided hearing loss is of particular importance to the otolaryngologist[14] and is discussed in greater depth elsewhere in this text. Failure of older adults to respond appropriately to amplification suggests defective executive function, and should be interpreted as requiring further testing. "Speech-in-noise" or other specialized audiometry testing should be employed in the evaluation of older patients with evidence of mild cognitive decline or evidence of poor auditory rehabilitation following aiding. Perhaps even more pertinent is newer evidence suggesting early amplification may retard cognitive decline—a topic beyond the scope of this chapter.

Assessment of Social Support

Historically, in the United States and in many cultures today, elderly people benefited from the support of their children and extended family. However, dramatic changes in U.S. culture including smaller families, mobile society, and two-income families mean that many elderly have no nearby family members to care for them. When their children have left home older people often relocate to "adult communities" remote from family and friends. As they age and require increasing levels of support, they may—or may not—be able to access support from community infrastructure and friends. In many such communities, support for the elderly is by other elderly—an obviously time-limited arrangement. As a result, some assessment of support is necessary for all elderly patients. This should include documentation of family member availability, community resources, primary care and other physicians, and assessment of travel needs and modalities. It is not uncommon to encounter patients in their 90s still driving to their appointments despite high levels of frailty and mild cognitive decline. It is not the intent of this chapter to address otolaryngologist involvement in deciding the wisdom of such behaviors, but clearly there is an expectation that any concerns be communicated not only to the patient, but also to the family and primary care provider.

Eliciting Patient Goals

The goals and expectations of older adults usually differ from those of younger adults. These include independence, mobility, ability to communicate with family and friends, and avoidance of being alone, issues that younger people take for granted. One of the primary goals of most adults (old or young) is what geriatricians term compression of morbidity.[15] Aging is accompanied by the recognition that life is time-limited, and that sooner or later all must die. However, gradual decline may not be inevitable because illness and functional ability may be modifiable such that disability is compressed into the shortest possible time prior to death (**Fig. 4.1**). Older patients are not so much afraid of dying as they are afraid of prolonged disability. Elicitation and identification of specific goals is a critical component of assessment of an older patient. Open discussion with the patient and caregiver (if available) should be undertaken at the first consultation, and the discussion should be reopened whenever difficult decisions arise. The goal of compression of morbidity may lead to decisions to avoid invasive procedures that have the potential

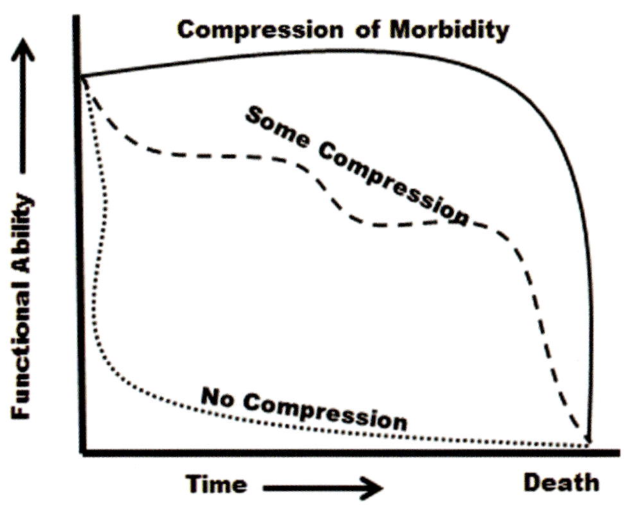

Fig. 4.1 Compression of morbidity.

to lead to long-term disability—or, conversely, may suggest early, aggressive intervention to extend useful, rewarding life even when the intervention may be accompanied by risk of earlier demise. This sort of decision making defies application of standard guidelines and mandates open, forthright discussion. Most older adults have no difficulty in making such decisions if the choices are clear and unambiguous. Unfortunately, predicting outcomes for a specific individual is a daunting task, regardless of age. Such discussions must include a frank disclosure of uncertainty when it exists, as well as clear openness on the part of the physician to accept and work with decisions made knowledgeably by each older patient.

Summary

Assessment of the older adult patient should be viewed as a more complex process than that used in the evaluation of younger patients. In addition to the typical medical evaluation of the presenting symptom or concern, the otolaryngologist should assess several age-related characteristics. Decisions regarding diagnostic tests and treatment plans should begin with assessment of patient goals and expectations and must take into account patient comorbidities, medications with possible interactions, and support systems. Finally, it is critical that an assessment of physical and cognitive functioning be obtained to assist in treatment decision making.

All of these assessments take extra time. However, the time invested by the otolaryngologist is rewarded by reductions in unanticipated treatment-related morbidity as well as improved patient and caregiver satisfaction.

References

1. Institute of Medicine. Retooling for an Aging America: Building the Healthcare Workforce. Washington, DC: National Academies Press; 2008
2. Stuck AE, Siu AL, Wieland GD, Adams J, Rubenstein LZ. Comprehensive geriatric assessment: a meta-analysis of controlled trials. Lancet 1993;342(8878):1032–1036
3. Saliba D, Elliott M, Rubenstein LZ, et al. The Vulnerable Elders Survey: a tool for identifying vulnerable older people in the community. J Am Geriatr Soc 2001;49(12):1691–1699
4. Makary MA, Segev DL, Pronovost PJ, et al. Frailty as a predictor of surgical outcomes in older patients. J Am Coll Surg 2010;210(6):901–908
5. Adams P, Ghanem T, Stachler R, Hall F, Velanovich V, Rubinfeld I. Frailty as a predictor of morbidity and mortality in inpatient head and neck surgery. JAMA Otolaryngol Head Neck Surg 2013;139(8):783–789
6. Balducci L. Aging, frailty, and chemotherapy. Cancer Contr 2007;14(1):7–12
7. Centers for Disease Control. Timed Get Up and Go Test. http://www.cdc.gov/homeandrecreationalsafety/pdf/steadi/timed_up_and_go_test.pdf. Accessed January 21, 2014
8. Studenski S, Perera S, Patel K, et al. Gait speed and survival in older adults. JAMA 2011;305(1):50–58
9. Rantanen T, Guralnik JM, Foley D, et al. Midlife hand grip strength as a predictor of old age disability. JAMA 1999;281(6):558–560
10. American Geriatrics Society 2012 Beers Criteria Update Expert Panel. American Geriatrics Society updated Beers Criteria for potentially inappropriate medication use in older adults. J Am Geriatr Soc 2012;60(4):616–631
11. Panel on Prevention of Falls in Older Persons, American Geriatrics Society and British Geriatrics Society. Summary of the Updated American Geriatrics Society/British Geriatrics Society clinical practice guideline for prevention of falls in older persons. J Am Geriatr Soc 2011;59(1):148–157
12. Folstein MF, Folstein SE, McHugh PR. "Mini-mental state": A practical method for grading the cognitive state of patients for the clinician. J Psychiatr Res 1975;12(3):189–198
13. Standardized Mini-Mental State Examination. http://www.health.gov.bc.ca/pharmacare/adti/clinician/pdf/ADTI%20SMMSE-GDS%20Reference%20Card.pdf. Accessed January 31, 2014
14. Lin FR, Yaffe K, Xia J, et al; Health ABC Study Group. Hearing loss and cognitive decline in older adults. JAMA Intern Med 2013;173(4):293–299
15. Fries JF. Aging, natural death, and the compression of morbidity. N Engl J Med 1980;303(3):130–135

5 Operative Evaluation of the Geriatric Patient

Natalie Justicz and Jeanne Hatcher

■ Introduction

The American population is aging. In the next 25 years, the population of Americans age 65 years or older will double to ~ 72 million.[1] Older Americans are more likely to need surgery than their younger counterparts. About half of adults age 65 and older will undergo a major surgical procedure.[2] In the past 30 years, though, surgeries in the 65 and older cohort have increased by more than demographic trends alone might predict; in addition to emergent surgeries, patients in the 65 and older age group are becoming increasingly comfortable with elective surgeries to improve quality of life or treat disease burden.

In the field of otolaryngology, 14.3% of the patient population was age 65 or older in 2004, compared with 17.9% in 2010.[3] The common pathologies in geriatric patients differ from those in younger age groups: 73% of geriatric diagnoses are otologic in nature, compared with just 32% of diagnoses in patients age 18 to 45 years.[3] As the baby boomer generation ages, the percentage of the American population over 65 grows. These geriatric patients are more likely to undergo surgical procedures than previous generations, and these surgeries are increasingly more likely to be in the field of otolaryngology. In response to these changing dynamics, the American Society of Geriatric Otolaryngology was founded in 2007.

■ Surgery in the Elderly

The decision to operate in the geriatric population should be made with careful consideration and evaluation of potential risks and benefits. Despite the low-risk profile of numerous surgeries, the elderly are more likely to experience complications than their younger counterparts.[4] Surgery is performed more frequently in the geriatric population, at a rate of 190 procedures per 100,000 for patients 65 and over, compared with 136 per 100,000 for those ages 40 to 64.[2] Geriatric patients are more likely to require emergent surgery than younger patients,[5] and nonelective procedures have higher rates of morbidity and mortality than elective operations. Elective surgery requires careful planning to minimize perioperative morbidity and mortality: preoperative evaluation, perioperative monitoring, and postoperative management.

Head and neck surgery requires the same careful evaluation as other operative procedures. However, several unique considerations apply. For example, head and neck cancer may drastically affect both functionality and quality of life, and many head and neck cancer patients may be candidates for relatively aggressive cancer therapy.[6] Both surgical and nonsurgical treatments may be worth exploring in the face of a large cancer burden, even if the patient has a relatively poor prognosis, because these procedures may lead to improvement in quality of life or symptom control.[7] Geriatric patients with few comorbidities and generally good fitness have long-term outcomes similar to younger counterparts after aggressive head and neck cancer therapy. Age should not define their cancer treatment nor preclude geriatric patients from standard management.[7]

■ General Considerations

The goals of treatment vary between patients. When deciding on an elective operation, it is important to elicit patient preferences and properly evaluate understanding of the procedure. This process should include a discussion of quality of life with and without surgical intervention as well as nonoperative treatment options. If surgical intervention is chosen, further counseling centers around the likelihood of achieving the desired surgical result, the estimated degree of symptom improvement, the risk of negative outcomes, and the expected postoperative course.[8]

Understanding the patient's support system is critical in evaluation for elective surgery. Some geriatric patients have an extensive support network, whereas others live alone and have little help available. Depending on the postoperative needs of a particular patient, care may be required from family, friends, or home health workers. Geriatric patients undergoing head and neck reconstruction are more likely to be discharged to a nursing or other care facility when compared with younger patients. In a study of 450 patients undergoing head and neck reconstruction, 14.1% were unable to return home after surgery. Patients age 71 or older were 5 times less likely to return home than their younger counterparts; those 81 or older were 13 times less likely.[9] An early analysis of psychosocial support can help with determining the long-term success of surgery and recovery. This is an especially valuable conversation for geriatric patients and those with significant comorbidities.[9]

Every adult is assumed to be responsible for his or her own medical decision making, and most geriatric patients maintain the capacity to consent to a procedure. In obtaining consent from a geriatric patient for surgery, a physician must ensure that (1) the patient is capable of giving consent and (2) there are no barriers to consent that cannot be easily overcome or reversed. Physicians must aim to preserve a patient's autonomy while also being mindful that geriatric patients are more likely to have impaired cognition or physical ailments such as hearing or vision loss that can affect communication. Geriatric patients may also be physically, financially, or socially dependent on the people around them, complicating the consent process.[10] If it is not clear that a patient has the level of understanding necessary to consent, a simple test such as a Mini-Mental State Examination (MMSE) can be performed to assess cognition, but a poor performance does not necessarily mean that a patient lacks capacity to consent to a surgical procedure.[11] Whenever possible, patients should participate in their informed consent process.

If a patient has a designated health care proxy, the informed consent process changes. Surrogate decision makers may act in the best interest of the patient if the patient is unable to consent. Caution should be used in these situations to ensure that the surrogate decision maker is acting in accordance with both the patient's wishes and his or her best interest. If a patient obviously lacks capacity and is in need of emergent surgery, medical care may be provided in the absence of consent if it is in the patient's best interest and the patient's wishes are not known. However, emergent situations do not override existing health care directives.

Shuman and colleagues promote an honest discussion of realistic surgical outcomes before head and neck cancer treatment or surgery. Given that medical or surgical stresses may lead to a change in functional status and a loss of decision-making capacity, they suggest that patients help identify surrogate decision makers in this preoperative period. Additionally, patients should outline their preferences in regard to life-sustaining interventions such as mechanical ventilation and airway management, code status, and artificial hydration and nutrition.[7] It is best if these decisions are documented in the form of a living will, durable power of attorney, or formal establishment of a health care surrogate.

By understanding the patient's treatment goals and psychosocial support, the physician can provide the best patient-centric care. Once these myriad considerations are adequately addressed in the geriatric patient, it is appropriate to proceed into the preoperative assessment, a more quantitatively driven process for evaluating a patient's appropriateness for undergoing surgery.

Normal Physiological Changes and Complicating Medical Comorbidities

Certain metabolic changes predictably impact the physiological reserve of the older adult, leading to normal alterations in every organ system.[12] This should not be confused with medical comorbidities that are frequently seen in older adults. These comorbidities can be just as, if not more, important in preoperative assessment than chronological age. Both normal physiological changes as well as comorbid conditions will be factors in preoperative assessment.

According to Centers for Disease Control and Prevention (CDC) data, two out of every three older Americans suffer from multiple chronic conditions.[1] Every patient who is considering elective surgery must be assessed for overall health. These concurrent chronic conditions include arthritis, asthma, chronic respiratory disease, heart disease, and high blood pressure. It is now uncommon to have just one chronic condition; for example, only 9.3% of adults with diabetes have no other chronic health conditions.[1] Those with ongoing medical problems are also more likely to suffer from mental illness and cognitive impairments.

Medication Assessment and Polypharmacy

In preparation for surgery the medications that a patient takes need to be elucidated and perhaps adapted. Prescription polypharmacy (using five or more prescription medications concurrently) has increased to 12% in the past few years. Geriatric patients are especially affected: of those 65 and older, 90% use at least 1 drug per week, 40% use 5 or more medications, and nearly 20% use 10 or more medications per week.[12–14] The most common medications are those used for treatment of cardiovascular disease (60%), arthritis (51%), diabetes (20%), chronic obstructive pulmonary disease (COPD) (11%), and asthma (10%). Some of these medications, including aspirin, diuretics, statins, β-blockers, angiotensin-converting enzyme (ACE) inhibitors, and warfarin, are of particular concern due to effects on heart rate, blood pressure, and clot formation.[14]

Functional Status

In the normal aging process, metabolic function is well preserved under basal conditions.[15] Functional reserve is a measurement of tolerance of an increased physiological burden and gradually decreases with age, though it varies based on genetics, lifestyle choices, and the presence of comorbidities.[15] Undergoing a surgical procedure can stress and potentially exceed existing homeostasis, leading to a functional decline. Functional status is often measured by activities of daily living (ADLs) and instrumental activities of daily living (IADLs). ADLs represent the tasks necessary for self-care, whereas IADLs are the activities fundamental to living independently.[16]

Nutrition and Frailty

Nutritional status may worsen with age. Though this is not a normal part of aging, it is relatively common. Several factors in the geriatric population may contribute to poor nutritional status. These include inadequate dietary intake due to dementia, dysphagia, and even decreased access to or desire for food. Some medications may also affect appetite.[8] Frailty has been described by Fried et al as a clinical syndrome in which three or more of the following criteria are present: unintentional weight loss (10 lb in the past year), weakness, slow walking speed, low physical activity, and self-reported exhaustion,. Frailty is increasingly prevalent with age, with 6.9% of adults aged 65 and older meeting frailty criteria. It is distinct from comorbidity and disability but is independently predictive of fall risk, hospitalization, and mortality.[17]

Cognitive Changes

As we age, normal cognitive changes include minor memory loss but can be complicated by dementia or delirium. There is some debate over whether surgical procedures can unmask or precipitate dementia, though its presence at baseline is known to predict poor outcomes.[18] Robinson et al examined the impact of impaired cognition (evaluated via Mini-Cog testing) on postoperative outcomes in geriatric patients undergoing major elective surgeries and found complications to be more prevalent in those with a history of impaired cognition.[18] Delirium is distinct from dementia, defined as a waxing and waning level of consciousness often accompanied by confusion, agitation, and disorganized thought processes. It may occur in patients with or without dementia.

Pulmonary Changes

As we age, pulmonary reserve decreases. This is characterized by a decrease in pulmonary perfusion and elastic recoil, as well as parameters such as forced expiratory volume and forced vital capacity.[19] Asthma and COPD are two relatively common medical conditions that further impact lung function.

Cardiovascular Changes

Aging is associated with numerous molecular and physiological changes in the heart muscle that affect energy usage, excitation–contraction coupling, and cell maintenance (**Tables 5.1** and **5.2**).[20] These underlying biochemical changes in turn lead to changes in cardiac function, eventually leading to decreased contractility and stiffening of myocytes and vascular structures. Systolic blood pressure increases in response to this arterial impedance, which drives left ventricular afterload and leads to left ventricular hypertrophy (**Fig. 5.1**).[20]

Renal Changes

Glomerular filtration rate (GFR), the best measurement of renal function, slowly decreases with age. A true measurement of GFR is complicated and expensive, thus measurements of creatinine clearance (CrCl) are used. Baseline serum creatinine may slowly increase with age, but used in isolation it is not a reliable marker for renal function.[21] In the middle-aged population, an increase in serum creatinine may demonstrate renal impairment, but in the geriatric population serum creatinine may return to normal because of an age-dependent decrease in muscle mass leading to a decrease in creatinine production. Patients diagnosed with diabetes or hypertension or those who have recently undergone imaging with contrast dye are more likely to demonstrate renal insufficiency.

Table 5.1 Age-related changes in cardiac morphology and function

Morphology	Decrease in myocyte number, increase in myocyte size, decrease in matrix connective tissue, increase in left ventricular wall thickness, decrease in conduction fiber density, decrease in sinus node cell number
Function	Decrease in intrinsic contractility, increase in myocardial contraction time, decrease in myocardial contraction velocity, increase in myocardial stiffness, increase in ventricular filling pressures, increase in left atrial pressure/size, increase in action potential time, decrease in coronary flow reserve, decrease in β-adrenoceptor-mediated modulation of inotropy and chronotropy

Used with permission from Priebe HJ. The aged cardiovascular risk patient. Br J Anaesth 2000;85(5):763–778.

Table 5.2 Age-related changes in vascular morphology and function

Morphology	Increase in diameter and stiffness of large elastic arteries, increase in medial and intimal thickness, increase in endothelial variant cells, increase in elastolytic and collagenolytic activity, change in vascular cell proliferation/migration, change in vascular wall matrix
Function	Decrease in β-adrenoceptor; flow-dependent, endothelium-dependent, and atrial natriuretic-peptide-mediated vasodilation; decrease in nitric oxide production/effect; increase in vascular impedance; increase in pulse wave velocity; early reflected pulse waves

Used with permission from Priebe HJ. The aged cardiovascular risk patient. Br J Anaesth 2000;85(5):763–778.

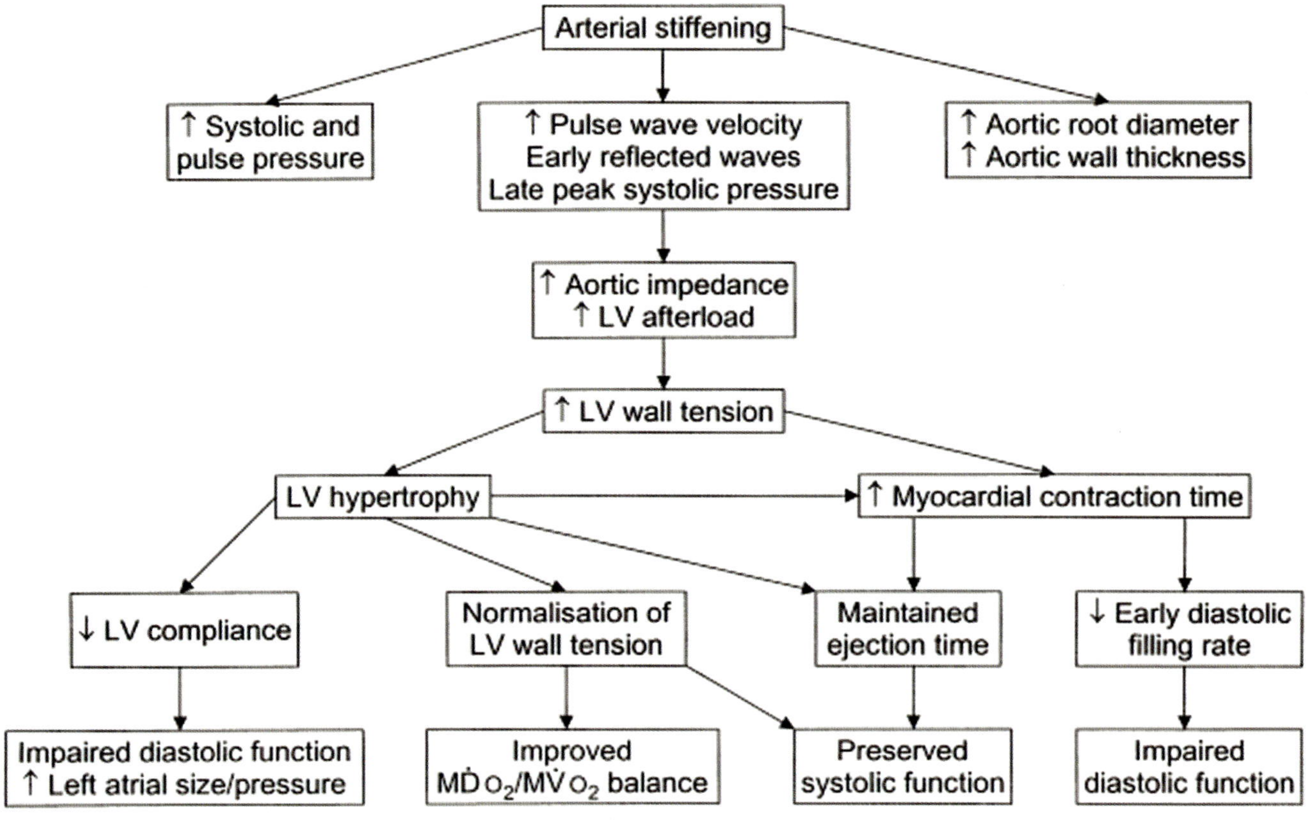

Fig. 5.1 Cardiac adjustments to arterial stiffening during aging. LV, left ventricular; MDO_2, myocardial oxygen delivery. MVO_2, myocardial oxygen demand. (Used with permission from Priebe HJ. The aged cardiovascular risk patient. Br J Anaesth 2000;85(5):763–778.)

Hepatic Changes

Hepatic function changes with age, with a reduction in hepatic blood flow of ~ 40% between the ages of 25 and 65. Due to the reduction in blood flow, anesthetic medications like lidocaine, as well as opioid medications like fentanyl, take longer to be cleared from the bloodstream.[12]

Preoperative Assessment

If elective surgery is indicated in the geriatric patient, a preoperative assessment is necessary. Because physiological reserve decreases with age and may be further complicated by medical comorbidities, it is important to establish baseline metrics and monitor comorbidities before proceeding to surgery. There is no absolute consensus on appropriate "routine" preoperative tests. The National Institute for Health and Care Excellence (NICE) is one source for guidelines on preoperative testing recommendations for adults over 60.[22] These guidelines help to provide a framework for necessary laboratory work and imaging and are a summation of clinician consensus rather than a definitive evidence base.[22]

Appropriate assessment relies on information gleaned from the patient's medical records, history, and physical examination, with some additional screening tests.[23] In collecting laboratory data or imaging, considerations for specific testing include (1) assessing a preexisting health problem or medical comorbidity, (2) identifying unexpected conditions, (3) predicting perioperative complications, and (4) providing a baseline for later comparisons. An overzealous laboratory workup may unmask abnormalities in an asymptomatic, low-risk geriatric population.[2] See **Table 5.3** for a summary of preoperative testing.

Functional Status Evaluation

Research has shown that maximum functional status decline occurs 1 week after surgery. Average time to recover back to baseline ranges from 3 weeks for a normal Mini-Mental State Exam to as long as 6 months to have full IADLs and achieve relatively complete independence.[24] Recovery further varies depending on preoperative physical condition. By preparing surgical patients in the preoperative evaluation about the length of time often required to return to baseline status, preparations can be made for psychosocial support, rehabilitation, and recovery.

Table 5.3 Preoperative assessment

Target population	What to obtain	Purpose
All patients	Ask: "Have you lost 10 or more pounds without trying?" Laboratories: – Complete metabolic panel[a] – Complete blood count	Identify nutritional deficiencies – Evaluate for electrolyte abnormalities, nutritional deficiencies, renal and liver dysfunction – Evaluate for anemia
Known liver disease or affecting medications	PT/PTT, INR	– Evaluate for changes in coagulation
Major surgery, expected ICU stay, or known cardiopulmonary disease	Chest X-ray	– Baseline image for future comparison, evaluate for enlarged cardiac silhouette, lung hyperinflation, pulmonary edema
Intermediate-risk surgery Known cardiopulmonary disease, diabetes, or renal insufficiency	ECG	– Provide cardiac baseline – Evaluate for infarction, rhythm changes
Other testing to consider	– Pulmonary function testing – Swallow study – Type and screen, type and cross	– Poorly characterized dyspnea, known obstructive lung disease and unsure control – Frailty, malnutrition, known dysphagia – Major surgery, anemia

Abbreviations: ECG, electrocardiogram; INR, international normalized ratio; PT, prothrombin time; PTT, partial thromboplastin time.

[a] Complete metabolic panel—sodium, potassium, calcium, chloride, bicarbonate, blood urea nitrogen, creatinine, glucose, total protein, albumin, aspartate aminotransferase, alanine transaminase, alkaline phosphatase.

Nutrition and Frailty

Recent weight loss raises concern for poor nutritional status. Poor preoperative nutritional status has been shown to negatively impact surgical outcomes and lead to perioperative complications.[2] Some studies have demonstrated a decrease in perioperative complications if oncological patients are given nutritional supplementation preoperatively.[2] This can be evaluated by obtaining serum albumin and prealbumin levels. Low serum hemoglobin may indicate anemia, potentially caused by vitamin deficiency and poor nutritional status.

Frailty can be assessed in several ways. The modified frailty index (MFI) has been adapted for otolaryngology, using data from the American College of Surgeons (ACS) National Surgical Quality Improvement Program (NSQIP).[25] Otolaryngological patients generally have low frailty. However, the MFI is associated with morbidity and mortality: five or more positive variables can raise mortality 10-fold and increase complications from 10 to 40% (**Table 5.4**).[25]

Table 5.4 Modified frailty index (MFI)

History of diabetes mellitus
Nonindependent functional status
History of chronic obstructive pulmonary disease or pneumonia
History of congestive heart failure
History of myocardial infarction
History of percutaneous coronary intervention, stenting, or angina
History of hypertension requiring medication
History of peripheral vascular disease or ischemic rest pain
History of impaired sensorium
History of transient ischemic attack or cerebrovascular accident
History of cerebrovascular accident with neurological deficit

Used with permission from Adams P, Ghanem T, Stachler R, Hall F, Velanovich V, Rubinfeld I. Frailty as a predictor of morbidity and mortality in inpatient head and neck surgery. JAMA Otolaryngol Head Neck Surg 2013;139(8):783–789.

Note: Scoring: 1 point per variable, with 5 or more significant for increased complications and mortality.

Cognitive Assessment

There are several testing options to evaluate dementia. In the geriatric population, the MMSE is consistent and easily administered (**Table 5.5**).[26] Delirium is more difficult to quantify. Patients with dementia will be more likely to experience delirium. Other complicating factors that may increase the likelihood of delirium in geriatric otolaryngological patients include pain medications (e.g., narcotic pain medication, benzodiazepines, anticholinergics), electrolyte abnormalities, and being in the intensive care unit.[27]

Pulmonary Assessment

In a recent literature review, postoperative pulmonary complications were more frequently seen in those of advanced age, with an American Society of Anesthesiologists (ASA) score of 2 or more, and who were functionally dependent. Undergoing head and neck surgery alone increases risk as well. Evidence supports obtaining a chest X-ray as well as serum albumin to better stratify pulmonary risk preoperatively.

Cardiovascular Assessment

For noncardiac geriatric surgical patients, chest X-rays (CXRs), electrocardiograms (ECGs), and nonstress testing may not be routinely indicated for every patient. However, depending on an individual patient's surgery and functional status, these tests may become necessary.

Many older adults have a history of ischemic heart disease, atrial fibrillation, heart failure, hyperlipidemia, diabetes, or stroke, all of which can complicate any type of surgery. These disorders may also be diagnosed for the first time during a preoperative assessment and may need management before surgery can proceed.

The American College of Cardiology (ACC) and American Heart Association (AHA) have published guidelines to help assess both prior cardiac and noncardiac patients for elective, noncardiac surgery. For patients undergoing elective surgery, cardiac risk factors include a history of ischemic heart disease, decompensated heart failure, or cerebrovascular disease, as well as diabetes mellitus or renal insufficiency. The presence of unstable coronary symptoms, decompensated heart failure, significant arrhythmias, or severe valvular disease indicate major clinical risk and may delay or cancel elective surgery.[28] The treatment algorithm produced by the ACC helps to provide a framework for evaluation of the noncardiac surgical patient, taking into account functional status, urgency of the surgical procedure,

Table 5.5 Mini-Mental State Examination (MMSE) Sample Items

Orientation to Time	"What is the date?"
Registration	"Listen carefully. I am going to say three words. You say them back after I stop. Ready? Here they are... APPLE (pause), PENNY (pause), TABLE (pause). Now repeat those words back to me." [Repeat up to 5 times, but score only the first trial.]
Naming	"What is this?" [Point to a pencil or pen.]
Reading	"Please read this and do what it says." [Show examinee the words on the stimulus form.] CLOSE YOUR EYES

Reproduced by special permission of the Publisher, Psychological Assessment Resources, Inc., 16204 North Florida Avenue, Lutz, Florida 33549, from the Mini-Mental State Examination, by Marshal Folstein and Susan Folstein, Copyright 1975, 1998, 2001 by Mini Mental LLC, Inc. Published 2001 by Psychological Assessment Resources, Inc. Further reproduction is prohibited without permission of PAR, Inc. The MMSE can be purchased from PAR, Inc. by calling +1-813-968-3003.

and prior cardiovascular conditions. ACC/AHA guidelines from 2007 stratify head and neck surgery into the intermediate risk category, with a cardiac risk of 1 to 5% (**Fig. 5.2**).

Renal Assessment

Renal function testing is part of the preoperative workup for any geriatric patient, because many of the anesthetic and analgesic medications used in the perioperative period are renally excreted. Serum blood urea nitrogen and creatinine are usually adequate for screening purposes. More specific testing may be needed in those with abnormal results or a known history of renal disease, hypertension, or diabetes. Consultation with a nephrologist for any concerns should be considered, particularly with elective surgery.

Hepatic Assessment

Serum albumin is a measurement of synthetic liver function and is routinely measured in all operative patients. A coagulation profile may be considered with known or identified liver disease or for major procedures.[8]

Other Preoperative Concerns

For any patient undergoing a head and neck procedure, it is also important to establish a preoperative plan for securing the airway. For patients in whom the normal head and neck anatomy may be distorted by disease process, radiation, or prior surgical procedures, an awake fiberoptic intubation or tracheotomy may be necessary. Have an open discussion with your anesthesia team to make the plan clear and thus

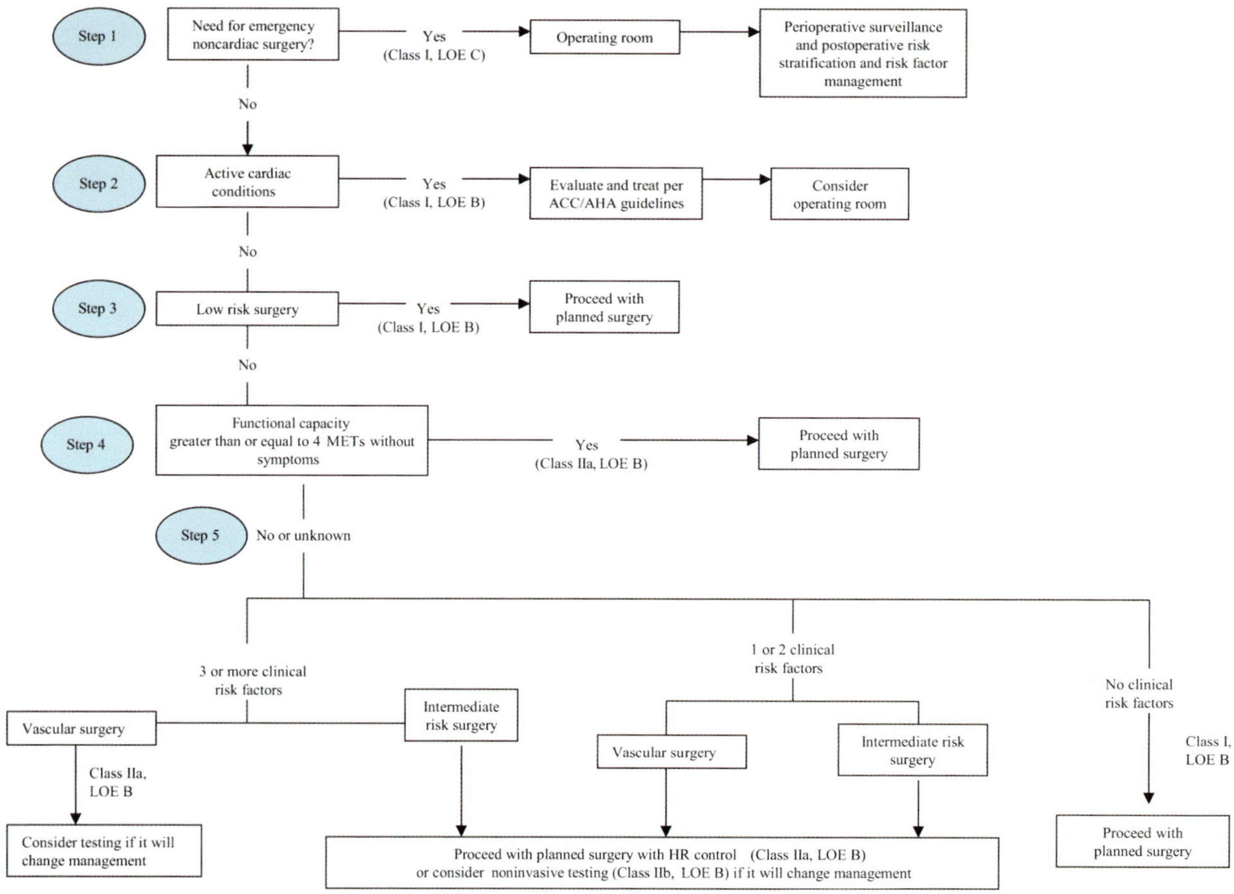

Fig. 5.2 Cardiac evaluation and care algorithm for noncardiac surgery based on active clinical conditions, known cardiovascular disease, or cardiac risk factors for patients ≥ 50 years of age. (Used with permission from ACC/AHA 2007 guidelines on perioperative cardiovascular evaluation and care for noncardiac surgery.)

safe for your patient. Also, remember that postoperative planning begins preoperatively. As discussed earlier, anticipate the need for nursing care or assistance in the recovery period and allow your patient and his or her support network to adjust and make any arrangements.

Intraoperative Considerations

Anesthesia is an integral part of surgery and becomes more complex with age. Because metabolism changes with age, pharmacokinetics is affected, leading to an increased incidence of complications and toxicity.[2] In the older patient, there is a decrease in gastrointestinal motility and blood flow to the gut, as well as the previously discussed alterations in renal and hepatic function. Drug distribution will also change as lean muscle mass and total body water decrease and body fat increases. Free drug fraction may increase due to decreased albumin and protein binding, also contributing to change in drug distribution. For medications with a narrow therapeutic index such as warfarin, this can lead to adverse drug events and an increased risk of bleeding.[12] Decreased total body water will also shift drug levels of anesthetic induction agents such as propofol and long-acting benzodiazepines, thus making dose adjustments necessary. In addition to pharmacokinetic differences, metabolic changes also affect thermoregulation. Intraoperative hypothermia is more common in geriatric patients and affects the distribution of many commonly given peri-operative medications. Hypothermia may be combated through body warmers and room temperature adjustments.[29]

Anesthetic agents can decrease renal perfusion intraoperatively due to hypotension and thus glomerular filtration rate. Renally excreted drugs such as muscle relaxants and opioids will thus increase in serum concentration. Cisatracurium and remifentanil are degraded by serum enzymes and will not be affected. Poor pulmonary function will alter inhalational agent elimination, as will the increase in body fat for certain agents. Decreased hepatic blood flow will consequently decrease first-pass metabolism, increasing serum levels of medications with high first-pass metabolism. Anesthetic agents with high extraction ratios include fentanyl, lidocaine, meperidine, ketamine, and propofol.[30] In the postoperative period, this also makes the elderly more susceptible to the effects of morphine and other opioids.

Postoperative Monitoring and Complications

Delirium

Delirium is a concern for any geriatric patient in the postoperative period. The best way to identify postoperative delirium is by establishing a baseline assessment, especially in those with dementia.[31] Several medications can heighten or worsen delirium, particularly opiates and benzodiazepines. Conversely, inadequately controlled pain can also cause delirium. Pain management should include regular pain and sedation scoring, or nonverbal scoring systems if appropriate.[32] The use of pain assessment charts can reduce postoperative complications.[32] Depending on the severity of the patient's pain and its potential contribution to delirium, it may be appropriate to consult a pain care service. Dehydration and electrolyte abnormalities are both risk factors and can be more difficult to manage in those with head and neck cancer and require parenteral nutrition. The Cochrane Database has identified environmental factors such as sleep regularity and immobility that negatively contribute to delirium.[31] Aside from environmental controls, prophylactic low-dose haloperidol has shown benefit; it is also the first option for treatment of delirium, should it occur, to decrease the duration and severity.

Falls

Fall risk may be judged preoperatively as part of a frailty screen or more independently by the timed Get Up and Go test to evaluate mobility and balance.[33] In the postoperative period, those with a history of difficulty with the Get Up and Go or new trouble with ambulating may be referred for postoperative physical therapy. Complete assessment of mobility with an evaluation from a physical therapist is also essential in determining needs at discharge: durable medical equipment, 24 hour assistance, or a regular therapy regimen.

Infection and Wound Care

Three of the most common postoperative infections in geriatric patients are urinary tract infection (UTI), pneumonia, and surgical site wound infection, which all represent an important source of morbidity and mortality.[33] UTIs may be caused by prolonged catheterization, of which the elderly are at greater risk because of concomitant incontinence or immobility.[2] Like delirium, a UTI may present as confusion. Early catheter removal or complete avoidance of catheterization are best to prevent UTIs. Pneumonia risk is heightened by the use of nasogastric tubes, dementia, and immobility.[2] Both early mobilization and incentive spirometry or other activities such as deep breathing and coughing are suggested. Surgical site infection (SSI) is heightened in geriatric patients, leading to longer hospitalizations and more frequent readmissions, making vigilant wound care necessary.[33] Treatment of SSI may require incision and drainage or the use of antibiotics in systemic cases.[33]

Venous Thromboembolism

Both age and postsurgical immobility are risk factors for the development of venous thromboembolism (VTE). Although early ambulation can help prevent both deep venous thrombosis and pulmonary embolism, in the early postoperative period patients may be too weak to ambulate. Mechanical prophylaxis via sequential compression devices or pharmacological prophylaxis via heparin (either unfractionated or low-molecular-weight) are alternatives to decrease the incidence of VTE.

Cardiac Complications

As in the preoperative period, the ACC/AHA guidelines can be useful in identifying patients of concern for cardiovascular complications. In all postoperative patients β-blockers should be continued unless otherwise contraindicated as described in the Surgical Care Improvement Project.[34] Statins should also be continued.[31] Up to 8% of patients undergoing noncardiac surgery may suffer from postoperative atrial fibrillation, the most common postoperative arrhythmia. This is typically, though not always, a transient and reversible phenomenon.[35] Advanced age, male gender, and a history of heart failure or valvular disease are shared risk factors for both postoperative and permanent atrial fibrillation.[35]

Pulmonary Complications

There is an aging-related decline in the usual protective reflexes in the oropharynx, which predisposes all geriatric patients to aspiration, especially those with head and neck abnormalities.[31] In particular, patients with Parkinson disease or swallowing disorders at baseline are at especially high risk.[31] In the postoperative period, it is imperative that recommended guidelines for nothing by mouth (NPO) are followed and that sedatives are provided only when necessary. Speech-language pathologists (SLPs) may be consulted to help evaluate management of dysphagia. If eventual improvement in dysphagia is anticipated, compensations or short-term adjustments may be made. These include food, liquid, or environmental changes aimed at maintaining nutritional status until the patient is more fully recovered. If dietary modifications, swallow maneuvers, and postural adjustments are not sufficient, more intense rehabilitation strategies are available.[36]

In the postoperative period, pain, drowsiness, and immobilization can all contribute to shallow breathing and the development of atelectasis or other pulmonary complications.[31] Light movement and activity should be encouraged as soon as the patient is able. This also decreases the risk of pneumonia, one of the more common perioperative infections.[2]

Renal Failure

Geriatric patients typically have a lower GFR than younger patients. The geriatric patient may have reduced renal function, even if this is not clinically apparent, and a decreased ability to deal with fluid overload or, conversely, fluid depletion.[37] During the anesthesia or the hospital course, fluid overload may stress the cardiorespiratory reserve.[37] Fluid status can be monitored via charting of fluid balance or more invasive monitoring such as central venous pressure. Nonsteroidal anti-inflammatory drugs (NSAIDS) should be given with care, because they inhibit the normal prostaglandin-induced methods of vasodilation, contributing to fluid retention and renal insufficiency.[38]

■ Rehabilitation and Disposition

As discussed earlier in this chapter, preparation for postoperative needs, for both the patient and the family, helps to establish expectations and facilitate planning. Early mobilization in the postoperative period helps to facilitate recovery,[32] and patients, if able, should be encouraged to ambulate. Physical therapy consultation should be obtained to facilitate this safely if necessary. The recovery process may last several months. It begins in an acute care setting but may also include a rehabilitation or subacute care facility.[19] It is important, and can be established through proactive counseling, that discharge to a nursing care facility does not represent any sort of failure on the part of the patient or the health care team. Physical and occupational therapists as well as SLPs can greatly contribute to both short-term and long-term postoperative care.[32] Through case management, social workers, and the patient's family and friends working collaboratively, the best recovery can be attained.

■ Conclusions

Perioperative care and evaluation of geriatric patients is complex. Though with careful preoperative evaluation, intraoperative monitoring, and postoperative planning, morbidity and mortality can be reduced. Consultation with geriatricians may also optimize care, assisting with preoperative decision making, postoperative treatment of delirium, and management of polypharmacy, as well as discharge planning. It is also important to continue conversations with patients that promote patient-centric decisions in all aspects of care in the perioperative period.

■ References

1. Centers for Disease Control and Prevention. The State of Aging and Health in America. 2013. http://www.cdc.gov/aging/help/dph-aging/state-aging-health.html
2. Beliveau MM, Multach M. Perioperative care for the elderly patient. Med Clin North Am 2003;87(1):273–289
3. Creighton FX Jr, Poliashenko SM, Statham MM, Abramson P, Johns MM III. The growing geriatric otolaryngology patient population: a study of 131,700 new patient encounters. Laryngoscope 2013;123(1):97–102 doi: 10.1002/lary.23476
4. Polanczyk CA, Marcantonio E, Goldman L, et al. Impact of age on perioperative complications and length of stay in patients undergoing noncardiac surgery. Ann Intern Med 2001; 134(8):637–643
5. Seymour DG, Vaz FG. A prospective study of elderly general surgical patients: II. Post-operative complications. Age Ageing 1989;18(5):316–326
6. Shuman AG, Korc-Grodzicki B, Shklar V, Palmer F, Shah JP, Patel SG. A new care paradigm in geriatric head and neck surgical oncology. J Surg Oncol 2013;108(3):187–191 doi: 10.1002/jso.23370
7. Shuman AG, Patel SG, Shah JP, Korc-Grodzicki B. Optimizing perioperative management of geriatric patients with head and

neck cancer. Head Neck 2014;36(5):743–749. doi: 10.1002/hed.23347

8. Walke LM, Rosenthal RA. Preoperative evaluation of the older surgical patient. In: Rosenthal RA, Katlic MR, Zenilman ME, eds. Principles and Practice of Geriatric Surgery. 2nd ed. New York, NY: Springer; 2011:267–288
9. Hatcher JL, Bell EB, Browne JD, Waltonen JD. Disposition of elderly patients after head and neck reconstruction. JAMA Otolaryngol Head Neck Surg 2013;139(11):1236–1241 doi: 10.1001/jamaoto.2013.5054
10. Ivashkov Y, Van Norman GA. Informed consent and the ethical management of the older patient. Anesthesiol Clin 2009;27(3):569–580
11. Paillaud E, Ferrand E, Lejonc JL, Henry O, Bouillanne O, Montagne O. Medical information and surrogate designation: results of a prospective study in elderly hospitalised patients. Age Ageing 2007;36(3):274–279
12. Barnett SR. Polypharmacy and perioperative medications in the elderly. Anesthesiol Clin 2009;27(3):377–389
13. Patterns of medication use in the United States 2006: A Report from the Slone Survey. http://www.bu.edu/slone/files/2012/11/SloneSurveyReport2006.pdf
14. Qato DM, Alexander GC, Conti RM, Johnson M, Schumm P, Lindau ST. Use of prescription and over-the-counter medications and dietary supplements among older adults in the United States. JAMA 2008;300(24):2867–2878 doi: 10.1001/jama.2008.892
15. Lewis MC. Alterations in metabolic functions and electrolytes. In: Silverstein JH, Rooke GA, Reves JG, McLeskey CH, eds. Geriatric Anesthesiology. 2nd ed. New York, NY: Springer; 2008:97–106
16. Silverstein JH. The practice of geriatric anesthesia. In: Silverstein JH, Rooke GA, Reves JG, McLeskey CH, eds. Geriatric Anesthesiology. 2nd ed. New York, NY: Springer; 2008:3–14
17. Fried LP, Tangen CM, Walston J, et al; Cardiovascular Health Study Collaborative Research Group. Frailty in older adults: evidence for a phenotype. J Gerontol A Biol Sci Med Sci 2001;56(3):M146–M156
18. Robinson TN, Wu DS, Pointer LF, Dunn CL, Moss M. Preoperative cognitive dysfunction is related to adverse postoperative outcomes in the elderly. J Am Coll Surg 2012;215(1):12–17, discussion 17–18
19. Seshamani M, Kashima ML. Special considerations in managing geriatric patients. In: Flint PW, Haughey BH, Lund VJ, et al, eds. Cummings Otolaryngology: Head & Neck Surgery. 5th ed. Philadelphia, PA; Mosby Elsevier; 2010:230–238
20. Priebe HJ. The aged cardiovascular risk patient. Br J Anaesth 2000;85(5):763–778
21. Péquignot R, Belmin J, Chauvelier S, et al. Renal function in older hospital patients is more accurately estimated using the Cockcroft-Gault formula than the modification diet in renal disease formula. J Am Geriatr Soc 2009;57(9):1638–1643
22. Reynolds TM; National Institute for Health and Clinical Excellence; Clinical Scince Reviews Committee of the Association for Clinical Biochemistry. National Institute for Health and Clinical Excellence guidelines on preoperative tests: the use of routine preoperative tests for elective surgery. Ann Clin Biochem 2006;43(Pt 1):13–16
23. García-Miguel FJ, Serrano-Aguilar PG, López-Bastida J. Preoperative assessment. Lancet 2003;362(9397):1749–1757
24. Lawrence VA, Hazuda HP, Cornell JE, et al. Functional independence after major abdominal surgery in the elderly. J Am Coll Surg 2004;199(5):762–772
25. Adams P, Ghanem T, Stachler R, Hall F, Velanovich V, Rubinfeld I. Frailty as a predictor of morbidity and mortality in inpatient head and neck surgery. JAMA Otolaryngol Head Neck Surg 2013;139(8):783–789 10.1001/jamaoto.2013.3969
26. Borson S, Scanlan JM, Watanabe J, Tu SP, Lessig M. Simplifying detection of cognitive impairment: comparison of the Mini-Cog and Mini-Mental State Examination in a multiethnic sample. J Am Geriatr Soc 2005;53(5):871–874
27. Vaurio LE, Sands LP, Wang Y, Mullen EA, Leung JM. Postoperative delirium: the importance of pain and pain management. Anesth Analg 2006;102(4):1267–1273
28. Fleisher LA, Beckman JA, Brown KA, et al; American College of Cardiology/American Heart Association Task Force on Practice Guidelines (Writing Committee to Revise the 2002 Guidelines on Perioperative Cardiovascular Evaluation for Noncardiac Surgery); American Society of Echocardiography; American Society of Nuclear Cardiology; Heart Rhythm Society; Society of Cardiovascular Anesthesiologists; Society for Cardiovascular Angiography and Interventions; Society for Vascular Medicine and Biology; Society for Vascular Surgery. ACC/AHA 2007 guidelines on perioperative cardiovascular evaluation and care for noncardiac surgery: a report of the American College of Cardiology/American Heart Association Task Force on Practice Guidelines (Writing Committee to Revise the 2002 Guidelines on Perioperative Cardiovascular Evaluation for Noncardiac Surgery): developed in collaboration with the American Society of Echocardiography, American Society of Nuclear Cardiology, Heart Rhythm Society, Society of Cardiovascular Anesthesiologists, Society for Cardiovascular Angiography and Interventions, Society for Vascular Medicine and Biology, and Society for Vascular Surgery. Circulation 2007;116(17):e418–e499
29. Moorthy SS, Radpour S. Management of anesthesia in geriatric patients undergoing head and neck surgery. Ear Nose Throat J 1999;78(7):496–498
30. LacKamp AN, Sieber FE. Physiologic response to anesthesia in the elderly. In: Rosenthal RA, Katlic MR, Zenilman ME, eds. Principles and Practice of Geriatric Surgery. New York, NY: Springer; 2011:291–304
31. Sieber FE, Barnett SR. Preventing postoperative complications in the elderly. Anesthesiol Clin 2011;29(1):83–97
32. Dodds C, Foo I, Jones K, Singh SK, Waldmann C. Peri-operative care of elderly patients—an urgent need for change: a consensus statement to provide guidance for specialist and non-specialist anaesthetists. Perioper Med (Lond) 2013;2(1):6
33. Lagoo-Deenadayalan SA, Newell MA, Pofahl WE. Common perioperative complications in older patients. In: Rosenthal RA, Katlic MR, Zenilman ME, eds. Principles and Practice of Geriatric Surgery. New York, NY: Springer; 2011:361–376
34. Potenza B, Deligencia M, Estigoy B, et al. Lessons learned from the institution of the Surgical Care Improvement Project at a teaching medical center. Am J Surg 2009;198(6):881–888 doi: 10.1016/j.amjsurg.2009.08.015
35. Mayson SE, Greenspon AJ, Adams S, et al. The changing face of postoperative atrial fibrillation prevention: a review of current medical therapy. Cardiol Rev 2007;15(5):231–241
36. Sura L, Madhavan A, Carnaby G, Crary MA. Dysphagia in the elderly: management and nutritional considerations. Clin Interv Aging 2012;7:287–298
37. Murray D, Dodds C. Perioperative care of the elderly. Cont Educ Anaesth Crit Care Pain 2004;4(6):193–196
38. Whelton A, Watson AJ. Nonsteroidal anti-inflammatory drugs: effects on kidney function. In: Clinical Nephrotoxins: Renal Injury from Drugs and Chemicals. New York, NY: Springer; 1998:203–216

6 Age-Related Hearing Loss

Kourosh Parham, Frank R. Lin, and Brian W. Blakley

Introduction

With advances in health care, life expectancy is increasing. Aging is associated with multiple related medical problems which have been referred to as geriatric syndromes.[1] These syndromes typically interact with one another, have more than one cause, and broadly impact functional status of the geriatric patient. Sensory problems, such as impairments of vision, balance, and hearing, are well recognized geriatric syndromes, with hearing loss being the most common sensory problem among older adults.

In 2012, the U.S. Census Bureau projected that the U.S. population aged 65 and older will outnumber the population younger than 18 by 2038.[2] It is projected that, in 2015, 15% (47 million) and 2% (6 million) of the population will be 65 and 85 years old and older, respectively; but by 2060, the percent distribution will increase to 22% (92 million) and 4% (18 million), respectively. Studies based on the National Health and Nutrition Examination Survey (NHANES) show that an increasing proportion of the population suffers from hearing loss, reaching more than 80% of those older than 85 years.[3] Age-related hearing loss (ARHL) is, by far, the leading cause of hearing loss in developed countries.[4]

By definition, ARHL is a progressive disorder. Another term commonly used for this disorder is *presbycusis*. New York otologist St. John Roosa is credited with being the first to describe it as "a physiological . . . rather than a pathological, change in the ear . . . analogous to presbyopia, and . . . termed presbykousis."[5] The term is derived from the Greek *presbus* (elder) and *acouste* (to hear). Today, our understanding of this disorder has expanded to include pathological processes in the cochlea and the brain that were not suspected in the late 19th century. Whereas the peripheral pathology is universally accepted, our understanding of changes in the central auditory pathways and the global implications of these changes for management of patients with ARHL is continuing to evolve.

Presentation

Although onset is variable and dependent on several contributing factors, often the earliest symptoms of ARHL appear late in middle age. By this time, cochlear changes have progressed to affect hearing sensitivity in the frequency range that makes up our daily communication sounds. Patients commonly misunderstand similar-sounding words and tend to use context to compensate for this early deficit. In general, consonants are higher pitched than vowels and are spoken more softly than vowels. Age-related high-frequency hearing loss will result in difficulty hearing consonants and makes it easier for background noise to mask. Because consonants convey most of the information in a word, inability to hear them effectively will result in deterioration of speech intelligibility. Furthermore, consonants serve to separate syllables and words from one another. Therefore, with disruption of these breakpoints, words tend to run together and sound "mumbled." Because voices of children and women tend to have a higher pitch, the initial complaints might be about the low volume and quality of a grandchild's voice.

Over the years, as disruption of cochlear function extends toward the lower frequency regions, functional consequences become more substantial. With age-related cognitive changes ranging from slowed processing to frank impairment, the ability to use context efficiently to compensate for hearing deficits diminishes. Hearing in noisy or reverberant environments and accented or fast-paced speech become more challenging. A common complaint arising from these disruptions in speech intelligibility is "I can hear the words, but I can't understand them." Patients resort to varied strategies to cope. These strategies are influenced by several factors, including personality traits. When individuals have an external locus of control, complaints such as "my grandchildren mumble" are common. On the other hand, those with an internal locus of control display maladaptive strategies such as withdrawal from family conversations.

In general, evaluation and management of hearing loss require insights into the contributing pathophysiological conditions. However, management of age-related disorders is far more complex and challenging because these disorders, including hearing loss, rarely present in isolation. It is estimated that 50 to 75% of adults over age 65 have multiple chronic health conditions. Improving care of these individuals is a priority for the Department of Health and Human Services, and they are a focus of Healthy People 2020.[6] Toward this goal, effort is being directed toward integrated care for older individuals with multimorbidity.[7] This effort is compelling because persons with combined disabilities are at increased risk of cardiovascular and all-cause mortality.[8]

The diagnosis of ARHL is based on patient history, physical examination, and a battery of audiological and other testing. Pathophysiology of ARHL is that of a progressive and insidious process, with affected individuals frequently less aware of their communication difficulties than the people around them. In longitudinal studies, deterioration of hearing is reported to be continuous and gradual for the majority of people, ranging from 1 to 6 dB/decade,[9–11] although this rate may increase up to 9 dB/decade in older individuals.[9] Because of the insidious nature of this disorder, patients often present reluctantly to the clinician, at the insistence of family members.

Besides speech sounds, other important high-frequency warning sounds (alarms, ringing tones, turn signals, etc.) also become more difficult to hear. The common scenario in which a grandparent wearing a digital watch is unaware of the beeping high-pitched alarm is one typical example. Reduced ability to hear alarms raises concern about safety. For example, older individuals with hearing loss have been shown to be at increased risk of motor vehicle accidents while driving.[12] There are also social ramifications to this attribute of age-related hearing loss. Difficulties hearing on the telephone, particularly cell phones in which quality of sound may fluctuate with the strength of the network signal, serve as a barrier to their effective use as an alternative to face-to-face communication. The use of high-pitched ring tones by adolescents to communicate via cell phones takes advantage of the inability of the older listeners to detect these sounds in structured settings such as classrooms. Older listeners are also typically unaware of unpleasant high-pitched noise emitted by some electronic devices and chargers, as well as antiloitering devices.

Besides difficulty in hearing communication sounds and alarms, other auditory functions are also impaired. For example, age and hearing loss also impact localization performance. A large body of evidence shows that the accuracy to localize sound sources declines with age, resulting in front–back confusions, especially for spectrally restricted sounds.[13–15] Localization accuracy and acuity of acoustic stimuli decline with age and result in a blurred representation of sound sources.[16] These deficits are attributed to age-related increase in the neural temporal jitter in the central auditory system that affects the accurate processing of timing information, which is crucial to acuity in representation of sound source position.

As hearing loss severity increases, overall functional status diminishes among older individuals.[17,18] It has long been speculated that inability to communicate effectively, and potential decreased overall functional status, will lead to social isolation. For example, hearing impairment has been shown to be associated with poorer scores in social functioning assessments in older Australians.[19] Similarly, poorer self-reported hearing scores predicted deterioration in social support among a large cohort of Dutch seniors.[20] A recent study by Mick et al, in which cross-sectional data for adults 60 to 84 years old were extracted from the 1999 to 2006 cycles of the U.S. NHANES, revealed that greater hearing loss is associated with increased odds of being socially isolated in women aged 60 to 69 years.[21] This association was not affected by use of hearing aids. Based on their results, Mick et al conjectured that females may rely more heavily than males on verbal communication; therefore, hearing loss might impair their ability to receive emotional support to a greater degree than males. Social isolation has significant implications for the well-being of geriatric patients: lonely or isolated older adults are at greater risk for all-cause mortality and development and progression of cardiovascular disease, and lonely older individuals are more than twice as likely to develop Alzheimer disease (AD).[22] As noted earlier, hearing loss in older individuals was shown to be associated with increased all-cause mortality in the Australian Blue Mountains Hearing Study.[8] Increased all-cause mortality is believed to be mediated by three variables: disability in walking, cognitive impairment, and self-rated health. Thus, besides the insidious nature of the disorder, the isolation associated with hearing loss may be another factor that leads to delayed presentation and diagnosis, primarily because there is little pressure to seek care for communication difficulties.

Inherent difficulties in communication that result in compounding psychosocial effects such as isolation may precipitate psychiatric disorders such as depression. Whether hearing loss can contribute to depression has been a subject of debate. "Limited" and "'pervasive" degrees of depression were reported in 69% of community-dwelling elders with hearing impairment compared with 31% of non-hearing-impaired individuals.[23] Davis and colleagues reported that hearing-impaired elders were 1.79 times more likely than non-hearing-impaired subjects to be depressed.[9] Consistent with this view,

ARHL tends be associated with late-onset depression but not with early-onset depression.[24] In a meta-analysis of published literature, the relationship between chronic diseases and risk for depression in old age was examined by calculating odds risk (OR) and relative risk (RR) for prevalence and incidence rates of depression, respectively.[25] Loss of hearing was among a few chronic diseases, including stroke, loss of vision, cardiac disease, or chronic lung disease, that had both a significant OR and a significant RR for increased depression in old age.

On the other hand, the Nord-Trøndelag Hearing Loss Study with data from over 50,000 Norwegians aged 20 to 101 found substantial effects of hearing loss on symptoms of anxiety, depression, self-esteem, and subjective well-being in young and middle-aged persons, but not the older persons.[26] Similarly, the Longitudinal Aging Study Amsterdam, in a 4-year follow-up study of older hearing-impaired subjects, found that although hearing loss was associated with loneliness, it was not associated with depression.[27]

In a cross-sectional study of Americans aged 50 and above, dual sensory loss, vision loss only, and hearing loss only were significantly associated with depression after age, gender, poverty, education, functional impairment, bed days, self-rated health, social support, and social activities were controlled for.[28] In contrast, in an English longitudinal study, controlling for health-related variables, including the number of medical conditions and functional disability renders insignificant the association between sensory loss in both vision and hearing with both the onset and the persistence of depression in older persons.[29]

If depression is indeed a consequence of hearing loss and isolation, that may further reduce the likelihood of patients with ARHL seeking medical attention. Given its psychosocial implications, it has been recommended that clinicians maintain a low threshold for suspecting hearing loss in older patients, particularly when they present with comorbidities like anxiety, depression, or apparent cognitive decline.[30]

Another symptom that affects the well-being of patients with sensorineural hearing loss is tinnitus. About 85% of patients visiting an otologist have tinnitus.[31] The incidence of tinnitus increases with age: tinnitus affects 15% of the general population and 33% of geriatric persons.[32] In a longitudinal study of Swedish men and women in their 70s, 15% had continuous tinnitus, and 42% had occasional tinnitus, without any difference in the prevalence of tinnitus between men and women.[33] It is not surprising that tinnitus commonly accompanies ARHL.[34] This latter entity has been referred to as presbytinnitus.[35] Presence of tinnitus by itself is not an independent risk factor for depression,[36] but older individuals who perceive their tinnitus to be a problem or who have problems with tinnitus when going to bed often display depression symptoms.[37] In patients who also have ARHL, tinnitus can be a source of emotional and sleep disorders, difficulties in concentration, and social problems.[34] Tinnitus has been divided broadly into two groups based on age of onset: early- and late-onset.[38] The two differ not only with regard to prevalence but also with regard to tinnitus-related distress, with late-onset sufferers being more distressed. Resting state electroencephalography source-localized activity and connectivity comparing the two groups revealed increased activity and functional connectivity in the late-onset group, supporting intrinsic differences in tinnitus-related neural activity, which may have implications for management.[39]

In geriatric patients, the presence of tinnitus is associated with reduced systolic and diastolic blood pressure, reduced left ventricular ejection fraction, and increased brain natriuretic peptide (BNP) plasma levels.[40] These finding suggest that tinnitus is associated with worse control of congestive heart failure in geriatric patients and may have important clinical implications for the early identification of patients who need more aggressive management of heart failure. These findings also lend support to the notion that hemodynamic imbalance can contribute to cochlear impairment in general and tinnitus in particular.

Risk Factors

Several factors have been recognized as contributing to the development of ARHL. These might be broadly classified into two categories: intrinsic and extrinsic. Intrinsic factors are host factors and are primarily genetic (including sex and race), but also include health comorbidities (hypertension, diabetes, and stroke). Extrinsic factors in the environment include occupational and leisure noise exposure, smoking, ototoxic medications, socioeconomic status, and other factors. A more practical classification of risk factors is based on whether they can be modified to reduce their impact on ARHL. From this perspective, at the present time, genetic factors are not modifiable. In contrast, disease processes and environmental factors are believed to be modifiable such that their control could delay or minimize hearing loss.

Genetic Factors

Individuals with ARHL often report a family history of hearing loss among parents, siblings, and close relatives. Therefore, it has been presumed that ARHL has a genetic component that influences the age of onset and severity of the loss. Challenges in separation of environmental from genetic factors have made it difficult to assess the contribution of genetics to ARHL. Several lines of evidence, including animal research, large population-based cohort studies, and gene studies using linkage and association analysis have led to estimations of heritability and identified several genetic foci that are thought to be contributory.

Similarities between the auditory systems of mice and humans have allowed researchers to use mice as a model for better understanding of ARHL. Specifically, mutation of the *Ahl1* gene (age-related hearing loss gene 1), mapped to chromosome 10, is associated with elevated hearing thresholds at high frequencies in middle- and older-aged inbred mice.[41] Cadherin 23 is the gene associated with this locus and has been localized to stereocilia.[42] Based on this finding, it is hypothesized that cadherin 23 plays a critical role in signal transduction in the inner ear. More recently, four other genes on the mouse chromosome 10 have been implicated.[43–46] Using a genetically heterogeneous population of mice, several polymorphisms affecting ARHL and its modulation by noise have been defined, which included chromosome 10.[47] The homologous genes regulating ARHL have yet to be identified in humans.

Large-population-based cohorts have proven useful in detecting the role of inheritance in ARHL. In the Framingham cohort, heritability of ARHL phenotypes was estimated to be 0.35 to 0.55.[48] In that study, hearing levels in genetically unrelated and genetically related individuals with sensory and strial presbycusis were compared. The sensory presbycusis phenotype (described later in the chapter) showed a familial aggregation of hearing threshold levels, which was greatest for mother–daughter pairs, sister pairs, and brother pairs. The correlations for the father–child pairs were not significant, which was suggestive of extrinsic factors playing a larger role in the father's hearing loss patterns. The strial presbycusis phenotype (described later in the chapter) demonstrated a strong familial association in the sister–sister and mother–daughter pairs. Overall, the heritability estimates suggest that 35 to 55% of the variance of the sensory presbycusis phenotype and 25 to 42% of the strial presbycusis phenotype are attributable to genes. The results of this study demonstrated that in a large group of biologically related people, hearing sensitivity is more similar than in a group in the same general environment but who are unrelated. A subsequent study in this population examined the genetic linkage between measures from audiometric examinations and markers from a genomewide scan.[49] The scan identified multiple chromosomal locations with evidence of linkage to presbycusis, with some of these locations corresponding with genes implicated in congenital deafness. The analysis revealed three distinct regions on chromosome 11 (2, 79, 143 cM), as well as a region on chromosomes 10 (171 cM), 14 (126 cM), and 18 (116 cM) that showed evidence of linkage.

Heritability of audiometric shape parameters and the familial aggregation of different types of presbycusis were investigated in siblings.[50] The authors found higher heredity for severe types of presbycusis compared with moderate or mild types, and low heredity for "concavity."

The association between the magnitude of hearing loss and self-reported family history was explored in a study conducted in a population 50 years or older in Sydney, Australia.[51] The prevalence of hearing loss was 33%, with 68.2% classified as mild and 31.8% classified as moderate to severe. Of the 2,669 subjects, 46.7% gave a family history of hearing loss. Participants who reported a family history of hearing loss were younger than those who reported no family history. Participants with increased severity of hearing loss were also more likely to report a family history of hearing loss among parents or siblings. After adjusting for known risk factors (age, sex, history of noise exposure, diabetes, smoking) a positive family history was shown to be strongly associated with hearing loss. This association was true regardless of whether the loss was reported in the mother, father, or siblings. The findings from this study support a strong association between family history and presbycusis, with the association seemingly stronger with more severe hearing loss. Strong associations were found between maternal family history and moderate to severe hearing loss in women and paternal family history and moderate to severe hearing loss in men.

A study of monozygotic and dizygotic twins explored the relative importance of genetic and environmental factors in self-reported reduced hearing among an older Danish population.[52] That study showed that probandwise concordance rates (probability of disease for one twin given that the partner is affected) and odds ratios (the increased risk of reduced hearing for one twin given the presence vs. the absence of reduced hearing in the partner twin) were higher in the monozygotic twin pairs than in the dizygotic twin pairs, indicating a heritable effect. The heritability was estimated to be 40%.

Members of the National Academy of Sciences–National Research Council (NAS-NRC) twin panel underwent a linkage analysis for presbycusis.[53] This study highlighted a region of chromosome 3 mapped to the *DFNA18* locus and showed a heritability of 61% for presbycusis. Individuals carrying two mutations of gap junction gene, *GJB2*, are at increased risk of developing early presbycusis.[54]

In another effort to identify specific ARHL genes, a genetic association study was performed with 2,418 samples from across nine European countries.[55] One gene, the grainyhead-like 2 gene (*GRHL2*), was found to be associated with ARHL in this population.[55] In contrast, no positive association was found between *GRHL2* polymorphisms and ARHL in Han Chinese.[56] Therefore, population differences might be a key factor in genetic expression.

Mitochondrial DNA mutations also have been implicated in the development of presbycusis. Mitochondrial function is essential for tissues with high metabolic activity such as the cochlea. Mutations in the mitochondrial genome accumulate with age; and once they reach a threshold level, oxidative phosphorylation and tissue function are compromised. Bai and colleagues reported that the Common Deletion (CD, a 4,977 base pair deletion most commonly associated with aging) was found in a higher frequency in temporal bones from individuals known to have been affected by presbycusis compared with those unaffected.[57] Consistent with this finding, Markaryan and colleagues reported that with increasing age, the quantity of the CD increased and that the amount of the CD directly and significantly correlated with the severity of hearing loss at 8,000 Hz.[58] Mitochondrial mutation and deletion have been shown to contribute to the development of ARHL in a rodent model of presbycusis.[59] On the other hand, ARHL in humans was not associated with mitochondrial mutations in a large sample of 200 patients with ARHL.[60]

Oxidative stress is one possible mechanism for the aging process,[61] and cochlear oxidative stress has been implicated in mouse models of ARHL.[62,63] The dismutase 2 (*SOD2*) gene encodes a ubiquitous mitochondrial superoxide dismutase enzyme (manganese superoxide dismutase [MnSOD]) crucial for maintenance of reactive oxygen species homeostasis and has been implicated in the pathology of aging. *SOD2* expression is reported to increase along a basal-to-apical gradient in cochlear spiral ganglion cells in a manner consistent with the known gradient of hair cell loss in ARHL.[64] A genetic association between different polymorphisms in the *SOD2* gene and noise-induced hearing loss has also been described.[65] A role of common *SOD2* promoter variation on *SOD2* promoter regulation has been described, and *SOD2* has been linked to ARHL risk in men, further implicating mitochondrial genes.[66]

Antioxidant enzymes include those involved in glutathione metabolism, such as glutathione S-transferase (GST) and *N*-acetyltransferase (NAT), which are involved in the metabolism and detoxification of cytotoxic and carcinogenic compounds as well as reactive oxygen species (ROS). Individuals carrying polymorphisms of GSTM1, GSTT1 null genotype,[67] and a NAT mutant allele[68] are at increased risk of developing presbycusis. In fact, individuals with the GSTT1 null genotypes are almost three times more likely to develop presbycusis.[67] The association of audiometric patterns and polymorphisms of antioxidant enzymes have also been explored in ARHL.[69] Mutant alleles for GSTT1 are more likely to have a high-frequency, steeply sloping audiogram, suggesting that the basal turn of the cochlea is susceptible to GSTT1-regulated oxidative stress.

On the threshold of the era of personalized medicine, identification of specific genetic factors may render gene therapy a possible treatment for presbycusis. For example, the introduction of the developmental gene *Math1* has resulted in the recovery of hearing abilities of mature deaf mice.[70] In the more proximate future, however, knowledge of genetic susceptibility may allow individuals with a family history of presbycusis to take preventive measures from a young age to help avoid or delay the development of hearing loss by addressing modifiable risk factors for ARHL. Steps that could particularly help these at-risk individuals include healthier diet, not smoking, minimization of noise exposure, and management of aggravating comorbidities such as diabetes and vascular disease.

Modifiable Risk Factors

The influence of genetics is likely to be modulated by a set of nongenetic factors. Cross-sectional studies have identified several associations between chronic health conditions and hearing loss, although longitudinal analyses have failed to support consistently the association of some of these risk factors with incidence of ARHL. Cardiovascular disease[71–75] and diabetes[76–80] are well recognized as risk factors. Hypertension is also linked to hearing loss in some studies,[11,81] but not consistently.[82] Older persons with moderate-to-severe hearing loss have a significantly higher likelihood of reporting previous stroke; but unlike sudden hearing loss, age-related hearing loss is not predictive of increased risk of stroke, at least over a 5-year follow-up.[83] Chronic kidney disease[76,84] and systemic inflammation may contribute to progression of ARHL,[85] although the latter may affect ARHL more actively in its early phases.[86] A common thread among these disorders is vascular disease/arteriosclerosis. Along this line, it has been suggested that hearing loss precedes clinical manifestations of ischemic heart disease and may be an important “early marker” of a vascular or generalized arteriosclerotic process.[87]

Although these conditions are risk factors for prevalence of hearing loss (cross-sectional studies), they are not always found to be predictive of incidence of hearing loss (longitudinal studies).[11] Some studies may fail to implicate these risk factors because they are only weakly associated with hearing loss such that their effect is obscured by other factors.[82]

Besides systemic disorders, otologic disease can also impact hearing in the aged. In one study, chronic otitis media was found in 13.8% of the cases, otosclerosis in 3.8%, and Ménière disease in 1.3%.[88] A more recent study found the prevalence of middle-ear diseases resulting in conductive or mixed hearing loss to be 6.1 to 10.3%, 1 to 3% for otosclerosis and 1.2% for Ménière disease.[89] Hearing impairment in Ménière disease appeared to increase linearly with the duration of the disease for patients < 50 years of age; but in older subjects, the effect of the duration of the disease decreased.[90] The difference that occurred at the onset of the disease remained until presbycusis in the better ear reached the hearing level of the worse ear. There is an increase in the prevalence of otosclerosis in those older than 60 years of age, reaching its peak in the age group above 80 years (**Fig. 6.1**).[91] A significant deterioration in the hearing level has been reported in otosclerotic ears as a function of age,[91] but the rate of age-related sensorineural hearing loss in stapedectomy-treated ears is similar to that expected from presbycusis.[91–93] Demineralization of the cochlea has been associated with sensorineural hearing loss in bone diseases, including Paget disease and cochlear otosclerosis. The extent to which Paget disease and cochlear otosclerosis interact with ARHL to affect hearing has not been described. An association between femoral neck bone mass and ARHL in a population of rural women aged 60 to 85 years has been reported.[94] This finding suggests that demineralization of the otic capsule in conjunction with age-related bone mass loss might be one biological factor contributing to hearing loss in the geriatric population. However, no consistent relationship was found between bone density and hearing sensitivity in a population-based sample.[95]

Besides disease-related risk factors, there is also a set of modifiable environmental factors that have been identified. Noise exposure and cigarette smoking[73,81,96,97] are the best established risk factors. Smoking-related worsening of hearing loss with age is likely mediated by vascular disease. Those with a history of noise exposure typically display more accelerated ARHL,[98–100] although vulnerability to deleterious effects of noise exposure is not uniform across the population,[101] and not all studies are in agreement on the effect of noise on ARHL.[10,102] There is experimental evidence that early noise exposure can lead to accelerated age-related hearing loss in a mouse model.[103] Among older adults, a history of exposure to workplace noise raises the risk of cardiovascular disease and angina, and severe exposure was associated with incident stroke (OR 3.44).[104] Long-time smokers with occupational noise exposure tend to have a higher risk of permanent sensorineural hearing loss (SNHL).[105]

Another recognized risk factor is history of exposure to ototoxic drugs. For example, chemotherapeutic agents such as cisplatin are used commonly in management of oncological disease, the incidence of which increases with age. Persons over 70 account for 45% of newly diagnosed malignancies.[106] Not surprisingly, many cancer patients have ARHL before introduction of chemotherapeutic regimens.[107] All markers of oxidant stress, lipid peroxidation, glutathionylation, and nitrosylation of proteins increase, whereas the measures of antioxidant defenses, mitochondrial apoptosis-inducing factor, and superoxide dismutase 2 (SOD2) decrease with age.[108] Similarly, ototoxicity in general is believed to involve accumulation of ROS, leading to apoptosis.[109,110] Therefore, at least theoretically, the dual demand on the antioxidant scavenger system might be expected to lead to poorer hearing outcomes.[111] It is not known whether a synergistic interaction between ARHL and cisplatin ototoxicity is present. There is only one study that hints at possible outcomes. Older patients appear to show significantly greater incidence of audiometric

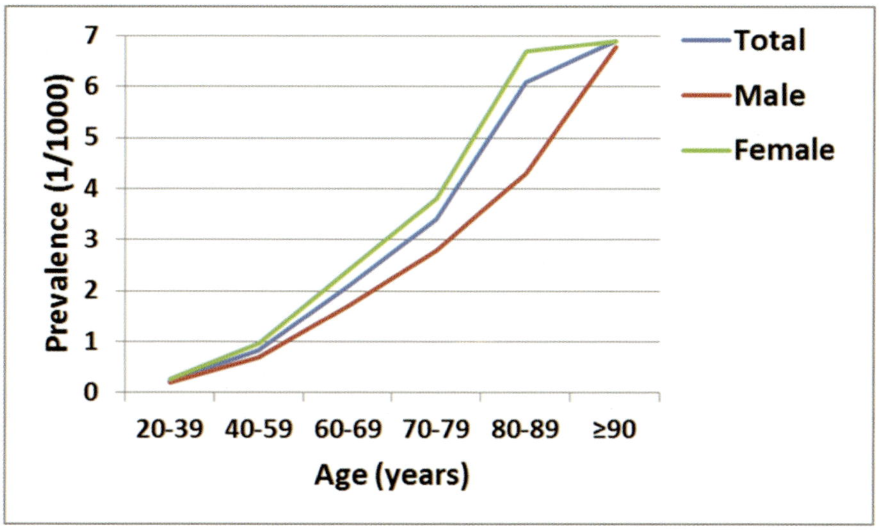

Fig. 6.1 Prevalence estimates for otosclerosis as a function of age and gender.

changes after cisplatin treatment.[112] However, this study did not have adequate controls to be conclusive. The experimental finding that intratympanic dexamethasone has otoprotectant properties against cisplatin-induced ototoxicity might imply that the antioxidant scavenger system might have sufficient reserve to prevent a negative interaction between ARHL and ototoxins.[111]

Because oxidative stress has been linked to ARHL, several studies have examined whether an antioxidant-rich diet can delay the progression of ARHL in animal models of presbycusis, with mixed results.[113–115] Caloric restriction has been shown to suppress apoptosis in the cochlea and prevent presbycusis in a mouse model.[116] Diet and nutrition certainly appear to influence human ARHL. Increased levels of dietary vitamin E and A (antioxidants) are associated with a reduced likelihood of prevalent hearing loss, but they do not affect risk of incident hearing loss in 5 year follow-up.[117] There is an inverse association between higher dietary intake of long-chain omega-3 fatty acids and regular weekly fish consumption.[118] Overall, healthy diets tend to be associated with better high-frequency thresholds in adults.[119] High body mass index[97] and central obesity, as measured by waist circumference, is an independent risk factor for age-related hearing loss in women older than 55.[120] Moderate alcohol consumption is inversely correlated with hearing loss in the high, as well as in the low frequencies.[97]

Chronic sun exposure, as measured by facial wrinkles, is positively associated with age-related hearing loss.[121] Sunlight, a source of ultraviolet radiation, may be a source of systemic oxidative stress, which may be an underlying mechanism for presbycusis. Chronic sun exposure is more likely to produce hearing loss in those with low levels of antioxidants but without occupational noise exposure.[121] Chronic low-level lead exposure may be an important risk factor for ARHL.[122] On the other hand, higher educational attainment appears to be negatively associated with hearing impairment.[123]

People born in more recent years are less likely to have hearing impairment at a given age than those born in earlier years.[124] Over a typical generational span of 20 years, the prevalence of hearing impairment declined by 42% and 23% for men and women, respectively. This birth cohort effect likely is secondary to increased awareness of deleterious effects of noise and is consistent with the view that environmental and modifiable factors may be associated with the development of hearing impairment. Given concern about early exposure to noise resulting in accelerated age-related hearing loss,[103] the decline in hearing impairment may be reversed with the popularity of personal listening devices among youth today. Indeed, the users of these devices have been demonstrated to exhibit elevated extended high-frequency (9–16 kHz) audiometric thresholds and reduced otoacoustic emission amplitudes, an early finding of noise-induced hearing loss.[125]

Relationship of Audiogram Characteristics to Cochlear Pathology

Audiometric evaluation for ARHL relies principally on the pure-tone threshold audiogram. It should be acknowledged that a standard audiometric evaluation is not a purely sensory test. Patient decisions about having heard a signal are governed by a set of self-generated rules that lie along a continuum from stringent to lenient. A patient who adopts a strict approach will respond only when absolutely certain that a signal was heard. In contrast, when lenient rules are adopted the patient will respond whenever presence of a signal is suspected. The decision variables reflect the central processes within listeners that mediate all stimulus-response tasks. The notion of a cognitive component for threshold testing (i.e., "did I hear the tone or not") is supported by Gates and colleagues, who reported that pure-tone thresholds were worse in those with poorer executive function scores when they compared normal subjects to those with mild memory impairment but without other signs of dementia and to those with an established diagnosis of AD.[126]

For the purpose of the present discussion, cognitive implications of threshold testing will be set aside to focus on peripheral processes of ARHL. As highlighted in the preceding discussion, there are numerous factors that can affect hearing in old age and reflect history of genes, noise exposure, vascular health, diet, medications, and other factors. Therefore, it is not surprising that patients with ARHL do not present with a characteristic audiometric pattern or onset in a fixed age range. Whereas the conventional audiogram evaluates hearing thresholds up to 8 kHz, testing higher frequencies (i.e., extended high frequency) allows detection of elevated hearing thresholds at a younger age.[10,127,128] This suggests that ARHL is a progressive sensorineural degenerative process whose onset may actually precede "old age."

Given the diversity in presentation of ARHL, types of ARHL have been classified based on audiometric profile (**Fig. 6.2**). Perhaps the best-known scheme is that of Schuknecht, who correlated postmortem cochlear histopathology and pure-tone threshold audiogram findings to propose four main types of presbycusis: neural—associated with spiral ganglion loss; metabolic—associated with stria vascularis changes; sensory—associated primarily with hair cell loss; and conductive—not associated with a clear pathological correlate.[129,130]

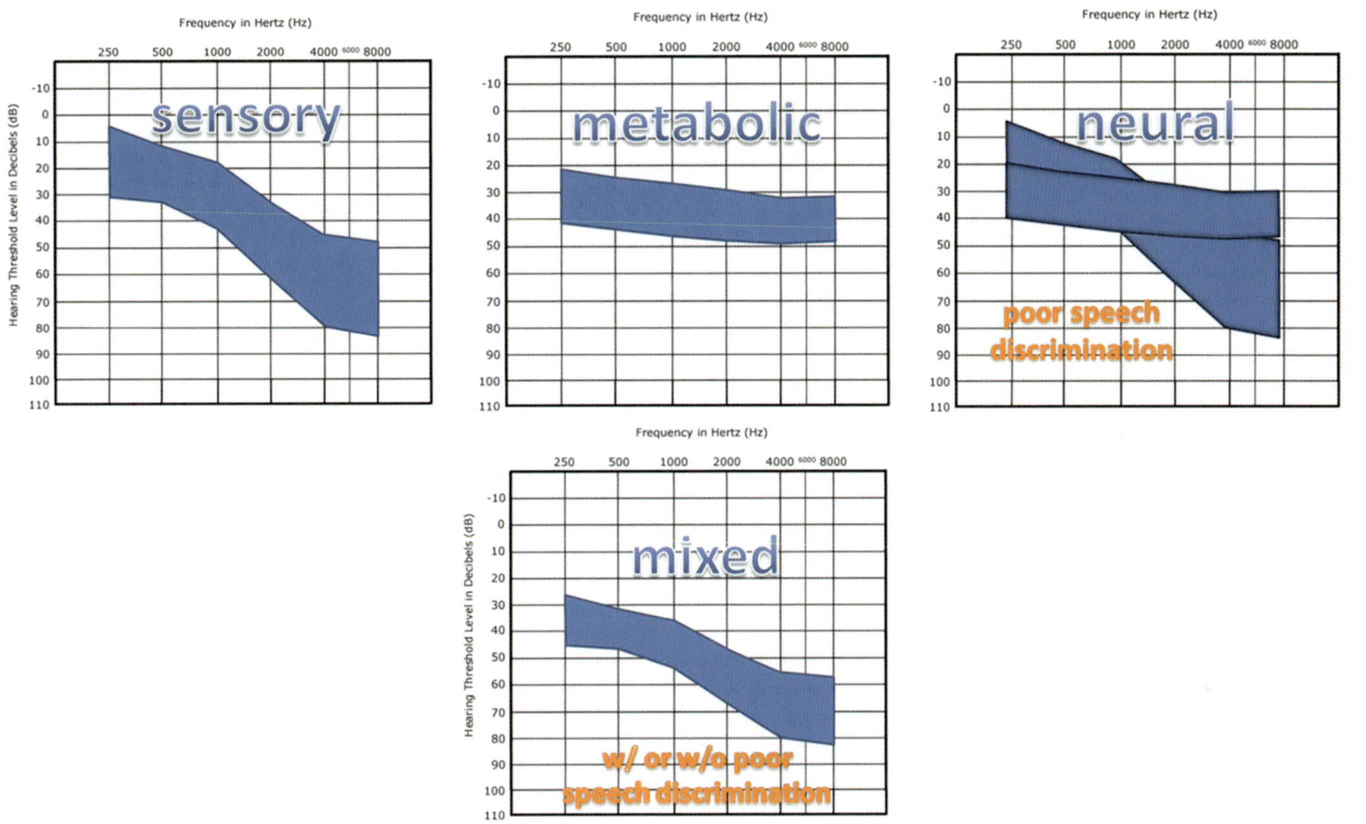

Fig. 6.2 Schematic representation of common audiometric patterns in age-related hearing loss.

Sensory presbycusis appears to be from disruption or loss of outer hair cells, in the basal turn of the cochlea. Histologically, as hair cells and supporting cells undergo apoptosis, flattening and atrophy of the organ of Corti are seen. Microscopic examination of cochlear tissue reveals accumulation of lipofuscin intracellularly, a marker of senescence. The audiogram associated with sensory presbycusis typically shows a sharply sloping, high-frequency loss extending beyond the speech frequency range, with a slow, symmetric and bilateral progression of hearing loss over the years.

Neural presbycusis is associated with a loss of spiral ganglion cells and axons within the spiral osseous lamina, beginning in the basal turn of the cochlea. The organ of Corti in this type of presbycusis may show little sign of age-related degeneration. These changes disrupt transmission of the electrochemical signal from the cochlea into the auditory pathway via cranial nerve (CN) VIII, as reflected in increased thresholds of compound action potentials and dyssynchronous neural activity, which may be related to synaptic abnormalities.[131] Classically, audiograms of patients with neural presbycusis show a moderate downward slope into higher frequencies with gradual worsening over time. A severe loss in speech discrimination out of proportion to the threshold loss is often described, making amplification difficult due to poor comprehension.

Strial or *metabolic presbycusis* occurs with deterioration or atrophy of the stria vascularis. It is slowly progressive and often genetic within families. Functionally, the stria can be thought of as the "battery" of the cochlea that maintains endolymphatic potential. Audiograms classically associated with strial presbycusis show a flat loss with slow progression and good speech discrimination with no loudness recruitment. Although structurally intact, the function of the hair cells and consequently the spiral ganglion is disrupted by the inability to maintain endolymphatic potential. Significant improvement is possible with hearing aid amplification because speech discrimination is not usually affected. Strial loss usually occurs in small, focal lesions in the extreme ends of the apex and lower basal turns of the cochlea, but it can spread to involve larger segments or diffuse strial loss. Localized areas with only 20 to 30% loss may not result in much functional change, but > 50% loss leads to decreased endolymphatic potential and poor cochlear amplification with loss of gain (20 dB in the cochlear apex up to 60 dB in the base).

Mechanical (or conductive) *presbycusis* is a category of age-related hearing impairment that was interpreted as arising from stiffening of the basilar membrane and atrophy of the spiral ligament. Histologically, several structural deformities suggest disruption of cochlear mechanics. Spiral ligament atrophy occurs most commonly in the apical turn and least often in the basal turn. Severe deterioration and cystic degeneration may lead to full detachment of the organ of Corti from the lateral cochlear wall. Audiograms in mechanical presbycusis typically have an upward slope toward the high frequencies, with preserved speech discrimination.

Vascular and *noise-induced presbycusis* are among other proposed categories of presbycusis that reflect threshold elevations correlated to hypertension, cardiac disease, and stroke, or threshold elevations related to the intensity, duration, and frequency of noise exposure. In clinical practice, most cases of presbycusis do not separate into a specific type but have mixtures of these pathologies (mixed presbycusis), and ~ 25% of all cases of presbycusis show none of the foregoing characteristics. This latter group was classified as *indeterminate* presbycusis.[130] Based on histological observations, Schucknecht and Gacek highlighted the importance of stria vascularis atrophy and neuronal losses over sensory cell losses.[130]

Other studies looking specifically at these classic categories have failed to establish a correlation between a pure-tone threshold pattern and structural abnormalities in the cochlea.[132] For example, flat audiograms were associated with strial atrophy in Schucknecht's scheme. However, Nelson and Hinojosa reported that this audiographic pattern was infrequently associated with strial atrophy, and more often occurred with outer hair cell loss alone or in combination with inner hair cell and spiral ganglion loss.[132] In contrast, the classic downward-sloping audiogram has been associated with the extent of degeneration of the stria vascularis, inner and outer hair cells, and spiral ganglion cells.[133] Ultrastructural features such as deformation of the cuticular plate in surviving hair cells[134] or a peripheral neurite loss pattern[135] may need to be considered in a full characterization of cochlear changes in presbycusis. Regardless of the debate on cochlear pathology–audiogram correlation, the notion that presbycusis arises from disruption of one or more of the key cochlear functional elements, including the inner and outer hair cells, spiral ganglion cells, and stria vascularis is widely accepted (**Fig. 6.3**).

Efforts at classification of audiograms of patients with age-related hearing loss can be aided by findings from animal models.[136] The gerbil model of presbycusis has demonstrated that age-related hearing loss is not a sensory but a metabolic disorder. That is, hair cell losses are attributed to noise exposure; and in the absence of noise damage, age-related strial

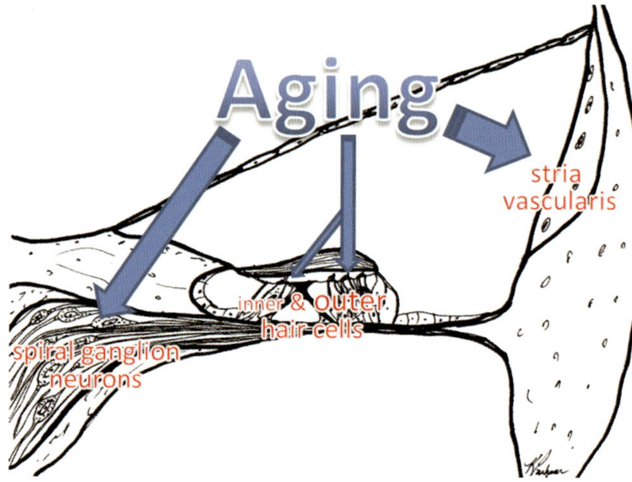

Fig. 6.3 Primary targets of the aging process in the cochlea that significantly impact hearing.

changes result in decreased endocochlear potential, which reduces cochlear sensitivity to a greater extent in the basal cochlea than in the apex. Using physiological findings in quiet-aged and furosemide-exposed gerbils as the conceptual framework, the main audiometric phenotypes (sensory, metabolic, and mixed sensory/metabolic) are believed to be consistent with predictions from animal findings associated with sensory and strial pathology.[136]

Central Presbycusis

Peripheral changes are expected to produce secondary central changes. This would be consistent with a model of "maladaptive" neural plasticity in which degeneration of spiral ganglion afferents[133] induces slow secondary neural loss further up the auditory pathway. Well-described peripheral auditory declines in the cochlea have been shown in mouse models of presbycusis to have direct and indirect consequences on the loss of neurons in the central auditory nuclei and potential reorganization of tonotopic mapping in the primary auditory cortex and multiple associated cortices.[137–141] In older human listeners, there is a linear relationship between hearing thresholds and gray matter volume in the primary auditory cortex, suggesting that even moderate declines in peripheral auditory acuity lead to a systematic downregulation of neural activity during the processing of higher-level aspects of speech and may also contribute to loss of gray matter volume in the primary auditory cortex.[142] In fact, individual differences in hearing sensitivity appear to predict the degree of language-driven neural recruitment during auditory sentence comprehension in the bilateral superior temporal gyri (including primary auditory cortex), thalamus, and brainstem for older listeners.[142]

However, not all of the central changes are due to hearing loss. For example, by controlling for hearing loss, one study demonstrated that age alone substantially reduces spatial release from masking.[143] The finding that aging can affect the ability to use spatial and spectrotemporal cues to separate competing speech streams suggests age-related changes in the cortical and/or subcortical structures essential for spatial hearing are independent of hearing loss and points to the importance of central processing.

Perception comes from the Latin word *percepio* (to receive) and implies organization of sensory input. Perception leads to cognition, which comes from the Latin word *cognoscere* (to learn or know), implying interpretation and assigning meaning. To move from signal detection to signal recognition and interpretation requires cognitive processing, which occurs through interaction of subcortical auditory pathways and multiple cortical regions. These interactions are collectively referred to as central auditory processing. Central auditory processing is used for successful completion of more challenging auditory tasks such as detection of a signal in background noise. Such tasks become more complex in understanding speech, during which the listeners must perceive and attend to relevant speech features, such as the pitch, timing, and timbre of the speaker's voice. Background or competing noise increases complexity of the task, further taxing central mechanisms. Performance of these tasks would be expected to be influenced by age-related changes in central auditory processing, as well as in cognitive function.

Although cognitive skills such as processing speed, memory functioning, and ability to divide attention diminish with age, older adults with normal hearing can compensate successfully for degradations in speech perception.[144] It is believed that this compensation arises from linguistic skills and a lifetime of accumulated vocabulary. In addition, slowed speech bestows additional restoration benefit because it provides older listeners more time to process noisy speech and to use available cues from the speech signal more effectively. It is believed that older people use context effectively[145] toward this goal. On the other hand, older listeners with sensorineural hearing loss demonstrate deficits in the ability to compensate for degraded speech, and the severity of this deficit appears to be determined by the severity of the hearing loss.[146] Saija and colleagues suggest that newly demonstrated top-down restoration skills of older individuals may lead to the development of new cognitive training methods to cope with complex listening environments of everyday life,[144] as in perception of interrupted speech.[147]

Functional magnetic resonance imaging (fMRI) has identified a core sentence-processing area located in the perisylvian region of the left cerebral hemisphere and an associated network of brain regions that support the working memory and other resources needed for comprehension of long or syntactically complex sentences in normal healthy older adults.[148] This finding suggests that brain plasticity and compensatory neural recruitment contribute to maintenance of language comprehension with age. There are specific differences in activation of the auditory pathways observed through fMRI testing of speech listening in young and old listeners.[149] Geriatric listeners show decreased activation of the auditory cortex compared with younger listeners, with even greater differences during speech listening in white noise compared with quiet listening. Specific sites of decreased activation included the anterior and posterior regions of the superior temporal gyrus bilaterally with particularly distinct differences within the posterior left superior temporal gyrus. Corpus callosum degeneration and resulting decreased interhemispheric neural transfer has also been implicated in asymmetric interaural responses during dichotic listening, with right-ear dominance frequently resulting.[149]

Further support for compensatory age-related changes in auditory processing comes from a recent study correlating hearing in quiet and noise with cortical structures evaluated with magnetic resonance imaging (MRI).[150] In older adults, a decline in the relative volume and cortical thickness of the prefrontal cortex was associated with a declining ability to perceive speech in a naturalistic environment. This finding is consistent with the decline–compensation hypothesis, which states that a decline in sensory processing caused by cognitive aging can be accompanied by an increase in the recruitment of more general cognitive areas as a means of compensation.[150] These compensatory mechanisms were also investigated using fMRI to compare neural processing of degraded speech between young and older adults.[151] Older adults adapted to degraded speech at the same rate as young listeners, although their overall comprehension of degraded speech was lower, driven by a reduced dynamic range. Neurally, both older and young adults relied on the left anterior insula for degraded more than clear speech. However, older adults relied on the middle frontal gyrus in addition to a core speech comprehension network. Once again, these findings lead to the conclusion that older adults recruit cognitive control networks as a compensatory mechanism.[151] The foregoing studies suggest that older listeners appear to be able to compensate for the impact of aging per se on the brain, so long as age-related pathological processes such as significant peripheral threshold elevations and possibly cerebrovascular and cognitive disorders (yet to be discussed) are not present.

In one of the earliest studies of central presbycusis, the progressive loss in central auditory competence measured by simultaneous binaural challenges and frequency and temporal distortion tests correlated with age.[152] It was suggested that central presbycusis, in addition to the peripheral form, further compounds hearing disorders in older patients and accounts for hearing disability in noise or speech competitive environments. Although some of the difficulties of hearing in noisy environments can be accounted for by loss of peripheral sensitivity, age-related deficits in interhemispheric information processing also contribute.[153] In older individuals when speech-in-noise perception is poor, deficiencies in the subcortical spectrotemporal representation of speech, including low-frequency spectral magnitudes and the timing of transient response peaks, can be demonstrated.[154]

A recent authoritative review emphasized that accumulating evidence supports the existence of central presbycusis as a multifactorial condition that involves age- and/or disease-related changes in the auditory system and in the brain.[155] Dysfunction of central auditory processing is believed to contribute more significantly to the pathology of late presbycusis,[126] making up a large component of presbycusis in people over 70 years of age.[156]

Some patients with central auditory processing disorder perform better with a single hearing aid in the better ear than with binaural aids.[157] In noise, 71% of geriatric patients perform better with one hearing aid, rather than two.[158] This might be due to an imbalance or asynchrony in binaural signal or a cognitive processing deficit and serves to highlight the importance of dichotic tests when evaluating any older patient with hearing loss.

Given the preceding implications of central presbycusis, the standard approach of treating ARHL through compensation of peripheral functional deficits (i.e., hearing aids and cochlear implants) may not be optimal. Some have promoted a more comprehensive management strategy for ARHL consisting of diagnostic evaluation that goes beyond conventional audiometric testing and includes measures of central auditory function, such as dichotic tasks and speech-in-noise testing.[159] A more comprehensive approach is expected to bestow substantial advantages on rehabilitation of the geriatric patient with ARHL.[160]

Although a better understanding of central presbycusis is compelling because of its profound implications for auditory rehabilitation, the importance of this age-related process is further highlighted by the implications of the inherent relationship between central presbycusis and cognitive function. Gates and colleagues have shown that poor performance on the Synthetic Sentence Identification with an Ipsilateral Competing Message (SSI-ICM), one measure of central processing disorder, is common in people with AD.[161] Using the SSI-ICM, in another study, a subset of older people from the Framingham Heart Study with normal cognitive screening test results on the Mini-Mental State Examination were identified to have very poor performance on the SSI-ICM (< 50% correct), yet normal word recognition in each ear. In this subset, the odds ratio for later diagnosis of dementia was over 12. This finding was interpreted as a common mechanism for AD and central processing disorder. Gates and colleagues reasoned that, because executive functioning is abnormal in people with AD and that many of the elements involved in central auditory processing, such as short-term memory, attention to task, and inhibition of unwanted signals, might involve executive functioning and undertook an examination of executive functioning and central auditory processing in another cohort. In that cohort, the significant relation of central auditory test results and the neuropsychiatric tests persisted even after adjustment for age, education, and pure-tone hearing thresholds, as well as, exclusion of AD cases.[126] The prevalence of a poor central auditory test (including SSI-ICM) was 33% for the cognitively normal group, 80% for the memory-impaired group, and 90% for the AD group.

In summary, all "hearing" is a cognitive activity and difficult hearing environments (e.g., in the presence of background noise) can overload the cognitive aspects of understanding, especially when age and disease limit cognitive resources. Attention to central processes in evaluation of hearing loss has the potential to refine the current approach to rehabilitation and should include cognitive screening.

Epidemiological Impact of Hearing Loss in Older Adults

As already noted, a growing number of epidemiological and clinical research studies have demonstrated strong associations between hearing impairment and measures of cognitive functioning and health outcomes. A conceptual model through which ARHL could be mechanistically associated with these downstream outcomes that are critical to aging and public health is depicted in **Fig. 6.4**. Investigating the potential mechanisms that underlie these associations begins with an understanding that age-related hearing loss reflects progressive damage to cochlear structures from aging and other factors (e.g., noise, vascular risk factors) that results in poorer encoding of sound by the cochlea. Earlier, we identified common factors that could underlie a simple correlation between hearing and aging outcomes, such as age, vascular risk factors (e.g., diabetes, smoking), and demographic or social factors (e.g., education). In contrast, mechanistic pathways through which hear-

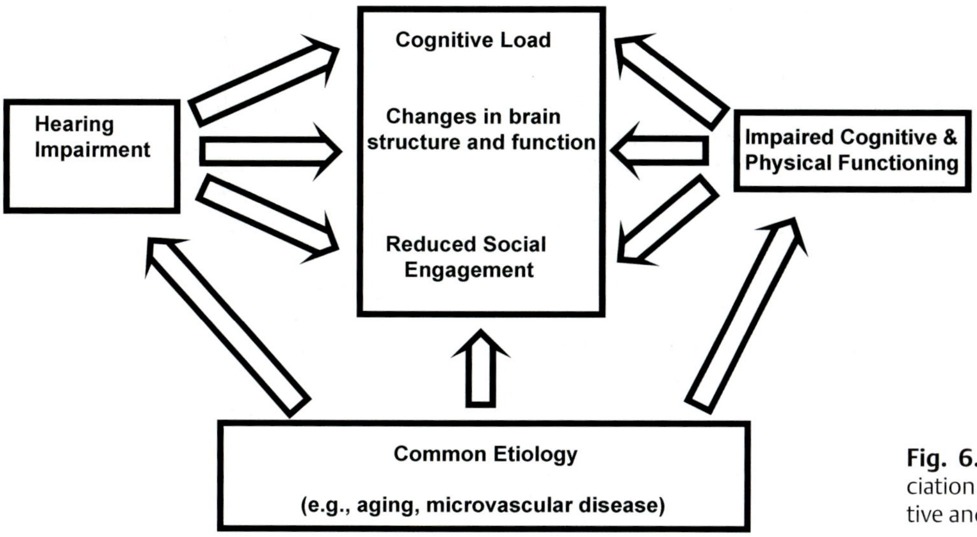

Fig. 6.4 Conceptual model of the association of hearing impairment with cognitive and physical functioning in older adults

ing impairment could contribute to poorer functioning include the effect of hearing impairment on cognitive load, brain structure, and decreased social engagement.

Mechanistic Pathways

Cognitive Load

Hearing impairment results in poor fidelity and distorted encoding of complex sounds (e.g., speech) in the cochlea.[162] The effect of poor peripheral encoding of sound is demonstrated by studies in which a degraded auditory signal requires greater cognitive resources for auditory perceptual processing to the detriment of other cognitive processes, such as working memory.[163–169] Neuroimaging studies have also demonstrated compensatory recruitment of regions in the prefrontal and temporoparietal cortex to maintain auditory speech processing in older adults.[142,148] The increased auditory processing required for a distorted speech sound for an individual with hearing loss would affect the cognitive resources available for the performance of other tasks consistent with a resource capacity model.[170] Importantly, such a cognitive load would always be present, given that hearing and cortical processing of sound are evolutionarily evolved processes that remain constantly active (e.g., monitoring of environmental sound cues). This cognitive "dual task" imposed by hearing impairment could, therefore, impact cognitive abilities as well as aspects of physical functioning that are dependent on attentional resources (e.g., gait, balance, driving).

Brain Structure and Function

Another pathway through which hearing impairment could contribute to impaired cognitive and physical functioning is through effects on brain structure. Neuroimaging studies have demonstrated that hearing loss is associated with reduced volumes in the primary auditory cortex[142,171,172] and loss of integrity of central auditory white matter tracks.[171,173–175] The basis of these associations remains unknown but may be related to alterations in the degree of neural activation provided by an impoverished auditory signal with subsequent changes in cortical reorganization and brain morphometry.[142] In animal models, cochlear impairments are known to be associated with both tonotopic reorganization of the auditory cortex[176–178] and morphological changes in central neuronal structures.[179] Interestingly, degraded fidelity of peripheral encoding of sound likely results in recruitment and activation of broader neural networks needed for auditory processing,[148,180,181] suggesting that peripheral hearing loss may carry cascading consequences for other regions of the brain and brain function. Under such a model, hearing impairment may constitute a "second hit" on the brain and thereby adversely affect cognitive performance and increase the risk of dementia in parallel to brain pathology caused by amyloid-b accumulation, neurofibrillary tangles, and microvascular disease. In support of this hypothesis, a recent neuroimaging study demonstrated that individuals with hearing impairment have accelerated rates of whole brain atrophy as well as specific volume declines in the right superior, middle, and inferior temporal gyri over a mean 6.4 years of follow-up.[182] These temporal regions are intriguing because they are important not only for spoken language processing,[183] but also for semantic memory and sensory integration and are involved in the early stages of mild cognitive impairment or early AD.[184]

Social Engagement

A final pathway through which hearing impairment could affect downstream outcomes is through effects on social engagement. Verbal communication is particularly susceptible to the effects of hearing loss given the inherent properties of spoken language. The components of spoken language consisting of the linguistic subsystems of phonology, semantics, and syntax are often encoded subtly in the auditory stream (e.g., *Sunday* and *someday* are phonetically similar but have markedly different meanings in conversation). Presbycusis leads to decrements in auditory sensitivity and loss of frequency resolution, which compromise an individual's access to these fine auditory cues.[162] These effects result in degraded verbal comprehension and impaired communication, particularly in situations with poor signal-to-noise ratio where effective communication is most critical (e.g., conversing with friends/family at dinner, participating in a meeting).[185–189] Degraded communication can subsequently lead to impaired social functioning as demonstrated in several studies of older adults.[190–195] Social relationships have powerful effects on physical and mental health that have been recognized since Durkheim first described the relationship between social integration and suicide in 1897.[196] Subsequent prospective studies have consistently implicated a causal effect of poor social relationships on all-cause mortality,[197–199] cognitive decline,[200–205] dementia,[206–212] heart disease,[213–215] physical functioning,[216–219] institutionalization,[220,221] gene expression profiles,[222,223] and depression.[224–226] A conceptual framework developed by Berkman et al to explain these effects hypothesizes that an individual's social network provides opportunities for social support, social influence, social engagement, person-to-person contact, and access to resources.[227]

Epidemiological Outcomes

Cognitive Functioning

Most previous epidemiological studies of hearing and cognition have demonstrated positive associations between hearing and cognition,[228–235] but some studies have shown no association.[236,237] Heterogeneity in study results is likely attributable to differences in how hearing and cognition have been defined and measured in each study.[238] Recent epidemiological studies have used objective audiometric assessments of hearing, both auditory and nonauditory tests of cognition, and have adjusted for multiple confounders (e.g., age, vascular risk factors). In two recent cross-sectional studies,[239,240] the magnitude of the association of a 25 dB hearing loss (equivalent to shifting from normal to a mild hearing loss) with executive functioning was equivalent to ~ 7 years of aging. In subsequent longitudinal studies, greater hearing loss was also associated with accelerated rates of decline on both nonauditory and auditory tests such that individuals with hearing loss had a 30 to 40% faster rate of cognitive decline compared with those individuals with normal hearing over a 6 year period.[241] Finally, hearing impairment has been found to be independently associated with a substantially increased risk of incident dementia.[240,242] Compared with individuals with normal hearing, those individuals with a mild, moderate, and severe hearing impairment, respectively, had a two-, three-, and fivefold increased risk of incident dementia over > 10 years of follow-up.[240]

Physical Functioning

Recent studies have demonstrated independent associations between hearing impairment and impaired daily functioning,[17,192,243,244] mobility (e.g., gait speed[245,246] and falls[247,248]), and mortality.[249,250] In contrast, other reports have indicated that there is no significant association between hearing and physical functioning and activity.[251,252] Heterogeneity in study results is likely explained by subjective measurement or varying definitions of hearing. Similar mechanisms linking hearing and cognition could mediate these observed associations. Individuals with hearing impairment may perform less physical activity due to a greater likelihood of social isolation (and thus a lesser likelihood of exercise in a social setting) than individuals with normal hearing.[253] Studies have also demonstrated that impaired hearing can contribute to cognitive load[168] and can therefore affect attentional and cognitive resources[82,239] that are important for maintaining posture and balance.[254,255] Finally, impaired hearing could restrict an individual's ability to monitor the auditory environment effectively (e.g., hearing footfalls and other auditory cues that provide orientation to the physical environment) and thereby affect an individual's likelihood of performing physical activities.

Role of Hearing Rehabilitative Therapies

These epidemiological analyses of the association of hearing impairment with cognitive and physical functioning have adjusted for known confounders (e.g., age, education, diabetes). Although there is still likely to be residual confounding from some unmeasured common pathological factor (e.g., inflammation), the consistency and robustness of these results across multiple studies and independent datasets strongly suggest that there are mechanistic pathways through which hearing loss directly or indirectly impacts cognitive and physical functioning in older adults. The most salient question, therefore, is whether hearing rehabilitative therapies could potentially mitigate these effects regardless of the mechanistic pathway. Results from observational epidemiological studies have generally demonstrated nonsignificant trends toward a protective effect with hearing aid use, but such results remain difficult to interpret. Individuals with hearing impairment who choose to use hearing aids and other technologies are likely to be healthier and of higher socioeconomic status (creating a positive bias of seeing a protective effect) but at the same time are also likely to have more severe hearing problems (leading to a negative bias) than individuals with hearing impairment who don't use hearing aids. Answering this question, therefore, will require a definitive, randomized, controlled trial (RCT) of current best-practices hearing loss treatment (counseling/education, provision of hearing aid and other assistive devices) versus watchful waiting in a large cohort of older adults with untreated hearing impairment. Only one RCT of hearing aids focused on broader downstream outcomes has ever been performed, and this moderately sized RCT of veterans performed over 20 years ago demonstrated positive effects of hearing aids on cognition and other functional domains at 4 months posttreatment.[256] Trials incorporating more representative cohorts and technology (e.g., digital hearing aids and other assistive devices paired with counseling and education), following patients for several years, and providing observations of the effects of hearing rehabilitation on cognitive, physical, and social functioning have never been performed. A substantial advantage of such an RCT is that a well-designed and carefully planned trial can definitively answer the critical public health question at hand (does treating hearing loss reduce the risk of dementia?) while also providing the data to explore the various mechanistic pathways that underlie these associations.

Surgical Treatment of Conductive Hearing Loss in the Geriatric Patient

As already noted, ARHL can occur superimposed on other otologic disorders. This section is concerned with surgical treatments for conductive hearing loss in this subset of geriatric patients. Other treatments such as surgery to control cholesteatomas, infection, cochlear implants, or vestibular schwannomas are discussed elsewhere. Although the major issues are similar between older and younger otology patients, there are a few considerations that are of key importance in the geriatric patient.

First, there are some standard audiometric concepts that are of particular concern in older adults. For otologic surgery, the key considerations are hearing thresholds, word recognition (speech discrimination), and air–bone gap. The size of this air–bone gap assesses the physical contribution of the tympanic membrane and middle ear to hearing loss and represents the maximum potential improvement that surgery can achieve. Although variable, as sensorineural thresholds decline, word recognition also declines. Word recognition scores do not particularly deteriorate as the air–bone gap increases, though, and this is of key interest for otologic surgery in the older adult. Some geriatric patients have word recognition scores that are disproportionately worse than one would expect from the bone thresholds. These patients may also have a large air–bone gap and have elevated bone thresholds. Surgery may reduce the air–bone gap, but this may be of little use to the patient if word recognition is poor. Surgery is not advisable for this subset of patients. Poor word recognition may be a major reason that many hearing-impaired people do not use hearing aids. Neither surgery nor hearing aids can substantially improve word recognition. People want to hear mostly to participate in conversation, but there is no reliable treatment for impaired word recognition. Word recognition scores < 60% are considered poor.[257]

Traditionally, stapedectomy, tympanoplasty, and ossiculoplasty of various types have made up the bulk of major otologic surgery for conductive hearing loss. Otosclerosis is usually diagnosed in middle age, so most patients undergo stapedectomy earlier in life. For this reason, revision stapedectomy is more likely in the older adult.[258,259] Proportionately more geriatric patients undergo stapedectomy/stapedotomy procedures for other indications, such as tympanosclerosis or other forms of stapes fixation. Bone may be soft in older patients, so complications such as prosthesis erosion or fracture of the incus may be more common in the older adult. Tympanoplasty may be indicated in certain geriatric patients for the same indications as in younger individuals, but revision surgery is more likely in the older adult than primary surgery because eustachian tube problems usually start early in life. Tympanostomy tube insertion and even cerumen removal can be considered surgical procedures and should not be overlooked because these procedures may improve hearing in many people. There are no major differences in technique that apply only to older people, but some general considerations are important.

Bone-anchored hearing aids (BAHAs) are surgically implanted bone conduction hearing aids.

Results do not appear to differ between older or younger patients.[260,261]

Is age a factor in surgical treatment of hearing loss? It is difficult to find a paper that reports a significant difference in hearing outcome based on age alone. Sensorineural thresholds matter and they covary with age. Comorbidities matter, and they increase with age. For stapedectomy, Meyer and Lambert reported that results were similar in the older and younger adults.[258] It would seem that unless there are individual medical concerns, surgical treatment of hearing loss in the older patient is similar to treatment in younger patients. There are no randomized trials of surgical treatment for hearing loss specific to the geriatric population, possibly reflecting a lack of need to differentiate between older and younger patients. Age alone is not a valid reason to decline surgical treatment of conductive hearing loss. Obviously, many older patients have medical problems that must be considered and may be risk factors for surgery. These include factors, such as impaired vision, frailty, or preexisting increased fall risk, that could influence postoperative course, which may include dizziness and at least temporary hearing impairment. Individual preference and tolerance for surgery may be factors in patients' decision making as well. In fact, most conductive hearing losses in geriatric patients are mixed losses with a significant sensorineural component that cannot be corrected with surgery.

Hearing aids are nonsurgical options for treatment of hearing loss. Many older adults decide against having any treatment; nevertheless, hearing aids can be worthwhile.[262] Older patients may have high expectations for hearing aids,[263,264] but many hearing-impaired candidates do not use them.[265–272] Cited reasons for low usage rates include cost, difficulty using them, occlusion effect. These seem inadequate to explain fully the low usage rates. Many patients purchase hearing aids and then put them in a drawer; so cost does not always seem to drive usage.[273] These people say, "The hearing aid just doesn't work for me." They must be right, at least for their specific aid and level of training in use. For some reason, a hearing aid does not meet their needs.[274] For some patients, an aid may have been fitted poorly; but audiometric reasons seem to offer the most likely explanation for low usage. Temporal processing abilities are disproportionately reduced in the geriatric patient (see Central Presbycusis earlier in the chapter).[266,275–277] The most likely audiometric reason that hearing aids do not meet expectations may be poor word recognition.[278] The lesson for surgeons is to be careful, because many of the reasons that hearing aids are not effective for some people are the same reasons that surgery is less effective in those same people.

There are two main advantages of surgical options for the geriatric patient:

1. Otologic procedures are usually of short duration, are well tolerated, and can often be performed under local anesthesia.
2. Significant improvement in hearing quality can result if patient selection is appropriate.

Pitfalls and considerations include the following:

1. Late-age onset of conductive hearing loss is unusual. Otosclerosis typically begins in teen years, and chronic eustachian tube issues are typically lifelong problems that do not arise primarily in the older adult unless a tumor is present. If patients present with new, conductive hearing loss for the first time after the age of 60, we need to be suspicious that there may be an important etiology.
2. Conductive hearing loss occurs in the geriatric patient, but there is usually a significant sensorineural component as well. Surgery and amplification can both improve thresholds, but neither can improve speech discrimination appreciably. Failure to consider preoperative speech recognition (e.g., word recognition score $< 60\%$) may be the most common error in surgical judgment in otologic surgery in the older patient.
3. Another audiometric consideration for surgery is the shape of the audiogram. The sloping, high-frequency loss that is typically seen in ARHL[133] is more difficult for fitting a hearing aid than a flat loss. Surgery may also create a high-frequency loss. It is appropriate to ask whether a hearing aid will still be required if surgery is successful. If so, surgery may still be reasonable, but it is critically important that the patient and surgeon understand the goal of surgery in advance and that the patient is aware a hearing aid will be required postoperatively.
4. Consider comorbidities carefully. Although there are recognized risk criteria for anesthesia, surgically specific issues are important, as well.
   a. Bone strength and density might be of concern for some prostheses or procedures, particularly if crimping is involved, as in stapedectomy. In placing BAHAs, one should consider the possibility that the screw may not osseointegrate properly. It may be wise not to abbreviate the traditional 6-week wait time between surgery for BAHA placement and activation of the device, because bone density may be inadequate in the older patient.

b. Healthy older patients do not have increased infection rates overall, but evidence of poor healing from other procedures or injuries in an individual can be a valid reason to decline surgery in some geriatric patients. Otologic surgery is not life-saving and should not involve significant risk to life, especially if other treatment options exist.
c. Many older patients have some cognitive decline, so the surgeon must be sure that the patient understands the risks and potential benefits and, most important, that he or she understands the rationale and does not have unrealistic expectations.

5. A hearing aid usage trial should be encouraged in elderly patients because it is easily reversible and may predict surgical success. Before embarking on surgical treatment for failed hearing aid use, the surgeon must be sure that the reasons for hearing aid failure are not also going to cause the surgery to fail.
6. Tinnitus treatment is not certain. Many older patients are troubled by tinnitus and hope that surgery will improve both the hearing and the tinnitus. Although this is a widely held belief, evidence that hearing correction improves tinnitus is not strong.[279,280] Many patients who undergo surgery for tinnitus are disappointed.
7. Be gentle with geriatric patients. They have greater difficulty compensating for dizziness than young patients. They may require more recuperation time in the hospital. They need more explanation. They need more time.
8. Psychological concerns can be crucial in preoperative older patients. This is part of the true art of medicine. Patients who will never be happy or who play manipulative psychological games—and there are many of these—should be identified. They are generally to be avoided unless they can come to appreciate their problems preoperatively.

In summary, surgical treatment of conductive hearing loss in older patients without medical contraindications can be successful if performed for the right indications. Particular attention should be paid to speech discrimination scores. Geriatric patients may require more explanation and more recovery time.

Acknowledgment

The authors gratefully acknowledge George A. Gates, MD, for his leadership in age-related hearing loss research and review of this manuscript.

References

1. Inouye SK, Studenski S, Tinetti ME, Kuchel GA. Geriatric syndromes: clinical, research, and policy implications of a core geriatric concept. J Am Geriatr Soc 2007;55(5):780–791
2. U.S. Census Bureau. 2012 National Population Projections. 2012. http://www.census.gov/population/projections/data/national/2012/summarytables.html. Accessed February 14, 2014
3. Lin FR, Niparko JK, Ferrucci L. Hearing loss prevalence in the United States. Arch Intern Med 2011;171(20):1851–1852
4. Dobie RA. The burdens of age-related and occupational noise-induced hearing loss in the United States. Ear Hear 2008; 29(4):565–577
5. Schacht J, Hawkins JE. Sketches of otohistory. Part 9: presby[a]cusis. Audiol Neurootol 2005;10(5):243–247
6. U.S. Department of Health and Human Services. Healthy People 2020. 2010. http://www.healthypeople.gov/2020/topicsobjectives2020/overview.aspx?topicId=31. Accessed February 1, 2014
7. Boyd CM, McNabney MK, Brandt N, et al. Guiding principles for the care of older adults with multimorbidity: an approach for clinicians: American Geriatrics Society Expert Panel on the Care of Older Adults with Multimorbidity. J Am Geriatr Soc 2012;60(10):E1–E25
8. Karpa MJ, Gopinath B, Beath K, et al. Associations between hearing impairment and mortality risk in older persons: the Blue Mountains Hearing Study. Ann Epidemiol 2010;20(6):452–459
9. Davis AC, Ostri B, Parving A. Longitudinal study of hearing. Acta Otolaryngol Suppl 1990;476:12–22
10. Lee FS, Matthews LJ, Dubno JR, Mills JH. Longitudinal study of pure-tone thresholds in older persons. Ear Hear 2005;26(1):1–11
11. Kiely KM, Gopinath B, Mitchell P, Luszcz M, Anstey KJ. Cognitive, health, and sociodemographic predictors of longitudinal decline in hearing acuity among older adults. J Gerontol A Biol Sci Med Sci 2012;67(9):997–1003
12. Ivers RQ, Mitchell P, Cumming RG. Sensory impairment and driving: the Blue Mountains Eye Study. Am J Public Health 1999;89(1):85–87
13. Abel SM, Giguère C, Consoli A, Papsin BC. The effect of aging on horizontal plane sound localization. J Acoust Soc Am 2000;108(2):743–752
14. Chandler DW, Grantham DW. Minimum audible movement angle in the horizontal plane as a function of stimulus frequency and bandwidth, source azimuth, and velocity. J Acoust Soc Am 1992;91(3):1624–1636
15. Neher T, Laugesen S, Jensen NS, Kragelund L. Can basic auditory and cognitive measures predict hearing-impaired listeners' localization and spatial speech recognition abilities? J Acoust Soc Am 2011;130(3):1542–1558

16. Freigang C, Schmiedchen K, Nitsche I, Rübsamen R. Free-field study on auditory localization and discrimination performance in older adults. Exp Brain Res 2014;232(4): 1157–1172
17. Bess FH, Lichtenstein MJ, Logan SA, Burger MC, Nelson E. Hearing impairment as a determinant of function in the elderly. J Am Geriatr Soc 1989;37(2):123–128
18. Gopinath B, Schneider J, McMahon CM, Teber E, Leeder SR, Mitchell P. Severity of age-related hearing loss is associated with impaired activities of daily living. Age Ageing 2012;41(2):195–200
19. Chia EM, Wang JJ, Rochtchina E, Cumming RR, Newall P, Mitchell P. Hearing impairment and health-related quality of life: the Blue Mountains Hearing Study. Ear Hear 2007; 28(2):187–195
20. Pronk M, Deeg DJ, Smits C, et al. Prospective effects of hearing status on loneliness and depression in older persons: identification of subgroups. Int J Audiol 2011;50(12): 887–896
21. Mick P, Kawachi I, Lin FR. The association between hearing loss and social isolation in older adults. Otolaryngol Head Neck Surg 2014;150(3):378–384
22. Valtorta N, Hanratty B. Loneliness, isolation and the health of older adults: do we need a new research agenda? J R Soc Med 2012;105(12):518–522
23. Herbst KG, Humphrey C. Hearing impairment and mental state in the elderly living at home. BMJ 1980;281(6245): 903–905
24. Kalayam B, Meyers BS, Kakuma T, et al. Age at onset of geriatric depression and sensorineural hearing deficits. Biol Psychiatry 1995;38(10):649–658
25. Huang CQ, Dong BR, Lu ZC, Yue JR, Liu QX. Chronic diseases and risk for depression in old age: a meta-analysis of published literature. Ageing Res Rev 2010;9(2):131–141
26. Tambs K. Moderate effects of hearing loss on mental health and subjective well-being: results from the Nord-Trøndelag Hearing Loss Study. Psychosom Med 2004;66(5): 776–782
27. Pronk M, Deeg DJ, Kramer SE. Hearing status in older persons: a significant determinant of depression and loneliness? Results from the longitudinal aging study Amsterdam. Am J Audiol 2013;22(2):316–320
28. Capella-McDonnall ME. The effects of single and dual sensory loss on symptoms of depression in the elderly. Int J Geriatr Psychiatry 2005;20(9):855–861
29. Chou KL. Combined effect of vision and hearing impairment on depression in older adults: evidence from the English Longitudinal Study of Ageing. J Affect Disord 2008;106(1-2): 191–196
30. Huang Q, Tang J. Age-related hearing loss or presbycusis. Eur Arch Otorhinolaryngol 2010;267(8):1179–1191
31. Sataloff J, Sataloff RT, Lueneburg W. Tinnitus and vertigo in healthy senior citizens without a history of noise exposure. Am J Otol 1987;8(2):87–89
32. Seidman MD, Jacobson GP. Update on tinnitus. Otolaryngol Clin North Am 1996;29(3):455–465
33. Rosenhall U, Karlsson AK. Tinnitus in old age. Scand Audiol 1991;20(3):165–171
34. Ferreira LM, Ramos Júnior AN, Mendes EP. Characterization of tinnitus in the elderly and its possible related disorders. Braz J Otorhinolaryngol 2009;75(2):249–255
35. Claussen CF, ed. Presbyvertigo, Presbyataxie, Presbytinnitus. German ed. Berlin, Germany: Springer Verlag; 1984
36. Dobie RA. Depression and tinnitus. Otolaryngol Clin North Am 2003;36(2):383–388
37. Loprinzi PD, Maskalick S, Brown K, Gilham B. Association between depression and tinnitus in a nationally representative sample of US older adults. Aging Ment Health 2013;17(6): 714–717
38. Schlee W, Kleinjung T, Hiller W, Goebel G, Kolassa IT, Langguth B. Does tinnitus distress depend on age of onset? PLoS ONE 2011;6(11):e27379
39. Song JJ, De Ridder D, Schlee W, Van de Heyning P, Vanneste S. "Distressed aging": the differences in brain activity between early- and late-onset tinnitus. Neurobiol Aging 2013; 34(7):1853–1863
40. Borghi C, Cosentino ER, Rinaldi ER, et al. Tinnitus in elderly patients and prognosis of mild-to-moderate congestive heart failure: a cross-sectional study with a long-term extension of the clinical follow-up. BMC Med 2011;9:80
41. Johnson KR, Erway LC, Cook SA, Willott JF, Zheng QY. A major gene affecting age-related hearing loss in C57BL/6J mice. Hear Res 1997;114(1-2):83–92
42. Noben-Trauth K, Zheng QY, Johnson KR. Association of cadherin 23 with polygenic inheritance and genetic modification of sensorineural hearing loss. Nat Genet 2003;35(1): 21–23
43. Drayton M, Noben-Trauth K. Mapping quantitative trait loci for hearing loss in Black Swiss mice. Hear Res 2006;212(1-2): 128–139
44. Mashimo T, Erven AE, Spiden SL, Guénet JL, Steel KP. Two quantitative trait loci affecting progressive hearing loss in 101/H mice. Mamm Genome 2006;17(8):841–850
45. Zheng QY, Ding D, Yu H, Salvi RJ, Johnson KR. A locus on distal chromosome 10 (ahl4) affecting age-related hearing loss in A/J mice. Neurobiol Aging 2009;30(10):1693–1705
46. Noben-Trauth K, Latoche JR, Neely HR, Bennett B. Phenotype and genetics of progressive sensorineural hearing loss (Snhl1) in the LXS set of recombinant inbred strains of mice. PLoS ONE 2010;5(7):e11459
47. Schacht J, Altschuler R, Burke DT, et al. Alleles that modulate late life hearing in genetically heterogeneous mice. Neurobiol Aging 2012;33(8):e15–e29
48. Gates GA, Couropmitree NN, Myers RH. Genetic associations in age-related hearing thresholds. Arch Otolaryngol Head Neck Surg 1999;125(6):654–659
49. DeStefano AL, Gates GA, Heard-Costa N, Myers RH, Baldwin CT. Genomewide linkage analysis to presbycusis in the Framingham Heart Study. Arch Otolaryngol Head Neck Surg 2003;129(3):285–289
50. Demeester K, van Wieringen A, Hendrickx JJ, et al. Heritability of audiometric shape parameters and familial aggregation of presbycusis in an elderly Flemish population. Hear Res 2010;265(1-2):1–10
51. McMahon CM, Kifley A, Rochtchina E, Newall P, Mitchell P. The contribution of family history to hearing loss in an older population. Ear Hear 2008;29(4):578–584
52. Christensen K, Frederiksen H, Hoffman HJ. Genetic and environmental influences on self-reported reduced hearing in the old and oldest old. J Am Geriatr Soc 2001;49(11): 1512–1517
53. Garringer HJ, Pankratz ND, Nichols WC, Reed T. Hearing impairment susceptibility in elderly men and the DFNA18 locus. Arch Otolaryngol Head Neck Surg 2006;132(5): 506–510
54. Rodriguez-Paris J, Ballay C, Inserra M, et al. Genetic analysis of presbycusis by arrayed primer extension. Ann Clin Lab Sci 2008;38(4):352–360
55. Van Laer L, Van Eyken E, Fransen E, et al. The grainyhead like 2 gene (GRHL2), alias TFCP2L3, is associated with age-related hearing impairment. Hum Mol Genet 2008;17(2): 159–169
56. Lin YH, Wu CC, Hsu CJ, Hwang JH, Liu TC. The grainyhead-like 2 gene (GRHL2) single nucleotide polymorphism is not asso-

ciated with age-related hearing impairment in Han Chinese. Laryngoscope 2011;121(6):1303–1307

57. Bai U, Seidman MD, Hinojosa R, Quirk WS. Mitochondrial DNA deletions associated with aging and possibly presbycusis: a human archival temporal bone study. Am J Otol 1997; 18(4):449–453

58. Markaryan A, Nelson EG, Hinojosa R. Quantification of the mitochondrial DNA common deletion in presbycusis. Laryngoscope 2009;119(6):1184–1189

59. Crawley BK, Keithley EM. Effects of mitochondrial mutations on hearing and cochlear pathology with age. Hear Res 2011;280(1-2):201–208

60. Bonneux S, Fransen E, Van Eyken E, et al. Inherited mitochondrial variants are not a major cause of age-related hearing impairment in the European population. Mitochondrion 2011;11(5):729–734

61. Sohal RS, Weindruch R. Oxidative stress, caloric restriction, and aging. Science 1996;273(5271):59–63

62. Staecker H, Zheng QY, Van De Water TR. Oxidative stress in aging in the C57B16/J mouse cochlea. Acta Otolaryngol 2001;121(6):666–672

63. Riva C, Donadieu E, Magnan J, Lavieille JP. Age-related hearing loss in CD/1 mice is associated to ROS formation and HIF target proteins up-regulation in the cochlea. Exp Gerontol 2007;42(4):327–336

64. Ying YL, Balaban CD. Regional distribution of manganese superoxide dismutase 2 (Mn SOD2) expression in rodent and primate spiral ganglion cells. Hear Res 2009;253(1-2): 116–124

65. Chang NC, Ho CK, Wu MT, Yu ML, Ho KY. Effect of manganese-superoxide dismutase genetic polymorphisms IVS3-23T/G on noise susceptibility in Taiwan. Am J Otolaryngol 2009;30(6):396–400

66. Nolan LS, Cadge BA, Gomez-Dorado M, Dawson SJ. A functional and genetic analysis of SOD2 promoter variants and their contribution to age-related hearing loss. Mech Ageing Dev 2013;134(7-8):298–306

67. Bared A, Ouyang X, Angeli S, et al. Antioxidant enzymes, presbycusis, and ethnic variability. Otolaryngol Head Neck Surg 2010;143(2):263–268

68. Unal M, Tamer L, Doğruer ZN, Yildirim H, Vayisoğlu Y, Camdeviren H. N-acetyltransferase 2 gene polymorphism and presbycusis. Laryngoscope 2005;115(12):2238–2241

69. Angeli SI, Bared A, Ouyang X, Du LL, Yan D, Zhong Liu X. Audioprofiles and antioxidant enzyme genotypes in presbycusis. Laryngoscope 2012;122(11):2539–2542

70. Izumikawa M, Minoda R, Kawamoto K, et al. Auditory hair cell replacement and hearing improvement by Atoh1 gene therapy in deaf mammals. Nat Med 2005;11(3):271–276

71. Gates GA, Cobb JL, D'Agostino RB, Wolf PA. The relation of hearing in the elderly to the presence of cardiovascular disease and cardiovascular risk factors. Arch Otolaryngol Head Neck Surg 1993;119(2):156–161

72. Torre P III, Cruickshanks KJ, Klein BE, Klein R, Nondahl DM. The association between cardiovascular disease and cochlear function in older adults. J Speech Lang Hear Res 2005;48(2):473–481

73. Agrawal Y, Platz EA, Niparko JK. Prevalence of hearing loss and differences by demographic characteristics among US adults: data from the National Health and Nutrition Examination Survey, 1999-2004. Arch Intern Med 2008;168(14): 1522–1530

74. Hull RH, Kerschen SR. The influence of cardiovascular health on peripheral and central auditory function in adults: a research review. Am J Audiol 2010;19(1):9–16

75. Helzner EP, Patel AS, Pratt S, et al. Hearing sensitivity in older adults: associations with cardiovascular risk factors in the health, aging and body composition study. J Am Geriatr Soc 2011;59(6):972–979

76. Kakarlapudi V, Sawyer R, Staecker H. The effect of diabetes on sensorineural hearing loss. Otol Neurotol 2003;24(3): 382–386

77. Bainbridge KE, Hoffman HJ, Cowie CC. Risk factors for hearing impairment among U.S. adults with diabetes: National Health and Nutrition Examination Survey 1999-2004. Diabetes Care 2011;34(7):1540–1545

78. Austin DF, Konrad-Martin D, Griest S, McMillan GP, McDermott D, Fausti S. Diabetes-related changes in hearing. Laryngoscope 2009;119(9):1788–1796

79. Cheng YJ, Gregg EW, Saaddine JB, Imperatore G, Zhang X, Albright AL. Three decade change in the prevalence of hearing impairment and its association with diabetes in the United States. Prev Med 2009;49(5):360–364

80. Mitchell P, Gopinath B, McMahon CM, et al. Relationship of Type 2 diabetes to the prevalence, incidence and progression of age-related hearing loss. Diabet Med 2009;26(5):483–488

81. Brant LJ, Gordon-Salant S, Pearson JD, et al. Risk factors related to age-associated hearing loss in the speech frequencies. J Am Acad Audiol 1996;7(3):152–160

82. Lin FR. Hearing loss and cognition among older adults in the United States. J Gerontol A Biol Sci Med Sci 2011;66(10): 1131–1136

83. Gopinath B, Schneider J, Rochtchina E, Leeder SR, Mitchell P. Association between age-related hearing loss and stroke in an older population. Stroke 2009;40(4):1496–1498

84. Vilayur E, Gopinath B, Harris DC, Burlutsky G, McMahon CM, Mitchell P. The association between reduced GFR and hearing loss: a cross-sectional population-based study. Am J Kidney Dis 2010;56(4):661–669

85. Verschuur CA, Dowell A, Syddall HE, et al. Markers of inflammatory status are associated with hearing threshold in older people: findings from the Hertfordshire Ageing Study. Age Ageing 2012;41(1):92–97

86. Nash SD, Cruickshanks KJ, Zhan W, et al. Long-term assessment of systemic inflammation and the cumulative incidence of age-related hearing impairment in the epidemiology of hearing loss study. J Gerontol A Biol Sci Med Sci 2014;69(2):207–214

87. Susmano A, Rosenbush SW. Hearing loss and ischemic heart disease. Am J Otol 1988;9(5):403–408

88. Lim DP, Stephens SD. Clinical investigation of hearing loss in the elderly. Clin Otolaryngol Allied Sci 1991;16(3): 288–293

89. Rosenhall U, Hederstierna C, Idrizbegovic E. Otological diagnoses and probable age-related auditory neuropathy in "younger" and "older" elderly persons. Int J Audiol 2011; 50(9):578–581

90. Kotimäki J, Sorri M, Muhli A. Prognosis of hearing impairment in Ménière's disease. Acta Otolaryngol Suppl 2001;545: 14–18

91. Sakihara Y, Parving A. Clinical otosclerosis, prevalence estimates and spontaneous progress. Acta Otolaryngol 1999; 119(4):468–472

92. Dornhoffer JL, Bailey HA Jr, Graham SS. Long-term hearing results following stapedotomy. Am J Otol 1994;15(5): 674–678

93. Soudry E, Sulkes J, Attias J, Nageris BI. Bone conduction in otosclerosis—operated versus non-operated ears. J Basic Clin Physiol Pharmacol 2007;18(3):189–199

94. Clark K, Sowers MR, Wallace RB, Jannausch ML, Lemke J, Anderson CV. Age-related hearing loss and bone mass in a population of rural women aged 60 to 85 years. Ann Epidemiol 1995;5(1):8–14

95. Helzner EP, Cauley JA, Pratt SR, et al. Hearing sensitivity and bone mineral density in older adults: the Health, Aging and Body Composition Study. Osteoporos Int 2005;16(12): 1675–1682
96. Cruickshanks KJ, Klein R, Klein BE, Wiley TL, Nondahl DM, Tweed TS. Cigarette smoking and hearing loss: the epidemiology of hearing loss study. JAMA 1998;279(21):1715–1719
97. Fransen E, Topsakal V, Hendrickx JJ, et al. Occupational noise, smoking, and a high body mass index are risk factors for age-related hearing impairment and moderate alcohol consumption is protective: a European population-based multicenter study. J Assoc Res Otolaryngol 2008;9(3):264–276, discussion 261–263
98. Gates GA, Schmid P, Kujawa SG, Nam B, D'Agostino R. Longitudinal threshold changes in older men with audiometric notches. Hear Res 2000;141(1-2):220–228
99. Rosenhall U. The influence of ageing on noise-induced hearing loss. Noise Health 2003;5(20):47–53
100. Xiong M, Yang C, Lai H, Wang J. Impulse noise exposure in early adulthood accelerates age-related hearing loss. Eur Arch Otorhinolaryngol 2014;271(6):1351–1354
101. Biassoni EC, Serra MR, Richtert U, et al. Recreational noise exposure and its effects on the hearing of adolescents. Part II: development of hearing disorders. Int J Audiol 2005; 44(2):74–85
102. Ciorba A, Benatti A, Bianchini C, et al. High frequency hearing loss in the elderly: effect of age and noise exposure in an Italian group. J Laryngol Otol 2011;125(8):776–780
103. Kujawa SG, Liberman MC. Acceleration of age-related hearing loss by early noise exposure: evidence of a misspent youth. J Neurosci 2006;26(7):2115–2123
104. Gopinath B, Thiagalingam A, Teber E, Mitchell P. Exposure to workplace noise and the risk of cardiovascular disease events and mortality among older adults. Prev Med 2011;53(6):390–394
105. Wild DC, Brewster MJ, Banerjee AR. Noise-induced hearing loss is exacerbated by long-term smoking. Clin Otolaryngol 2005;30(6):517–520
106. National Cancer Institute. Surveillance, Epidemiology, and End Results Program (SEER). Revision History of the SEER Cancer Statistics Review (CSR), 1975–2010. 2013. http://seer.cancer.gov/csr/1975_2010/. Accessed February 1, 2014
107. Nagy JL, Adelstein DJ, Newman CW, Rybicki LA, Rice TW, Lavertu P. Cisplatin ototoxicity: the importance of baseline audiometry. Am J Clin Oncol 1999;22(3):305–308
108. Jiang H, Talaska AE, Schacht J, Sha SH. Oxidative imbalance in the aging inner ear. Neurobiol Aging 2007;28(10): 1605–1612
109. Rybak LP, Ramkumar V. Ototoxicity. Kidney Int 2007; 72(8):931–935
110. Rybak LP, Mukherjea D, Jajoo S, Ramkumar V. Cisplatin ototoxicity and protection: clinical and experimental studies. Tohoku J Exp Med 2009;219(3):177–186
111. Parham K. Can intratympanic dexamethasone protect against cisplatin ototoxicity in mice with age-related hearing loss? Otolaryngol Head Neck Surg 2011;145(4):635–640
112. Laurell G, Borg E. Ototoxicity of cisplatin in gynaecological cancer patients. Scand Audiol 1988;17(4):241–247
113. Bielefeld EC, Coling D, Chen GD, et al. Age-related hearing loss in the Fischer 344/NHsd rat substrain. Hear Res 2008; 241(1-2):26–33
114. Someya S, Xu J, Kondo K, et al. Age-related hearing loss in C57BL/6J mice is mediated by Bak-dependent mitochondrial apoptosis. Proc Natl Acad Sci USA 2009;106(46): 19432–19437
115. Sha SH, Kanicki A, Halsey K, Wearne KA, Schacht J. Antioxidant-enriched diet does not delay the progression of age-related hearing loss. Neurobiol Aging 2012;33(5):e15–e16
116. Someya S, Yamasoba T, Weindruch R, Prolla TA, Tanokura M. Caloric restriction suppresses apoptotic cell death in the mammalian cochlea and leads to prevention of presbycusis. Neurobiol Aging 2007;28(10):1613–1622
117. Gopinath B, Flood VM, McMahon CM, et al. Dietary antioxidant intake is associated with the prevalence but not incidence of age-related hearing loss. J Nutr Health Aging 2011;15(10):896–900
118. Gopinath B, Flood VM, Rochtchina E, McMahon CM, Mitchell P. Consumption of omega-3 fatty acids and fish and risk of age-related hearing loss. Am J Clin Nutr 2010;92(2):416–421
119. Spankovich C, Le Prell CG. Healthy diets, healthy hearing: National Health and Nutrition Examination Survey, 1999-2002. Int J Audiol 2013;52(6):369–376
120. Hwang JH, Wu CC, Hsu CJ, Liu TC, Yang WS. Association of central obesity with the severity and audiometric configurations of age-related hearing impairment. Obesity (Silver Spring) 2009;17(9):1796–1801
121. Michikawa T, Nishiwaki Y, Asakura K, et al. Sunlight exposure may be a risk factor of hearing impairment: a community-based study in Japanese older men and women. J Gerontol A Biol Sci Med Sci 2013;68(1):96–103
122. Park SK, Elmarsafawy S, Mukherjee B, et al. Cumulative lead exposure and age-related hearing loss: the VA Normative Aging Study. Hear Res 2010;269(1-2):48–55
123. Zhan W, Cruickshanks KJ, Klein BE, et al. Modifiable determinants of hearing impairment in adults. Prev Med 2011; 53(4-5):338–342
124. Zhan W, Cruickshanks KJ, Klein BE, et al. Generational differences in the prevalence of hearing impairment in older adults. Am J Epidemiol 2010;171(2):260–266
125. Sulaiman AH, Husain R, Seluakumaran K. Evaluation of early hearing damage in personal listening device users using extended high-frequency audiometry and otoacoustic emissions. Eur Arch Otorhinolaryngol 2014;271(6):1463–1470
126. Gates GA, Gibbons LE, McCurry SM, Crane PK, Feeney MP, Larson EB. Executive dysfunction and presbycusis in older persons with and without memory loss and dementia [published correction available in Cogn Behav Neurol 2011;24(1):39. Note: McCusrry, Susan M corrected to McCurry, Susan M] . Cogn Behav Neurol 2010;23(4):218–223
127. Monteiro de Castro Silva I, Feitosa MA. High-frequency audiometry in young and older adults when conventional audiometry is normal. Braz J Otorhinolaryngol 2006;72(5): 665–672
128. Stenklev NC, Laukli E. Presbyacusis-hearing thresholds and the ISO 7029. Int J Audiol 2004;43(5):295–306
129. Schuknecht HF. Further Observations on the Pathology of Presbycusis. Arch Otolaryngol 1964;80:369–382
130. Schuknecht HF, Gacek MR. Cochlear pathology in presbycusis. Ann Otol Rhinol Laryngol 1993;102(1 Pt 2):1–16
131. Gates GA, Mills JH. Presbycusis. Lancet 2005;366(9491): 1111–1120
132. Nelson EG, Hinojosa R. Presbycusis: a human temporal bone study of individuals with flat audiometric patterns of hearing loss using a new method to quantify stria vascularis volume. Laryngoscope 2003;113(10):1672–1686
133. Nelson EG, Hinojosa R. Presbycusis: a human temporal bone study of individuals with downward sloping audiometric patterns of hearing loss and review of the literature. Laryngoscope 2006;116(9 Pt 3, Suppl 112):1–12
134. Scholtz AW, Kammen-Jolly K, Felder E, Hussl B, Rask-Andersen H, Schrott-Fischer A. Selective aspects of human

pathology in high-tone hearing loss of the aging inner ear. Hear Res 2001;157(1-2):77–86

135. Chen MA, Webster P, Yang E, Linthicum FH Jr. Presbycusic neuritic degeneration within the osseous spiral lamina. Otol Neurotol 2006;27(3):316–322

136. Dubno JR, Eckert MA, Lee FS, Matthews LJ, Schmiedt RA. Classifying human audiometric phenotypes of age-related hearing loss from animal models. J Assoc Res Otolaryngol 2013;14(5):687–701

137. Willott JF, Hunter KP, Coleman JR. Aging and presbycusis: effects on 2-deoxy-D-glucose uptake in the mouse auditory brain stem in quiet. Exp Neurol 1988;99(3):615–621

138. Willott JF, Jackson LM, Hunter KP. Morphometric study of the anteroventral cochlear nucleus of two mouse models of presbycusis. J Comp Neurol 1987;260(3):472–480

139. Willott JF, Parham K, Hunter KP. Response properties of inferior colliculus neurons in middle-aged C57BL/6J mice with presbycusis. Hear Res 1988;37(1):15–27

140. Willott JF, Parham K, Hunter KP. Response properties of inferior colliculus neurons in young and very old CBA/J mice. Hear Res 1988;37(1):1–14

141. Willott JF, Aitkin LM, McFadden SL. Plasticity of auditory cortex associated with sensorineural hearing loss in adult C57BL/6J mice. J Comp Neurol 1993;329(3):402–411

142. Peelle JE, Troiani V, Grossman M, Wingfield A. Hearing loss in older adults affects neural systems supporting speech comprehension. J Neurosci 2011;31(35):12638–12643

143. Gallun FJ, Diedesch AC, Kampel SD, Jakien KM. Independent impacts of age and hearing loss on spatial release in a complex auditory environment. Front Neurosci 2013;7:252

144. Saija JD, Akyürek EG, Andringa TC, Başkent D. Perceptual restoration of degraded speech is preserved with advancing age. J Assoc Res Otolaryngol 2014;15(1):139–148

145. Kathleen Pichora-Fuller M. Use of supportive context by younger and older adult listeners: balancing bottom-up and top-down information processing. Int J Audiol 2008; 47(Suppl 2):S72–S82

146. Başkent D, Eiler CL, Edwards B. Phonemic restoration by hearing-impaired listeners with mild to moderate sensorineural hearing loss. Hear Res 2010;260(1-2):54–62

147. Benard MR, Başkent D; MR B. Perceptual learning of interrupted speech. PLoS ONE 2013;8(3):e58149

148. Wingfield A, Grossman M. Language and the aging brain: patterns of neural compensation revealed by functional brain imaging. J Neurophysiol 2006;96(6):2830–2839

149. Hwang JH, Li CW, Wu CW, Chen JH, Liu TC. Aging effects on the activation of the auditory cortex during binaural speech listening in white noise: an fMRI study. Audiol Neurootol 2007;12(5):285–294

150. Wong PC, Ettlinger M, Sheppard JP, Gunasekera GM, Dhar S. Neuroanatomical characteristics and speech perception in noise in older adults. Ear Hear 2010;31(4):471–479

151. Erb J, Obleser J. Upregulation of cognitive control networks in older adults' speech comprehension. Front Syst Neurosci 2013;7:116

152. Welsh LW, Welsh JJ, Healy MP. Central presbycusis. Laryngoscope 1985;95(2):128–136

153. Martin JS, Jerger JF. Some effects of aging on central auditory processing. J Rehabil Res Dev 2005;42(4, Suppl 2): 25–44

154. Anderson S, Kraus N. Sensory-cognitive interaction in the neural encoding of speech in noise: a review. J Am Acad Audiol 2010;21(9):575–585

155. Humes LE, Dubno JR, Gordon-Salant S, et al. Central presbycusis: a review and evaluation of the evidence. J Am Acad Audiol 2012;23(8):635–666

156. Gates GA, Feeney MP, Mills D. Cross-sectional age-changes of hearing in the elderly. Ear Hear 2008;29(6):865–874

157. Chmiel R, Jerger J. Hearing aid use, central auditory disorder, and hearing handicap in elderly persons. J Am Acad Audiol 1996;7(3):190–202

158. Henkin Y, Waldman A, Kishon-Rabin L. The benefits of bilateral versus unilateral amplification for the elderly: are two always better than one? J Basic Clin Physiol Pharmacol 2007;18(3):201–216

159. Parham K, Lin FR, Coelho DH, Sataloff RT, Gates GA. Comprehensive management of presbycusis: central and peripheral. Otolaryngol Head Neck Surg 2013;148(4):537–539

160. Gates GA. Central presbycusis: an emerging view. Otolaryngol Head Neck Surg 2012;147(1):1–2

161. Gates GA, Cobb JL, Linn RT, Rees T, Wolf PA, D'Agostino RB. Central auditory dysfunction, cognitive dysfunction, and dementia in older people. Arch Otolaryngol Head Neck Surg 1996;122(2):161–167

162. Pickles JO. An Introduction to the Physiology of Hearing. Bingley, UK: Emerald Group Publishing; 2008

163. Tun PA, McCoy S, Wingfield A. Aging, hearing acuity, and the attentional costs of effortful listening. Psychol Aging 2009;24(3):761–766

164. Pichora-Fuller MK, Schneider BA, Daneman M. How young and old adults listen to and remember speech in noise. J Acoust Soc Am 1995;97(1):593–608

165. Rabbitt PM. Channel-capacity, intelligibility and immediate memory. Q J Exp Psychol 1968;20(3):241–248

166. Rabbitt P. Mild hearing loss can cause apparent memory failures which increase with age and reduce with IQ. Acta Otolaryngol Suppl 1990;476:167–175, discussion 176

167. McCoy SL, Tun PA, Cox LC, Colangelo M, Stewart RA, Wingfield A. Hearing loss and perceptual effort: downstream effects on older adults' memory for speech. Q J Exp Psychol A 2005;58(1):22–33

168. Wingfield A, Tun PA, McCoy SL. Hearing loss in older adulthood: what it is and how it interacts with cognitive performance. Curr Dir Psychol Sci 2005;14(3):144–148

169. Wingfield A, McCoy SL, Peelle JE, Tun PA, Cox LC. Effects of adult aging and hearing loss on comprehension of rapid speech varying in syntactic complexity. J Am Acad Audiol 2006;17(7):487–497

170. Kahneman D. Attention and Effort. Englewood Cliffs, NJ: Prentice-Hall; 1973

171. Husain FT, Medina RE, Davis CW, et al. Neuroanatomical changes due to hearing loss and chronic tinnitus: a combined VBM and DTI study. Brain Res 2011;1369:74–88

172. Eckert MA, Cute SL, Vaden KI Jr, Kuchinsky SE, Dubno JR. Auditory cortex signs of age-related hearing loss. J Assoc Res Otolaryngol 2012;13(5):703–713

173. Chang Y, Lee SH, Lee YJ, et al. Auditory neural pathway evaluation on sensorineural hearing loss using diffusion tensor imaging. Neuroreport 2004;15(11):1699–1703

174. Lin Y, Wang J, Wu C, Wai Y, Yu J, Ng S. Diffusion tensor imaging of the auditory pathway in sensorineural hearing loss: changes in radial diffusivity and diffusion anisotropy. J Magn Reson Imaging 2008;28(3):598–603

175. Miao W, Li J, Tang M, et al. Altered white matter integrity in adolescents with prelingual deafness: a high-resolution tract-based spatial statistics imaging study. AJNR Am J Neuroradiol 2013;34(6):1264–1270

176. Kakigi A, Hirakawa H, Harel N, Mount RJ, Harrison RV. Tonotopic mapping in auditory cortex of the adult chinchilla with amikacin-induced cochlear lesions. Audiology 2000;39(3):153–160

177. Cheung SW, Bonham BH, Schreiner CE, Godey B, Copenhaver DA. Realignment of interaural cortical maps in asymmetric hearing loss. J Neurosci 2009;29(21):7065–7078
178. Schwaber MK, Garraghty PE, Kaas JH. Neuroplasticity of the adult primate auditory cortex following cochlear hearing loss. Am J Otol 1993;14(3):252–258
179. Gröschel M, Götze R, Ernst A, Basta D. Differential impact of temporary and permanent noise-induced hearing loss on neuronal cell density in the mouse central auditory pathway. J Neurotrauma 2010;27(8):1499–1507
180. Davis MH, Johnsrude IS. Hearing speech sounds: top-down influences on the interface between audition and speech perception. Hear Res 2007;229(1-2):132–147
181. Peelle JE, Johnsrude IS, Davis MH. Hierarchical processing for speech in human auditory cortex and beyond. Front Hum Neurosci 2010;4:51
182. Lin FR, Ferrucci L, An Y, et al. Association of hearing impairment with brain volume changes in older adults. Neuroimage 2014;90(Jan):84–92
183. Peelle JE. The hemispheric lateralization of speech processing depends on what "speech" is: a hierarchical perspective. Front Hum Neurosci 2012;6:309
184. Chételat G, Landeau B, Eustache F, et al. Using voxel-based morphometry to map the structural changes associated with rapid conversion in MCI: a longitudinal MRI study. Neuroimage 2005;27(4):934–946
185. Gordon-Salant S. Hearing loss and aging: new research findings and clinical implications. J Rehabil Res Dev 2005; 42(4, Suppl 2):9–24
186. Wiley TL, Cruickshanks KJ, Nondahl DM, Tweed TS, Klein R, Klein BE. Aging and word recognition in competing message. J Am Acad Audiol 1998;9(3):191–198
187. Halling DC, Humes LE. Factors affecting the recognition of reverberant speech by elderly listeners. J Speech Lang Hear Res 2000;43(2):414–431
188. Humes LE, Watson BU, Christensen LA, Cokely CG, Halling DC, Lee L. Factors associated with individual differences in clinical measures of speech recognition among the elderly. J Speech Hear Res 1994;37(2):465–474
189. Dubno JR, Dirks DD, Morgan DE. Effects of age and mild hearing loss on speech recognition in noise. J Acoust Soc Am 1984;76(1):87–96
190. Brink P, Stones M. Examination of the relationship among hearing impairment, linguistic communication, mood, and social engagement of residents in complex continuing-care facilities. Gerontologist 2007;47(5):633–641
191. Kramer SE, Kapteyn TS, Kuik DJ, Deeg DJ. The association of hearing impairment and chronic diseases with psychosocial health status in older age. J Aging Health 2002;14(1): 122–137
192. Strawbridge WJ, Wallhagen MI, Shema SJ, Kaplan GA. Negative consequences of hearing impairment in old age: a longitudinal analysis. Gerontologist 2000;40(3):320–326
193. Resnick HE, Fries BE, Verbrugge LM. Windows to their world: the effect of sensory impairments on social engagement and activity time in nursing home residents. J Gerontol B Psychol Sci Soc Sci 1997;52(3):S135–S144
194. Weinstein BE, Ventry IM. Hearing impairment and social isolation in the elderly. J Speech Hear Res 1982;25(4): 593–599
195. Thomas A, Herbst KG. Social and psychological implications of acquired deafness for adults of employment age. Br J Audiol 1980;14(3):76–85
196. Durkheim E. Suicide. New York, NY: Free Press; [1897], 1951
197. Seeman TE. Social ties and health: the benefits of social integration. Ann Epidemiol 1996;6(5):442–451
198. House JS, Landis KR, Umberson D. Social relationships and health. Science 1988;241(4865):540–545
199. Broadhead WE, Kaplan BH, James SA, et al. The epidemiologic evidence for a relationship between social support and health. Am J Epidemiol 1983;117(5):521–537
200. Barnes DE, Cauley JA, Lui LY, et al. Women who maintain optimal cognitive function into old age. J Am Geriatr Soc 2007;55(2):259–264
201. Béland F, Zunzunegui MV, Alvarado B, Otero A, Del Ser T. Trajectories of cognitive decline and social relations. J Gerontol B Psychol Sci Soc Sci 2005;60(6):320–P330
202. Holtzman RE, Rebok GW, Saczynski JS, Kouzis AC, Wilcox Doyle K, Eaton WW. Social network characteristics and cognition in middle-aged and older adults. J Gerontol B Psychol Sci Soc Sci 2004;59(6):278–284
203. Barnes LL, Mendes de Leon CF, Wilson RS, Bienias JL, Evans DA. Social resources and cognitive decline in a population of older African Americans and whites. Neurology 2004; 63(12):2322–2326
204. Zunzunegui MV, Alvarado BE, Del Ser T, Otero A. Social networks, social integration, and social engagement determine cognitive decline in community-dwelling Spanish older adults. J Gerontol B Psychol Sci Soc Sci 2003;58(2):S93–S100
205. Bassuk SS, Glass TA, Berkman LF. Social disengagement and incident cognitive decline in community-dwelling elderly persons. Ann Intern Med 1999;131(3):165–173
206. Saczynski JS, Pfeifer LA, Masaki K, et al. The effect of social engagement on incident dementia: the Honolulu-Asia Aging Study. Am J Epidemiol 2006;163(5):433–440
207. Karp A, Paillard-Borg S, Wang HX, Silverstein M, Winblad B, Fratiglioni L. Mental, physical and social components in leisure activities equally contribute to decrease dementia risk. Dement Geriatr Cogn Disord 2006;21(2):65–73
208. Wang HX, Karp A, Winblad B, Fratiglioni L. Late-life engagement in social and leisure activities is associated with a decreased risk of dementia: a longitudinal study from the Kungsholmen project. Am J Epidemiol 2002;155(12): 1081–1087
209. Scarmeas N, Levy G, Tang MX, Manly J, Stern Y. Influence of leisure activity on the incidence of Alzheimer's disease. Neurology 2001;57(12):2236–2242
210. Fratiglioni L, Wang HX, Ericsson K, Maytan M, Winblad B. Influence of social network on occurrence of dementia: a community-based longitudinal study. Lancet 2000; 355(9212):1315–1319
211. Helmer C, Damon D, Letenneur L, et al. Marital status and risk of Alzheimer's disease: a French population-based cohort study. Neurology 1999;53(9):1953–1958
212. Bickel H, Cooper B. Incidence and relative risk of dementia in an urban elderly population: findings of a prospective field study. Psychol Med 1994;24(1):179–192
213. Vogt TM, Mullooly JP, Ernst D, Pope CR, Hollis JF. Social networks as predictors of ischemic heart disease, cancer, stroke and hypertension: incidence, survival and mortality. J Clin Epidemiol 1992;45(6):659–666
214. Ruberman W, Weinblatt E, Goldberg JD, Chaudhary BS. Psychosocial influences on mortality after myocardial infarction. N Engl J Med 1984;311(9):552–559
215. Reed D, McGee D, Yano K, Feinleib M. Social networks and coronary heart disease among Japanese men in Hawaii. Am J Epidemiol 1983;117(4):384–396
216. Strawbridge WJ, Camacho TC, Cohen RD, Kaplan GA. Gender differences in factors associated with change in physical functioning in old age: a 6-year longitudinal study. Gerontologist 1993;33(5):603–609

217. Roos NP, Havens B. Predictors of successful aging: a twelve-year study of Manitoba elderly. Am J Public Health 1991;81(1):63–68
218. Mor V, Murphy J, Masterson-Allen S, et al. Risk of functional decline among well elders. J Clin Epidemiol 1989;42(9): 895–904
219. Palmore EB, Nowlin JB, Wang HS. Predictors of function among the old-old: a 10-year follow-up. J Gerontol 1985;40(2):244–250
220. Freedman VA, Berkman LF, Rapp SR, Ostfeld AM. Family networks: predictors of nursing home entry. Am J Public Health 1994;84(5):843–845
221. Steinbach U. Social networks, institutionalization, and mortality among elderly people in the United States. J Gerontol 1992;47(4):S183–S190
222. Cole SW, Hawkley LC, Arevalo JM, Cacioppo JT. Transcript origin analysis identifies antigen-presenting cells as primary targets of socially regulated gene expression in leukocytes. Proc Natl Acad Sci USA 2011;108(7):3080–3085
223. Cole SW, Hawkley LC, Arevalo JM, Sung CY, Rose RM, Cacioppo JT. Social regulation of gene expression in human leukocytes. Genome Biol 2007;8(9):R189
224. Glass TA, De Leon CF, Bassuk SS, Berkman LF. Social engagement and depressive symptoms in late life: longitudinal findings. J Aging Health 2006;18(4):604–628
225. Kawachi I, Berkman LF. Social ties and mental health. J Urban Health 2001;78(3):458–467
226. Oxman TE, Berkman LF, Kasl S, Freeman DH Jr, Barrett J. Social support and depressive symptoms in the elderly. Am J Epidemiol 1992;135(4):356–368
227. Berkman LF, Glass T, Brissette I, Seeman TE. From social integration to health: Durkheim in the new millennium. Soc Sci Med 2000;51(6):843–857
228. Uhlmann RF, Larson EB, Rees TS, Koepsell TD, Duckert LG. Relationship of hearing impairment to dementia and cognitive dysfunction in older adults. JAMA 1989;261(13): 1916–1919
229. Valentijn SA, van Boxtel MP, van Hooren SA, et al. Change in sensory functioning predicts change in cognitive functioning: results from a 6-year follow-up in the maastricht aging study. J Am Geriatr Soc 2005;53(3):374–380
230. Ohta RJ, Carlin MF, Harmon BM. Auditory acuity and performance on the mental status questionnaire in the elderly. J Am Geriatr Soc 1981;29(10):476–478
231. Granick S, Kleban MH, Weiss AD. Relationships between hearing loss and cognition in normally hearing aged persons. J Gerontol 1976;31(4):434–440
232. Thomas PD, Hunt WC, Garry PJ, Hood RB, Goodwin JM, Goodwin JS. Hearing acuity in a healthy elderly population: effects on emotional, cognitive, and social status. J Gerontol 1983;38(3):321–325
233. Gussekloo J, de Craen AJ, Oduber C, van Boxtel MP, Westendorp RG. Sensory impairment and cognitive functioning in oldest-old subjects: the Leiden 85+ Study. Am J Geriatr Psychiatry 2005;13(9):781–786
234. Lindenberger U, Baltes PB. Sensory functioning and intelligence in old age: a strong connection. Psychol Aging 1994;9(3):339–355
235. Tay T, Wang JJ, Kifley A, Lindley R, Newall P, Mitchell P. Sensory and cognitive association in older persons: findings from an older Australian population. Gerontology 2006;52(6): 386–394
236. Gennis V, Garry PJ, Haaland KY, Yeo RA, Goodwin JS. Hearing and cognition in the elderly. New findings and a review of the literature. Arch Intern Med 1991;151(11):2259–2264
237. Anstey KJ, Luszcz MA, Sanchez L. Two-year decline in vision but not hearing is associated with memory decline in very old adults in a population-based sample. Gerontology 2001;47(5):289–293
238. Gallacher J. Hearing, cognitive impairment, and aging: a critical review. Rev Clin Gerontol 2004;14:199–209
239. Lin FR, Ferrucci L, Metter EJ, An Y, Zonderman AB, Resnick SM. Hearing loss and cognition in the Baltimore Longitudinal Study of Aging. Neuropsychology 2011;25(6):763–770
240. Lin FR, Metter EJ, O'Brien RJ, Resnick SM, Zonderman AB, Ferrucci L. Hearing loss and incident dementia. Arch Neurol 2011;68(2):214–220
241. Lin FR, Yaffe K, Xia J, et al; Health ABC Study Group. Hearing loss and cognitive decline in older adults. JAMA Intern Med 2013;173(4):293–299
242. Gallacher J, Ilubaera V, Ben-Shlomo Y, et al. Auditory threshold, phonologic demand, and incident dementia. Neurology 2012;79(15):1583–1590
243. Wallhagen MI, Strawbridge WJ, Shema SJ, Kurata J, Kaplan GA. Comparative impact of hearing and vision impairment on subsequent functioning. J Am Geriatr Soc 2001;49(8): 1086–1092
244. Hickson L, Wood J, Chaparro A, Lacherez P, Marszalek R. Hearing impairment affects older people's ability to drive in the presence of distracters. J Am Geriatr Soc 2010;58(6): 1097–1103
245. Viljanen A, Kaprio J, Pyykkö I, Sorri M, Koskenvuo M, Rantanen T. Hearing acuity as a predictor of walking difficulties in older women. J Am Geriatr Soc 2009;57(12):2282–2286
246. Li L, Simonsick EM, Ferrucci L, Lin FR. Hearing loss and gait speed among older adults in the United States. Gait Posture 2013;38(1):25–29
247. Viljanen A, Kaprio J, Pyykkö I, et al. Hearing as a predictor of falls and postural balance in older female twins. J Gerontol A Biol Sci Med Sci 2009;64(2):312–317
248. Lin FR, Ferrucci L. Hearing loss and falls among older adults in the United States. Arch Intern Med 2012;172(4):369–371
249. Karpa MJ, Gopinath B, Beath K, et al. Associations between hearing impairment and mortality risk in older persons: the Blue Mountains Hearing Study. Ann Epidemiol 2010; 20(6):452–459
250. Fisher D, Li CM, Chiu MS, et al. Impairments in hearing and vision impact on mortality in older people: the AGES-Reykjavik Study. Age Ageing 2014;43(1):69–76
251. Lin MY, Gutierrez PR, Stone KL, et al; Study of Osteoporotic Fractures Research Group. Vision impairment and combined vision and hearing impairment predict cognitive and functional decline in older women. J Am Geriatr Soc 2004; 52(12):1996–2002
252. Rudberg MA, Furner SE, Dunn JE, Cassel CK. The relationship of visual and hearing impairments to disability: an analysis using the longitudinal study of aging. J Gerontol 1993;48(6):M261–M265
253. Mulrow CD, Aguilar C, Endicott JE, et al. Association between hearing impairment and the quality of life of elderly individuals. J Am Geriatr Soc 1990;38(1):45–50
254. Shumway-Cook A, Woollacott M. Attentional demands and postural control: the effect of sensory context. J Gerontol A Biol Sci Med Sci 2000;55(1):M10–M16
255. Woollacott M, Shumway-Cook A. Attention and the control of posture and gait: a review of an emerging area of research. Gait Posture 2002;16(1):1–14
256. Mulrow CD, Aguilar C, Endicott JE, et al. Quality-of-life changes and hearing impairment. A randomized trial. Ann Intern Med 1990;113(3):188–194

257. Lee KJ. Essential Otolaryngology. 8th ed. New York, NY: McGraw-Hill; 2003:36
258. Meyer TA, Lambert PR. Primary and revision stapedectomy in elderly patients. Curr Opin Otolaryngol Head Neck Surg 2004;12(5):387–392
259. Langman AW, Lindeman RC. Revision stapedectomy. Laryngoscope 1993;103(9):954–958
260. van der Pouw CT, Mylanus EA, Cremers CW. Percutaneous implants in the temporal bone for securing a bone conductor: surgical methods and results. Ann Otol Rhinol Laryngol 1999;108(6):532–536
261. Tringali S, Grayeli AB, Bouccara D, et al. A survey of satisfaction and use among patients fitted with a BAHA. Eur Arch Otorhinolaryngol 2008;265(12):1461–1464
262. Mondelli MF, Souza PJ. Quality of life in elderly adults before and after hearing aid fitting. Braz J Otorhinolaryngol 2012;78(3):49–56
263. Schum DJ. Perceived hearing aid benefit in relation to perceived needs. J Am Acad Audiol 1999;10(1):40–45
264. Kricos PB, Lesner SA, Sandridge SA. Expectations of older adults regarding the use of hearing aids. J Am Acad Audiol 1991;2(3):129–133
265. Parving A, Philip B. Use and benefit of hearing aids in the tenth decade—and beyond. Audiology 1991;30(2):61–69
266. Meister H, von Wedel H. Demands on hearing aid features—special signal processing for elderly users? Int J Audiol 2003;42(Suppl 2):S58–S62
267. Kyle JG, Wood PL. Changing patterns of hearing-aid use and level of support. Br J Audiol 1984;18(4):211–216
268. Knudsen LV, Oberg M, Nielsen C, Naylor G, Kramer SE. Factors influencing help seeking, hearing aid uptake, hearing aid use and satisfaction with hearing aids: a review of the literature. Trends Amplif 2010;14(3):127–154
269. Leek MR, Molis MR, Kubli LR, Tufts JB. Enjoyment of music by elderly hearing-impaired listeners. J Am Acad Audiol 2008;19(6):519–526
270. Pacala JT, Yueh B. Hearing deficits in the older patient: "I didn't notice anything." JAMA 2012;307(11):1185–1194
271. Riko K, McShane D, Hyde ML, Alberti PW. Hearing aid usage in occupational hearing loss claimants. J Otolaryngol 1990;19(1):25–30
272. Sorri M, Luotonen M, Laitakari K. Use and non-use of hearing aids. Br J Audiol 1984;18(3):169–172
273. Newman CW, Hug GA, Wharton JA, Jacobson GP. The influence of hearing aid cost on perceived benefit in older adults. Ear Hear 1993;14(4):285–289
274. Pothier DD, Bredenkamp C. Hearing aid insertion: correlation between patients' confidence and ability. J Laryngol Otol 2006;120(5):378–380
275. Pickora-Fuller MK. Processing speed and timing in aging adults: psychoacoustics, speech perception, and comprehension. Int J Audiol 2003;42(Suppl 1):S59–S67
276. Kuk FK, Tyler RS. Relationship between consonant recognition and subjective ratings of hearing aids. Br J Audiol 1990;24(3):171–177
277. Marshall L. Auditory processing in aging listeners. J Speech Hear Disord 1981;46(3):226–240
278. Thompson ME. Speech discrimination skills in the elderly: a critical review. J Otolaryngol 1987;16(6):354–361
279. Trotter MI, Donaldson I. Hearing aids and tinnitus therapy: a 25-year experience. J Laryngol Otol 2008;122(10): 1052–1056
280. Peifer KJ, Rosen GP, Rubin AM. Tinnitus: etiology and management. Clin Geriatr Med 1999;15(1):193–204, viii

7 Regenerative Therapies for Sensorineural Hearing Loss: Current Research Implications for Future Treatment

Cynthia L. Chow and Samuel P. Gubbels

Introduction

Hearing impairment is one of the most common maladies affecting older adults. Almost two thirds of individuals 70 years of age and older have some level of hearing loss.[1] The prevalence of hearing loss increases over time and is generally associated with aging; however, it is often untreated.[2] Hearing loss can cause difficulty communicating with others, localizing sound, and perceiving warnings, all contributing to a poorer quality of life.[3] The National Institute on Deafness and Other Communication Disorders estimates there are nearly 36 million adults in the United States with some degree of hearing loss, most cases of which are caused by the loss of cochlear sensory hair cells.[4] Cochlear hair cells are highly specialized mechanosensory receptors that are responsible for converting mechanical sound information into an electrical signal, amplifying it and transmitting it to the brain via auditory nerve fibers. In humans and other higher vertebrates, the inability of cochlear hair cells to regenerate after damage is the primary reason for the permanence of hearing loss. This chapter describes the multiple approaches being taken in pursuit of novel regenerative treatments for sensorineural hearing loss in addition to discussing the most critical challenges in the field.

Background

The organ of Corti is highly organized and consists of many cell types, including cochlear hair cells, supporting cells, and auditory nerve fibers (**Fig. 7.1**). At birth, the human cochlea contains ~ 15,000 sensory hair cells. There are two types of sensory hair

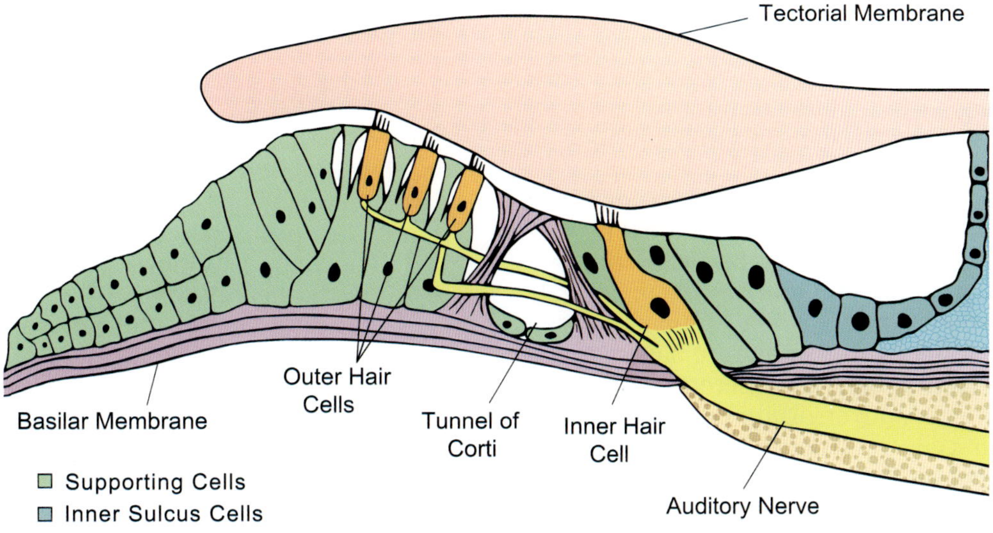

Fig. 7.1 The organization of the organ of Corti. Outer hair cells and inner hair cells are arranged in a 3:1 ratio surrounded by supporting cells. Stereocilia on the apical portion of the hair cells are embedded in the tectorial membrane. Outer and inner hair cells are properly innervated at the base and attach to auditory nerve fibers, which send the auditory signal to the brain for processing.

cells—inner hair cells and outer hair cells—both of which are important for hearing. Inner hair cells are responsible for converting sound information into an electrical signal, whereas outer hair cells are responsible for amplifying the signal. Auditory nerve fibers are responsible for sending sound information from cochlear hair cells to the brain for processing. Loss or damage of cochlear hair cells and auditory nerve fibers has been estimated to account for ~ 80% of cases of hearing loss.[5]

Currently, amplification devices and cochlear implants are the primary treatment options available for individuals with sensorineural hearing loss. Although these treatment options can return some hearing capability, the results vary between individuals. In addition, both hearing aids and cochlear implants require lifelong device usage, and they generally do not restore normal hearing qualities. As such, other approaches for restoring more normal cochlear function are actively being explored.

Hair Cell Regeneration

In mammals, it is known that skin and bone marrow cells are continually replenished throughout life.[6,7] Furthermore, taste buds and olfactory bulb interneurons are constantly renewed in adult mammals[8–11]; however, such regeneration is not seen in the mammalian cochlea. It was previously thought that auditory hair cell regeneration did not occur in any context until 1988 when investigators found functional recovery of hearing due to regenerated hair cells after noise trauma in birds.[12–14] The mammalian inner ear was thought to lack this regenerative capacity to replace damaged hair cells until 1993, when investigators found evidence of hair cell regeneration in the vestibular sensory epithelia of adult mammals.[15,16] Although replacement of vestibular hair cells was observed, the newly regenerated cells occurred infrequently, and the amount of functional recovery that the regenerated cells may produce has been questioned.[17]

In the avian inner ear, hair cell regeneration begins after an auditory insult. Subsequent signaling after the insult begins a process whereby supporting cells divide and differentiate into immature hair cells and supporting cells.[18–20] Alternatively, supporting cells may transform directly into immature hair cells,[19,21,22] a process referred to as transdifferentiation. Using molecular, genetic and environmental cues, these immature hair cells continue to become morphologically distinct as they mature over the course of several weeks.[23,24] When compared with that of birds, fish, and amphibians, the cochlear sensory epithelium in mammals appears to have lost its ability to regenerate after hair cell loss. Exactly why this loss of regenerative ability has occurred with evolution remains unclear. Regardless, many investigators have focused attention on using what is known of mammalian hair cell development to guide efforts focused on regenerating hair cells after loss.

Treatments based on regenerating lost or damaged tissue are inevitably complex, and efforts to regenerate hair cells in the mammalian cochlea are subject to unique challenges beyond those seen in other organs. First, one needs to consider the complexity of an auditory hair cell. Hair cells are morphologically distinct, with a round base and thinner apex. They contain small hair cell-like bundles called stereocilia, which extend from the apex of the cell and are embedded in the tectorial membrane. These hair cell bundles are mechanosensitive, responding to ionic flow, which transforms sound vibrations into electrical impulses. The electrical signal is then sent to the brain via auditory nerve fibers for further processing. Because of this, proper neural integration needs to be established to transmit sound information to the brain. Moreover, the cochlea has a distinct cytoarchitecture that is highly organized. This cytoarchitectural organization of the cochlea is critical to its proper function. Newly generated hair cells would need to integrate in the proper location within the cochlea and furthermore within the auditory sensory epithelium (the organ of Corti) to encode sound information accurately. Last, the cochlea is a delicate, membranous, and fluid-filled structure that is surrounded by dense otic capsular bone, making surgical access to the organ of Corti challenging. Efforts to outline meaningful regenerative therapies for hearing loss in humans need to address these unique challenges, and numerous laboratories worldwide are actively engaged in this exciting area of research.

Mechanisms for Avian Hair Cell Regeneration

Currently, there are two proposed mechanisms for cochlear hair cell regeneration in the avian inner ear: supporting cell proliferation and transdifferentiation. Cell proliferation is referred to as the growth and division of cells, during which a supporting cell reenters the cell cycle giving rise to two daughter cells that differentiate into one supporting cell and one hair cell. When cochlear hair cells are destroyed, they send a signal to neighboring supporting cells to activate proliferation.[18,25] This signal prompts supporting cells to migrate through the sensory epithelium, reenter the cell cycle, and generate a daughter hair cell and a supporting cell.[15] Alternatively, hair cells may be generated via supporting cell transdifferentiation, during which a differentiated cell is transformed into another cell type without cell cycle reentry.[26] In this approach, neighboring supporting cells are converted to hair cells via nonmitotic mechanisms with consequent depletion of the supporting cell population.

As applied to the mammalian inner ear, it is not clear how these mechanisms of regeneration might affect the organization, structure, and functional integrity of the organ of Corti.[27,28] If supporting cells don't replace themselves as they transdifferentiate into hair cells, the cytoarchitecture and function of the organ of Corti might be compromised. As such, a method to regenerate hair cells in the mammalian inner ear that does not lead to depletion of the cohort of endogenous supporting cells would seem logically preferable to one that relies on transdifferentiation alone. It is possible, however, that the mammalian inner ear has some tolerance to a level of depletion of the supporting cell population if it provides a healthy, functional cohort of hair cells. Ongoing research in this area through the approaches described here will likely provide insight into these unanswered questions in the years to come.

Regenerative Approaches for the Treatment of Hearing Loss

There are several approaches being taken in the pursuit of novel, regenerative treatments for hearing loss, each having unique potential benefits and challenges. These approaches can generally be grouped into four categories:

1. Gene transfer
2. Pharmacotherapies
3. Exogenous delivery of stem cells
4. Promotion of endogenous stem cells

Gene Transfer

Gene transfer has become an attractive avenue for regenerating hair cells by introducing a gene of interest to cells. To date, several studies expressing various genes of interest have produced promising results, which are discussed next.

Atoh1

The expression of the basic helix-loop-helix transcription factor *Atoh1* is one of the first indicators of hair cell differentiation in the cochlea.[29–32] In developing mammals, *Atoh1* is expressed in prosensory patches that give rise to the auditory sensory epithelia and is both necessary and sufficient for hair cell development and formation.[31–33] Mice without the *Atoh1* gene lack sensory hair cells in the auditory and vestibular portions of the inner ear.[29,31,32] In contrast, when *Atoh1* is overexpressed in cultured cochlear explants, supernumerary hair cells are generated.[33] Moreover, *Atoh1* has been found to be upregulated during hair cell fate specification in the adult chicken during hair cell regeneration.[34] Collectively, these findings speak to the critical role that *Atoh1* plays in determining hair cell fate specification within the inner ear.

Investigators have introduced *Atoh1*-expressing viral vectors into the organs of Corti of a variety of different rodent species. Kawamoto and colleagues showed that delivery of *Atoh1*-expressing adenoviral vectors to the organ of Corti of mature, normal-hearing guinea pigs results in expression of the gene product in the organ of Corti and in some nonsensory locations (ectopic expression in cells outside of the organ of Corti) within the cochleae.[35] Cells expressing the exogenously delivered *Atoh1* also expressed the hair cell marker myosin VIIa and displayed immature stereociliary bundles at the apex of the cell. In addition, these newly formed hair cells appeared to attract axons extended from the auditory nerve on some level. From this, the authors of this study concluded that cells in the normal-hearing adult mammalian inner ear are capable of generating new hair cells upon *Atoh1* misexpression.

Taking this a step further, Izumikawa and colleagues delivered an *Atoh1*-expressing adenovirus to the organs of Corti of deafened mature guinea pigs.[36] Animals transfected with the virus showed new hair cell formation in the organ of Corti and in some ectopic locations in the cochlea. The authors also reported a significant improvement in auditory brainstem response thresholds in the ears of animals transfected with *Atoh1*. Cross-section analysis revealed that some of the cells displayed a mixed phenotype, having both hair cell and supporting cell features. As a whole, the source of the newly generated hair cells was unclear; however, it was hypothesized they arose from transdifferentiated and proliferated cells within the damaged regions that had been transfected with the *Atoh1*-expressing adenovirus.

In 2008, Gubbels and colleagues established a method to conduct gain-of-function studies in the developing inner ear using an in utero gene transfer technique.[37] Plasmids encoding *Atoh1* and green fluorescent protein (GFP) were microinjected into the otic vesicle of mice on embryonic day 11.5 and examined on embryonic day 18.5 and later time points. Ears that received *Atoh1* demonstrated supernumerary hair cell formation throughout the cochlea. Cells that formed secondary to the delivery of exogenous *Atoh1* expressed myosin VIIa and displayed stereociliary bundles. Moreover, they attracted neuronal processes and expressed the ribbon synapse marker carboxy-terminal binding protein 2. Postnatal electrophysiological analysis of the cells generated from in utero transfer of *Atoh1* revealed age-appropriate basolateral conductances and mechanoelectrical transduction properties. These results demonstrate that it is possible to generate cochlear hair cells by *Atoh1* misexpression after in utero gene transfer. Moreover, this study showed that the generated hair cells are functional on a cellular level and establish connections with the central auditory network.

Collectively, these studies suggest that a gene transfer approach using transcription factors known to be critical for hair cell development can generate hair cells in normal and deafened cochleae of both adult and developing rodents. Furthermore, these studies demonstrate that the newly generated hair cells are able to associate with the nearby auditory nerve and are functional on a cellular and possibly even an organ system level. It remains unclear if this type of approach leads to depletion of the supporting cell population and, if so, its implications. In addition, the long-term viability of hair cells generated through *Atoh1* gene transfer is similarly unclear. Regardless, *Atoh1* gene transfer–based approaches represent a promising and active area of investigation in the pursuit of novel, regenerative therapies for hearing loss.

Cell Cycle Modulators

Modulating genes that have a role in cell cycle regulation is another molecular approach being pursued to achieve hair cell regeneration. Although mammalian supporting cells are generally quiescent in vivo, several studies have reported that these cells have the capacity to reenter the cell cycle and generate hair cell–like cells in vitro.[38–43] The concept of this approach is that by altering the cell cycle of residual supporting cells following hair cell loss, proliferation may ensue, with subsequent differentiation of the progeny into hair and supporting cells.

It is well established that during development, cell cycle exit continues progressively along the cochlear duct from the apex to the base, starting on embryonic day 12 and completing by embryonic day 14 in mice.[29,44–46] While this is occurring, cochlear cells begin to express hair cell markers, including *Atoh1*, myosin VI, and myosin VIIa.[29,31,32] At a similar developmental time, supporting cells begin to express the cyclin-dependent kinase inhibitor p27kip1.[44,46] The expression of p27kip1 has been shown to coincide with the cell cycle exit of hair cell and supporting cell progenitors.[29,44,47] P27kip1 is continually expressed in supporting cells, which may be responsible, to some degree, for maintaining the quiescent state of supporting cells.[46] Alternatively, hair cells rapidly downregulate p27kip1 during differentiation, expressing the cyclin-dependent kinase inhibitor p19Ink4d instead,[46,48] which is thought to maintain them in a quiescent state (see later discussion).

Modulation of the expression of cell cycle inhibitors, such as p27kip1, may hold promise as a potential means for promoting some level of regeneration of hair cells in the mammalian inner ear. P27kip1 appears to play a significant role in the inability of mammalian hair cells to regenerate after damage.[47,49] In the cochlea, P27kip1 is regulated at both transcriptional and posttranscriptional levels.[44] Mice deficient for p27kip1 have supernumerary hair cells and supporting cells, most of which are located in the apical region of the cochlea.[47] In addition, auditory brainstem response thresholds obtained from these mice were significantly elevated compared with controls, suggesting severe to profound hearing loss. The significant elevation in auditory brainstem response thresholds is thought to occur from excess hair cells and supporting cells disrupting the spatial organization and mechanical properties of the basilar membrane.[47,49] In another study, White and colleagues examined the regenerative capacity of supporting cells isolated from the postnatal mouse.[41] The authors found that postmitotic supporting cells are capable of transdifferentiating into new hair cells in vitro. In the first experiment, the ability of postmitotic supporting cells to reenter the cell cycle was examined by isolating supporting cells expressing green fluorescent protein under a p27kip1 promoter and culturing them in vitro. After 2 days, 60% of green fluorescent protein (p27kip1) positive cells downregulated expression of p27kip1, whereas 38% of these cells incorporated BrdU, signifying that these cells had reentered the cell cycle. Additional analysis determined that these cells were then able to differentiate into hair cells. A small number of these cells expressed the hair cell marker myosin VI. These results demonstrate that postnatal supporting cells from mice have the ability to divide and differentiate into hair cells via mitotic and nonmitotic means. Collectively, these studies suggest that modulation of p27kip1 in supporting cells may establish a method, or part of a method, to regenerate hair cells following their loss.

Although p27kip1 expression coincides with cell cycle exit, it is not essential for this occurrence.[50] This suggests there are other genes that play a more central function in regulating cell cycle exit. Retinoblastoma (RB) 1 is another type of cell cycle regulator, which plays a role in holding inner ear hair cells in a state of quiescence and may represent a potential target for enabling regeneration to occur in the mammalian organ of Corti. The RB1 gene is a tumor suppressor involved in regulating cell cycle exit, differentiation, and survival. Although hair cells in the vestibular and auditory portions of the inner ear generally undergo similar processes during development and differentiation, RB1 appears to play different roles in these regions.[51,52] In 2005, Sage and colleagues found that targeted deletion of RB1 in the developing mouse utricle leads to proliferation of vestibular hair cells,[53] suggesting a potential role for alteration of RB1 as a means to achieve regeneration of hair cells in the future. More recently, inactivation of RB protein in postmitotic supporting cells resulted in cell cycle reentry, with a subsequent increase in the number of supporting cells in the neonatal mouse cochlea.[54] Moreover, some of the nuclei of proliferating supporting cells were intermittently observed in the hair cell layer above their normal position, similar to supporting cells undergoing regeneration in the avian auditory epithelium. There was no evidence of newly generated hair cells from supporting cells, suggesting that there may be a potential role involving other signaling factors to facilitate the continued differentiation of the newly generated cells into hair cells. One concern in the application of this type of strategy lies in the risk of tumor formation with manipulation of tumor suppressor genes such as RB1. As such, additional investigation will be needed to determine if efforts aimed at targeted alteration in the expression or function of genes, such as RB1, could be pursued safely as a potential therapeutic strategy for hair cell regeneration in the future.

Following hair cell formation, a mechanism to maintain the postmitotic status and continued viability of the cells is necessary to prevent their degeneration. The cyclin-dependent kinase inhibitor p19Ink4d is a factor that appears to sustain the postmitotic status of hair cells.[48] During development, mice deficient for p19Ink4d develop in a normal manner; however, hair cell loss is observed beginning on postnatal day 17.[48] In these mice, it appears that hair cells attempt to reenter the cell cycle, causing them to die by programmed cell death. As already discussed, hair cells rapidly downregulate p27kip1 during differentiation,[46] suggesting that p19Ink4d alone is responsible for maintaining the postmitotic state of the hair cells.[48] For the purpose of newly generated hair cells, continued maintenance is a constant process, and failure to regulate this accurately can have adverse effects on hearing. Accordingly, future efforts aimed at regenerating hair cells in the deafened cochlea will need to take into account the ongoing need for maintenance of the newly generated hair cells to ensure their permanence.

Collectively, studies evaluating gene transfer–based approaches for the treatment of hearing loss have produced promising results. Additional investigation is necessary to characterize key genes and cell cycle modulators that have been found to be critical for hair cell regeneration in animal and cell culture models. Furthermore, it is essential to determine if direct transdifferentiation of supporting cells into hair cells leads to a depletion of supporting cells, which might disrupt the cytoarchitecture of the organ of Corti. Moreover, the long-term viability of hair cells generated through gene transfer is similarly unclear. In addition, determining a safe and effective method to deliver genetic material into the inner ear remains a critical challenge. It is plausible that genes of interest could be introduced to the inner ear through transtympanic delivery to the middle ear with subsequent transport or diffusion through the round window membrane to the cochlea. Alternatively, direct injection of a gene of interest to the scalar fluids of the inner ear might ultimately be required for meaningful delivery within the cochlea. The ability of the gene to penetrate all areas of the cochlea would need to be determined in addition to ensuring that no further damage results from these delivery approaches to the inner ear. Beyond the challenges of gene delivery on an organ basis, genetic material needs to be transported across the cell membrane for subsequent transcription to take place. Methods to accomplish this include packaging the gene in a viral vector that has tropism for the supporting cells of the organ of Corti, usage of electrical pulsations (electroporation) to drive the genetic material through the cell membrane or potentially packaging the genetic material in a lipid-based carrier that fuses with the cell membrane to release the gene of interest into the cytoplasm. Although these cellular delivery mechanisms are plausible approaches for gene delivery to the inner ear, a viral-based method for gene delivery appears to be the most logical candidate and the approach used in scientific studies on cochlear gene transfer to date.[35–37] Although many questions remain to be answered, gene transfer–based approaches for the treatment of hearing loss remain a promising and attractive area of investigation.

Pharmacotherapy

Pharmacotherapeutics focuses on the use of drugs to modulate signaling pathways or gene expression in a cell. In regard to hearing loss, these drugs may target specific cellular pathways that signal supporting cells to divide, or target the regulation of specific genes such as *Atoh1* in attempts to generate new hair cells. In concept, these synthetic molecules with biological activities could potentially be given systemically, transtympanically, or by intracochlear administration to effect the generation of hair cells after loss, potentially avoiding some of the challenges associated with other approaches for hair cell regeneration.

The Notch signaling pathway is one potential target for pharmacotherapeutically mediated efforts toward hair cell regeneration. This signaling pathway is responsible for establishing, at least in part, the hair cell–supporting cell mosaic of the organ of Corti during inner ear development.[55–60] During development, Notch activation in supporting cells upregulates Hes and Hey transcription factors, which inhibit *Atoh1* expression.[60–63] Thus Notch activation suppresses hair cell differentiation in supporting cells, thereby regulating the number of hair cells and supporting cells.[60] In addition, Notch expression appears to increase during hair cell regeneration in the avian inner ear.[64] Because of this, investigators have hypothesized that disrupting the Notch signaling pathway might promote hair cell generation. During embryonic development, the absence of the Notch ligand Jagged1 resulted in a severe reduction of hair cells in both the auditory and the vestibular portions of the inner ears of mice, indicating that it is required for the prosensory inductive function of Notch.[65] Other studies that inactivated the Notch ligands Delta1 and Jagged2 reported a greater number of hair cells relative to control cochleae, in addition to an increase in the number of supporting cells, suggesting Notch signaling may also play a role in regulating hair and supporting cell proliferation.[65,66] Several other studies have also reported that during development, disruption of Notch signaling can lead to a cellular conversion from a supporting cell fate to a hair cell fate.[65–70] Collectively, these studies suggest that careful manipulation of Notch signaling in supporting cells may provide an avenue for regenerating hair cells following auditory insult.

One of the first reports of pharmacological inhibition of Notch signaling treated deafened guinea pigs using a γ-secretase inhibitor.[71] In this study, the authors reported that a small number of hair cells were generated following γ-secretase administration, with newly generated cells expressing the hair cell marker myosin VIIa. More recently, pharmacological inhibition of Notch signaling using other types of small molecule γ-secretase inhibitors has been shown to cause partial recovery of hearing thresholds in mice exposed to noise trauma.[72] In this study, pharmacological inhibition of Notch signaling with LY411575 in deafened mice resulted in transdifferentiation of supporting cells into cochlear hair cells and partial restoration of hearing verified by auditory brainstem response testing. The supporting cells did not appear to reenter the cell cycle following γ-secretase administration, indicating that hair cells were generated through transdifferentiation. Of note, both of these studies used direct delivery of γ-secretase inhibitors to the scala tympani, which represents one potential advantage to a pharmacotherapeutic approach. In contrast, other approaches for hair cell regeneration such as gene transfer and cell transplantation (to be described) are more likely to require intracochlear delivery methods, which have a higher potential risk for hearing loss. In general, for this approach to become clinically relevant, the ability of the drug to penetrate all regions of the cochlea and prevent ectopic hair cell formation needs to be explored further. In addition, generating hair cells in proper locations within the organ of Corti while avoiding depletion of the supporting cell population will need to be accomplished. Although more investigation is needed, the foregoing studies demonstrate that pharmacotherapeutic targeting of Notch signaling may enable meaningful regeneration of hair cells in the deafened cochlea in the future.

Exogenous Stem Cells

One promising approach in regenerative therapies involves the use of stem cells as a substrate to generate mature cell types of interest with subsequent transplantation. There has been great progress with this approach for regeneration of tissue in other organ systems, with several ongoing clinical trials aimed at treating macular dystrophy and macular degeneration.[73,74] With regard to the inner ear, several laboratories are attempting to generate cochlear hair cells in vitro using types of pluripotent stem cells such as embryonic stem cells (ESCs) and induced pluripotent stem cells (iPSCs). Pluripotent stem cells are defined as undifferentiated, self-renewing cells that have the ability to generate mature cell types from all three germ layers. Embryonic stem cells are a type of pluripotent cell derived from the inner cell mass of a blastocyst ~ 5 to 7 days after fertilization (**Fig. 7.2**). Induced pluripotent stem cells are also pluripotent; however, they are derived from fully differentiated adult cells (**Fig. 7.2**), typically fibroblasts from a skin punch biopsy that have been reprogrammed into a state of pluripotency by treatment with combinations of transcription factors. During development, pluripotent cells of the inner cell mass of a blastocyst undergo sequential differentiation, becoming more specialized and tissue-specific as the organism matures. The process of differentiation of pluripotent stem cells (ESCs or iPSCs) in culture to generate mature cell types recapitulates the process of development on some level. As applied to the goal of generating hair cells from pluripotent stem cells, the process of differentiating ESCs or iPSCs requires recapitulating inner ear, and subsequently hair cell, development in culture (**Fig. 7.3**). Several studies have reported successful differentiation of mouse pluripotent stem cells into otic progenitor cells and hair cell-like cells, whereas reports of achieving the same goal using human stem cells are more limited.[75,76]

Differentiation of Pluripotent Stem Cells into Hair Cell-Like Cells

In 2010, Oshima and colleagues published a stepwise guidance protocol using mouse ESCs and iPSCs to generate mechanosensitive hair cell-like cells.[77]

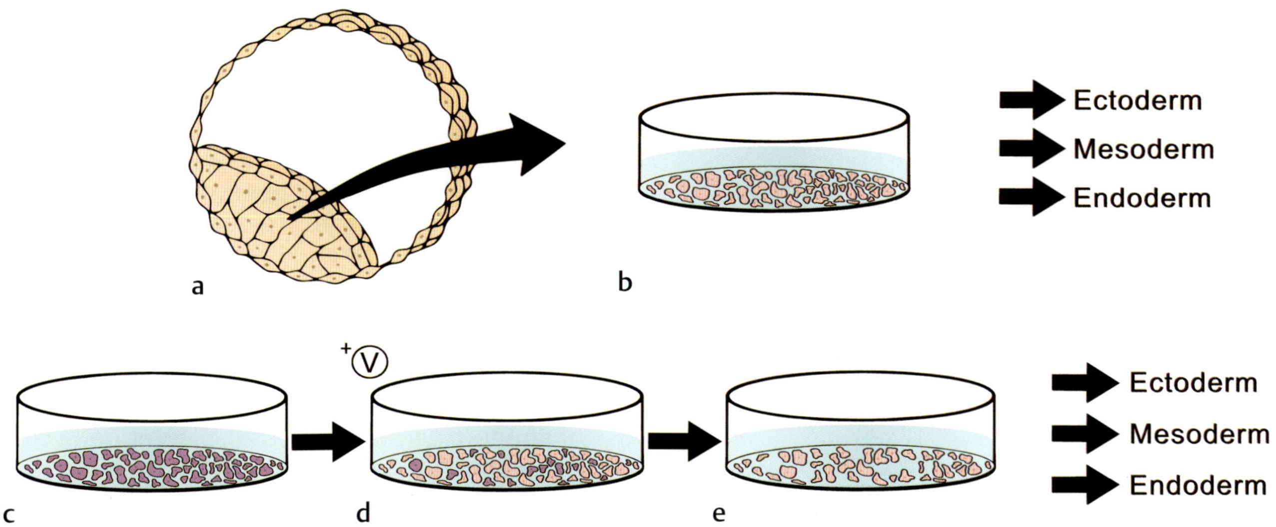

Fig. 7.2 (**a, b**) Generation of embryonic stem cells and (**c–e**) induced pluripotent stem cells. In generation of human embryonic stem cells, (**a**) cells are isolated from the inner cell mass of a blastocyst 5–7 days after fertilization and (**b**) cultured in vitro. These cells have the potential to differentiate into all cell types in the body. In generation of human-induced pluripotent stem cells, (**c**) adult cells are isolated from a donor, typically fibroblasts of a skin punch biopsy, and cultured in vitro. (**d**) Genes associated with pluripotency (*Oct ¾*, *Sox 2*, *Klf4*, and *c-Myc* or *Oct ¾*, *Sox 2*, *Nanog*, and *LIN28*) are delivered into the cells via viral vectors. (**e**) Cells expressing markers associated with pluripotency (pink) are isolated and continually cultured. As with embryonic stem cells, these cells have the potential to differentiate into all cell types in the body.

The protocol uses principles of early development to direct the differentiation of pluripotent stem cells along ectoderm and otic lineages, respectively. Hair cell-like cells generated from this protocol displayed stereociliary hair bundles similar to hair cells of the postnatal mouse inner ear. Furthermore, these cells responded to mechanical stimulation and displayed electrophysiological properties similar to immature inner ear hair cells. More recently, Koehler and colleagues reported a three-dimensional in vitro model to generate inner ear sensory epithelia from mouse pluripotent stem cells.[78] Unlike the previous report, their model did not use mitotically inactivated chicken utricle stromal cells to guide the differentiation process; rather, they employed a defined, three-dimensional culture system to provide the necessary cues for hair cell differentiation. These intriguing studies provide a basis for using pluripotent stem cells to gain a deeper insight into the mechanisms underlying inner ear development, in addition to generating hair cells in vitro for disease modeling, molecular diagnostics, and drug discovery. Furthermore, these studies provide a method to generate populations of mouse inner ear progenitor and hair cell-like cells to be used in the pursuit of stem cell transplantation–based treatment approaches for hearing loss. Although progress in generating hair cells from human pluripotent stem cells has been forthcoming,[75,76] additional studies will be needed to refine techniques so that the hair cell-like cells generated from human stem cells have morphological refinement and functionality comparable with those seen in the mouse ESC and iPSC studies discussed earlier.

Cell Transplantation to the Organ of Corti

There have been several reports to date investigating the ability of stem cells to integrate into cochlear tissues upon inner ear transplantation.[79–88] Multiple types of stem cells and methods for transplantation have been explored using both normal-hearing and acutely deafened cochleae. One of the first reports of stem cell delivery to the inner ear of mammals was published in 2001 by investigators in Japan.[79] Neural stem cells were prepared from hippocampal tissues and injected into the scala tympani of newborn rat cochleae. Two to 4 weeks following transplantation, the authors reported grafted cell survival, with some resembling hair cells along the organ of Corti. Other studies transplanting stem cells into the damaged cochlea have described evidence of grafted cell survival and some integration into the sensory epithelia of the inner ear. In one study, investigators transplanted mouse fetal neural stem cells into the inner ears of mice following ototoxic injury.[80] Grafted cells were identified in the cochlear, vestibular, and spi-

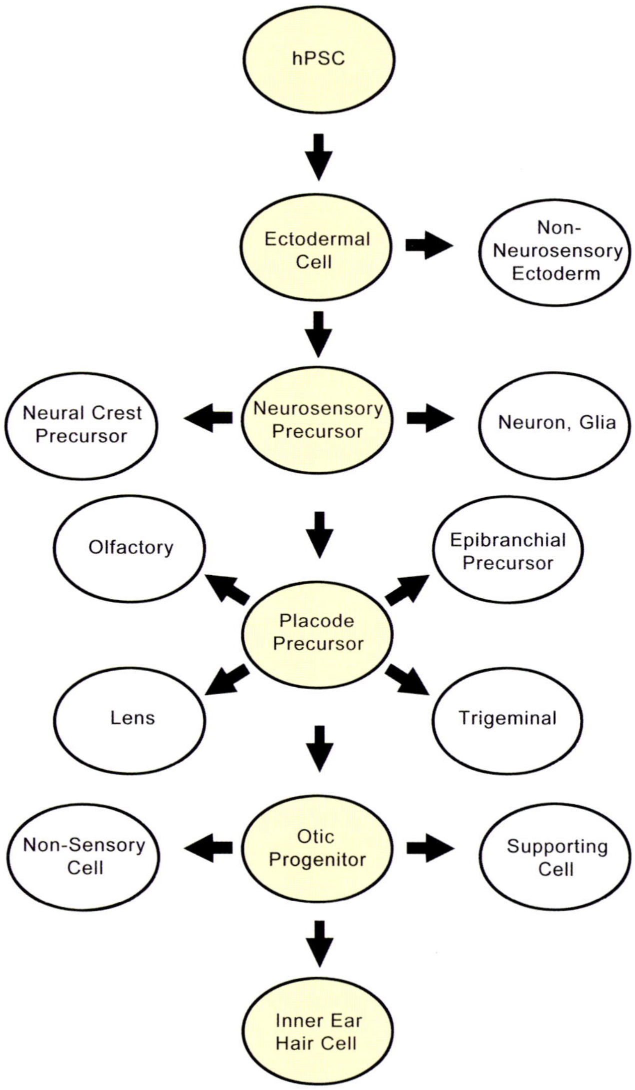

Fig. 7.3 Cell fate decisions in differentiating pluripotent stem cells to an inner ear hair cell-like cell. The highlighted lineage decisions recapitulate those made by inner ear hair cells during normal development. Discrete modifications of the cell culture environment during pluripotent stem cell differentiation act to guide the cells through these fate decisions to ultimately generate an enriched population of mature inner ear hair (or supporting) cells.

ral ganglion portions of the inner ear. Surprisingly, transplanted cells that integrated into the vestibular sensory epithelia expressed hair cell markers; however, this was not observed in grafted cells in the cochlear sensory epithelia. In addition, migration of transplanted cells was not observed in nondamaged control cochleae, suggesting that the molecular microenvironment of the acutely damaged mammalian cochlea may aid in the migration and integration of grafted cells. Building on this work, another group of investigators reported that neural stem cells transplanted into the sound-damaged inner ear were able to migrate throughout the cochlea.[81] The authors reported that the grafted neural stem cells in the organ of Corti expressed the hair cell markers myosin VIIa, oncomodulin, and calbindin. In addition, some of the grafted cells in the spiral ganglion exhibited a comparable phenotype to spiral ganglion neurons. In aggregate, the findings of these studies suggest that grafted stem cells can survive in the adult cochlea after transplantation for as long as 4 months in some cases. Despite the evidence of grafted cell survival,[82–87] there have been a limited number of reports demonstrating sensory integration and/or differentiation of grafted cells into hair or supporting cells after transplantation in the adult mammalian cochlea.[17,79–81,88] As such, a great deal of further investigation will be needed to identify stem cell or host-related factors that could be modified to allow for more successful integration of transplanted cells into the organ of Corti as hair cells.

Although stem cell transplantation into the adult mammalian cochlea has been met with limited success, several investigators have reported that mouse stem cells transplanted into the developing avian inner ear have the capacity to generate hair-cell-like cells. In one study, investigators generated otic progenitor-like cells in vitro from mouse ESCs, which were subsequently transplanted into the developing inner ear of chick embryos.[89] The investigators reported that these otic progenitor cells were able to integrate into the avian auditory sensory epithelium and differentiate into cells expressing hair cell markers. More recently, another team of investigators used an alternative method to differentiate mouse ESC into hair cell-like cells.[90] Consistent with the previous report, when transplanted into the otic vesicle of developing chick embryos, these cells were found to incorporate in the correct location and function as host cells in the inner ear. Together, these studies demonstrate that mouse stem cells are capable of engraftment and differentiation under appropriate conditions when transplanted into the developing chick inner ear. This suggests that the microenvironment of the developing inner ear presents transplanted stem cells, even those from another species, with the signaling necessary to allow for engraftment and terminal differentiation as hair cells. Identification of host-related factors present in the developing inner ear that permit successful engraftment of transplanted stem cells may influence the future development of strategies whereby deafened adult mammalian cochleae may be modified or primed in some way to allow for subsequent engraftment of transplanted stem cells. Clearly, a great deal of research will be needed to realize the potential of stem cell transplantation as a regenerative therapy for hearing loss in the future; however, steady progress continues to be made in this area.

Cell Transplantation to the Auditory Nerve

In 2006, Corrales and colleagues transplanted neuronal progenitor cells derived from mouse ESCs into the cochlear nerve trunk of gerbils after experimentally induced damage to the auditory nerve.[91] The transplanted cells were found to occupy substantial portions of the space previously occupied by spiral ganglion cells. Moreover, the cells were able to survive and extend processes throughout the cochlear nerve area, making contact with cochlear hair cells in the organ of Corti. From this study it appears that transplanted neuronal progenitor cells have the potential to survive, terminally differentiate, and morphologically specialize in an animal model of auditory neuronal degeneration. More recently, restoration of auditory brainstem response thresholds following lesioning of the rodent auditory nerve was reported using otic progenitor cells derived from human ESCs.[76] In vitro, human ESCs were directed toward an otic progenitor fate using the signaling molecules fibroblast growth factor 3 and 10. Using these growth factors, human pluripotent cells were able to differentiate into hair cell-like cells and functional auditory neurons in vitro. The authors transplanted the human ESC-derived neural progenitor–like cells into the spiral ganglion region of gerbils after deafening them by destroying the host auditory neurons. Analysis of the transplanted cells revealed that they were able to engraft, differentiate, and improve auditory brainstem response thresholds relative to deafened but untreated control animals. These studies demonstrate the ability of stem cell–derived neural progenitors to integrate successfully, terminally differentiate as auditory neurons, and ultimately improve auditory thresholds upon transplantation. Given these reports, the potential of stem cell transplantation for auditory nerve–related hearing loss may offer more immediate promise as a regenerative therapy when compared with stem cell transplantation into the cochlea.

Cell transplantation may be a viable treatment option in the future to replace damaged or lost cells in the inner ear; however, critical issues will need to be addressed to achieve this goal. First, an in vitro method to generate adequate and consistent numbers of hair cell progenitors from human pluripotent stem cells needs to be established to supply the cochlea with a sufficient number of cells to replace those that are damaged or have been lost. Because there are many types of pluripotent stem cells being used in this pursuit, the most effective cell type(s) would also need to be determined. Moreover, it is essential to identify the factors that are most critical for successful integration and terminal differentiation of grafted cells as hair cells to translate this approach to humans. Likewise, the transplanted cells also need to migrate to correct locations along the basilar membrane, avoiding the occurrence of ectopic or supernumerary hair cells to maintain the precise organization of the organ of Corti. In addition, grafted cells need to establish proper integration and neuronal circuitry for normal function. Furthermore, a safe and effective method to deliver cells to the organ of Corti must be established to ensure that it is not further damaged by the transplantation procedure itself. Last, transplanted cells face the possibility of immune responses that may ultimately lead to their rejection by the host, so immunosuppressive therapy may prove to be necessary. Although it remains to be determined if exogenous stem cells have the therapeutic potential to improve hearing ability, studies to date have provided promising results that may one day contribute to making this a viable treatment option.

Endogenous Stem Cells

The presence and potential of cells with stem cell–like properties in the mammalian inner ear is the topic of ongoing investigation in several laboratories. Mammalian organs with the capacity to regenerate generally contain a population of adult stem cells, which are responsible for preserving and repairing the tissue in which they are found.[92–94] These cells differ from pluripotent stem cells in that they are multipotent, meaning they are only able to differentiate into tissue-specific cell types, not all cell types. When an adult stem cell divides, one of the resulting daughter cells replaces itself as an adult stem cell, whereas the other daughter cell becomes a tissue-specific progenitor cell. Thus adult stem cells act as a self-repair system, repopulating themselves as adult stem cells in addition to replacing the damaged or destroyed tissue.

Adult stem cells are found in a variety of organs and tissues, including the central nervous system, skin, bone marrow, and gut. Increasing evidence suggests that the inner ear may also possess a niche of stem cells. In one study, cells with a high proliferative potential and capacity to self-renew were isolated from the vestibular portion of the adult mouse inner ear.[95] These inner ear–derived cells demonstrated the ability to form spheres, one feature of stem cells. When cultured in vitro, these cells showed the capacity to differentiate into cells expressing mature hair cell markers. In addition, when these sphere-derived cells were transplanted into the developing inner ear of chicken embryos, they were capable of differentiating into hair cell-like cells.

In another study evaluating the presence of adult stem cells in the mouse inner ear, investigators isolated stem cells from cochlear and vestibular tissues in mice 1 to 4 months of age.[96] Differences in the capacity for sphere formation were observed, with stem cells from the vestibular sensory epithelia displaying a higher capacity for sphere formation compared with those isolated from the cochlear sensory epithelia. In addition, the sphere-forming ability of the cochlear sensory epithelia rapidly decreased from the second to the third postnatal week, whereas the sphere-forming ability of the vestibular sensory epithelia declined more slowly and into adulthood. As already stated, the mammalian vestibular organ has some capacity to replace lost hair cells,[15,16] whereas the cochlea appears to lack this regenerative potential. Results from this study suggest that stem cell–like cells may be responsible for the persistence of some regenerative potential observed in the vestibular sensory epithelium. In addition, the inability of the cochlear sensory epithelium to regenerate might be due to a reduction in the number or potential of the tissue-specific stem cell population in the organ of Corti.

Although there are reports of low/undetectable progenitor cells in the adult mammalian inner ear, other lines of investigation suggest that stem cell compartments may persist within the mature cochlea. The intermediate filament protein nestin is expressed in proliferating tissues and is widely regarded as a marker of mitotically active cells and neural stem cells.[97–100] As such, nestin is commonly used to identify cells with stem cell characteristics in developing and adult tissues.[97] Several studies have reported the existence of nestin-expressing cells in the inner ears of mice; however, their presence and location differ between reports.[101–103] In the first report, nestin expression was observed in supporting cells below the inner and outer hair cells in the immature mouse cochlea, in addition to some mild expression in the outer hair cells; however, in the early adult mouse, nestin expression was downregulated and localized to only a few cells under the outer hair cell layer.[101] In another study, nestin expression was observed in supporting cells near the inner hair cell layer, with some mild expression in a few inner and outer hair cells in the immature cochlea.[102] In the mature inner ear, nestin expression was found to be limited to only the spiral ganglion. Most recently, nestin expression was found in supporting cells lateral to the outer hair cell region.[103] This expression was observed throughout the whole cochlea in newborn mice; however, the number of nestin-expressing cells decreased as the cochlea matured. Of interest, the authors reported that there appeared to be an increase in the number of nestin-expressing cells following noise trauma.[103] Collectively, the presence of nestin-expressing cells in the murine inner ear raises the possibility of the persistence of a population of stem cell-like cells within the mammalian cochlea. Further work exploring their exact presence, localization, and overall function is essential to understand any therapeutic potential that they may possess.

More recently, Lgr5, a Wnt target gene, has emerged as another area of interest for hair cell regeneration.[40,104,105] Lgr5 is a stem cell marker found in multiple proliferating adult tissues.[106–109] During embryonic development, Lgr5 is expressed in nascent hair cells and supporting cells and is later downregulated as the cells mature, with expression limited to the third row of Deiters cells in the mature organ of Corti.[104] Analysis of these cells by other investigators revealed that they give rise to hair cell lineages in vivo and in vitro.[40] In this study, Lgr5-expressing cells were isolated and cultured in vitro and found to self-renew and differentiate into cells expressing the hair cell marker myosin VIIa. In vivo, these cells were able to give rise to hair cells. In agreement with the previous report, Lgr5 expression was downregulated to the third row of Deiters cells; however, inner pillar cells also appeared to retain this expression as well. Additional analysis revealed these Lgr5-expressing cells proliferate and generate hair cells under certain experimental conditions in neonatal mice.[105] Evidence that these cells are able to reenter the cell cycle and proliferate offers the advantage that these cells could replenish both hair cells and supporting cells in the damaged mammalian cochlea. It remains unclear at this point how long the population of Lgr5-expressing cochlear stem cells persist into adulthood. As with nestin expression, further investigation of these cells is needed to determine their therapeutic potential as a means for regenerating cochlear hair cells.

In summary, the presence of endogenous stem cells in the mammalian inner ear presents the possibility of local therapy aimed at recruiting and directing these cells to repopulate the organ of Corti with functional cochlear hair cells after the native population of hair cells has been lost or damaged. Some studies on the topic have reported that, over time, the number and/or viability of multipotent stem cells in the cochlea decreases.[96,101–104] Consequently, there exists the possibility that, by the time these cells are needed for most patients with acquired causes of hearing loss, they no longer exist. Accordingly, further research is warranted to determine the function, location, and persistence into adulthood of cochlear stem cells to better define their potential as the basis for a novel therapeutic approach for hearing loss.

Conclusion

The past 30 years of research have provided a better understanding of the mechanisms underlying inner ear development, avian cochlear hair cell regeneration, pluripotent stem cell differentiation, cell transplantation, the presence of endogenous stem cells, and the potential therapeutic application of gene transfer and pharmacotherapies for hearing loss. Although much has been learned about the use of exogenous stem cells, inner ear stem cells, gene transfer, and pharmacotherapies for the replacement of damaged cells, these approaches for the treatment of hearing loss are still in experimental stages. There are many intricate components, and therefore challenges, involved in the process of auditory nerve and cochlear hair cell regeneration. As such, it is possible that a combination of the approaches described here or others not yet evident will yield novel, clinically meaningful treatments for hearing loss in the future. Although there are no clinical trials in this field to date for adults with hearing loss, several recent discoveries using cell culture and animal models give hope that otolaryngologists will have novel, regenerative therapeutic options for the management of sensorineural hearing loss in the future.

Challenges of Regenerative Therapy

- Challenges facing all approaches
  - Identifying the safest and most efficient method to access the cochlea
  - Repopulating the cochlea with an adequate amount of cells
  - Avoidance of generating hair cells outside of the organ of Corti
  - Maintenance of newly generated cells
  - Reestablishment of neuronal circuitry
- Gene-based treatment and pharmacotherapies
  - Generation of replacement hair cells without significantly compromising the supporting cell population
  - Insuring that treatment does not compromise the cytoarchitecture of the organ of Corti
  - Unregulated cell proliferation carries the risk of tumor formation
- Exogenous stem cells
  - Determine the timing of transplantation relative to damage for optimal success
  - Proper migration, integration, and terminal differentiation of transplanted cells into the organ of Corti as hair cells
  - Immune rejection of transplanted cells
- Endogenous stem cells
  - Identifying if endogenous cochlear stem cells persist into adulthood and maintain potency to become hair cells
  - Determining the spatial and temporal organization of adult stem cells in the cochlea
  - Identifying a method for allowing cochlear stem cells, if present, to enter the cell cycle, proliferate, and replace lost hair cells

Key Points

- Multiple approaches such as the following are being taken in pursuit of regenerative treatments for sensorineural hearing loss:
  - Gene transfer
  - Pharmacotherapies
  - Exogenous delivery of stem cells
  - Promotion of endogenous stem cells
- All approaches are still in experimental stages with no clinical trials to date in adults.
- Each approach has its own unique advantages and disadvantages.
- A combination of these approaches may be necessary for successful treatment of sensorineural hearing loss in the future.

Acknowledgments

Samuel Gubbels receives support (KL2 award and Type I pilot) from the Clinical and Translational Science Award (CTSA) program, previously through the National Center for Research Resources (NCRR) grant 1UL1RR025011, and now by the National Center for Advancing Translational Sciences (NCATS), grant 9U54TR000021. The content is solely the responsibility of the authors and does not necessarily represent the official views of the NIH. SG also receives support from NIH/NIDCD 1 R03 DC012432-01, 1 R01 DC013912-01, as well as P30 HD003352.

References

1. Lin FR, Thorpe R, Gordon-Salant S, Ferrucci L. Hearing loss prevalence and risk factors among older adults in the United States. J Gerontol A Biol Sci Med Sci 2011;66(5):582–590
2. Dillon CF, Gu Q, Hoffman HJ, Ko CW. Vision, hearing, balance, and sensory impairment in Americans aged 70 years and over: United States, 1999-2006. NCHS Data Brief 2010; 31(31):1–8
3. Arlinger S. Negative consequences of uncorrected hearing loss—a review. Int J Audiol 2003;42(Suppl 2):S17–S20
4. National Institute on Deafness and Other Communication Disorders. Quick Statistics. 2010. http://www.nidcd.nih.gov/health/statistics/Pages/quick.aspx. Accessed December 16, 2013
5. Davis AC. Hearing disorders in the population: first phase findings of the MRC National Study of Hearing. In: Lutman ME, Haggard MP, eds. Hearing Science and Hearing Disorders. New York, NY: Academic Press 1983; 35-60
6. Morrison SJ, Spradling AC. Stem cells and niches: mechanisms that promote stem cell maintenance throughout life. Cell 2008;132(4):598–611
7. Watt FM, Lo Celso C, Silva-Vargas V. Epidermal stem cells: an update. Curr Opin Genet Dev 2006;16(5):518–524
8. Miura H, Kusakabe Y, Harada S. Cell lineage and differentiation in taste buds. Arch Histol Cytol 2006;69(4): 209–225
9. Altman J. Autoradiographic and histological studies of postnatal neurogenesis. IV. Cell proliferation and migration in the anterior forebrain, with special reference to persisting neurogenesis in the olfactory bulb. J Comp Neurol 1969; 137(4):433–457
10. Lois C, Alvarez-Buylla A. Long-distance neuronal migration in the adult mammalian brain. Science 1994;264(5162): 1145–1148
11. Kornack DR, Rakic P. The generation, migration, and differentiation of olfactory neurons in the adult primate brain. Proc Natl Acad Sci USA 2001;98(8):4752–4757
12. Corwin JT, Cotanche DA. Regeneration of sensory hair cells after acoustic trauma. Science 1988;240(4860):1772–1774
13. Ryals BM, Rubel EW. Hair cell regeneration after acoustic trauma in adult Coturnix quail. Science 1988;240(4860): 1774–1776
14. Smolders JW. Functional recovery in the avian ear after hair cell regeneration. Audiol Neurootol 1999;4(6):286–302
15. Warchol ME, Lambert PR, Goldstein BJ, Forge A, Corwin JT. Regenerative proliferation in inner ear sensory epithelia from adult guinea pigs and humans. Science 1993; 259(5101):1619–1622
16. Forge A, Li L, Corwin JT, Nevill G. Ultrastructural evidence for hair cell regeneration in the mammalian inner ear. Science 1993;259(5101):1616–1619
17. Groves AK. The challenge of hair cell regeneration. Exp Biol Med (Maywood) 2010;235(4):434–446
18. Bhave SA, Stone JS, Rubel EW, Coltrera MD. Cell cycle progression in gentamicin-damaged avian cochleas. J Neurosci 1995;15(6):4618–4628
19. Duncan LJ, Mangiardi DA, Matsui JI, Anderson JK, McLaughlin-Williamson K, Cotanche DA. Differential expression of unconventional myosins in apoptotic and regenerating chick hair cells confirms two regeneration mechanisms. J Comp Neurol 2006;499(5):691–701
20. Stone JS, Choi YS, Woolley SM, Yamashita H, Rubel EW. Progenitor cell cycling during hair cell regeneration in the vestibular and auditory epithelia of the chick. J Neurocytol 1999; 28(10-11):863–876
21. Roberson DW, Alosi JA, Cotanche DA. Direct transdifferentiation gives rise to the earliest new hair cells in regenerating avian auditory epithelium. J Neurosci Res 2004;78(4): 461–471
22. Adler HJ, Raphael Y. New hair cells arise from supporting cell conversion in the acoustically damaged chick inner ear. Neurosci Lett 1996;205(1):17–20
23. Duckert LG, Rubel EW. Ultrastructural observations on regenerating hair cells in the chick basilar papilla. Hear Res 1990;48(1-2):161–182
24. Duckert LG, Rubel EW. Morphological correlates of functional recovery in the chicken inner ear after gentamycin treatment. J Comp Neurol 1993;331(1):75–96
25. Warchol ME. Cell density and N-cadherin interactions regulate cell proliferation in the sensory epithelia of the inner ear. J Neurosci 2002;22(7):2607–2616
26. Beresford WA. Direct transdifferentiation: can cells change their phenotype without dividing? Cell Differ Dev 1990; 29(2):81–93
27. Colvin JS, Bohne BA, Harding GW, McEwen DG, Ornitz DM. Skeletal overgrowth and deafness in mice lacking fibroblast growth factor receptor 3. Nat Genet 1996;12(4):390–397
28. Fritzsch B, Beisel KW, Hansen LA. The molecular basis of neurosensory cell formation in ear development: a blueprint for hair cell and sensory neuron regeneration? BioEssays 2006;28(12):1181–1193
29. Chen P, Johnson JE, Zoghbi HY, Segil N. The role of Math1 in inner ear development: Uncoupling the establishment of the sensory primordium from hair cell fate determination. Development 2002;129(10):2495–2505
30. Lumpkin EA, Collisson T, Parab P, et al. Math1-driven GFP expression in the developing nervous system of transgenic mice. Gene Expr Patterns 2003;3(4):389–395
31. Woods C, Montcouquiol M, Kelley MW. Math1 regulates development of the sensory epithelium in the mammalian cochlea. Nat Neurosci 2004;7(12):1310–1318
32. Bermingham NA, Hassan BA, Price SD, et al. Math1: an essential gene for the generation of inner ear hair cells. Science 1999;284(5421):1837–1841
33. Zheng JL, Gao WQ. Overexpression of Math1 induces robust production of extra hair cells in postnatal rat inner ears. Nat Neurosci 2000;3(6):580–586
34. Cafaro J, Lee GS, Stone JS. *Atoh1* expression defines activated progenitors and differentiating hair cells during avian hair cell regeneration. Dev Dyn 2007;236(1):156–170
35. Kawamoto K, Ishimoto S, Minoda R, Brough DE, Raphael Y. Math1 gene transfer generates new cochlear hair cells in mature guinea pigs in vivo. J Neurosci 2003;23(11): 4395–4400
36. Izumikawa M, Minoda R, Kawamoto K, et al. Auditory hair cell replacement and hearing improvement by *Atoh1* gene therapy in deaf mammals. Nat Med 2005;11(3):271–276
37. Gubbels SP, Woessner DW, Mitchell JC, Ricci AJ, Brigande JV. Functional auditory hair cells produced in the mammalian cochlea by in utero gene transfer. Nature 2008;455(7212): 537–541
38. Chai R, Kuo B, Wang T, et al. Wnt signaling induces proliferation of sensory precursors in the postnatal mouse cochlea. Proc Natl Acad Sci USA 2012;109(21):8167–8172
39. Doetzlhofer A, White P, Lee YS, Groves A, Segil N. Prospective identification and purification of hair cell and supporting cell progenitors from the embryonic cochlea. Brain Res 2006;1091(1):282–288

40. Shi F, Kempfle JS, Edge AS. Wnt-responsive Lgr5-expressing stem cells are hair cell progenitors in the cochlea. J Neurosci 2012;32(28):9639–9648
41. White PM, Doetzlhofer A, Lee YS, Groves AK, Segil N. Mammalian cochlear supporting cells can divide and trans-differentiate into hair cells. Nature 2006;441(7096):984–987
42. Savary E, Hugnot JP, Chassigneux Y, et al. Distinct population of hair cell progenitors can be isolated from the postnatal mouse cochlea using side population analysis. Stem Cells 2007;25(2):332–339
43. Sinkkonen ST, Chai R, Jan TA, et al. Intrinsic regenerative potential of murine cochlear supporting cells. Sci Rep 2011; 1:26
44. Lee YS, Liu F, Segil N. A morphogenetic wave of p27Kip1 transcription directs cell cycle exit during organ of Corti development. Development 2006;133(15):2817–2826
45. Ruben RJ. Development of the inner ear of the mouse: a radioautographic study of terminal mitoses. Acta Otolaryngol 1967;(Suppl 220):1–44
46. Chen P, Segil N. p27(Kip1) links cell proliferation to morphogenesis in the developing organ of Corti. Development 1999;126(8):1581–1590
47. Löwenheim H, Furness DN, Kil J, et al. Gene disruption of p27(Kip1) allows cell proliferation in the postnatal and adult organ of corti. Proc Natl Acad Sci USA 1999;96(7): 4084–4088
48. Chen P, Zindy F, Abdala C, et al. Progressive hearing loss in mice lacking the cyclin-dependent kinase inhibitor Ink4d. Nat Cell Biol 2003;5(5):422–426
49. Kanzaki S, Beyer LA, Swiderski DL, et al. p27(Kip1) deficiency causes organ of Corti pathology and hearing loss. Hear Res 2006;214(1-2):28–36
50. Chen ZY. Cell cycle, differentiation and regeneration: where to begin? Cell Cycle 2006;5(22):2609–2612
51. Huang M, Sage C, Tang Y, et al. Overlapping and distinct pRb pathways in the mammalian auditory and vestibular organs. Cell Cycle 2011;10(2):337–351
52. Sage C, Huang M, Vollrath MA, et al. Essential role of retinoblastoma protein in mammalian hair cell development and hearing. Proc Natl Acad Sci USA 2006;103(19):7345–7350
53. Sage C, Huang M, Karimi K, et al. Proliferation of functional hair cells in vivo in the absence of the retinoblastoma protein. Science 2005;307(5712):1114–1118
54. Yu Y, Weber T, Yamashita T, et al. In vivo proliferation of postmitotic cochlear supporting cells by acute ablation of the retinoblastoma protein in neonatal mice. J Neurosci 2010; 30(17):5927–5936
55. Kimble J, Simpson P. The LIN-12/Notch signaling pathway and its regulation. Annu Rev Cell Dev Biol 1997;13: 333–361
56. Louvi A, Artavanis-Tsakonas S. Notch signalling in vertebrate neural development. Nat Rev Neurosci 2006;7(2):93–102
57. Lanford PJ, Lan Y, Jiang R, et al. Notch signalling pathway mediates hair cell development in mammalian cochlea. Nat Genet 1999;21(3):289–292
58. Eddison M, Le Roux I, Lewis J. Notch signaling in the development of the inner ear: lessons from Drosophila. Proc Natl Acad Sci USA 2000;97(22):11692–11699
59. Lewis J. Rules for the production of sensory cells. Ciba Found Symp 1991;160:25–39, discussion 40–53
60. Kiernan AE. Notch signaling during cell fate determination in the inner ear. Semin Cell Dev Biol 2013;24(5):470–479
61. Zine A, Aubert A, Qiu J, et al. Hes1 and Hes5 activities are required for the normal development of the hair cells in the mammalian inner ear. J Neurosci 2001;21(13):4712–4720
62. Li S, Mark S, Radde-Gallwitz K, Schlisner R, Chin MT, Chen P. Hey2 functions in parallel with Hes1 and Hes5 for mammalian auditory sensory organ development. BMC Dev Biol 2008;8:20
63. Lanford PJ, Shailam R, Norton CR, Gridley T, Kelley MW. Expression of Math1 and HES5 in the cochleae of wildtype and Jag2 mutant mice. J Assoc Res Otolaryngol 2000;1(2): 161–171
64. Stone JS, Rubel EW. Delta1 expression during avian hair cell regeneration. Development 1999;126(5):961–973
65. Brooker R, Hozumi K, Lewis J. Notch ligands with contrasting functions: Jagged1 and Delta1 in the mouse inner ear. Development 2006;133(7):1277–1286
66. Kiernan AE, Cordes R, Kopan R, Gossler A, Gridley T. The Notch ligands DLL1 and JAG2 act synergistically to regulate hair cell development in the mammalian inner ear. Development 2005;132(19):4353–4362
67. Doetzlhofer A, Basch ML, Ohyama T, Gessler M, Groves AK, Segil N. Hey2 regulation by FGF provides a Notch-independent mechanism for maintaining pillar cell fate in the organ of Corti. Dev Cell 2009;16(1):58–69
68. Hayashi T, Kokubo H, Hartman BH, Ray CA, Reh TA, Bermingham-McDonogh O. Hesr1 and Hesr2 may act as early effectors of Notch signaling in the developing cochlea. Dev Biol 2008;316(1):87–99
69. Takebayashi S, Yamamoto N, Yabe D, et al. Multiple roles of Notch signaling in cochlear development. Dev Biol 2007;307(1):165–178
70. Yamamoto N, Tanigaki K, Tsuji M, Yabe D, Ito J, Honjo T. Inhibition of Notch/RBP-J signaling induces hair cell formation in neonate mouse cochleas. J Mol Med (Berl) 2006;84(1):37–45
71. Hori R, Nakagawa T, Sakamoto T, Matsuoka Y, Takebayashi S, Ito J. Pharmacological inhibition of Notch signaling in the mature guinea pig cochlea. Neuroreport 2007;18(18): 1911–1914
72. Mizutari K, Fujioka M, Hosoya M, et al. Notch inhibition induces cochlear hair cell regeneration and recovery of hearing after acoustic trauma. Neuron 2013;77(1):58–69
73. Picanço-Castro V, Moreira LF, Kashima S. Covas DT. Can pluripotent stem cells be used in cell-based therapy? Cell Reprogram 2014;16(2):98-107
74. Pan CK, Heilweil G, Lanza R, Schwartz SD. Embryonic stem cells as a treatment for macular degeneration. Expert Opin Biol Ther 2013;13(8):1125–1133
75. Ronaghi M, Nasr M, Ealy M, et al. Inner ear hair cell-like cells from human embryonic stem cells. Stem Cells Dev 2014; 23(11):1275–1284
76. Chen W, Jongkamonwiwat N, Abbas L, et al. Restoration of auditory evoked responses by human ES-cell-derived otic progenitors. Nature 2012;490(7419):278–282
77. Oshima K, Shin K, Diensthuber M, Peng AW, Ricci AJ, Heller S. Mechanosensitive hair cell-like cells from embryonic and induced pluripotent stem cells. Cell 2010;141(4):704–716
78. Koehler KR, Mikosz AM, Molosh AI, Patel D, Hashino E. Generation of inner ear sensory epithelia from pluripotent stem cells in 3D culture. Nature 2013;500(7461):217–221
79. Ito J, Kojima K, Kawaguchi S. Survival of neural stem cells in the cochlea. Acta Otolaryngol 2001;121(2):140–142
80. Tateya I, Nakagawa T, Iguchi F, et al. Fate of neural stem cells grafted into injured inner ears of mice. Neuroreport 2003; 14(13):1677–1681
81. Parker MA, Corliss DA, Gray B, et al. Neural stem cells injected into the sound-damaged cochlea migrate throughout the cochlea and express markers of hair cells, supporting cells, and spiral ganglion cells. Hear Res 2007;232(1-2):29–43

82. Coleman B, Hardman J, Coco A, et al. Fate of embryonic stem cells transplanted into the deafened mammalian cochlea. Cell Transplant 2006;15(5):369–380
83. Hildebrand MS, Dahl HH, Hardman J, Coleman B, Shepherd RK, de Silva MG. Survival of partially differentiated mouse embryonic stem cells in the scala media of the guinea pig cochlea. J Assoc Res Otolaryngol 2005;6(4):341–354
84. Hu Z, Wei D, Johansson CB, et al. Survival and neural differentiation of adult neural stem cells transplanted into the mature inner ear. Exp Cell Res 2005;302(1):40–47
85. Naito Y, Nakamura T, Nakagawa T, et al. Transplantation of bone marrow stromal cells into the cochlea of chinchillas. Neuroreport 2004;15(1):1–4
86. Sakamoto T, Nakagawa T, Endo T, et al. Fates of mouse embryonic stem cells transplanted into the inner ears of adult mice and embryonic chickens. Acta Otolaryngol Suppl 2004; (551):48–52
87. Tamura T, Nakagawa T, Iguchi F, et al. Transplantation of neural stem cells into the modiolus of mouse cochleae injured by cisplatin. Acta Otolaryngol Suppl 2004; (551):65–68
88. Han Z, Yang JM, Chi FL, et al. Survival and fate of transplanted embryonic neural stem cells by *Atoh1* gene transfer in guinea pigs cochlea. Neuroreport 2010;21(7):490–496
89. Li H, Roblin G, Liu H, Heller S. Generation of hair cells by stepwise differentiation of embryonic stem cells. Proc Natl Acad Sci USA 2003;100(23):13495–13500
90. Ouji Y, Ishizaka S, Nakamura-Uchiyama F, Yoshikawa M. In vitro differentiation of mouse embryonic stem cells into inner ear hair cell-like cells using stromal cell conditioned medium. Cell Death Dis 2012;3:e314
91. Corrales CE, Pan L, Li H, Liberman MC, Heller S, Edge AS. Engraftment and differentiation of embryonic stem cell-derived neural progenitor cells in the cochlear nerve trunk: growth of processes into the organ of Corti. J Neurobiol 2006;66(13):1489–1500
92. Leblond CP, Clermont Y, Nadler NJ. The pattern of stem cell renewal in three epithelia (esophagus, intestine and testis). Proc Can Cancer Conf 1967;7:3–30
93. Shihabuddin LS, Ray J, Gage FH. Stem cell technology for basic science and clinical applications. Arch Neurol 1999;56(1): 29–32
94. Weissman IL. Stem cells: units of development, units of regeneration, and units in evolution. Cell 2000;100(1): 157–168
95. Li H, Liu H, Heller S. Pluripotent stem cells from the adult mouse inner ear. Nat Med 2003;9(10):1293–1299
96. Oshima K, Grimm CM, Corrales CE, et al. Differential distribution of stem cells in the auditory and vestibular organs of the inner ear. J Assoc Res Otolaryngol 2007;8(1):18–31
97. Lendahl U, Zimmerman LB, McKay RD. CNS stem cells express a new class of intermediate filament protein. Cell 1990;60(4):585–595
98. Sejersen T, Lendahl U. Transient expression of the intermediate filament nestin during skeletal muscle development. J Cell Sci 1993;106(Pt 4):1291–1300
99. Kachinsky AM, Dominov JA, Miller JB. Intermediate filaments in cardiac myogenesis: nestin in the developing mouse heart. J Histochem Cytochem 1995;43(8):843–847
100. Suzuki S, Namiki J, Shibata S, Mastuzaki Y, Okano H. The neural stem/progenitor cell marker nestin is expressed in proliferative endothelial cells, but not in mature vasculature. J Histochem Cytochem 2010;58(8):721–730
101. Lopez IA, Zhao PM, Yamaguchi M, de Vellis J, Espinosa-Jeffrey A. Stem/progenitor cells in the postnatal inner ear of the GFP-nestin transgenic mouse. Int J Dev Neurosci 2004;22(4): 205–213
102. Smeti I, Savary E, Capelle V, Hugnot JP, Uziel A, Zine A. Expression of candidate markers for stem/progenitor cells in the inner ears of developing and adult GFAP and nestin promoter-GFP transgenic mice. Gene Expr Patterns 2011; 11(1-2):22–32
103. Watanabe R, Morell MH, Miller JM, et al. Nestin-expressing cells in the developing, mature and noise-exposed cochlear epithelium. Mol Cell Neurosci 2012;49(2):104–109
104. Chai R, Xia A, Wang T, et al. Dynamic expression of Lgr5, a Wnt target gene, in the developing and mature mouse cochlea. J Assoc Res Otolaryngol 2011;12(4):455–469
105. Shi F, Hu L, Edge AS. Generation of hair cells in neonatal mice by b-catenin overexpression in Lgr5-positive cochlear progenitors. Proc Natl Acad Sci USA 2013;110(34): 13851–13856
106. Barker N, van Es JH, Kuipers J, et al. Identification of stem cells in small intestine and colon by marker gene Lgr5. Nature 2007;449(7165):1003–1007
107. Barker N, Huch M, Kujala P, et al. Lgr5(+ve) stem cells drive self-renewal in the stomach and build long-lived gastric units in vitro. Cell Stem Cell 2010;6(1):25–36
108. Jaks V, Barker N, Kasper M, et al. Lgr5 marks cycling, yet long-lived, hair follicle stem cells. Nat Genet 2008;40(11): 1291–1299
109. Ootani A, Li X, Sangiorgi E, et al. Sustained in vitro intestinal epithelial culture within a Wnt-dependent stem cell niche. Nat Med 2009;15(6):701–706

8 Hearing Aids: Considerations in the Geriatric Population

Amanda Kantor, Erica Miele, John Luckhurst, Mary Hawkshaw, and Robert T. Sataloff

Introduction

Hearing loss is the most common sensory deficit in the elderly.[1] Hearing loss can impair communication, thus creating loneliness, isolation, dependence, frustration, and even communication disorders.[1] When left untreated, hearing loss can substantially impair quality of life. *Audiological rehabilitation*, *auditory rehabilitation*, and *aural rehabilitation* are often used interchangeably to describe a patient's management process designed for individuals who experience deficits in communication, as reported by Weinstein.[2] Functional capabilities must be assessed on an individual basis due to wide variations in characterizing elderly adults. Chronological age is not a reliable predictor of physical, social, or mental status; therefore, it is important to understand how individuals view themselves. The impact of hearing loss varies by the degree of loss and the individual's personality and activity level. The effects of hearing loss cannot be restricted to pathology alone because the mechanics of the ear cannot be isolated from the social aspects of hearing. The personality effects of hearing loss are largely dependent on an individual's character, including mental, spiritual, societal, and economic resources. These components determine one's reaction to hearing loss and the level of handicap it generates. Rehabilitation in the elderly must include a comprehensive approach to assessment and a multidimensional intervention. The purpose of rehabilitation with older adults, regardless of the severity or type of impairment, is to assist in recovering lost physical, psychological, and social skills.

The entire auditory system undergoes considerable change as the aging process progresses. Specific conditions may affect the type of aural rehabilitation to provide. For example, older adults develop changes of the outer ear and external auditory canal due to thinning of the epithelium, atrophy of subcutaneous tissue, and decline in secretory abilities of the glands. Hence certain types of hearing aids or audiological testing may not be appropriate due to changes in the ear structure. Although outer and middle ear pathologies are monitored under the care of a physician, the audiologist should be aware of any such issues. It is important to consider age-related changes in the brain when determining auditory rehabilitation in the elderly population. Aging is associated with progressive losses in function across multiple systems, including sensation, cognition, memory control, and affect. Age-related modifications in the central nervous system are associated with declines in the ability to perform selected cognitive and sensorimotor tasks; decreased functional capacity; and alterations in gait control, learning, and memory.[3] These deficits may affect the patient's ability to respond to aural rehabilitation strategies.

Hearing loss may be severe in older persons, whether from causes associated with aging or owing to other etiologies. More severe-to-profound losses may be associated with a change in personality and lifestyle due to the challenges that listening presents. Elderly individuals with hearing loss also find listening in the presence of multiple speakers or background noise especially difficult because their ability to detect signals in noise diminishes with age. All too often, the elderly person begins to believe that the inability to hear and understand a conversation is due to deterioration of the brain (intellectual impairment). Family, friends, and stereotypes of the elderly population may reinforce this belief. People may ignore the hearing-impaired person in group conversations and assume that the person does not know what is going on. Stereotypes of aging, such as physical and mental slowing, further undermine the elderly person's weakened self-confidence and hasten his or her withdrawal from society. The isolation caused by hearing loss can contribute to delay in elderly individuals' seeking medical attention to address their hearing handicap.

There is a significant relationship between hearing and speech. The ear is sensitive to a certain frequency range, and speech falls within that range. Speech can be divided into two types of sounds:

vowels and consonants. Roughly, vowels fall into the frequencies below 1,500 Hz, and consonants above 1,500 Hz. Vowels are relatively powerful sounds, whereas consonants are weaker sounds and are dropped often in everyday speech or not pronounced clearly. In essence, low-frequency speech sounds provide the listener with a sense of volume, whereas higher-frequency speech sounds provide meaning and clarity. Most commonly, older adults experience a hearing loss configuration that reflects comparatively good low-frequency hearing and poorer high-frequency hearing. High-frequency sensorineural hearing loss often causes deterioration of a person's ability to understand speech. Speech recognition ability can be correlated with the aging process.[4] In some cases, diminished speech understanding is due to peripheral hearing loss. This type of loss typically presents with the ability to hear speech but not understand it. A second cause of trouble understanding speech is central auditory processing issues, such that age-related changes or other changes in the auditory pathways of the brainstem or portions of the auditory cortex degrade the speech signal.[5] Individuals with hearing loss may ask people to speak louder in an attempt to achieve better speech clarity. Unfortunately, "louder" is not always the answer. Loudness may actually reduce discrimination ability due to distortion of the speech signal. Distortion occurs more frequently in people with high-frequency hearing losses because overall loudness also amplifies the low-frequency sounds, such as vowels, which they usually hear at a normal or close to normal volume. Speaking in a louder voice creates overpowering vowels with relatively weaker consonants and does not improve the clarity of speech. These factors must be assessed and are critical to proper hearing aid selection.

Before a hearing aid is recommended, it is necessary to determine whether the patient will be helped by it enough to justify purchasing one. Hearing aids are generally not covered by Medicare; however, Medicaid or private insurance plans may cover the cost of hearing aids in whole or in part. Regardless of insurance type, patients must be offered the same services, the cost of the services must be equitable, and national procedure codes must be used for requesting reimbursement. It is important to assist the elderly patient in figuring out what his or her specific insurance will cover, if anything, before proceeding with purchasing hearing aids. For those patients that have served in the military, it is advisable to obtain amplification through the Veteran's Administration because hearing aids and other assistive devices are fully covered through veteran's benefits. Both economic factors and individual hearing loss should be taken into account. This is particularly important in a sensorineural impairment in which the problem is more one of discrimination than of amplification. Typically, high-frequency sensorineural hearing loss is attributed to presbycusis—age-related hearing loss that is associated with the cochlear degenerative process of aging. Humes et al reported that the hearing loss of older adults is greatest in the frequency region (≥ 2,000 Hz) for which the amplitude of speech is the lowest.[6]

Beyond presbycusis, there are also medical causes of hearing loss, including infection, autoimmune disease, medication effects, and many other conditions. These causes should always be evaluated by a physician, and medical causes of hearing impairment generally should be treated in conjunction with auditory rehabilitation and amplification for every patient. A patient being considered for a hearing aid should undergo otologic evaluation first.

Hearing Aid Considerations

Hearing aids, assistive listening devices, and implantable devices may be helpful for older adults with hearing loss and communication issues. A hearing aid is a portable personal amplifying system used to compensate for a loss of hearing. Almost all hearing-impaired patients are candidates for a hearing aid, although some will receive greater benefits from their aids than others. Any patient who is motivated to use a hearing aid deserves a thorough evaluation and a trial with an appropriate instrument. Assistive listening devices include amplified telephones, television amplifiers, and other such tools that can increase signal intensity for the listener. Implantable devices can include bone-anchored hearing aids, cochlear implants, and the auditory brainstem implant. Hearing aids are appropriate for the vast majority of patients, and this chapter does not address cochlear implants or auditory brainstem implants.

According to Kochkin, the average age of new hearing aid users is 71.1 years.[7] Of the 34 million people with hearing loss in the United States, only 25% use hearing instruments, which suggests that over 25 million people are living with untreated/unaided hearing loss.[8] Despite recent advances in hearing aid technology and miniaturization of hearing aids, negative attitudes persist. Before fitting a hearing aid in an older adult, various factors must be considered, such as communication, physical, psychological, and sociological factors. Some of the issues older adults face when considering use of hearing aids include the following:

1. Experience with hearing aids
2. Financial considerations
3. Attitudes toward hearing aids
4. Degree of hearing loss
5. Lack of need

6. Visual/manual dexterity issues
7. Recommendations from professionals
8. Recommendations from family and friends
9. Stigma
10. Trust
11. Lack of knowledge.

The audiologist is responsible for informing patients fully about the entire process and providing realistic expectations, counseling, and support before fitting a hearing aid.

Prefitting Assessment

The audiologist must administer tests to determine whether a hearing loss is present and, if so, the nature of the hearing loss. Threshold measures used in conjunction with otoscopy and immittance testing can help determine the need for medical or surgical remediation. If a condition requires immediate medical attention, the patient should be referred to the appropriate medical professional. Regardless of any degree or nature of impairment, medical clearance for hearing aids from a physician should always be obtained. If no medically treatable condition is present, the severity of hearing impairment, symmetry, configuration, type of hearing loss, and speech perception should be documented. Once medical contraindications are ruled out and the patient is determined to be a candidate for amplification, the audiologist must discuss thoroughly the nature of the hearing loss, its consequences, and realistic expectations, and must evaluate personal factors and the patient's motivational level to use amplification.[2]

The patient should be given a clear explanation of the hearing problem and why he or she has trouble hearing or understanding speech. Patients should understand the difference between hearing difficulty and understanding difficulty, and how amplification affects both. The problems that might easily lead the patient to develop frustration and behavioral changes should be explained clearly so that these problems can be met forthrightly and intelligently. The goal of aural rehabilitation is to prevent or mitigate psychosocial changes and quality-of-life impairments that may result from hearing loss.

Psychological adjustment for each patient involves giving the patient more penetrating insight into the "personality problems" that are already in evidence or likely to develop as a result of hearing loss. Therapy should not use a predetermined technique but must be designed to meet the needs of the specific hearing-impaired individual. Frequently, it is advisable to implement aural rehabilitation not only with the patient, but also with the patient's spouse or family because it is impossible to separate a person's individual problems from family problems. The patient must be encouraged to associate with friends and not become isolated because of difficulties in communication. It must be impressed on individuals that using residual hearing effectively allows them to enjoy life and interact as usual with only minor modifications. Use of questionnaires can be very helpful during the prefitting assessment. The Hearing Handicap Inventory for the Elderly Screening Version described by Weinstein (HHIE-S) is a good tool for determining patients' perception of their hearing loss.[2] The HHIE-S is a 10-item questionnaire developed to assess how an individual perceives the social and emotional effects of hearing loss. A higher HHIE-S score suggests a greater handicapping effect of a hearing impairment.[2] The information obtained from this questionnaire can help the audiologist tailor counseling and intervention strategies.

As discussed previously, speech discrimination problems experienced by older adults often have a central auditory or cognitive basis. Because this issue has been identified, part of amplification candidate selection should include a test battery that at least screens for central auditory processing disorder (CAPD). A relationship between sensorineural hearing loss and cognitive impairment has also been identified.[9] It can be difficult to separate cognitive and central auditory effects from peripheral effects in the elderly. Recent data suggest that central auditory dysfunction may be an early manifestation of more general cognitive impairment and therefore may be a contributing factor to poor performance of older adults.[10]

Physical Factors

In the elderly, vision status, manual dexterity, ear/ear canal variables, and overall health status should affect the hearing aid decision process.[2] Vision problems may dictate the choice of hearing aid design, style, and type of signal processing. Otologic issues such as excessive wax buildup, active infections, stenosis of the external auditory canal, or unusual growths (such as exostoses) can inhibit the insertion of a hearing aid or limit the effectiveness of a specific style of hearing aid. Patients with a tendency to accumulate excess earwax should be acquainted with options for controlling earwax so that it doesn't affect hearing aid performance. Wax buildup inside of a hearing aid can impair the overall sound quality. Acute middle ear problems such as active infection or effusion can also contraindicate hearing aid use until the problem is resolved. Acute otitis externa will prevent use of a hearing aid until the infection is cleared as determined by their physician. In all cases of suspected medical pathology, patients should be urged to seek medical intervention.

Today's digital hearing aids are considerably smaller than the older technology. Smaller hearing aids can pose a challenge for many older adults who may suffer from poor vision, reduced manual dexterity, diminished tactile sensitivity, or reduced fine motor coordination.[2] Most state-of-the-art hearing aids are digital and adapt their settings automatically for best listening in various environments. This feature can be useful, especially for patients with dexterity issues, because it bypasses the need for manual hearing aid control. Additionally, the adaptive feature can make hearing aids more serviceable for patients with cognitive or memory issues. When selecting a hearing aid, assessment of these factors may be helpful. For example, those elderly patients that may experience reduced mobility, tactile sensitivity, and tremors may have exceptional difficulty changing the small hearing aid batteries; batteries generally need to be changed on a weekly basis. If batteries are left unchanged, the hearing aid itself is no longer of any use and will likely sit in the ear as an earplug rather than an assistive device. Additionally, visual issues that occur in the elderly population can further create a barrier in proper care for amplification devices. It is crucial to give a family member or caregiver the responsibility of caring for the device in terms of changing the batteries as well as general cleaning. Manual dexterity can be measured using the Nine-Hole Pegboard Test, which is designed to evaluate fine-motor coordination and finger dexterity.[2] Visual-motor coordination and touch recognition may affect successful use of amplification and should also be evaluated.

Acclimatization

The concept of acclimatization must be discussed and addressed with the patient as part of the counseling. It is critical to allow ample time for auditory and cognitive acclimatization to hearing aids, especially in the case of overall auditory deprivation, or switching from a monaural to binaural array. Arlinger et al reported that acclimatization to hearing aids is associated with improvement in auditory performance over time, and acclimatization usually results in a 3 to 5% improvement in speech recognition ability.[11] Factors impacting acclimatization include time course, age of patient, degree/configuration of hearing loss, previous experience, training effects, and the amount of audibility that it restores. Specifically, results have shown a significant acclimatization effect in a group of elderly individuals that were fitted monaurally with a linear algorithm.[12] Although linear processing is less common in today's hearing aid fittings, this further brings up the question of whether a monaural fitting is more appropriate in the elderly population.

Hearing Aid Arrangement: Monaural versus Binaural

In the case of bilateral hearing loss, choosing to invest in one versus two hearing aids is a decision that must be considered thoroughly. In general, binaural amplification is associated with increased speech understanding, improved directional hearing, improved spatial organization, and signal redundancy.[13] Although many audiologists would consider binaural amplification to be the preferable option in the case of bilateral hearing loss, there is variable evidence regarding success in monaural versus binaural hearing aid fittings.[12]

It is accepted generally that a binaural fitting will provide the greatest localization and speech perception in both quiet and noise. Most studies indicate that binaural fittings help improve binaural squelch, head shadow effects, and binaural redundancy.[14] Binaural amplification can also prevent auditory deprivation, a phenomenon described as a decrease over time in auditory performance associated with the reduced availability of acoustic information.[11]

In the case of elderly patients, however, this approach may not always be optimal. Contrary to these findings, other studies have suggested that binaural fittings can actually be more detrimental to the elderly user. In some cases, auditory processing disorders can present with binaural interference, making binaural speech perception worse than best-ear abilities.[15] Additionally, it has been found that elderly individuals often exhibit reduced speech intelligibility when aided binaurally as opposed to monaurally. This is referred to as the Binaural Interference Effect. Unless it is determined during the evaluation that the patient exhibits binaural interference, a binaural fitting should still be considered because the majority of patients will benefit from binaural amplification. Subjective reports or dichotic listening tasks are more helpful in determining this than typical audiometric speech tests, which have limited diagnostic value. It may take 6–12 weeks for an older adult to acclimate to binaural amplification, especially if one ear has been unaided for a lengthy period of time.[2]

Cox et al found that specific hearing loss parameters (severity, configuration) were not predictors of a monaural versus binaural preference.[16] The investigators found that patients who preferred a monaural fit attributed this to comfort and quality. Patients who preferred a binaural fit attributed this to restoration of balance, clarity of sounds, and comfort. Nearly all hearing aid manufacturers and audiologists implement a trial period for hearing aids, allowing flexibility for the patient and audiologist to determine the fitting arrangement that provides the greatest benefit. Audiologists and otologists should remain alert for binaural interference in older patients and should not hesitate to recommend removal of one hearing aid if binaural amplification does not provide the expected result.

Hearing Aid Technology

Old hearing aid technology did very little to improve a person's ability to understand but improved the ability to hear by making sounds louder. Recent hearing aid technology targets sensorineural losses with poorer discrimination, improving the amount of benefit individuals can receive from a hearing aid, although not necessarily truly improving discrimination ability. In addition to advances in technology, there is also a lot of flexibility regarding discretion. Many companies offer multiple color options so that the patient can choose if they want their hearing aid to match the tone of their skin or hair. Modern technology and color options have made hearing aids more appealing.

One of the most important things that a hearing aid does for people with hearing loss is it permits the individual to hear sounds with greater ease, reducing the strain of listening. Although the individual may not necessarily be able to understand more with an aid than without one, the device may relieve tension, fatigue, and some of the complications of a hearing impairment.

Over-the-Counter Hearing Aids

Amplification systems are often available over the counter at a considerably reduced price in comparison to those dispensed by a licensed professional. Although these may seem appealing due to their reduced cost and accessibility, these devices should be used with caution. This option may be beneficial for a select number of elderly patients that present with a relatively flat hearing loss and require only some additional gain for speech clarity. In this case, an over-the-counter amplification system may provide the needed benefit at a lower cost. Although a basic amplifier may work for a small percentage of elderly patients, they often do not take into account individual frequency and gain requirements and will often produce more distortion and discomfort rather than offering any noticeable benefit. Patients in these cases may end up wearing a device that is inappropriate for their audiological needs. For some, the poor performance experienced from these devices may deter them from trying other amplification altogether. Another unfortunate outcome may be that the patient often spends unnecessary costs before deciding to purchase devices from a licensed professional.

Body-Worn Hearing Aid

Given today's microtechnology, the body aid is no longer dispensed. The body aid is a large, high-powered instrument worn on the body and connected to the ear via an earmold. Body aids offer a wide range of amplification and are often used by patients with severe to profound hearing impairment (**Fig. 8.1**). The microphone, amplifier, and battery are located in the case, which is worn on the body or carried in a pocket. The receiver is connected to the amplifiers by a long wire and is attached directly to the earmold—a custom earpiece designed to collect sound into the ear. This separation of receiver and microphone helps eliminate acoustical feedback in high-amplification instruments. Body aids can be fit to losses of 40 to 110 dBHL. Given that newer technology can also fit a wide range of hearing losses, body aids are now obsolete. Additionally, newer technology contains numerous digital feedback suppression algorithms, eliminating the issue of feedback for patients with significant amplification needs.

Behind-the-Ear (BTE)

Behind-the-ear (BTE) hearing aids are currently the best choice for severe to profound hearing losses. All of the necessary components of the amplifying system, including the battery, are held in a single case that sits behind the ear. The amplified sound is then fed to the ear via a plastic tube attached to a custom ear mold. This design provides adequate separation of microphone and receiver to reduce acoustical feedback, which can be common in severe losses. These hearing aids can be adapted for mild to profound losses, making them very flexible.

In-the-Ear (ITE)

Previously, in-the-ear (ITE) hearing aids (**Fig. 8.2a**) were the most widely dispensed. In these types of instruments, the entire hearing aid system is actually housed inside the earmold shell. The aids can help in various cases of hearing loss, typically anywhere in the range from 25 to 80 dBHL. Additionally, various modifications can be made to accommodate different degrees and configurations of hearing loss. There are several styles of ITE instruments available: full-shell (**Fig. 8.2a**); half-shell (**Fig. 8.2b**); in-the-canal (ITC) (**Fig. 8.2c**); and completely-in-the-canal (CIC) (**Fig. 8.2b**), listed from largest to smallest, respectively. One drawback of the smaller ITE styles is that they cannot adequately provide as much amplification as the larger shells, making them inappropriate for more severe hearing loss. Generally, the larger the device, the larger the fitting range. For those with dexterity and cognitive issues, a larger ITE style

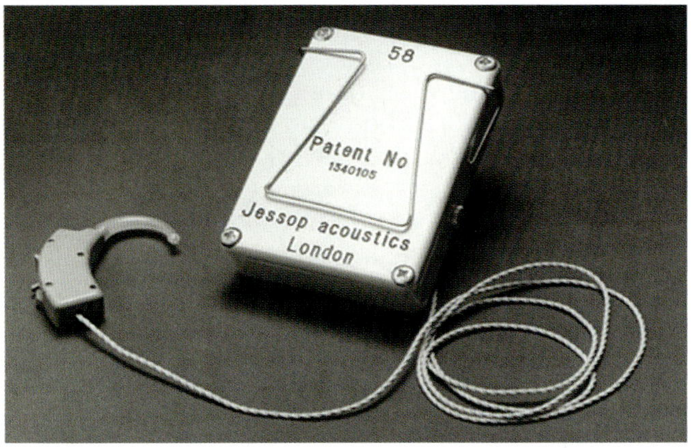

Fig. 8.1 Example of a typical body-worn hearing aid device.

is often preferable for ease of insertion and manipulation. Also, the batteries tend to be larger in larger devices, therefore maintenance of batteries is easier, and battery life may be longer.

Receiver-in-Canal (RIC) Hearing Aids

Receiver-in-canal (RIC) hearing aids (**Fig. 8.2d; Fig. 8.3**) are a newer style that looks very similar to open fit or slim tube BTE hearing aids. The difference is that the hearing aid's speaker is housed inside the ear canal. The hearing aid speaker's proximity to the tympanic membrane offers a sharper sound quality. Additionally, the small device that is seated behind the ear makes the device more appealing cosmetically as opposed to other styles. RIC hearing aids are popular due to their small size, discrete appearance, and ability to minimize occlusion. Minimizing occlusion creates a more natural sound quality for the patient. The devices also fit hearing losses from mild to severe. The popularity of these open-fit devices is attributable largely to feedback suppression systems.[17] Given the small size of these instruments, elderly patients with dexterity issues may have difficulty manipulating these devices, particularly with inserting and removing the aids.

Lyric

The Lyric (Phonak, Zurich, Switzerland) (**Fig. 8.4**) is a continuous-wear hearing aid designed for moderate to severe hearing loss. A specially trained audiologist or otologist inserts the device completely in the ear canal only 3 or 4 mm from the eardrum. The patient rarely touches the device, and it can remain in the ear for up to 4 months at a time because it is not affected by contact with water. Users can turn the device on and off and raise the volume using an external magnet. One advantage of this device is lack of handling and changing of batteries, which can be particularly helpful for those with both cognitive and dexterity issues. However, the device is more suited for those with mild hearing losses and is susceptible to damage due to wax or moisture given its deep insertion in the ear canal.

■ Hearing Aid Orientation

After the device has been fitted, the audiologist should educate the patient as to the hearing aid parts, and if possible, the patient's frequent com-

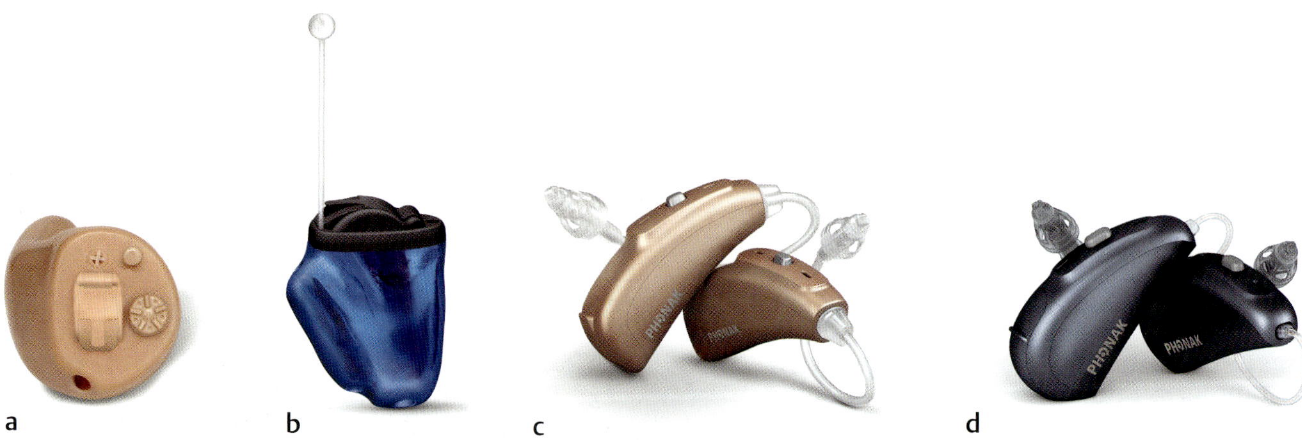

Fig. 8.2 (**a**) Custom full-shell in-the-ear (ITE) hearing aids; smaller models are typically called half-shell (HS) or in-the-canal (ITC) hearing aids. (**b**) Custom completely in the canal (CIC) hearing aids. (**c**) Behind-the-ear (BTE) hearing aids; these devices are coupled with custom earmolds. (**d**) An example of receiver-in-the-canal (RIC) hearing aids; also may be referred to as micro BTE hearing aids. (Republished from Phonak; with permission.)

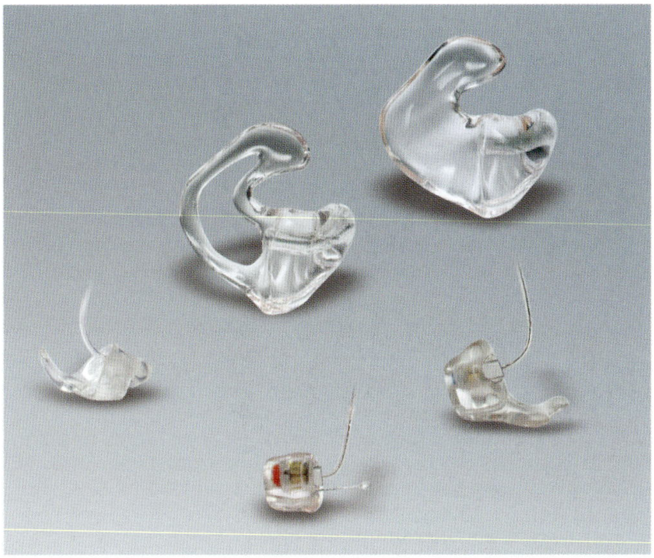

Fig. 8.3 Examples of various earmolds used to couple with behind-the-ear (BTE) or receiver-in-the-canal (RIC) hearing instruments. Size and style vary depending on individual factors such as degree of hearing loss and ear canal anatomy. (Republished from Siemens Hearing USA; with permission.)

munication partners should be oriented, as well. Patients require an understanding of the hearing aid features, overall use (including, but not limited to insertion, removal, program button, volume control), and general maintenance and care. Cognition, memory, and physical factors should be kept in mind when orienting an elderly person to a hearing aid. The older patient may require more and different reinforcement. The clinician should speak at a slow rate to ensure adequate speech understanding; however, it is advised that the clinician not adopt an exaggerated tone, because this can be misconstrued as condescending.

Smith and West discussed the importance of positive reinforcement when working with elderly hearing aid patients.[18] They also stressed emphasizing self-efficacy, even if it means presenting information in a very simple manner. The audiologist should be prepared with vision-enhancing aids such as a magnifying glass to ensure that the patient can see small components of the hearing aid. It can also be helpful to point out tactile landmarks such as the catch on the battery door. Sufficient time should be spent ensuring that the patient can insert/remove the hearing aids, change the batteries, and perform basic maintenance. Realistic expectations and a wearing schedule should be reviewed with the patient at this appointment as well.

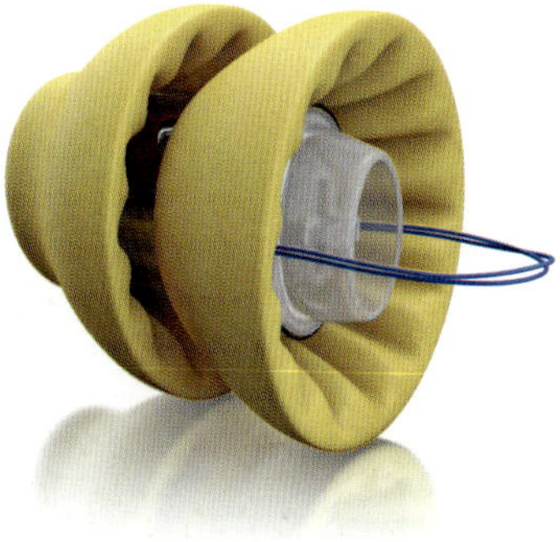

Fig. 8.4 An example of the only extended-wear hearing aid available, known as the Lyric (Phonak). (Republished from Phonak; with permission.)

Postfitting Process

Following the initial fitting, the patient should return for a postfitting appointment to ensure that the hearing aids have been used correctly. It is possible that the clinician may have to review the same procedures that were discussed in the fitting appointment. Postfitting questionnaires can help to determine benefit from the patient's perspective. If the patient is unsatisfied with the hearing aids at this point, the audiologist should determine why. There are many adjustments that can be made to the hearing aid circuitry. The audiologist should be prepared to counsel the patient and family as needed; modify the aids, change the number of aids worn, repeat counseling, and apply any intervention strategy needed to help elderly patients use hearing aids successfully.

Summary

Selecting amplification for any patient requires careful individualized consideration of numerous objective factors. These considerations become especially crucial when fitting the elderly population. Sensory deficits as well as issues with cognition, memory, and motor factors require extra care on both the part of the audiologist as well as the family or caregivers throughout the entire fitting process and thereafter. Counseling in particular becomes especially important, because there are various psychological effects due to hearing loss involved in addition to the hearing deficit itself. An individualized aural rehabilitation plan must be created to ensure that all needs of each individual are met.

References

1. Ciorba A, Bianchini C, Pelucchi S, Pastore A. The impact of hearing loss on the quality of life of elderly adults. Clin Interv Aging 2012;7:159–163
2. Weinstein B. Geriatric Audiology. 2nd ed. New York, NY: Thieme; 2013
3. Wong TP. Aging of the cerebral cortex. McGill J Med 2002; 6:104–113
4. Erber NP. Use of hearing aids by older people: influence of non-auditory factors (vision, manual dexterity). Int J Audiol 2003;42(Suppl 2):S21–S25
5. George ELJ, Zekveld AA, Kramer SE, Goverts ST, Festen JM, Houtgast T. Auditory and nonauditory factors affecting speech reception in noise by older listeners. J Acoust Soc Am 2007;121(4):2362–2375
6. Humes LE, Burk MH, Strauser LE, Kinney DL. Development and efficacy of a frequent-word auditory training protocol for older adults with impaired hearing. Ear Hear 2009;30(5): 613–627
7. Kochkin S. MarkeTrak VIII: The key influencing factors in hearing aid purchase intent. Hearing Review 2012;19(3):12–25
8. Kochkin S. MarkeTrak VIII: 25 year trends in the hearing health market. The Hearing Review 2009;16(11):12–31
9. Lin FR. Hearing loss and cognition among older adults in the United States. J Gerontol A Biol Sci Med Sci 2011;66(10): 1131–1136
10. Gates GA, Feeney MP, Mills D. Cross-sectional age-changes of hearing in the elderly. Ear Hear 2008;29(6):865–874
11. Arlinger S, Gatehouse S, Bentler RA, et al. Report of the Eriksholm Workshop on auditory deprivation and acclimatization. Ear Hear 1996;17(3, Suppl):87S–98S
12. Cox RM, Alexander GC, Johnson J, Rivera I. Cochlear dead regions in typical hearing aid candidates: prevalence and implications for use of high-frequency speech cues. Ear Hear 2011; 32(3):339–348
13. Ahlstrom JB, Horwitz AR, Dubno JR. Spatial benefit of bilateral hearing AIDS. Ear Hear 2009;30(2):203–218
14. Holmes AE. Bilateral amplification for the elderly: are two aids better than one? Int J Audiol 2003;42(Suppl 2):S63–S67
15. Jerger J, Silman S, Lew HL, Chmiel R. Case studies in binaural interference: converging evidence from behavioral and electrophysiologic measures. J Am Acad Audiol 1993;4(2): 122–131
16. Cox RM, Schwartz KS, Noe CM, Alexander GC. Preference for one or two hearing AIDS among adult patients. Ear Hear 2011;32(2):181–197
17. Ricketts T, Mueller G. Today's hearing aid features: Fluff or true hearing aid benefit? Paper presented at Audiology NOW, 23rd Annual Convention of the American Academy of Audiology; Chicago, IL; April 6-9, 2011
18. Smith SL, West RL. The application of self-efficacy principles to audiologic rehabilitation: a tutorial. Am J Audiol 2006;15(1):46–56

9 Cochlear Implantation in the Elderly

Daniel H. Coelho and Brian J. McKinnon

Introduction

Cochlear implantation (CI) has become a well-established means of addressing severe to profound sensorineural hearing loss in children and adults who cannot benefit from conventional amplification. It is understood to be both clinically effective and cost-effective,[1–3] and it is estimated that over 324,200 patients have received this medical device.[4] Nevertheless, although there is evidence supporting the benefits of CI in the general population, concern remains that there is insufficient evidence to support *geriatric* CI as appropriate, safe, effective, and cost-effective.[5] This chapter provides a broad description of the clinical challenges associated with CI and the potential benefits to recipients.

Epidemiology

Hearing loss is one of the most common disabilities in the elderly, the fastest-growing segment of our population. The U.S. population aged 65 and older will grow from 40.2 million in 2010 (13.5% of the population) to 88.5 million in 2050 (20.5%). One fifth of this 20% will be 85 and older. Studies based on the National Health and Nutrition Examination Survey (NHANES) show that an increasing proportion of the population has age-related hearing loss, reaching over 80% of those over 85 years of age.[6] For up to 10% of older patients with hearing loss, the impairment is so severe that conventional amplification devices fail to provide significant benefit.[7] Beyond speech perception, inability to communicate significantly impacts quality of life and overall well-being and is associated with cognitive impairment, dementia, personality changes, depression, and reduced functional status.[8,9]

Fortunately, as with younger patients, CI has proven to be an extremely effective intervention for older patients and is widely gaining in popularity. Several factors have contributed to the rapid increase in the number of elderly CI recipients. Chief among them is the growth in the overall population over the age of 65, increasing the absolute number of eligible recipients. In addition, not only does the incidence of hearing loss increases with age, but those with hearing loss will experience worsening of their hearing over time. The prevalence of hearing loss nearly doubles with every decade of age.[6] These factors, combined with a small but significant increase in awareness of this technology, have led to more patients opting for CI than ever before. Of all patients receiving CI, the over-65 age cohort is the fastest-growing segment, with the biggest growth in the over-80 subgroup.[6]

Despite the many elderly patients who have benefited from this life-changing technology, the rate of CI use in older adults who meet candidacy criteria is less than 5%.[6] Numerous myths and barriers exist—beliefs widely held by both the public and the medical communities. Among them are the perception that CI is exclusively for congenital hearing loss or children, CI is an untested/experimental technology, outcomes are poor for older adults, CI is not covered by insurance, the surgery poses an unacceptably high risk, or the device is too complicated to use, among others. Referral patterns likewise contribute to the bottleneck of access to CI. Few primary care providers screen for hearing loss at a new patient visit, with even fewer addressing hearing at follow-up visits.[10] In addition, some audiologists and otolaryngologists may have well intentioned though misplaced faith in conventional hearing aids, irrespective of a potential financial disincentive to refer.

Preoperative Considerations

Once an elderly patient has been identified audiologically as a candidate for CI, the process does not differ greatly from that for younger candidates. A thorough history must be obtained, with particular attention given to duration of hearing loss, especially severe-to-profound hearing loss. As with younger patients, speech performance outcomes are closely related to deafness duration and are critical in counseling patients and their family on reasonable expectations. Cognitive evaluations, although not common practice, can help guide assessment and counseling when appropriate.[11] Likewise, insofar as varying etiologies may have a higher risk of labyrinthine ossification (postmeningitic, posttraumatic, ototoxic, etc.), this, too, may influence both preoperative imaging choice and expected performance outcomes. Speech performance and expectations must be managed accordingly if traumatic or incomplete implantation is a possibility.

Careful attention must be paid to medical comorbidities. Although age itself is not a known risk factor for perioperative complications, the likelihood of coexisting cardiopulmonary pathology does increase with age. Medical optimization and clearance by the patient's primary care provider, cardiologist, pulmonologist, and care providers can be extremely helpful in assuring a successful procedure and recovery. Many older patients may be on aspirin, clopidogrel, warfarin, or other anticoagulative therapy. Collaborating with the prescribing physician can help to bridge the perioperative period, leading to a timely transition back to therapeutic anticoagulation.

Intraoperative Considerations

There is a pervasive, but erroneous, perception among both health care professionals and consumers that age is a significant risk factor for general anesthesia and for anesthetic and surgical complications. Current literature suggests that comorbidities and the American Society of Anesthesia (ASA) rating of physical status are more important than age as prognostic factors for adverse anesthetic outcome. Coexisting conditions of advanced age that potentially have an impact on the risk of anesthesia include cardiopulmonary insufficiency, arthritis, hepatorenal disease, endocrine dysfunction, nutritional status, and pharmacokinetic issues.[12]

Coelho et al reviewed 70 patients over the age of 70 undergoing CI and found that general anesthesia is well tolerated without significant risk in the majority of patients.[13] In their review of 50 patients 80 years or older, Carlson and colleagues found no higher rates of surgical complications when compared with younger CI recipients, though they did find a small but statistically significant higher risk of cardiovascular complications and hospital admission rate for this population.[14] Nonetheless, of great import to patients and physicians, there was no mortality associated with this elective procedure. This is not surprising: unlike other, nonelective surgeries that elderly patients frequently must undergo, CI usually requires only 1 to 2 hours to perform with ~ 1.5 to 2.5 hours of general anesthesia. Furthermore, the small incision and minimal blood loss do not result in significant hematologic or fluid imbalance.

Other studies have agreed that age alone is not an independent risk factor in geriatric populations, particularly in the nonemergent or outpatient procedures in geriatric populations. Lau and Brooks demonstrated that age itself is not a reliable predictor of unanticipated hospital admission after laparoscopic cholecystectomy.[15] In comparing age and ASA status, Trus and colleagues and Matin and colleagues independently found no increased risk contribution from age in patients older than 65 years who underwent laparoscopic reflux and urological surgery, respectively.[16,17]

Although "best anesthetic" technique has yet to be defined in patients with cardiovascular disease, hemodynamic stability and speed of recovery are impacted by choice of anesthesia. Kirkbride et al showed improved intraoperative blood pressure maintenance in older outpatients induced with the high-dose inhalation agent sevoflurane compared with those randomly assigned for intravenous propofol induction.[18] In addition to myocardial depressant effects of anesthetic agents, atelectasis associated with mechanical ventilation, and volume loading due to intravenous fluid administration contribute to cardiac and pulmonary complications, including congestive heart failure, hemodynamic instability, and pulmonary insufficiency. Cardiopulmonary complications can be reduced by minimizing intraoperative fluid administration and the duration and amount of anesthesia used. Elderly patients require up to 30% less minimum alveolar concentration of inhalational anesthetic compared with young adults.[19] The use of bispectral index (BIS) monitors may aid in the titration of anesthetic and improve early recovery.[20]

Postoperative Considerations

Surgical complications associated with CI are not increased in the elderly. Specifically, the older patient does not have a higher incidence of flap necrosis, improper electrode placement, infection, facial nerve stimulation or injury, or cerebrospinal fluid (CSF) leakage. In addition, no perioperative deaths have been reported.[14,21,22] Significant postoperative pain or nausea is rarely encountered, and patients frequently return to their normal routine within days. In fact, nausea and vomiting are less common in older than in younger adults.[23]

Postoperative urinary retention has been reported in patients with and without benign prostatic hypertrophy (BPH). Conversely, many CI patients with a history of BPH did not experience postoperative urinary retention.[13] The type of anesthesia administered (including analgesia and sedation) may play an important role in the development of postoperative urinary retention. Derangements of the sympathetic/parasympathetic balance result in increased bladder capacity and decreased rate of bladder contraction. Similarly, opioids relax the detrussor muscle and increase bladder capacity. Other indirect effects of anesthesia contribute to retention, including excessive intravenous volume administration, sedation leading to decreased awareness of bladder filling, and postoperative positioning or situations.[24] Because postoperative urinary retention is a rare complication of general anesthesia, the authors do not routinely place a Foley catheter.

In reviewing the published literature on surgical outcomes in elderly CI recipients, no studies reported a higher rate of device failure (hard or soft), infection, or extrusion. However, certain long-term situations unique to the geriatric population must be considered. For those implants not secured in a bony well or with bony tie-down sutures, the temporalis pocket serves as an important barrier to extrusion or anterior migration. Great care must be taken to avoid tearing the temporalis periosteum or creating an overly large subperiosteal pocket—both of which are more likely in the elderly population—and can result in postoperative migration of the receiver-stimulator. In addition, as patients age, and certainly during periods of poor health, lean body mass decreases.[25] Therefore, the external coil magnet may become too strong, resulting in inadvertent pressure necrosis. Close inspection at each programming session can help to identify this problem and prevent further injury.

Postoperative Audiological and Quality of Life Outcomes

With respect to postoperative rehabilitation, geriatric and younger adult cochlear implant users share similarities in terms of time frames between surgery and activation, the number of initial and follow-up sessions, and program strategies used. There appear to be no apparent differences in the factors used to guide geriatric and younger adult cochlear implant rehabilitation, with speech perception testing being the most important. Reported barriers for geriatric cochlear implant users receiving rehabilitation include reimbursement for services, limited time for rehabilitation services, and transportation.[11]

An excellent review[26] summarizes and details current postoperative audiological and quality of life (QOL) findings. There are several measures and instruments used to assess the audiological and QOL outcomes achieved by geriatric cochlear implant recipients, the complexity of which are beyond the scope of this chapter. The various measures and instruments make comparison of different studies difficult, and on occasion, impractical. Younger adults may have less restrictive candidate criteria, and cochlear implant candidate criteria can vary from country to country; many audiological and QOL outcome tests are specific to language, health system, or country. Although most audiological outcome testing is standardized, not all QOL outcomes instruments are, compounding the challenge. Lastly, there have been substantial advances in available technology over time, with concurrent improvement with CI outcomes, further complicating assessment of long-term performance, as well as comparison of current cochlear implant user outcomes with past cochlear implant user outcomes.

However, there are consistent trends being identified.[26] Geriatric cochlear implant users enjoy improved speech perception and have outcomes for speech perception in quiet that are comparable to younger cochlear implant users. Younger postlingual cochlear implant users do have better speech perception in noise than geriatric cochlear implant users, which may reflect a longer duration of hearing loss and poorer preoperative speech perception in the latter group. Geriatric patients tend to have a somewhat slower rate of speech perception gain. However, there is evidence of a strong correlation between length of daily cochlear implant use and speech perception performance. When preoperative speech perception was taken into account, age was not predictive of postoperative speech perception outcome.

Interestingly, unilateral geriatric cochlear implant users report a speech perception benefit similar to younger unilateral cochlear implant users, but less speech perception benefit was reported by bilateral geriatric cochlear implant users than by unilateral geriatric cochlear implant users or younger bilateral cochlear implant users.[26] Although many geriatric cochlear implant users reported continued challenges with telephone conversation, and conversation in noise and groups, larger speech perception gains have been seen in those who report increased social activity. Speech perception achievements appear stable over the long term, and speech perception may continue to improve.[26,27]

In aggregate, QOL outcomes of geriatric cochlear implant users, like speech perception, mirror those of younger cochlear implant users, though validated instruments were not used in many studies.[26] Greater QOL outcomes were seen with greater speech perception scores. Geriatric cochlear implant users show greater confidence and participation in social settings than they did preoperatively. Physical health and social support QOL scores were, in general, not improved. Overall, geriatric cochlear implant users and their families reported high levels of satisfaction and hearing benefits.

Although there is benefit to taking the data in aggregate, as been done here, it is worth taking a closer look at a more detailed level before leaving this topic. The studies that show subtle but significant differences are worthy of closer examination because they may provide insight into the physiology of normal aging. First, some studies show that performance is in fact slightly worse (but still excellent) in older individuals. Second, all geriatric implantees are not the same, and even when controlling for duration of deafness, the cohort over age 70 may not perform as well as those under age 70.[28] Third, the learning curve for older individuals may be different, taking them years to achieve speech recognition levels reached after only 1 year by younger matched adults.[29] Fourth, speech recognition in background noise may be impaired substantially in older individuals—a limitation that, unlike hearing in quiet, does not improve with time.[30] Fifth, similar to some studies in children but unlike matched adults, side may play a role in outcomes, with right side implantation resulting in improved speech perception.[31]

Economic assessment of efficacy further finds that geriatric CI compares favorably with pediatric and adult CI, despite shorter life expectancy,[32] and that rates of long-term use and nonuse compare favorably with children and adult recipients.[33–35] Nonetheless, funding and reimbursement issues are particularly relevant in this patient population. A RAND Corporation–funded study reviewed payments received for cochlear implants by providers and facilities in the United States and found substantial shortfalls in reimbursement.[36] With Medicare alone, the study determined that on average a hospital faced a $5,000 to $10,000 loss on every Medicare patient implanted, making the provision of CI to geriatric candidates economically tenuous.[37] Additionally, Medicare uses candidate criteria that are significantly more restrictive than those put forward by the Food and Drug Administration.[38] Such selection biases likely skew the outcomes data, underrepresenting the true benefit for older patients with moderate-to-severe hearing loss. Taken together, the lack of adequate reimbursement and the restrictive candidate criteria risk reduced access to CI for many geriatric patients who could benefit. Attempts to improve levels of reimbursement for cochlear implants are being impeded by the trend to control health care costs in the context of the current economic and political era, and the implementation of health care reform legislation, the Patient Protection and Affordable Care Act.[39]

Conclusion

An important question to consider asks not only what the geriatric patient can teach us about CI, but also what CI can teach us about the geriatric patient. The answers may lie within what is already known about CI. Cochlear implants have been studied sufficiently in the geriatric population to conclude that geriatric patients with severe-to-profound hearing loss achieve substantial and incontrovertible benefit from CI compared with no intervention or conventional hearing aids. In aggregate, many studies show that the benefit for older individuals (variably defined but generally older than 65) is comparable to that for younger matched adult controls.

Although geriatric CI candidates and recipients face many hurdles, there is growing evidence to support geriatric CI as appropriate, safe, effective, and cost-effective. Despite the evidence, access to CI and cochlear implant services will remain constrained due to restrictive candidate criteria and inadequate reimbursement. Efforts should be made to resolve these impediments so that CI can be made available to any geriatric patient likely to benefit from this remarkable technology.

References

1. Bond M, Elston J, Mealing S, et al. Effectiveness of multi-channel unilateral cochlear implants for profoundly deaf children: a systematic review. Clin Otolaryngol 2009;34(3):199–211
2. Bond M, Mealing S, Anderson R, et al. The effectiveness and cost-effectiveness of cochlear implants for severe to profound deafness in children and adults: a systematic review and economic model. Health Technol Assess 2009;13(44):1–330
3. Bond M, Elston J, Mealing S, et al. Systematic reviews of the effectiveness and cost-effectiveness of multi-channel unilateral cochlear implants for adults. Clin Otolaryngol 2010;35(2): 87–96
4. National Institute on Deafness and Other Communication Disorders. Cochlear implants. http://www.nidcd.nih.gov/health/hearing/pages/coch.aspx. Accessed February 21, 2014
5. Centers for Medicare and Medicaid Services. Effectiveness of Cochlear Implants in Adults with Sensorineural Hearing Loss. http://www.cms.gov/medicare-coverage-database/details/technology-assessments-details.aspx?TAId=80&bc=AAAQAAAAAAAA&. Accessed February 21, 2014
6. Lin FR. Hearing loss and cognition among older adults in the United States. J Gerontol A Biol Sci Med Sci 2011;66(10): 1131–1136
7. Havlik RJ. Aging in the eighties, impaired senses for sound and light in persons age 65 years and over. Adv Data 1986;125:1–7
8. Mulrow CD, Aguilar C, Endicott JE, et al. Association between hearing impairment and the quality of life of elderly individuals. J Am Geriatr Soc 1990;38(1):45–50
9. Cacciatore F, Napoli C, Abete P, Marciano E, Triassi M, Rengo F. Quality of life determinants and hearing function in an elderly population: Osservatorio Geriatrico Campano Study Group. Gerontology 1999;45(6):323–328
10. Yueh B, Shapiro N, MacLean CH, Shekelle PG. Screening and management of adult hearing loss in primary care: scientific review. JAMA 2003;289(15):1976–1985
11. Rossi-Katz J, Arehart KH. Survey of audiologic service provision to older adults with cochlear implants. Am J Audiol 2011;20(2):84–89
12. Beliveau MM, Multach M. Perioperative care for the elderly patient. Med Clin North Am 2003;87(1):273–289
13. Coelho DH, Yeh J, Kim JT, Lalwani AK. Cochlear implantation is associated with minimal anesthetic risk in the elderly. Laryngoscope 2009;119(2):355–358
14. Carlson ML, Breen JT, Gifford RH, et al. Cochlear implantation in the octogenarian and nonagenarian. Otol Neurotol 2010;31(8):1343–1349
15. Lau H, Brooks DC. Predictive factors for unanticipated admissions after ambulatory laparoscopic cholecystectomy. Arch Surg 2001;136(10):1150–1153
16. Trus TL, Laycock WS, Wo JM, et al. Laparoscopic antireflux surgery in the elderly. Am J Gastroenterol 1998;93(3): 351–353
17. Matin SF, Abreu S, Ramani A, et al. Evaluation of age and comorbidity as risk factors after laparoscopic urological surgery. J Urol 2003;170(4 Pt 1):1115–1120
18. Kirkbride DA, Parker JL, Williams GD, Buggy DJ. Induction of anesthesia in the elderly ambulatory patient: a double-blinded comparison of propofol and sevoflurane. Anesth Analg 2001;93(5):1185–1187
19. Gold MI, Abello D, Herrington C. Minimum alveolar concentration of desflurane in patients older than 65 yr. Anesthesiology 1993;79(4):710–714
20. Wong J, Song D, Blanshard H, Grady D, Chung F. Titration of isoflurane using BIS index improves early recovery of elderly patients undergoing orthopedic surgeries. Can J Anaesth 2002;49(1):13–18
21. Chatelin V, Kim EJ, Driscoll C, et al. Cochlear implant outcomes in the elderly. Otol Neurotol 2004;25(3):298–301
22. Alice B, Silvia M, Laura G, Patrizia T, Roberto B. Cochlear implantation in the elderly: surgical and hearing outcomes. BMC Surg 2013;13(Suppl 2):S1
23. Sinclair DR, Chung F, Mezei G. Can postoperative nausea and vomiting be predicted? Anesthesiology 1999;91(1): 109–118
24. Pertek JP, Haberer JP. [Effects of anesthesia on postoperative micturition and urinary retention]. Ann Fr Anesth Reanim 1995;14(4):340–351
25. Reife CM. Involuntary weight loss. Med Clin North Am 1995;79(2):299–313
26. Clark JH, Yeagle J, Arbaje AI, Lin FR, Niparko JK, Francis HW. Cochlear implant rehabilitation in older adults: literature review and proposal of a conceptual framework. J Am Geriatr Soc 2012;60(10):1936–1945
27. Dillon MT, Buss E, Adunka MC, et al. Long-term speech perception in elderly cochlear implant users. JAMA Otolaryngol Head Neck Surg 2013;139(3):279–283
28. Lin FR, Chien WW, Li L, Clarrett DM, Niparko JK, Francis HW. Cochlear implantation in older adults. Medicine (Baltimore) 2012;91(5):229–241
29. Herzog M, Schön F, Müller J, Knaus C, Scholtz L, Helms J. Long term results after cochlear implantation in elderly patients [in German]. Laryngorhinootologie 2003;82(7):490–493
30. Lenarz M, Sönmez H, Joseph G, Büchner A, Lenarz T. Cochlear implant performance in geriatric patients. Laryngoscope 2012;122(6):1361–1365
31. Budenz CL, Cosetti MK, Coelho DH, et al. The effects of cochlear implantation on speech perception in older adults. J Am Geriatr Soc 2011;59(3):446–453
32. Francis HW, Chee N, Yeagle J, Cheng A, Niparko JK. Impact of cochlear implants on the functional health status of older adults. Laryngoscope 2002;112(8 Pt 1):1482–1488
33. Choi JS, Contrera KJ, Betz JF, Blake CR, Niparko JK, Lin FR. Long-term use of cochlear implants in older adults: results from a large consecutive case series. Otol Neurotol 2014;35(5): 815–820
34. Contrera KJ, Choi JS, Blake CR, Betz JF, Niparko JK, Lin FR. Rates of long-term cochlear implant use in children. Otol Neurotol 2014;35(3):426–430
35. Bhatt YM, Green KM, Mawman DJ, et al. Device nonuse among adult cochlear implant recipients. Otol Neurotol 2005;26(2):183–187
36. Garber S, Ridgely MS, Bradley M, Chin KW. Payment under public and private insurance and access to cochlear implants. Arch Otolaryngol Head Neck Surg 2002;128(10):1145–1152
37. McKinnon BJ. Cochlear implant programs: balancing clinical and financial sustainability. Laryngoscope 2013;123(1): 233–238
38. Centers for Medicare and Medicaid Services. Medicare Benefit Policy Manual. Decision Memo for Cochlear Implantation (CAG-00107N). 4 April 2005. https://www.cms.gov/medicare-coverage-database/details/nca-decision-memo.aspx?NCAId=134&ver=15&NcaName=Cochlear+Implantation&NCDId=245&ncdver=1&IsPopup=y&bc=AAAAAAAAEAAA&. Accessed February 21, 2014
39. Pensak ML. Healthcare transformation: implications for implantation. Curr Opin Otolaryngol Head Neck Surg 2009; 17(5):333

10 Subjective Idiopathic Tinnitus in the Geriatric Population

Paul F. Shea and Brian J. McKinnon

Introduction

Tinnitus is the perception of sound in the absence of an external auditory stimulus; tinnitus can be distressing and annoying, contributing to disruption of sleep, anxiety, and depression.[1] It has been reported that 16% of the general population have experienced tinnitus to some extent.[1] About 25 to 30% of those who report tinnitus seek medical help; ~ 2 to 4% of all those with tinnitus report being unable to lead a normal life because of their tinnitus.[1] Nearly a quarter of geriatric patients report tinnitus, a finding that has been stable for some time; the rate of distress and negative impact is higher than in younger patients, and the perceived severity increases with later onset of tinnitus.[2–5]

Tinnitus can be separated into two broad categories, objective and subjective. Objective tinnitus can be heard by both the patient and the examiner. It is less common than subjective tinnitus and can be caused by somatosounds. Subjective tinnitus is perceived only by the patient and may be idiopathic or secondary to another disorder. Tinnitus is commonly associated with hearing loss, traumatic brain injury, ototoxicity, and other conditions.[1] When a diagnosis can be identified to which the tinnitus may be secondary, such as Ménière disease, otitis media, or cerumen impaction, treatment of the condition may provide improvement in the tinnitus.[6,7] A significant percentage of tinnitus patients with normal hearing have abnormalities of outer hair cell function that can be measured by otoacoustic emissions, as well as abnormal central activity measured by auditory brainstem responses,[8,9] and these cases are therefore not strictly idiopathic. Thus an effort should be made to identify any underlying conditions before making the diagnosis of idiopathic tinnitus. This review discusses subjective idiopathic tinnitus that is bothersome and that persists for longer than 6 months in the geriatric patient.

Evaluation

The evaluation of the geriatric patient with tinnitus does not differ significantly from that of other patients with hearing loss or tinnitus. A complete otolaryngological history is taken, and a physical examination is performed.[6,10] In the geriatric patient, attention should be paid to family medical history (particularly to hearing loss history) past and present noise exposure (both recreational and work related), use of hearing protection, past and current medications, previous surgery, and past hearing aid use. It should not be assumed that geriatric patients are inactive and free of ongoing noise exposure. A history of arthritis, head injury, or smoking is associated with an increased risk of developing tinnitus.[11] The concurrent complaint of anxiety and insomnia is also common in this population.[12,13]

A challenge in the evaluation of the geriatric tinnitus patient is the lack of a generally accepted instrument to document or describe the nature, severity, or quality of tinnitus. Visual analog scale scores can be used to assess loudness, pitch, and disturbance of the tinnitus. Questionnaires such as the Tinnitus Handicap Inventory and the Tinnitus Reaction can help with grading the tinnitus severity.[1,14] The Tinnitus Functional Index has the advantage of being able both to grade tinnitus severity and to measure effectiveness of tinnitus interventions.[1,15]

Physical examination should include meticulous otoscopy (ideally with magnification), and audiological testing. Auscultation should be performed in complaints of pulsatile tinnitus. Audiological testing should not be limited to routine audiometry and tympanometry; otoacoustic emission testing and auditory brainstem response can help identify possible causes, even in those with normal routine audiometry.[6,8,9] Laboratory tests such as autoimmune studies, tests for infectious causes (e.g., Lyme disease, syphilis), thyroid studies, hematocrit, blood chemistry, lipid profile, and others should be considered based on the level of suspicion created by the history and physical exam.[6,16]

Imaging is not performed routinely in elderly patients with symmetric hearing loss or tinnitus, nor in those with nonbothersome symmetric tinnitus without hearing loss. Imaging should be considered in patients with asymmetric hearing loss and tinnitus, asymmetric tinnitus without hearing loss, and pulsatile tinnitus.[6,10] An excellent algorithm for the evaluation of pulsatile tinnitus is described by Mattox and Hudgins.[17]

Management

Despite the immense amount of literature on the management of tinnitus, there is a dearth of studies of sufficient quality to permit specific recommendations regarding treatment.[1] Very little of the literature is specific to the management of tinnitus in the geriatric patient, and the studies that do exist are of insufficient quality to guide age-specific recommendations.

Currently there is no Food and Drug Administration (FDA)-approved pharmaceutical agent for tinnitus, and evidence-based pharmacological approaches are limited to the treatment of comorbidities such as depression, anxiety, and insomnia.[18] Many medications recommended to assist in the management of tinnitus (antidepressants, anticonvulsants, anxiolytics, and herbal preparations) may be inappropriate or unsafe in the geriatric patient, and some may exacerbate tinnitus.[1,19] Intratympanic medications studied in randomized, controlled trials have not shown benefit; in the case of lidocaine, no randomized, controlled trials have been performed,[1,18] and no conclusion can be drawn toward efficacy or safety. Novel therapies, such as acupuncture,[20,21] hold promise in the adult tinnitus population and await study in the geriatric tinnitus population, although benefit has not been established for hypnosis.[22–24]

Because cochlear implantation is not currently approved by the FDA for the management of tinnitus, this chapter does not review cochlear implantation for tinnitus management in the geriatric patient. However, it should be noted that tinnitus can improve in geriatric patients who undergo unilateral and bilateral cochlear implantation for severe to profound hearing loss.[25,26]

With the dearth of evidence supporting the safety or efficacy of pharmacological management of tinnitus, alternative therapies should be considered. In 2009, the UK Department of Health issued the Provision of Services for Adults with Tinnitus.[27] The recommendations included providing tinnitus patients with information/education, hearing aids, psychological support, relaxation therapy, cognitive behavioral therapy (CBT), sleep management, sound enrichment therapy, and habituation therapies.[27,28] These guidelines were not specific to the geriatric population and did not provide specific recommendations for assessing therapeutic benefit.[28] However, the guidelines do suggest a systematic and orderly approach to the management of the tinnitus patient. Of those therapies recommended by the guidelines, educational counseling and CBT appear to hold significant promise of benefit.

Progressive audiologic tinnitus management (PATM) is a form of educational counseling that is individualized to meet the needs of the patient, and it is modeled closely after similar programs used to manage chronic pain.[29] The program shifts the responsibility of tinnitus management from the provider to the patient. This is accomplished by helping patients gain an understanding of what tinnitus is, participate in decision making, develop and follow the plan of care, learn to manage the impact of the tinnitus on their daily life, and monitor their own progress. The plan of care may be modified as needed. Although geriatric-specific tinnitus research is not available, a component of PATM, CBT, has been studied in the geriatric tinnitus patient.

CBT can be combined with PATM or can be provided as a stand-alone therapy.[1,29,30] Described as a relatively brief psychological treatment approach directed at identifying and modifying maladaptive behaviors and cognition by means of behavior change and cognitive restructuring, CBT aims to decrease the psychological distress associated with tinnitus and is not targeted toward the loudness of tinnitus.[30] CBT can be provided as both individual and group therapy, and it appears to reduce the distress reported by geriatric tinnitus patients substantially.

Tinnitus retraining therapy (TRT) and sound therapy are commonly recommended in tinnitus patients,[1] though research specific to geriatric tinnitus patients is lacking. TRT (which the Provision of Services for Adults with Tinnitus guideline refers to as habituation therapy or simplified tinnitus retraining therapy) and sound therapy (also known as masking) have both been subjects of a Cochrane review.[31,32] Like many of the therapies mentioned previously, the Cochrane review could not make a determination on the efficacy of sound therapy due to the lack of good evidence in the literature.[31] A Cochrane review of TRT did identify a single, low-quality randomized, controlled trial suggesting TRT is more effective than masking[32]; other work has found CBT combined with TRT is beneficial.[33]

Tinnitus often occurs with hearing loss. Hearing aids have been the standard treatment of hearing loss for decades, particularly in geriatric patients, but are increasingly recognized for their role in the treatment of tinnitus as well. This is believed to be accomplished by several mechanisms. Amplification of speech diverts attention away from tinnitus, and amplification of other ambient sounds serves to partially mask tinnitus.[34] Hearing aids have also been developed that can deliver continuous masking noise, and others attempt to transpose the tinnitus with sound of a different frequency. A recent study demonstrated long-term benefit in tinnitus patients with linear octave frequency transposition (LOFT) hearing aids measured with a visual analog scale.[35] More studies are needed to determine which hearing aid programming strategies are most effective for the general and geriatric patients with hearing loss and tinnitus because there has been a lack of evidence supporting the use of hearing aids in the past.[24]

Conclusion

It is well established that geriatric patients find tinnitus disruptive, and with advancing time and age, tinnitus can become more intrusive and burdensome. The concern should be taken seriously, and the evaluation should be meticulous and thorough. The care of the geriatric tinnitus patient requires the recognition that there is little evidence to support aggressive medical or surgical therapy. Interventions making use of educational counseling, hearing aids, CBT, and sound therapy currently appear to hold the best chance of providing relief.

References

1. Pichora-Fuller MK, Santaguida P, Hammill A, et al. Evaluation and Treatment of Tinnitus: Comparative Effectiveness. Rockville, MD: Agency for Healthcare Research and Quality; 2013
2. Sataloff J, Sataloff RT, Lueneburg W. Tinnitus and vertigo in healthy senior citizens without a history of noise exposure. Am J Otol 1987;8(2):87–89
3. Negrila-Mezei A, Enache R, Sarafoleanu C. Tinnitus in elderly population: clinic correlations and impact upon QoL. J Med Life 2011;4(4):412–416
4. Schlee W, Kleinjung T, Hiller W, Goebel G, Kolassa IT, Langguth B. Does tinnitus distress depend on age of onset? PLoS ONE 2011;6(11):e27379
5. Song JJ, De Ridder D, Schlee W, Van de Heyning P, Vanneste S. "Distressed aging": the differences in brain activity between early- and late-onset tinnitus. Neurobiol Aging 2013;34(7):1853–1863
6. Sataloff RT. Tinnitus. In: Sataloff RT, Sataloff JT, eds. Hearing Loss. 4th ed. New York, NY: Taylor and Francis; 2005
7. Baguley D, McFerran D, Hall D. Tinnitus. Lancet 2013; 382(9904):1600–1607
8. Mokrian H, Shaibanizadeh A, Farahani S, et al. Evaluation of distortion and transient evoked otoacoustic emission in tinnitus patients with normal hearing. Iran J Otorhinolaryngol 2014;26(74):19–24
9. Singh S, Munjal SK, Panda NK. Comparison of auditory electrophysiological responses in normal-hearing patients with and without tinnitus. J Laryngol Otol 2011;125(7):668–672
10. McKinnon BJ. Hearing exam. In: Kountakis SE, ed. Encyclopedia of Otolaryngology, Head and Neck Surgery. New Delhi, India: Springer; 2013
11. Nondahl DM, Cruickshanks KJ, Huang GH, et al. Generational differences in the reporting of tinnitus. Ear Hear 2012; 33(5):640–644
12. Lasisi AO, Gureje O. Prevalence of insomnia and impact on quality of life among community elderly subjects with tinnitus. Ann Otol Rhinol Laryngol 2011;120(4):226–230
13. Ooms E, Vanheule S, Meganck R, Vinck B, Watelet JB, Dhooge I. Tinnitus severity and its association with cognitive and somatic anxiety: a critical study. Eur Arch Otorhinolaryngol 2012;269(11):2327–2333
14. Kamalski DM, Hoekstra CE, van Zanten BG, Grolman W, Rovers MM. Measuring disease-specific health-related quality of life to evaluate treatment outcomes in tinnitus patients: a systematic review. Otolaryngol Head Neck Surg 2010;143(2): 181–185
15. Meikle MB, Henry JA, Griest SE, et al. The tinnitus functional index: development of a new clinical measure for chronic, intrusive tinnitus. Ear Hear 2012;33(2):153–176
16. Crummer RW, Hassan GA. Diagnostic approach to tinnitus. Am Fam Physician 2004;69(1):120–126
17. Mattox DE, Hudgins P. Algorithm for evaluation of pulsatile tinnitus. Acta Otolaryngol 2008;128(4):427–431
18. Langguth B, Elgoyhen AB. Current pharmacological treatments for tinnitus. Expert Opin Pharmacother 2012;13(17): 2495–2509
19. American Geriatrics Society 2012 Beers Criteria Update Expert Panel. American Geriatrics Society updated Beers Criteria for potentially inappropriate medication use in older adults. J Am Geriatr Soc 2012;60(4):616–631
20. Park J, White AR, Ernst E. Efficacy of acupuncture as a treatment for tinnitus: a systematic review. Arch Otolaryngol Head Neck Surg 2000;126(4):489–492
21. Kim JI, Choi JY, Lee DH, Choi TY, Lee MS, Ernst E. Acupuncture for the treatment of tinnitus: a systematic review of randomized clinical trials. BMC Complement Altern Med 2012;12(12):97
22. Dobie RA. A review of randomized clinical trials in tinnitus. Laryngoscope 1999;109(8):1202–1211
23. Frank W, Konta B, Seiler G. Therapy of unspecific tinnitus without organic cause. GMS Health Technol Assess 2006;2: Doc17
24. Savage J, Cook S, Waddell A. Tinnitus. Clin Evid (Online) 2009;2009. pii: 0506
25. Olze H, Gräbel S, Förster U, et al. Elderly patients benefit from cochlear implantation regarding auditory rehabilitation, quality of life, tinnitus, and stress. Laryngoscope 2012;122(1): 196–203
26. Olze H, Gräbel S, Haupt H, Förster U, Mazurek B. Extra benefit of a second cochlear implant with respect to health-related quality of life and tinnitus. Otol Neurotol 2012;33(7): 1169–1175
27. Department of Health. Provision of Services for Adults with Tinnitus. A Good Practice Guide. London, UK: Central Office of Information; 2009

28. Hoare DJ, Gander PE, Collins L, Smith S, Hall DA. Management of tinnitus in English NHS audiology departments: an evaluation of current practice. J Eval Clin Pract 2012;18(2): 326–334
29. Henry JA, Zaugg TL, Myers PJ, Kendall CJ, Turbin MB. Principles and application of educational counseling used in progressive audiologic tinnitus management. Noise Health 2009;11(42):33–48
30. Andersson G, Porsaeus D, Wiklund M, Kaldo V, Larsen HC. Treatment of tinnitus in the elderly: a controlled trial of cognitive behavior therapy. Int J Audiol 2005;44(11):671–675
31. Hobson J, Chisholm E, El Refaie A. Sound therapy (masking) in the management of tinnitus in adults. Cochrane Database Syst Rev 2012;11(11):CD006371
32. Phillips JS, McFerran D. Tinnitus Retraining Therapy (TRT) for tinnitus. Cochrane Database Syst Rev 2010;17(3): CD007330
33. Cima RF, Maes IH, Joore MA, et al. Specialised treatment based on cognitive behaviour therapy versus usual care for tinnitus: a randomised controlled trial. Lancet 2012;379(9830): 1951–1959
34. Han BI, Lee HW, Kim TY, Lim JS, Shin KS. Tinnitus: characteristics, causes, mechanisms, and treatments. J Clin Neurol 2009;5(1):11–19
35. Peltier E, Peltier C, Tahar S, Alliot-Lugaz E, Cazals Y. Long-term tinnitus suppression with linear octave frequency transposition hearing aids. PLoS ONE 2012;7(12):e51915

11 Dizziness, Imbalance, and Age-Related Vestibular Loss in the Geriatric Population

Yuri Agrawal, Allan Rubin, and Stephen J. Wetmore

■ Introduction

Dizziness and imbalance are common conditions affecting the elderly population. They can be challenging to manage given that the symptoms can be nonspecific and may represent multiple underlying diagnoses. This chapter begins by defining dizziness and imbalance in the elderly and describing *age-related vestibular loss* (ARVL), which is of particular interest to the geriatric otolaryngologist. The chapter then reviews the epidemiology of dizziness, imbalance, and ARVL and discusses the physiological and pathological evidence for ARVL. Finally, the chapter reviews the evaluation and management of an older patient with dizziness and imbalance and closes with a discussion of falls risk assessment.

■ Definitions of Dizziness and Imbalance in the Geriatric Population

Dizziness connotes a subjective perception of disorientation or involuntary motion, which can occur during movement or at rest.[1] Dizziness can be subdivided further into the subtypes of vertigo and presyncopal lightheadedness. Vertigo is the false sensation that either the body or the environment is moving (usually spinning) and may be a symptom of vestibular, visual, or neurological impairment, psychological factors, or the use of multiple medications (polypharmacy). Vertigo that occurs in the elderly has been termed presbyvertigo. Presyncopal lightheadedness is the sensation of impending faint associated with transient diffuse cerebral hypoperfusion. Causal factors for lightheadedness include cardiovascular disease and orthostatic hypotension (e.g., resulting from excessive medication use or autonomic instability). Imbalance can be equated with disequilibrium, and it connotes a sense of postural instability generally associated with the trunk and legs without a sensation in the head.[2] Imbalance is usually described either while standing or walking and typically does not occur at rest. Imbalance results from neuromuscular impairment related to muscle weakness, loss of peripheral sensation or proprioception, and/or arthritis. The imbalance or disequilibrium that occurs with aging has been termed presbystasis or presbyequilibrium.

The typology of dizziness and imbalance is conceptualized in **Fig. 11.1** as a set of overlapping conditions. Age-related vestibular loss (ARVL), which is in the realm of geriatric otolaryngology, is also depicted. The vestibular system plays an integral role in maintaining the vestibulo-ocular and vestibulospinal reflexes (VOR and VSR). The VOR is important for stabilization of gaze during head movement, and VOR impairment manifests as dizziness (i.e., abnormal sensation of motion). The VSR is important for trunk and limb stabilization during head movement. VSR dysfunction manifests as postural instability. The VOR and VSR are depicted in **Fig. 11.1** as the overlap between ARVL and presbyvertigo and presbystasis, respectively. Interestingly, there is increasing recognition of the physiological importance of vestibuloautonomic projections. Vestibuloautonomic impairment has been associated with orthostatic hypotension.[3] Thus ARVL may also be a causal factor for the symptom of presyncopal lightheadedness. Emerging evidence is suggesting that a certain amount of ARVL is present in older individuals but may not be manifesting symptomatically as dizziness or imbalance.[4,5] This may be because the level of vestibular impairment has not crossed a critical threshold, or because an individual is able to compensate for the ARVL. ARVL is thus depicted in **Fig. 11.1** as asymptomatic or "subclinical" and symptomatic or "clinical."

As is evident in **Fig. 11.1**, multiple causative factors have been associated with dizziness and imbalance in the geriatric population. It is well known among researchers who study aging that geriatric conditions often result from numerous coexisting

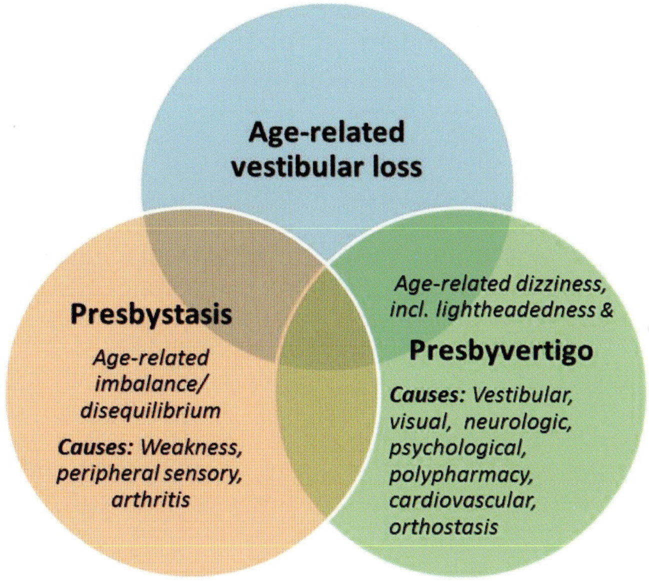

Fig. 11.1 Typology of age-related dizziness, imbalance, and vestibular loss. VOR, vestibulo-ocular reflex; VSR vestibulospinal reflex.

factors that may interact to have nonlinear, synergistic effects. Indeed, Tinetti and colleagues have described dizziness as a geriatric syndrome whereby symptoms result not from sole disease entities but from accumulated impairment in multiple systems.[6] As a corollary, the authors suggest that the management of geriatric syndromes requires multifactorial interventions, or alternatively a focus on improving functional outcomes irrespective of the complex web of etiologic factors.

Epidemiology of Dizziness, Imbalance, and Age-Related Vestibular Loss in the Geriatric Population

Estimates of the prevalence of dizziness and imbalance in the geriatric population depend largely on the definitions of dizziness and imbalance used, and on the populations surveyed. Definitions vary as noted previously. The populations surveyed can vary with respect to their age ranges, whether they are population-based or clinic-based, and what types of clinics are being studied (e.g., primary vs. specialty care). Several large population-based studies have found a 20 to 30% prevalence of dizziness and imbalance in the elderly population (age ≥ 65 years).[7–9] The prevalence of dizziness and imbalance rises steeply with age, with levels over 50% in the community-dwelling population over age 80.[10] A study in institutionalized nursing home residents observed a prevalence of dizziness and vertigo of 68%.[11] Among patients presenting to a primary care clinic, 24% reported dizziness and 17% identified dizziness as their major presenting complaint.[12] Within the otolaryngology clinic, one study of 131,000 consecutive patients found that 6% of patients over age 65 presented with vertigo or a presumed vestibular diagnosis.[13] Interestingly, this large-scale survey of otolaryngological practice found that visits from geriatric patients increased from 14.3% in 2004 to 17.9% in 2010. Moreover, this study noted that the five most common geriatric diagnoses were otologic (including hearing loss, external ear disorders, tinnitus, otitis media/eustachian tube disorders, and vertigo).

A landmark series of studies based in Germany estimated the population prevalence and incidence more specifically of vestibular vertigo (i.e., vertigo resulting from vestibular impairment). Community-dwelling participants in a national telephone survey were queried about symptoms of dizziness and vertigo. Those who reported moderate symptoms were administered a detailed neurotologic interview, from which vestibular vertigo was diagnosed based on symptoms of rotational vertigo, positional vertigo, or recurrent dizziness with nausea and oscillopsia or imbalance. Of note, the neurotologic interview was found to have good validity based on a gold standard of neurotology clinic–based diagnosis in establishing a vestibular diagnosis. The lifetime prevalence, 1-year prevalence, and incidence of vestibular vertigo were observed to be 7.8%, 4.9%, and 1.5%, respectively.[14] The 1-year prevalence of vestibular vertigo increased with age to 7.2% in those aged 60 to 69 and 8.8% in individuals over age 80. This study was among the first to estimate the population prevalence of ARVL.

A more recent study estimated the prevalence of vestibular impairment in the U.S. population using an objective, rather than subjective (self-report based), test. Data were drawn from the 2001–2004 National Health and Nutrition Examination Survey (NHANES). Vestibular function was assessed in NHANES using the modified Romberg test, whereby vestibular impairment was inferred from an inability to stand on a foam pad with eyes closed. Thirty-five percent of U.S. adults age 40 years and older had evidence of balance dysfunction based on this postural metric.[4] The odds of balance dysfunction increased significantly with age, such that 85% of individuals age 80 and above had evidence of balance dysfunction. These estimates are considerably higher than the prevalences of vestibular vertigo mentioned earlier from the German population. It is possible that the symptom of vestibular vertigo represents a component of *clinical* ARVL, whereas vestibular impairment based on the modified Romberg test represents *subclinical* ARVL.

Epidemiological analyses of dizziness, imbalance. and ARVL have also investigated risk factors for these conditions. Most studies have observed an increased prevalence of dizziness and imbalance in women.[1] Vestibular vertigo was also more prevalent in women.[15] However, the prevalence of vestibular impairment based on objective modified Romberg testing did not differ by gender.[4] Findings from a review of the most frequently reported causes of dizziness in primary care practice are presented in **Table 11.1**.[1] The review found that peripheral vestibular disease was the most common cause of dizziness, observed in 20 to 50% of cases. Peripheral vestibular diseases included benign paroxysmal positional vertigo (BPPV), labyrinthitis, and vestibular neuritis. Other common causes of dizziness were cardiovascular disease, systemic infection (leading to orthostatic hypotension), psychiatric disorders, metabolic disturbances, and use of multiple medications. A more recent epidemiological survey of the elderly population in England found that dizziness was associated with abnormal heart rhythm, hearing loss, vision loss, and low grip strength, whereas imbalance was associated with diabetes, arthritis, low grip strength, and vision loss.[8] With respect to vestibular vertigo, independent risk factors were depression, tinnitus, and cardiovascular risk factors, including hypertension and dyslipidemia.[14] Finally, independent risk factors for vestibular impairment as measured by the modified Romberg test included low socioeconomic status and diabetes mellitus.[4,16]

Epidemiological studies also have examined the impact of dizziness, imbalance, and ARVL on diverse outcomes, including falls, quality of life, health care utilization, and other economic outcomes. Dizziness has been associated with a two- to threefold increased risk of falling.[4,10] Specifically with respect to ARVL, the study from NHANES found that individuals with objective vestibular impairment who were also clinically symptomatic (i.e., reported dizziness) had a 12-fold increase in the odds of falling. In a small pilot study, older fallers were found to have significantly higher rates of peripheral vestibular dysfunction than older nonfallers.[17] A prospective study reported that elderly patients with vestibular asymmetry were significantly more likely to experience an incident fall.[18] Moreover, several studies have

Table 11.1 Most common causes of dizziness in primary care practice

Category	Percent	Examples
Peripheral vestibular disease	20–50	Benign paroxysmal positional vertigo (BPPV), labyrinthitis, vestibular neuritis
Cardiovascular disease	10–30	Arrhythmia, congestive heart failure, vasovagal conditions (e.g., carotid sinus hypersensitivity)
Systemic infection	10–20	Systemic viral and bacterial infection
Psychiatric conditions	5–15	Depression, anxiety, hyperventilation
Metabolic disturbances	5–10	Hypoglycemia, hyperglycemia, electrolyte disturbances, thyrotoxicosis, anemia
Medications	5–10	Antihypertensives, psychotropic medications

Data from Sloane PD, Coeytaux RR, Beck RS, Dallara J. Dizziness: state of the science. Ann Intern Med 2001;134(9 Pt 2):823–832.

observed an association between vestibular asymmetry and fall-related hip and wrist fracture risk.[19–21]

Quality of life measures assess general quality of life (e.g., the Short-Form Health Survey [SF-36]) as well as health-related quality of life (i.e., related to a specific health condition). Dizziness and vestibular vertigo have been associated with significantly poorer quality of life, in both the physical and the mental domains. One population-based study in Sweden found that dizziness was one of the most influential symptoms affecting general quality of life in older individuals.[22] The most widely used measures of dizziness- and imbalance-related quality of life are the Dizziness Handicap Inventory (DHI),[23] the Activities Balance Confidence (ABC) scale,[24] and the Falls Efficacy scale (which measures fear of falling).[25] Two studies that administered the DHI in patients presenting with dizziness to a primary care clinic and a specialized dizziness clinic found that over 60% of patients reported moderate to severe handicap associated with their dizziness in both clinical contexts.[26,27] With respect to health care utilization and economic outcomes, the German population-based study found that vestibular vertigo was more likely than nonvestibular vertigo to be associated with a medical consultation, sick leave, interruption of daily activities, and avoidance of leaving the house.[28] Similarly, a population-based study in the United States observed that 50% of older individuals with dizziness and balance problems saw at least one medical provider, and 35% saw three or more providers.[29] A single provocative longitudinal study found that patients with disequilibrium at baseline were at significantly increased risk only for new-onset cognitive decline compared with controls.[30]

The epidemiological data reviewed thus far suggest that dizziness, imbalance, and ARVL are prevalent in the population and have significant clinical, functional, and economic implications. Several final points deserve mention at the conclusion of this section. First, as has been highlighted by numerous authors, the goal of research on dizziness and imbalance in the geriatric population should be the development of evidence-based clinical practice guidelines for the effective diagnosis and management of these conditions.[1] To this end, the use of a common nomenclature is an important first step. Second, although dizziness and imbalance are prevalent in the geriatric population they are not universal. As one study specifically points out, not all individuals over age 90 had dizziness.[10] As such, dizziness and imbalance in the geriatric population may be considered "age-concomitant" rather than "age-dependent" conditions.[10] As a corollary, these conditions should be viewed as pathological, and efforts should be made to treat them. Finally, it follows that the potential scope of managing dizziness and imbalance in the geriatric population is enormous, likely far exceeding the capacity of geriatricians and otologists.[11] Thus it might be necessary to train other types of health care professionals such as nurses and physical therapists to assist more in managing these conditions.

Physiological and Pathological Evidence for Age-Related Vestibular Loss

As already described, there is epidemiological evidence that ARVL is prevalent in the geriatric population. The vestibular system consists of five organs: three semicircular canals (anterior or superior, posterior and horizontal, or lateral), and two otolith organs—the saccule and the utricle (**Fig. 11.2**). The semicircular canals detect angular head rotations along the planes of the canals, whereas the otoliths detect linear translations of the head, as well as head orientation with respect to gravity. The saccular neuroepithelium is oriented in a vertical direction and preferentially detects vertical linear head movements, whereas the utricular neuroepithelium is horizontally oriented and preferentially detects horizontal head movements.

In recent years, numerous vestibular physiological tests have been developed that allow for localization of dysfunction within the five organs of the vestibular system. The most widely used vestibular tests are caloric and rotational chair testing, which evaluate the function of the horizontal semicircular canal.[31] Recently, video-oculography techniques have made possible quantitative angular vestibulo-ocular reflex (AVOR) testing during head impulses to assess the function of each of the six semicircular canals.[32,33] The vestibular-evoked myogenic potential (VEMP) tests are gaining increasing popularity as measures of otolith function. The sound-evoked cervical VEMP (cVEMP) is a product of the sacculocollic reflex and is thought to specifically reflect saccular function.[34] The vibration-evoked ocular VEMP (oVEMP) has been suggested to selectively measure utricular function.[35]

Several classic studies have reported a decline in horizontal semicircular canal function with aging. Peterka and colleagues tested over 200 healthy subjects across a wide age range (7–81 years) and observed increased postural sway and decreased VOR gain to sinusoidal rotation with age.[36] Caloric responses, however, were not observed to change with age. Paige similarly observed declining VOR responses with age to high-amplitude and high-velocity sinusoidal rotations in 81 patients age 18 to 89.[37] The author concluded that "aging entails a progressive bilateral peripheral vestibular loss." Baloh and colleagues completed one of the only longitudinal studies of vestibular function in 57 normal older

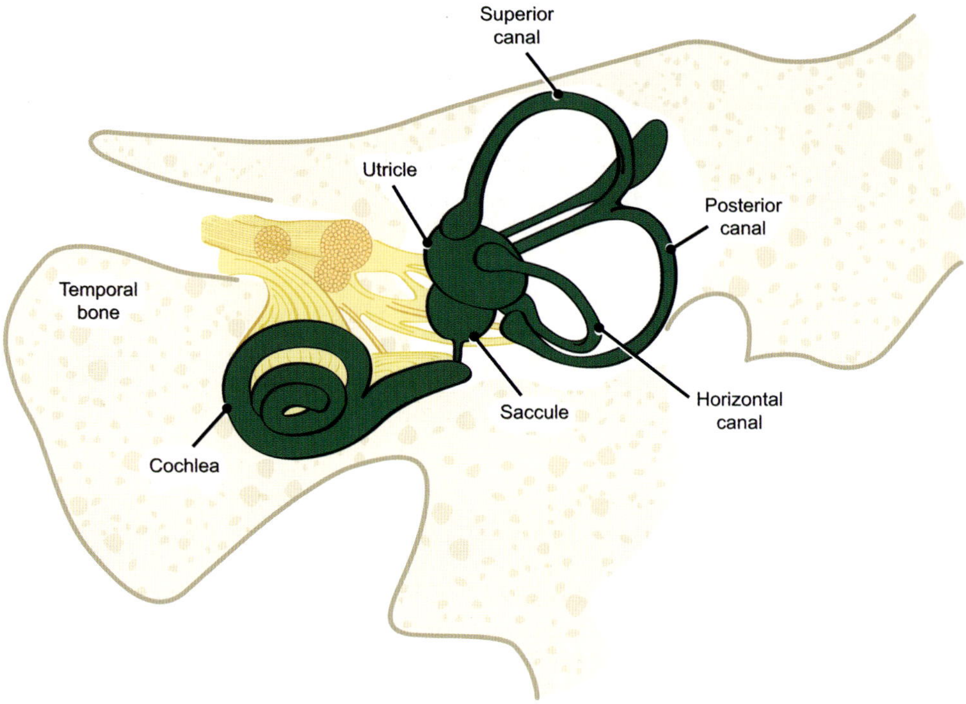

Fig. 11.2 Inner ear anatomy.

individuals who were followed annually for 5 years.[38] They observed a significant decrease over the 5 years in VOR gain to sinusoidal stimuli, again only at higher velocities.[5] Interestingly, none of the older individuals reported symptoms of dizziness or imbalance. It is possible that a threshold of ARVL must be crossed for the disease to move from being subclinical to clinical.

In addition to age-related declines in semicircular canal function, studies also suggest that otolith function decreases with age. Welgampola and Colebatch performed cVEMP testing in 70 adults age 25 to 85.[39] They observed decreasing click-evoked response amplitudes with age, notably a 25 to 30% decline in amplitude per decade from the sixth decade. Brantberg and colleagues measured tone-burst evoked cVEMPs in 1,000 consecutive patients seen in their clinic and observed a steady decline with age starting as early as age 40.[40] A pilot study of 50 healthy older individuals age 70 and over evaluated the five vestibular end-organs simultaneously to assess which if any organ was disproportionately affected.[41] The study observed that 80 to 90% of subjects had semicircular canal dysfunction, whereas only 50% of participants had abnormal saccular function and 20% had utricular impairment.

Histopathological analyses of human temporal bones also demonstrate the adverse effects of age, demonstrating declines in vestibular hair cell populations and progressive otoconial degeneration associated with aging.[42–44] Interestingly, findings from temporal bone specimens corroborate the foregoing physiological data, demonstrating a greater loss of vestibular hair cells in the cristae ampullares of the semicircular canals relative to the otolithic maculae.[45]

Evaluation and Management of an Older Patient with Dizziness and Imbalance

It is critical to take a systematic approach in the evaluation of an older patient with dizziness or imbalance. Some older individuals may report primarily vertigo, lightheadedness, or disequilibrium, which can suggest the predominance of certain underlying etiologies. However, it should be noted that older patients often have multiple concomitant impairments, such as low vision (e.g., from presbyopia or macular degeneration), cardiovascular disease (e.g., hypertension), muscle weakness, and arthritis, and the use of multiple medications. Although a particular impairment may predominate, it is possible that this impairment in combination with another deficit creates the clinical problem (i.e., the clinical problem is *multifactorial*). Accordingly, it is critical that the most common contributors to dizziness and imbalance in the elderly be addressed systematically *every time in every patient.*

The first step in the otolaryngologist's evaluation of an elderly patient with dizziness and imbalance is to obtain a history. This includes asking when the symptoms started, whether the symptoms are progressive, how the patient would further characterize the symptoms (vertigo, lightheadedness, and/or imbalance), whether the symptoms are constant versus episodic (if episodic whether the duration is seconds, minutes, hours, or days), and whether the episodes occur at rest or only during head movement, standing, or walking. Of the major vestibular diagnoses, BPPV is particularly common in older adults and bears special mention. Increased BPPV in the elderly may reflect age-related degeneration of the otoconial membrane, leading to abnormal seeding of otoconia in the endolymph.[46] A study of the German population observed a prevalence of 3.4% in individuals over age 60 and a cumulative lifetime incidence of almost 10% by age 80.[47] BPPV accounted for 39% of cases of vertigo in older patients presenting to neurotology clinics.[48] However, older patients do not always experience the classic presentation of BPPV—short episodes of rotatory vertigo associated with changes in head position. A study of 100 older patients presenting to general geriatric practices for chronic medical conditions found that 9% had unrecognized BPPV.[49] Moreover, patients with BPPV had significantly increased fall risk. Another study found that older patients with BPPV were more likely to experience postural instability.[50] Of note, this instability could be improved through canalith repositioning maneuvers.

The next step is to elicit a medical history to understand the multiple factors that might be contributing to the patient's dizziness. Specifically, the following conditions should be noted: (1) eye disorders (e.g., cataracts, macular degeneration, or glaucoma), (2) cardiovascular disease (e.g., hypertension, arrhythmias, syncope), (3) musculoskeletal disorders (e.g., arthritis, weakness), (4) peripheral sensory loss (e.g., neuropathy), (5) psychiatric disease (e.g., depression, anxiety), (6) cognitive impairment, and (7) systemic conditions (e.g., diabetes). If any unrecognized nonvestibular impairment is identified, an appropriate referral should be made. The otolaryngologist should also ask about a history of hearing loss. Emerging evidence is suggesting a link between hearing loss, imbalance, and elevated fall risk.[51]

The otolaryngologist should then review the patient's medications. Polypharmacy (i.e., the use of four or more medications) contributing to dizziness is a particular concern among older individuals. A study in the ambulatory adult population age 65 or older found that 44% of men and 57% of women take five or more medications.[52] Moreover, older adults metabolize drugs differently than younger adults and may be exposed to higher drug levels at the usual doses. An increase in the number of medications used in the elderly has been associated with an increased risk of impaired balance.[53] Certain classes of medications, including antihypertensive, psychotropic, and narcotic pain medications, have been associated with a particularly increased risk of dizziness and falls and have been termed fall risk–increasing drugs (FRIDs).[54–56] Several clinical tools have been developed to evaluate potentially inappropriate medication use in older patients. The Beers criteria is the most commonly used tool.[57] It contains of one list of medications that should be avoided independent of diagnosis, and a second list of medications that should be avoided considering the diagnosis. Further tools have been developed, including the Screening Tool of Older People's potentially inappropriate Prescriptions) (STOPP) criteria, which enumerate medications to be avoided by organ system, and the Screening Tool to Alert doctors to Right Treatments (START) criteria, which list medications that should be recommended in older patients according to condition in the absence of any contraindications.[57]

With respect to the physical examination, we recommend screening for orthostatic hypotension (a systolic blood pressure decrease of at least 20 mm Hg or a diastolic blood pressure decrease of at least 10 mm Hg within 3 minutes of standing). Evidence of orthostasis could indicate excessive dose of antihypertensive medications (among other conditions) and should prompt referral to the primary care provider or cardiologist. Eye movements should be assessed, particularly the cardinal movements of smooth pursuit, saccade, and vergence. Deficits may indicate brainstem or cerebellar pathology and should prompt a referral to a neurologist. Cerebellar function should also be assessed with maneuvers such as the finger-nose-finger test, the rapid alternating hand movement test and heel-to-shin test. Deficits in any of these tests may indicate cerebellar dysfunction and should prompt referral to a neurologist.

Clinical vestibular testing should include assessment for spontaneous nystagmus (which would indicate vestibular asymmetry), postheadshaking nystagmus (which would indicate a latent vestibular asymmetry), and the horizontal head impulse test (HIT) (which evaluates horizontal semicircular canal function). One study showed that 50% of older adults age 70 and older had an abnormal HIT.[58] Clinical testing should also include the Dix-Hallpike test to evaluate for BPPV, which, as mentioned previously, is very common in older individuals and is treatable. The Romberg test should be performed with eyes closed on foam to evaluate standing balance in the absence of vision and proprioceptive information (such that the patient is relying only on vestibular information).

The patient's gait should also be observed, to assess stability and the potential need for physical therapy and/or an assistive device. The timed up and go (TUG) test is an efficient and reproducible measure of fall risk. The patient is asked to stand from a seated position, walk 3 m, turn around, then return to sitting. Older adults who take longer than 14 seconds to complete the TUG are at significantly increased risk of falling.[59]

At present, the mainstays of management of the older patient with dizziness or imbalance seen in the otolaryngology clinic are management of polypharmacy, identification of nonvestibular contributors and appropriate referrals, management of hearing loss, home safety modification (including installing night lights and grab bars, removing throw rugs, and creating clear passageways within the home), use of assistive devices (cane and walker), and exercise programs (e.g., tai chi, or even light walking). For older patients with evidence of vestibular impairment, vestibular rehabilitation is the primary treatment. Vestibular rehabilitation is a program whereby patients learn to compensate for their vestibular loss by using visual or proprioceptive cues under the direction of a therapist.[60,61] Studies have shown that vestibular rehabilitation is as effective in older patients as in younger patients.[62] One randomized, controlled trial administered vestibular rehabilitation to a group of older patients with chronic dizziness seen in primary care clinics.[63] The study found that vestibular rehabilitation significantly reduced dizziness symptoms and improved postural stability and dizziness-related quality of life. This trial is among the first to administer vestibular rehabilitation in primary care patients who did not have a specific vestibular diagnosis (except perhaps ARVL). Further research is needed to establish the appropriate timing for vestibular rehabilitation. Evidence that vestibular function starts to decline in middle age suggests the potential benefit of vestibular exercises prior to the onset of significant vestibular loss.[11] This phenomenon has been termed prerehabilitation, or "prehab."[2] More recent studies have investigated the benefit of biofeedback prostheses in the treatment of vestibular impairment. The prostheses consist of body-worn devices that deliver sensory feedback (e.g., vibrotactile, auditory) to patients to orient the trunk during movement.[64–68] Early reports are promising that the prostheses effectively improve dizziness and imbalance. Additionally, the multichannel implantable vestibular prosthesis represents a potential new technology for the treatment of ARVL that is awaiting human trials.[69]

Finally, pharmacological therapies for dizziness should be used judiciously and sparingly in older individuals. The most commonly-used medications to treat dizziness are vestibular suppressants, which include antihistamines (e.g., meclizine), anticholinergics (e.g., scopolamine), and benzodiazepines (e.g., lorazepam).[70] Vestibular suppressants can be effective in reducing symptoms of vertigo and motion sickness. However, they have been shown to blunt the error signal that drives vestibular compensation.[71] As such, vestibular suppressants are not indicated in the setting of chronic, progressive vestibular impairment (e.g., ARVL) where compensation is critical. Moreover, vestibular suppressants have sedating effects and are metabolized and cleared more slowly in older individuals.[72] Thus they are not recommended in the elderly; indeed, antihistamines, anticholinergics, and benzodiazepines are listed in the Beers criteria. Interventions that challenge the vestibular system and foster compensation—such as vestibular therapy—are preferable to treat dizziness and imbalance in the elderly.

Falls Risk Assessment

The American Geriatrics Society (AGS) recommends that all patients older than age 65 with a history of falls or a balance and gait disorder should undergo multifactorial falls risk evaluation.[73] If the opportunity exists, otolaryngologists should consider joining or developing multidisciplinary teams that provide multifactorial falls risk evaluation to older patients. Such a multidisciplinary falls prevention clinic has been established at the first author's (YA's) institution. All patients seen in the clinic are given a standardized questionnaire (Appendix). The questionnaire was developed based on AGS guidelines and with input from a multidisciplinary group of providers at the institution, including geriatricians, neurologists, otolaryngologists, ophthalmologists, orthopedists, cardiologists, physiatrists, psychiatrists, and physical and occupational therapists. Notably, the questionnaire quantifies fall history with the use of a falls severity grading scale developed in the clinic.[74] Additionally, standard batteries such as the Geriatric Depression Scale, the Activities Balance Confidence Scale, the Lawton Instrumental Activities of Daily Living Scale, and the Falls Efficacy Scale are administered to measure the impact of imbalance and falls risk on the patient's functional status and quality of life.[24,25,75,76]

A standardized physical examination was also developed for patients seen in the falls prevention clinic (**Table 11.2**), using measures in wide clinical and research use such as the Balance Evaluations Systems Test (the Mini-BEST), the Scale for the Assessment and Rating of Ataxia (SARA), and the Montreal Cognitive Assessment (MOCA).[77–79] Vestibular testing is performed in all patients, including assessment of spontaneous nystagmus, gaze-evoked nystagmus, postheadshake nystagmus, visual VOR suppression,

Table 11.2 Standard physical examination administered in the Johns Hopkins Falls Prevention Clinic: physical therapy and occupational therapy components

Physical therapy component	Occupational therapy component
– Orthostatic vital signs – Contrast sensitivity – Vestibular and oculomotor testing using video-Frenzel lenses – Upper and lower extremity strength testing – Mini-BEST (Balance Evaluations Systems Test)	– Distal sensory testing (pinprick, joint proprioception, vibration) – Reflex testing (brachioradialis, patella, Achilles, Babinski) – Montreal Cognitive Assessment – Scale for the Assessment and Rating of Ataxia – Home assessment

Dix-Hallpike test, and HIT using video-oculography. We also evaluate the other key contributors to fall risk, including vision loss (specifically loss of contrast sensitivity),[80–82] peripheral sensory loss (particularly loss of joint proprioception),[83,84] muscle weakness (particularly of the lower limbs),[85,86] and neurocognitive decline (including loss of cerebellar and cognitive function).[87–89] All patients receive personalized counseling on home modification and the need for assistive devices and are prescribed a program of physical and/or occupational therapy as needed. The screening questionnaire is used to direct any specialty referrals (e.g., to neurology, otolaryngology, or ophthalmology).

Conclusion

As the population ages, increasingly otolaryngologists will be called on to manage the common geriatric problem of dizziness. This chapter reviews a nomenclature for dizziness and imbalance conditions in the elderly and emphasizes the need for a systematic approach to this multifactorial problem. Otolaryngologists should recognize the high prevalence of dizziness in the elderly, its potentially profound impact on quality of life and even length of life (shortened by fall injuries), and the availability of treatment to improve symptoms. Most older patients with dizziness can be helped, but first we must recognize them and treat them with enthusiasm and knowledge.

References

1. Sloane PD, Coeytaux RR, Beck RS, Dallara J. Dizziness: state of the science. Ann Intern Med 2001;134(9 Pt 2):823–832
2. Wetmore SJ, Eibling DE, Goebel JA, et al. Challenges and opportunities in managing the dizzy older adult. Otolaryngol Head Neck Surg 2011;144(5):651–656
3. Serrador JM, Schlegel TT, Black FO, Wood SJ. Vestibular effects on cerebral blood flow. BMC Neurosci 2009;10:119
4. Agrawal Y, Carey JP, Della Santina CC, Schubert MC, Minor LB. Disorders of balance and vestibular function in US adults: data from the National Health and Nutrition Examination Survey, 2001-2004. Arch Intern Med 2009;169(10):938–944
5. Baloh RW, Ying SH, Jacobson KM. A longitudinal study of gait and balance dysfunction in normal older people. Arch Neurol 2003;60(6):835–839
6. Tinetti ME, Williams CS, Gill TM. Dizziness among older adults: a possible geriatric syndrome. Ann Intern Med 2000;132(5):337–344
7. Gopinath B, McMahon CM, Rochtchina E, Mitchell P. Dizziness and vertigo in an older population: the Blue Mountains prospective cross-sectional study. Clin Otolaryngol 2009; 34(6):552–556
8. Stevens KN, Lang IA, Guralnik JM, Melzer D. Epidemiology of balance and dizziness in a national population: findings from the English Longitudinal Study of Ageing. Age Ageing 2008;37(3):300–305
9. Lin HW, Bhattacharyya N. Balance disorders in the elderly: epidemiology and functional impact. Laryngoscope 2012;122(8):1858–1861
10. Ekwall A, Lindberg A, Magnusson M. Dizzy—why not take a walk? Low level physical activity improves quality of life among elderly with dizziness. Gerontology 2009;55(6): 652–659
11. Tuunainen E, Poe D, Jäntti P, et al. Presbyequilibrium in the oldest old, a combination of vestibular, oculomotor and postural deficits. Aging Clin Exp Res 2011;23(5-6):364–371
12. Kao AC, Nanda A, Williams CS, Tinetti ME. Validation of dizziness as a possible geriatric syndrome. J Am Geriatr Soc 2001;49(1):72–75
13. Creighton FX Jr, Poliashenko SM, Statham MM, Abramson P, Johns MM III. The growing geriatric otolaryngology patient population: a study of 131,700 new patient encounters. Laryngoscope 2013;123(1):97–102
14. Neuhauser HK, von Brevern M, Radtke A, et al. Epidemiology of vestibular vertigo: a neurotologic survey of the general population. Neurology 2005;65(6):898–904
15. Neuhauser HK. Epidemiology of vertigo. Curr Opin Neurol 2007;20(1):40–46
16. Agrawal Y, Carey JP, Della Santina CC, Schubert MC, Minor LB. Diabetes, vestibular dysfunction, and falls: analyses from the National Health and Nutrition Examination Survey. Otol Neurotol 2010;31(9):1445–1450
17. Liston MB, Bamiou DE, Martin F, et al. Peripheral vestibular dysfunction is prevalent in older adults experiencing multiple non-syncopal falls versus age-matched non-fallers: a pilot study. Age Ageing 2014;43(1):38–43

18. Ekvall Hansson E, Magnusson M. Vestibular asymmetry predicts falls among elderly patients with multi- sensory dizziness. BMC Geriatr 2013;13(1):77
19. Kristinsdottir EK, Jarnlo GB, Magnusson M. Asymmetric vestibular function in the elderly might be a significant contributor to hip fractures. Scand J Rehabil Med 2000;32(2):56–60
20. Kristinsdottir EK, Nordell E, Jarnlo GB, Tjäder A, Thorngren KG, Magnusson M. Observation of vestibular asymmetry in a majority of patients over 50 years with fall-related wrist fractures. Acta Otolaryngol 2001;121(4):481–485
21. Nordell E, Kristinsdottir EK, Jarnlo GB, Magnusson M, Thorngren KG. Older patients with distal forearm fracture. A challenge to future fall and fracture prevention. Aging Clin Exp Res 2005;17(2):90–95
22. Grimby A, Rosenhall U. Health-related quality of life and dizziness in old age. Gerontology 1995;41(5):286–298
23. Jacobson GP, Newman CW. The development of the Dizziness Handicap Inventory. Arch Otolaryngol Head Neck Surg 1990;116(4):424–427
24. Powell LE, Myers AM. The Activities-specific Balance Confidence (ABC) Scale. J Gerontol A Biol Sci Med Sci 1995; 50A(1):M28–M34
25. Tinetti ME, Richman D, Powell L. Falls efficacy as a measure of fear of falling. J Gerontol 1990;45(6):239–243
26. Dros J, Maarsingh OR, Beem L, et al. Impact of dizziness on everyday life in older primary care patients: a cross-sectional study. Health Qual Life Outcomes 2011;9:44
27. Ten Voorde M, van der Zaag-Loonen HJ, van Leeuwen RB. Dizziness impairs health-related quality of life. Qual Life Res 2012;21(6):961–966
28. Neuhauser HK, Radtke A, von Brevern M, Lezius F, Feldmann M, Lempert T. Burden of dizziness and vertigo in the community. Arch Intern Med 2008;168(19):2118–2124
29. Roberts DS, Lin HW, Bhattacharyya N. Health care practice patterns for balance disorders in the elderly. Laryngoscope 2013;123(10):2539–2543
30. Kerber KA, Enrietto JA, Jacobson KM, Baloh RW. Disequilibrium in older people: a prospective study. Neurology 1998; 51(2):574–580
31. Proctor L, Dix R, Hughes D, Rentea R. Stimulation of the vestibular receptor by means of step temperature changes during continuous aural irrigation. Acta Otolaryngol 1975; 79(5-6):425–435
32. Aw ST, Haslwanter T, Halmagyi GM, Curthoys IS, Yavor RA, Todd MJ. Three-dimensional vector analysis of the human vestibuloocular reflex in response to high-acceleration head rotations. I. Responses in normal subjects. J Neurophysiol 1996;76(6):4009–4020
33. Macdougall HG, McGarvie LA, Halmagyi GM, Curthoys IS, Weber KP. The video Head Impulse Test (vHIT) detects vertical semicircular canal dysfunction. PLoS ONE 2013;8(4):e61488
34. Welgampola MS, Colebatch JG. Characteristics and clinical applications of vestibular-evoked myogenic potentials. Neurology 2005;64(10):1682–1688
35. Welgampola MS, Migliaccio AA, Myrie OA, Minor LB, Carey JP. The human sound-evoked vestibulo-ocular reflex and its electromyographic correlate. Clin Neurophysiol 2009;120(1): 158–166
36. Peterka RJ, Black FO, Schoenhoff MB. Age-related changes in human vestibulo-ocular reflexes: sinusoidal rotation and caloric tests. J Vestib Res 1990-1991;1(1):49–59
37. Paige GD. Senescence of human visual-vestibular interactions. 1. Vestibulo-ocular reflex and adaptive plasticity with aging. J Vestib Res 1992;2(2):133–151
38. Baloh RW, Enrietto J, Jacobson KM, Lin A. Age-related changes in vestibular function: a longitudinal study. Ann N Y Acad Sci 2001;942:210–219
39. Welgampola MS, Colebatch JG. Vestibulocollic reflexes: normal values and the effect of age. Clin Neurophysiol 2001; 112(11):1971–1979
40. Brantberg K, Granath K, Schart N. Age-related changes in vestibular evoked myogenic potentials. Audiol Neurootol 2007;12(4):247–253
41. Agrawal Y, Zuniga MG, Davalos-Bichara M, et al. Decline in semicircular canal and otolith function with age. Otol Neurotol 2012;33(5):832–839
42. Rauch SD, Velazquez-Villaseñor L, Dimitri PS, Merchant SN. Decreasing hair cell counts in aging humans. Ann N Y Acad Sci 2001;942:220–227
43. Walther LE, Westhofen M. Presbyvertigo-aging of otoconia and vestibular sensory cells. J Vestib Res 2007;17(2-3):89–92
44. Merchant SN, Velázquez-Villaseñor L, Tsuji K, Glynn RJ, Wall C III, Rauch SD. Temporal bone studies of the human peripheral vestibular system. Normative vestibular hair cell data. Ann Otol Rhinol Laryngol Suppl 2000;181:3–13
45. Rosenhall U. Degenerative patterns in the aging human vestibular neuro-epithelia. Acta Otolaryngol 1973;76(2): 208–220
46. Ishiyama G. Imbalance and vertigo: the aging human vestibular periphery. Semin Neurol 2009;29(5):491–499
47. von Brevern M, Radtke A, Lezius F, et al. Epidemiology of benign paroxysmal positional vertigo: a population based study. J Neurol Neurosurg Psychiatry 2007;78(7):710–715
48. Katsarkas A. Dizziness in aging: a retrospective study of 1194 cases. Otolaryngol Head Neck Surg 1994;110(3):296–301
49. Oghalai JS, Manolidis S, Barth JL, Stewart MG, Jenkins HA. Unrecognized benign paroxysmal positional vertigo in elderly patients. Otolaryngol Head Neck Surg 2000;122(5):630–634
50. Blatt PJ, Georgakakis GA, Herdman SJ, Clendaniel RA, Tusa RJ. The effect of the canalith repositioning maneuver on resolving postural instability in patients with benign paroxysmal positional vertigo. Am J Otol 2000;21(3):356–363
51. Lin FR, Ferrucci L. Hearing loss and falls among older adults in the United States. Arch Intern Med 2012;172(4): 369–371
52. Kaufman DW, Kelly JP, Rosenberg L, Anderson TE, Mitchell AA. Recent patterns of medication use in the ambulatory adult population of the United States: the Slone survey. JAMA 2002;287(3):337–344
53. Agostini JV, Han L, Tinetti ME. The relationship between number of medications and weight loss or impaired balance in older adults. J Am Geriatr Soc 2004;52(10):1719–1723
54. Hajjar ER, Cafiero AC, Hanlon JT. Polypharmacy in elderly patients. Am J Geriatr Pharmacother 2007;5(4):345–351
55. van der Velde N, Stricker BH, Pols HA, van der Cammen TJ. Withdrawal of fall-risk-increasing drugs in older persons: effect on mobility test outcomes. Drugs Aging 2007;24(8): 691–699
56. Woolcott JC, Richardson KJ, Wiens MO, et al. Meta-analysis of the impact of 9 medication classes on falls in elderly persons. Arch Intern Med 2009;169(21):1952–1960
57. Ryan C, O'Mahony D, Kennedy J, Weedle P, Byrne S. Potentially inappropriate prescribing in an Irish elderly population in primary care. Br J Clin Pharmacol 2009;68(6):936–947
58. Davalos-Bichara M, Agrawal Y. Normative results of healthy older adults on standard clinical vestibular tests. Otol Neurotol 2014;35(2):297–300
59. Alrwaily M, Whitney SL. Vestibular rehabilitation of older adults with dizziness. Otolaryngol Clin North Am 2011;44(2): 473–496, x
60. Brown KE, Whitney SL, Wrisley DM, Furman JM. Physical therapy outcomes for persons with bilateral vestibular loss. Laryngoscope 2001;111(10):1812–1817

61. Krebs DE, Gill-Body KM, Riley PO, Parker SW. Double-blind, placebo-controlled trial of rehabilitation for bilateral vestibular hypofunction: preliminary report. Otolaryngol Head Neck Surg 1993;109(4):735–741
62. Whitney SL, Wrisley DM, Marchetti GF, Furman JM. The effect of age on vestibular rehabilitation outcomes. Laryngoscope 2002;112(10):1785–1790
63. Yardley L, Donovan-Hall M, Smith HE, Walsh BM, Mullee M, Bronstein AM. Effectiveness of primary care-based vestibular rehabilitation for chronic dizziness. Ann Intern Med 2004;141(8):598–605
64. Kentala E, Vivas J, Wall C III. Reduction of postural sway by use of a vibrotactile balance prosthesis prototype in subjects with vestibular deficits. Ann Otol Rhinol Laryngol 2003;112(5):404–409
65. Wall C III, Kentala E. Control of sway using vibrotactile feedback of body tilt in patients with moderate and severe postural control deficits. J Vestib Res 2005;15(5-6):313–325
66. Goebel JA, Sinks BC, Parker BE Jr, Richardson NT, Olowin AB, Cholewiak RW. Effectiveness of head-mounted vibrotactile stimulation in subjects with bilateral vestibular loss: a phase 1 clinical trial. Otol Neurotol 2009;30(2):210–216
67. Hegeman J, Honegger F, Kupper M, Allum JH. The balance control of bilateral peripheral vestibular loss subjects and its improvement with auditory prosthetic feedback. J Vestib Res 2005;15(2):109–117
68. Basta D, Rossi-Izquierdo M, Soto-Varela A, et al. Efficacy of a vibrotactile neurofeedback training in stance and gait conditions for the treatment of balance deficits: a double-blind, placebo-controlled multicenter study. Otol Neurotol 2011;32(9):1492–1499
69. Della Santina CC, Migliaccio AA, Hayden R, et al. Current and future management of bilateral loss of vestibular sensation—an update on the Johns Hopkins Multichannel Vestibular Prosthesis Project. Cochlear Implants Int 2010;11(Suppl 2):2–11
70. Weerts AP, De Meyer G, Pauwels G, et al. Pharmaceutical countermeasures have opposite effects on the utricles and semicircular canals in man. Audiol Neurootol 2012;17(4):235–242
71. Zee DS. Perspectives on the pharmacotherapy of vertigo. Arch Otolaryngol 1985;111(9):609–612
72. Hain TC, Yacovino D. Pharmacologic treatment of persons with dizziness. Neurol Clin 2005;23(3):831–853, vii
73. Guideline for the prevention of falls in older persons. American Geriatrics Society, British Geriatrics Society, and American Academy of Orthopaedic Surgeons Panel on Falls Prevention. J Am Geriatr Soc 2001;49(5):664–672
74. Davalos-Bichara M, Lin FR, Carey JP, et al. Development and validation of a falls-grading scale. J Geriatr Phys Ther 2013; 36(2):63–67
75. Yesavage JA, Brink TL, Rose TL, et al. Development and validation of a geriatric depression screening scale: a preliminary report. J Psychiatr Res 1982-1983;17(1):37–49
76. Lawton MP, Brody EM. Assessment of older people: self-maintaining and instrumental activities of daily living. Gerontologist 1969;9(3):179–186
77. Franchignoni F, Horak F, Godi M, Nardone A, Giordano A. Using psychometric techniques to improve the Balance Evaluation Systems Test: the mini-BESTest. J Rehabil Med 2010; 42(4):323–331
78. Nasreddine ZS, Phillips NA, Bédirian V, et al. The Montreal Cognitive Assessment, MoCA: a brief screening tool for mild cognitive impairment. J Am Geriatr Soc 2005;53(4):695–699
79. Schmitz-Hübsch T, du Montcel ST, Baliko L, et al. Scale for the assessment and rating of ataxia: development of a new clinical scale [published correction available in Neurology 2006;67(2):299. Note: Fancellu, Roberto added]. Neurology 2006;66(11):1717–1720
80. Lord SR, Dayhew J. Visual risk factors for falls in older people. J Am Geriatr Soc 2001;49(5):508–515
81. Lord SR, Dayhew J, Howland A. Multifocal glasses impair edge-contrast sensitivity and depth perception and increase the risk of falls in older people. J Am Geriatr Soc 2002;50(11): 1760–1766
82. Lord SR, Smith ST, Menant JC. Vision and falls in older people: risk factors and intervention strategies. Clin Geriatr Med 2010;26(4):569–581
83. Lord SR, Clark RD, Webster IW. Physiological factors associated with falls in an elderly population. J Am Geriatr Soc 1991;39(12):1194–1200
84. Lord SR, Ward JA, Williams P, Anstey KJ. Physiological factors associated with falls in older community-dwelling women. J Am Geriatr Soc 1994;42(10):1110–1117
85. Lord SR, McLean D, Stathers G. Physiological factors associated with injurious falls in older people living in the community. Gerontology 1992;38(6):338–346
86. Lord SR, Sambrook PN, Gilbert C, et al. Postural stability, falls and fractures in the elderly: results from the Dubbo Osteoporosis Epidemiology Study. Med J Aust 1994;160(11):684–685, 688–691
87. Holtzer R, Wang C, Lipton R, Verghese J. The protective effects of executive functions and episodic memory on gait speed decline in aging defined in the context of cognitive reserve. J Am Geriatr Soc 2012;60(11):2093–2098
88. Verghese J, Lipton RB, Hall CB, Kuslansky G, Katz MJ, Buschke H. Abnormality of gait as a predictor of non-Alzheimer's dementia. N Engl J Med 2002;347(22):1761–1768
89. Verghese J, Robbins M, Holtzer R, et al. Gait dysfunction in mild cognitive impairment syndromes. J Am Geriatr Soc 2008; 56(7):1244–1251

JOHNS HOPKINS
MEDICINE
PHYSICAL MEDICINE AND REHABILITATION

FALLS PREVENTION CLINIC QUESTIONNAIRE

The Johns Hopkins Hospital
600 North Wolfe Street, Meyer 1130 Baltimore, MD 212877142
Appointments: (410) 6143234/ Fax: (410) 6140503

Thank you for arranging to visit our clinic.

Please complete this questionnaire before coming for your visit. It is confidential and will be part of your record. It asks for information about your current problems and your past medical history. This form will give us a better understanding of your problem, and will allow us to spend more time evaluating your problem and discussing treatment plans.

When you come for your first visit, please bring this completed form along with other medical information you or your doctor think is necessary. Should you have any questions, please do not hesitate to contact us at the number at the top of this page.

Thank you very much. We look forward to seeing you.

Johns Hopkins Falls Prevention Team

Name ______________________________ Date ______________

Birth date ______________ Age ________ Gender: ☐ Male ☐ Female

Race: ☐ Black or African American ☐ American Indian or Alaska native ☐ Asian
☐ Native Hawaiian or Pacific Islander ☐ White

Are you Hispanic or Latino: ☐ Yes ☐ No

Contact Information:

Home Phone: ________________ Work Phone: ________________

Email: ______________________________

Address: ____

I live with: ☐ Alone ☐ Spouse ☐ Family
☐ Other, please describe: ______________________________

Who referred you to us (name, address, phone)? ______________________________

____

Who is your primary care physician? ______________________________

Are there any other physicians involved in your care? Please list them below:

Name	Specialty	Phone Number

1. Past Medical History

Have you ever been told you have or had any of the following (check all that apply):

Cardiovascular

☐ High blood pressure
☐ Chest pain/angina
☐ Heart attack
☐ Rheumatic fever
☐ Blood clots/phlebitis
☐ High cholesterol

Gastrointestinal

☐ Ulcers
☐ Reflux
☐ Hepatitis
☐ Feeding tube (PEG)

Respiratory/Lung

☐ Emphysema
☐ Asthma
☐ Chronic bronchitis
☐ Allergies/hay fever
☐ Tracheostomy

Renal

☐ Kidney failure
☐ Hemodialysis
☐ Kidney stones

Neurological

☐ Stroke
☐ Hyperactivity
☐ Learning disability
☐ Attention problems
☐ Head injury
☐ Depression/anxiety
☐ Mental health problem
☐ Parkinson disease
☐ Seizures

Endocrine

☐ Diabetes
☐ Thyroid disease

☐ Osteoporosis
☐ Rheumatologic disease
☐ Hearing difficulties
☐ Vision problems
☐ Injuries
☐ Anemia
☐ Cancer where:

Please describe other health problems that you have: ______________________________

____

____

____

2. Medications

Allergies: ____

Current Medications: Please list all medications you are currently taking (including injections and skin patches), and when possible please provide the dosage:

____

____

3. Have you had any xrays, MRI or CT scans of your brain, neck or spine?

☐ No ☐ xray ☐ MRI ☐ CT scan ☐ Neck ☐ Back ☐ Brain

List and/or explain: ____

____

4. About your life

What is the highest degree you have earned?

□ High school □ Technical certificate □ Associate's □ Bachelor's □ Master's
□ Doctoral

What is your marital status? □ Married □ Single □ Divorced □ Widowed □ Separated
□ Other

If you have children, how many and how old?

____

Do you currently live in a: □ House □ Apartment □ Nursing facility
□ Other ________________

Are there any steps to get in the house/apartment?: □ Yes □ No
If yes, how many? ______________

Are there any steps inside the house/apartment?: □ Yes □ No
If yes, how many? ______________

Is there elevator access to other levels of your house/or to your apartment? □ Yes □ No

Is your house or apartment wheelchair accessible? □ Yes □ No

Do you smoke? (please include cigarettes, cigars or pipes) □ Yes □ No

If yes, how many packs per day? __________ For how many years? __________

If no, did you smoke formerly? □ Yes □ No
Packs per day? __________ For how many years? __________

Are you able to walk: □ Independently □ I use an assistive device Please choose below:
□ Cane □ Walker or Rollator □ Wheelchair
□ Other device, describe ____

5. About how you are feeling

Choose the best answer for how you have felt over the past week:

1. Are you basically satisfied with your life? ☐ Yes ☐ No
2. Have you dropped many of your activities and interests? ☐ Yes ☐ No
3. Do you feel that your life is empty? ☐ Yes ☐ No
4. Do you often get bored? ☐ Yes ☐ No
5. Are you in good spirits most of the time? ☐ Yes ☐ No
6. Are you afraid that something bad is going to happen to you? ☐ Yes ☐ No
7. Do you feel happy most of the time? ☐ Yes ☐ No
8. Do you often feel helpless? ☐ Yes ☐ No
9. Do you prefer to stay at home, rather than going out and doing new things? ☐ Yes ☐ No
10. Do you feel you have more problems with memory than most? ☐ Yes ☐ No
11. Do you think it is wonderful to be alive now? ☐ Yes ☐ No
12. Do you feel pretty worthless the way you are now? ☐ Yes ☐ No
13. Do you feel full of energy? ☐ Yes ☐ No
14. Do you feel that your situation is hopeless? ☐ Yes ☐ No
15. Do you think that most people are better off than you are? ☐ Yes ☐ No

6. About your falls

Hopkins Falls Grading Scale

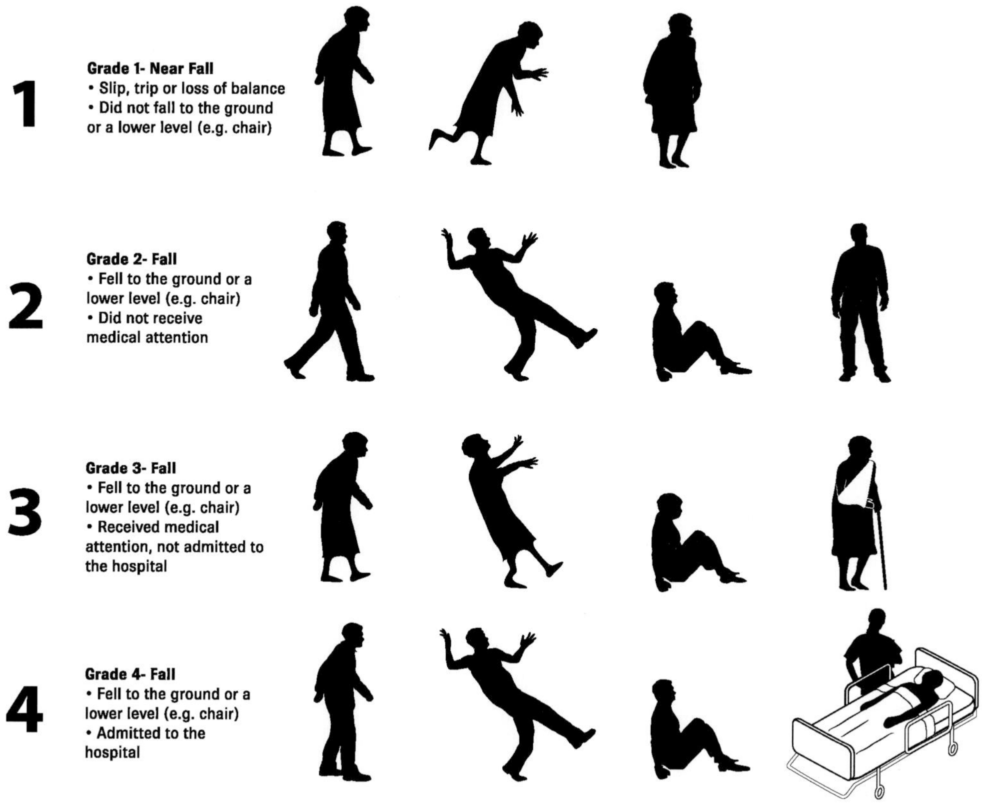

Using the picture above let us know how many falls you had:

	Number last year	Number in last 5 years
1. Near falls		
2. Falls did not require medical assistance		
3. Falls required medical assistance, but no hospital admission		
4. Falls required hospital admission		

If you experienced a fall in the last 5 years, please answer the following questions, otherwise skip to section 4.

Did any of your falls result in:

1. **Minor injury**—Treated at home resulted in pain, bruise or scrape. Used ice, wound cleaned at home: ☐ Yes ☐ No
2. **Moderate injury**—Required a doctor's evaluation resulting in stitches or other closure, splinting. A pulled muscle or tendon was diagnosed: ☐ Yes ☐ No
3. **Major injury**—Required a prolonged visit to the hospital and resulted in surgery, casting, head injury (skull fracture, brain bleed) or internal injury: ☐ Yes ☐ No

Please think of the worst fall you had. After falling:

1. Did you require medical assistance? ☐ Yes ☐ No
2. Did you call your physician? ☐ Yes ☐ No
3. Did you go to your physician's office? ☐ Yes ☐ No
4. Did you go to the emergency department? ☐ Yes ☐ No
5. Did you have surgery? ☐ Yes ☐ No
6. Did you have a broken bone requiring surgery? ☐ Yes ☐ No
7. Were you admitted to the hospital? ☐ Yes ☐ No
8. Were you in the hospital's intensive care unit? ☐ Yes ☐ No
9. Did you have any other treatment that you think is important? ☐ Yes ☐ No

Please describe the problem: ______________________________

____

The following questions are about the circumstances during which the fall occurred. During the fall were you/did you:

1. Changing positions (laying down to sitting, or sitting to standing) ☐ Yes ☐ No
2. Moving from the bed to a chair, or otherwise ☐ Yes ☐ No
3. Moving from one room to another inside the house ☐ Yes ☐ No
4. Walking up or down the stairs ☐ Yes ☐ No
5. Going from one room to the other in the dark ☐ Yes ☐ No
6. Taking a shower ☐ Yes ☐ No
7. Moving outside the house ☐ Yes ☐ No
8. Using alcohol ☐ Yes ☐ No
9. Using bifocal or multifocal eyeglasses ☐ Yes ☐ No
10. Having symptoms (shortness of breath, lightheaded, foot pain, etc.) ☐ Yes ☐ No
11. On a slippery surface (raining, snowing, liquid on the floor, etc.) ☐ Yes ☐ No
12. Trip over an object ☐ Yes ☐ No
13. Fall during day time ☐ Yes ☐ No
14. Fall during night time ☐ Yes ☐ No
15. Alone ☐ Yes ☐ No
16. With someone else in the same room ☐ Yes ☐ No
17. Being helped by someone (supporting or assisting in any way) ☐ Yes ☐ No
18. Have any other important circumstances at the time of the fall ☐ Yes ☐ No

Please describe the circumstances: ______________________________

____

7. SCREENING QUESTIONNAIRE

Question	No	Yes	If yes, please explain
7a. Do you have dizziness (includes imbalance, vertigo, room-spinning, light-headedness)? If yes, answer the following questions:			
7b. Does your dizziness include imbalance?			
7c. Does your dizziness include room-spinning or vertigo?			
7d. Has your dizziness been getting worse?			
7e. Does rolling over in bed or getting in or out of bed make you dizzy?			
7f. Does your dizziness last seconds?			
7g. Does your dizziness last minutes to hours?			
7h. Does your vision jump or blur while walking?			
7i. Do you experience sudden dizziness with loud sounds?			
7j. Do you experience dizziness with sneezing, coughing, straining?			
7k. Do you get dizzy/light-headed when you stand up quickly?			
7l. Is your dizziness triggered by certain foods/beverages?			
7m. Do you have a family history of dizziness or vertigo?			
7n. Have you lost consciousness when you were dizzy?			
7o. Do you have hearing loss or ringing in your ears?			

7p. Do you have headaches, head pressure, sinus pressure, visual changes, light sensitivity, sound sensitivity, or nausea?			
7q. Do you have difficulties with memory, attention, decision-making, i.e., cognitive changes?			
7r. Do emotional changes, sudden falling asleep cause you to fall?			
7s. Do you have slurred speech or difficulty swallowing?			
7t. Do you have shaking in your hands or recent change in handwriting?			
7u. Do you have bowel or bladder problems or erectile dysfunction?			
7v. Do you have weakness, numbness, tingling or pain running down your legs? Is it recent or chronic?			
7w. Do you have heart palpitations or an abnormal heart rhythm?			
7x. Do you have shortness of breath with walking?			
7y. Have you had a recent change in your vision?			
7z. Have you had a recent change in your glasses?			
7aa. Do you see double?			
7bb. Do you have low back pain?			
7cc. Do you have hip pain?			
7dd. Do you have knee pain?			

8. FEAR OF FALLING (Falls Efficacy Scale International)

For each activity below, please mark from 1–4 to show how concerned you are that you might fall if you did this activity. Please reply thinking about how you usually do the activity. If you currently don't do the activity (example: if someone does your shopping for you), please answer to show whether you think you would be concerned about falling IF you did the activity.

	Do you perform this activity?	Not at all concerned 1	Somewhat concerned 2	Fairly concerned 3	Very concerned 4
1. Cleaning the house (e.g. sweep, vacuum, dust)	□ Yes □ No				
2. Getting dressed or undressed	□ Yes □ No				
3. Preparing simple meals	□ Yes □ No				
4. Taking a bath or shower	□ Yes □ No				
5. Going to the shop	□ Yes □ No				
6. Getting in or out of a chair	□ Yes □ No				
7. Going up or down stairs	□ Yes □ No				
8. Walking around in the neighborhood	□ Yes □ No				
9. Reaching for something above your head or on the ground	□ Yes □ No				
10. Going to answer the telephone before it stops ringing	□ Yes □ No				
11. Walking on a slippery surface (e.g., wet or icy)	□ Yes □ No				
12. Visiting a friend or relative	□ Yes □ No				
13. Walking in a place with crowds	□ Yes □ No				
14. Walking on an uneven surface (e.g., rocky ground, poorly maintained pavement)	□ Yes □ No				
15. Walking up or down a slope	□ Yes □ No				
16. Going out to a social event (e.g., religious service, family gathering, or club meeting)	□ Yes □ No				

9. LAWTON SCALE—INSTRUMENTAL ACTIVITIES OF DAILY LIVING

Are you able to perform the following activities? For each activity, circle the item description that most closely resembles your functional level (either 0 or 1).

9a. Telephone use

9ai. Operates telephone on own initiative; looks up and dials numbers: ☐ **1**

9aii. Dials a few well-known numbers: ☐ **1**

9aiii. Answers telephone, but does not dial: ☐ **1**

9aiv. Does not use telephone at all: ☐ **0**

9b. Shopping

9bi. Takes care of all shopping needs independently: ☐ **1**

9bii. Shops independently for small purchases: ☐ **0**

9biii. Needs to be accompanied on any shopping trip: ☐ **0**

9biv. Completely unable to shop: ☐ **0**

9c. Food preparation

9ci. Plans, prepares and serves adequate meals independently: ☐ **1**

9cii. Prepares adequate meals if supplied with ingredients: ☐ **0**

9ciii. Heats, serves and prepares meals or prepares meals but does not maintain adequate diet: ☐ **0**

9civ. Needs to have meals prepared and served: ☐ **0**

9d. Housekeeping

9di. Maintains house alone or with occasional assistance (e.g., "heavy work domestic help"): ☐ **1**

9dii. Performs light daily tasks such as dish-washing, bed making: ☐ **1**

9diii. Performs light daily tasks but cannot maintain acceptable level of cleanliness: ☐ **1**

9div. Needs help with all home maintenance tasks: ☐ **1**

9dv. Does not participate in any housekeeping tasks: ☐ **0**

9e. Laundry

9ei. Does personal laundry completely: ☐ **1**

9eii. Launders small items; rinses stockings, etc.: ☐ **1**

9eiii. All laundry must be done by others: ☐ **0**

9f. Mode of transportation

9fi. Travels independently on public transportation or drives own car: ☐ **1**

9fii. Arranges own travel via taxi, but does not otherwise use public transportation: ☐ **1**

9fiii. Travels on public transportation when accompanied by another: ☐ **1**

9fiv. Travel limited to taxi or automobile with assistance of another: ☐ **0**

9fv. Does not travel at all: ☐ **0**

9g. Responsibility for own medication

9gi. Is responsible for taking medication in correct dosages at correct time: ☐ **1**

9gii. Takes responsibility if medication is prepared in advance in separate dosage: ☐ **0**

9giii. Is not capable of dispensing own medication: ☐ **0**

9h. Ability to handle finances

9hi. Manages financial matters independently (budgets, writes checks, pays rent and bills, goes to bank), collects and keeps track of income: ☐ **1**

9hii. Manages day-to-day purchases, but needs help with banking, major purchases, etc.: ☐ **1**

9hiii. Incapable of handling money: ☐ **0**

10. The Activities-Specific Balance Confidence (ABC) Scale

Instructions to Participants:

For each of the following, please indicate your level of confidence in doing the activity without losing your balance or becoming unsteady from choosing one of the percentage points on the scale from 0% to 100%. If you do not currently do the activity in question, try and imagine how confident you would be if you had to do the activity. If you normally use a walking aid to do the activity or hold onto someone, rate your confidence as it you were using these supports. If you have any questions about answering any of these items, please ask the administrator.

For each of the following activities, please indicate your level of self-confidence by choosing a corresponding number from the following rating scale:

0% 10 20 30 40 50 60 70 80 90 100%

no confidence completely confident

How confident are you that you will not lose your balance or become unsteady when you...

1. ...walk around the house? ____%
2. ...walk up or down stairs? ____%
3. ...bend over and pick up a slipper from the front of a closet floor ____%
4. ...reach for a small can off a shelf at eye level? ____%
5. ...stand on your tiptoes and reach for something above your head? ____%
6. ...stand on a chair and reach for something? ____%
7. ...sweep the floor? ____%
8. ...walk outside the house to a car parked in the driveway? ____%
9. ...get into or out of a car? ____%
10. ...walk across a parking lot to the mall? ____%
11. ...walk up or down a ramp? ____%
12. ...walk in a crowded mall where people rapidly walk past you? ____%
13. ...are bumped into by people as you walk through the mall? ____%
14. ... step onto or off an escalator while you are holding onto a railing? ____%
15. ... step onto or off an escalator while holding onto parcels such that you cannot hold onto the railing? ____%
16. ...walk outside on icy sidewalks? ____%

12 Sinonasal Disease in the Elderly

David R. Edelstein

Introduction

As the population in the United States ages, the number of patients with nasal and sinus disease and complaints will multiply. Between 2000 and 2030, the percentage of people over the age of 65 will increase from 12.4% of the population to 19.6%.[1] This is a dramatic increase in the elderly, and physicians need to begin to think of this group differently, since it has its own unique problems and challenges. This increase will continue during our lifetimes given that the 65 to 85 age group is projected to increase by 135% between 2000 and 2050.[2] In 1960, only 9% of the U.S. population was over the age of 65, whereas today 13% is.[3] Otolaryngologists will be treating many of the elderly based on the high prevalence of rhinitis, hay fever, asthma, chronic sinusitis, and hearing loss in this age group.

Many physicians have a difficult time thinking about aging of the nose and sinuses. We have been trained to appreciate the growth of the midface in the fetus and the development of the nose and dentition in childhood and adolescence. There has been little formal education, however, on the senescence of the midface, the skin of the nose, and the internal structures. Most of the literature on sinonasal disease was based on adults between the ages of 25 and 45, with little attention given to the aging of these structures over the age of 65.[4] Some of the problems, about which the elderly complain, are normal changes to the nose and respiratory tract. The fact that some of the nasal symptoms do not represent disease needs to be explained to the elderly patient, whose symptoms need to be treated depending on the level of patient anxiety and the severity of the problem. Many elderly patients are concerned that their symptoms, such as excessive rhinorrhea, represent the signs of worse problems and are happy to hear that their issues are a variation of normal and consequently require no therapy. Other patients need medications or sprays, but the side effects of the treatments need to be carefully reviewed so that new issues and complications do not arise. The nose and sinuses are often taken for granted until they become dysfunctional, but they present a coordinated respiratory and neurological organ that is affected by old age, other diseases of aging, and medications commonly taken by the elderly. The great advantage of electronic medical records is the ability to check that medications given for symptomatic relief do not interact with other essential drugs given to the elderly patient, such as cardiac medication and blood thinners. When there are interactions or questions, the elderly need to understand the treatment choices, and their primary care doctors should be involved in the decision-making process.

Our biases regarding treating the elderly also extend to our surgical decision trees. As the average life span extends from 85 to 90, the 20 to 25 years over the age of 65 will present many opportunities to examine the nose and sinuses and to consider surgical options. If a quarter of the population will soon be over the age of 60, how can we ignore the surgical issues that may affect this group? The methodology for surgical treatment needs to be modified from that of the average adult and expanded to include the special preoperative and postoperative problems facing the elderly surgical patient. For example, preoperative medications need to be reviewed to avoid day of surgery diabetic crises or hypertensive episodes. Likewise, avoidance of complications needs to be included in the surgical planning and the postoperative care. How often we see patients postoperatively may vary based on their frailty, family support, and ability to treat their nose and use postop medications.

How we treat the elderly and their aging noses and sinuses will determine how well they live given that chronic sinusitis is one of the critical negative factors affecting quality of life.[4] The care of the geriatric nose and sinuses is enhanced if the patient, the family, and the physician understand the differences between the normal and abnormal nose and sinuses. The goal of treatment is to help patients to understand their problems, recognize their options for therapy if they exist, appreciate any issues associated with the care options based on their age or infirmity, and make intelligent medical and surgical decisions. This chapter is about these challenges.

Growth, Development, and Aging Anatomy

The nose is an essential organ of respiration during our entire lives. At birth, we are obligate nasal breathers and will die of asphyxiation if we have bilateral choanal atresia and blockage at birth. The nose is very dynamic and needs to function from the moment of birth, when it is suctioned of meconium, and will be exposed to many noxious stimuli before death. It is a vehicle through which over 12,000 L of air pass per day.[5] Its purpose is not only to pass air, but also to warm, humidify, and clean the particles and bacteria in the air before it reaches the lungs. It serves to provide resistance or a type of positive end-expiratory pressure to keep the lungs expanded. It also provides a mechanism for olfaction. The sinuses lighten the face and hold the teeth, essential for proper nutrition. The midface serves as a buffer to protect the central nervous system and eyes from trauma.

The nose develops early in fetal development (between weeks 4 and 8) from the lateral nasal placodes. The simultaneous development of the facial bones and skull bring the nose into shape. Between weeks 11 and 12, the early ethmoidal infundibulum develops, and the lateral walls of the nose grow medially, giving room to the developing paranasal sinuses. By 15 to 16 weeks of fetal development, the three primordial turbinates will form. The nasal cartilages will eventually interlace, leading to the development of the nasal vestibule and valve. The lateral nasal wall is complete by 24 weeks. The rest of the midface follows in development, with significant interaction with the early upper alveolus and dental buds. Small changes in this early fetal development will not only change how the nose looks in childhood and adolescence, but also set the stage for the changes that occur in the geriatric nose and sinuses.

Growth is distinctive from development. Growth is what happens to the nose in childhood and adolescence. The basic structures are set, but the nose, midface, sinuses, and teeth develop up to adulthood at age 18. The nasal cartilages develop during childhood, and their appearance changes as the nasal bones grow and the dentition changes. The relationships of the nasal cartilages make up the nasal valve, which is the rate-limiting area for nasal breathing and airflow. As children grow, the cross-sectional area of the nose increases, and the size of the airway increases.[6,7] The nasal bones continue to develop until the face is mature and may accentuate any genetic predisposition to hump deformities or nasal drooping.

Nasal function is affected by the nasal structures and by aging. Many older facial plastic researchers have found that the nose lengthens with age and thus droops over the age of 65.[8,9] Some of these projects studied ethnic noses and others looked at cadaver dissections.[10] The oral surgical literature includes significant studies showing how the alveolus thins and reduces its bony support of the midface during aging.[11–13] This midfacial loss of support could explain the drooping of the nose, because there is no change in the nasal cartilage with aging.[14] "Normal Aging of the Nose in Adults" is a broad study that questioned the traditional teaching that the nose itself changes but found that there was a change in the facial and nasal cephalometrics with aging due more to changes in surrounding structures and less to nasal bony or cartilage weakness as traditionally thought.[15] The changes of the midface and nose may also occur with the loss of tensile strength in aging skin, giving the appearance of significant nasal deformity with aging.[16] The presumption that all elderly patients have newly drooping noses and thus need nasal reconstruction is probably false, and the nose needs to be looked at in the context of all of the surrounding facial and dental structures.

With aging, there are several changes to the skin, especially in the face and nose, because the face is the most exposed part of the body to sun and weather. Therefore, it tends to show more changes with age due to a variety of factors. The changes occur to the epidermis, the dermis, the skin appendages, and the subcutaneous tissue. The epidermis has a decrease in thickness and a reduction in melanocytes with age. This helps to thin the skin over the nose and highlights any trauma or imperfections of growth. It also shows the outlines of the nasal cartilages. The dermis has a reduction in fibroblasts, mast cells, and capillaries. This will reduce the strength of the skin over and around the nose. The reduction in the skin appendages such as the eccrine glands and hair follicles will further thin the nasal skin. The skin tension lines are enhanced with age, which may reduce the natural movements of the nose and affect the nasal valve.

Nasal Physiology in the Elderly

The normal nose serves many purposes, including respiration, nasal cleaning, sound resonance, airway resistance for the lower respiratory tract, and temperature regulation of inhaled air. Most of the studies on nasal physiology have been conducted either on children or on healthy young adults. For example, studies on airflow in the young adult demonstrate that the greatest flow is anterior to the inferior turbinate and along the middle meatus.[17] The resistance in the nose is made up of the nasal valve area with the intersection of the nasal vestibule, upper lateral cartilage, and anterior head of the inferior turbinate. This ratio and configuration have to work for a lifetime. However, the changes in the skin of the nose and lip and the regression of the teeth and alveolus may change how air flows into the older nose. The alar dilator muscle may also be reduced with age or by trauma in adulthood. Passive valvular collapse due to maximal inspiration may change transmural pressure and be affected by neuromuscular disease or muscle weakness of aging just as it is affected by facial palsies in young adulthood.

The inside of the nose is covered in respiratory mucosa except at the anterior nasal valve, where there is junctional squamous mucosa. This mucosa responds to a variety of stimuli, including temperature, moisture, emotion, hormones, and medication. Similarly, the capacitance vessels in the nasal septum and the inferior turbinates are also variable. This capacitance change at the nasal valve is the basis for the application of the Poiseuille principle in the nose. This principle states that pressure drops in a fluid or air flowing through a cylindrical pipe, in this case the anterior nose. The change in pressure is inversely related to the radius of the space to the fourth power.[18] Therefore, any small change in the nasal valve resulting from an increase or decrease in mucosal or erectile tissue, or any change in the muscular control of the alar, will change airflow to a significant degree. Thus small changes in mucosa from medication or muscular weakness due to neuromuscular disease or medication can affect airflow negatively. In normal geriatric adults, however, there is generally no change in the resistance of the nose and no significant change of airflow with old age.[15] In addition, normal elderly patients do have the potential for an increase in nasal airflow to make up for lower respiratory tract disease.

Compared with the nose, the lower respiratory tract shows significant changes in the elderly. The forced vital capacity, forced end expiratory volume, functional residual capacity, arterial pO_2 and perfusion progressively worsen with aging. The flow volume loop produced in the pulmonary function tests changes with aging. The forced expiratory volume in 1 second (FEV_1) is the volume that has been exhaled at the end of the first second of forced expiration. The elderly, if they are weak or infirm, cannot build up enough pressure, and this will reduce the FEV_1. The net effect of aging is to increase the work necessary for breathing and to decrease lung compliance.[19] The differences in aging in the lower respiratory tract can be judged by the changes in the effects of asthma in a younger versus older population. Madeo and colleagues have explained how asthma in the elderly leads to more hospitalization; is stimulated by more factors such as reflux, infection, and medication; usually needs continuous and not symptomatic therapy; and has a higher mortality than in younger adults. The authors contend that this may be made worse by a lower compliance with treatment protocols by the elderly patient with asthma.[20] It is unclear how the upper respiratory tract affects the lung capacity, but any limitation in the nose will be reflected in lower respiratory tract problems, and elderly patients with asthma complain bitterly if their nose is blocked.

The nose is also an important cleaning vehicle. The nose will pick up any bacteria and viruses or fungi in the air and pass them into the nasopharynx or stomach where they are broken down. The nose is a dirty environment, but the sinuses are sterile. There are many factors that help the nose remove particles from the airstream, including the particle size, airflow rate, air flow turbulence, the mucous lining of the nose, and mucociliary clearance of the nasal cilia. Many of the medications prescribed for elderly patients dry the nose and reduce the sol or gel layer of mucus. This may affect the movement of particles through the nose. Nevertheless, ciliary beat frequency, which is a prime mover for mucociliary flow, does not change with the normal aging of the nose.[15] This highlights the dynamic nature of the nasal lining, even with aging.

As the normal physiology of the nose changes with aging, the nasal symptoms of the elderly will vary. **Table 12.1** shows that the odds ratio of having the various symptoms changes for every decade from age 20 to 90. For example, as one ages, there is a 1.35% increase in postnasal drip for every decade. The other common symptoms that increase with age are nasal drainage, sneezing, cough, smell disorders, and gustatory rhinitis.[15] Sneezing is the primitive

Table 12.1 Symptoms by age: statistical significance and odds ratios

Symptom P	Value	Odds ratio
Postnasal drip	0.0065	1.35
Nasal drainage	0.0049	1.57
Sneezing	0.0041	1.40
Cough	0.0492	1.49
Smell disorders	0.0001	1.61
Gustatory rhinitis	0.0022	1.64

Reproduced with permission from Edelstein D. Aging of the normal nose in adults. Laryngoscope 1996;106(Suppl 81): 1–25.

defense mechanism relied on by the nose to clear noxious elements. One can think of it as the cough of the nose, and sneezes can achieve 65 mile per hour rates at their highest. Gustatory rhinitis is a type of vasomotor rhinitis, which increases with age, that manifests as a runny nose during eating. Generally this is an autonomic dysfunction in which the brain sees food and tries to turn on the saliva glands, but mistakenly turns on the Bowman glands and mucoserous glands of the nose instead.

Smell Disorders

The sense of smell is important in our everyday lives, as represented by the development of the perfume and deodorant industries. Smell is used as a protective mechanism to avoid noxious environments, rotting food, toxic gases, and dirty clothing. The nose is essential to the normal sense of smell, because olfactory epithelium grows in its roof at the cribriform plate and along the upper septum. Of all of the cranial nerves, olfaction is the first and the most primitive. The number of smells human beings can detect has been estimated to be ~ 10,000. The sense of smell is essential for the sense of taste, because taste is via other cranial nerves in the mouth and tongue and only detects bitter, sweet, salt, and sour elements.

All of our senses are reduced with aging, but none seems to cause as much anxiety as the loss of the sense of smell and taste. It has been estimated that we lose 1% of the sense of smell for every year we age over the age of 60.[21] This means that if the average life expectancy is 85, most elderly will have lost at least 25% of their sense of smell by the last year of life. The National Interview survey found that 40% of all the patients with a reduced sense of smell are over the age of 65.[22] Murphy et al have found that 62.5% of the elderly over the age of 80 had some smell impairment as defined by clinical olfactory testing.[23]

There are a variety of reasons for the reduced sense of smell in the elderly.[24] First, olfactory receptors may be reduced as a result of both aging and all of the infections and trauma that the upper nose may experience by late adulthood. Second, the olfactory bulb is an extension of the brain and thus may experience similar problems found in other parts of the brain due to demyelination during aging or the effects of Alzheimer disease or dementia. Third, many of the diseases affecting the elderly can also affect the sense of smell, including diabetes, hypothyroidism, liver disease, and renal failure. Fourth, medications and smoking have a profound effect on the nature of respiratory epithelium and neuroepithelium. Fifth, nutritional problems and malnutrition in the elderly can affect their sense of smell. Indeed, the rate of malnutrition in the elderly may be underestimated, partially because we often neglect to think of the risks of malabsorption of nutrients associated with inflammatory bowel disease, the use of proton pump inhibitors, and gastritis. Malnutrition may be greater in the elderly who are homebound or who have trouble taking care of themselves and can be present even among residents of nursing homes and rehabilitation centers, as evident in the reduction in weight and strength found in the elderly (**Table 12.2**).[25]

Olfactory neurons reproduce on a cycle of 1 to 2 months. This degeneration may be increased in the face of other neurological diseases such as Alzheimer and Parkinson disease. In some older patients, significant olfactory disturbances may be the earliest sign of intracranial and neurological deficits.[26] Neural changes occur in the anterior olfactory cortex and hippocampus in normal elderly patients.[27] Magnetic resonance studies of the elderly also show brain volume loss related to olfactory loss.[28] Serby has identified olfactory testing as a possible method to determine whether relatives of patients with Alzheimer disease are affected by the disease.[29]

The workup of olfactory disturbances in the elderly is not difficult for the average otolaryngologist. A detailed history is essential and should include a careful description of patients' sense of smell, starting with their everyday smells and working to a discussion of more complex smells. A simple question is whether they can taste and smell their coffee in the morning or the peel of an orange. Smells that are derived from or produce oils can be more stimulating to the olfactory epithelium. Coffee, garlic, ginger, orange, lemon, lime, and grapefruit are a few things common in the home and kitchen that will produce a longer-lasting sense of smell. An inability to smell these items is a significant sign of possible olfactory problems. For patients with a fluctuating sense of smell, the details of when and how they smell may help to determine the source and significance of the problem. This includes a fluctuation during seasons, which may be due to dry heat hurting the olfactory epithelium or due to inflammation from seasonal allergies. A good history will also include prior toxin exposure, smoking, trauma, nasal/sinus surgery, and occupation.

An examination of the nose and sinuses is important to the olfactory disturbance exam. This includes looking at the airflow patterns adjacent to the inferior and middle meatus because smell is directly related to airflow in the nose. The status of the osteomeatal complex will also give some idea if infection or irritation is the source of the smell disturbance. The presence of polyps could mean that there may be an excess of inflammatory cells, fungus, bacteria, or mucus, which can affect the roof of the nose. The examination of the nasopharynx may also give some insight by revealing infection, sphenoid drainage, or

Table 12.2 Causes of olfactory disturbances in the elderly patient

Neurologic		
Alzheimer disease	Parkinson disease	Syphilis
Meningitis	Temporal lobe epilepsy	Transient ischemic attack
Paget disease	Migraine	Amyotrophic lateral sclerosis
Hydrocephalus	Multiple sclerosis	Myasthenia gravis
Endocrine/metabolic		
Hypothyroidism	Panhypopituitarism	Cushing syndrome
Diabetes mellitus	Addison's disease	Sjogren syndrome
Infections		
Viral rhinitis	Upper respiratory infection	Rhinosinusitis
Fungal infection	Acquired immunodeficiency syndrome	Bronchiectasis
Influenza	Rickettsial	Lyme disease
Nutritional		
Alcoholism	Chronic renal failure	Liver cirrhosis
Vitamin deficiency	Zinc deficiency	Protein malnutrition
Gout	Whipple disease	Total parenteral nutrition
Psychiatric		
Schizophrenia	Depression	Anorexia nervosa
Hysteria	Severe anxiety	Seasonal affective disorder
Industrial exposure		
Acetone	Formaldehyde	Lead
Nickel	Potash	Coal
Paint solvent	Flour	Mercury
Pepper	Nitrous gases	Cement
Medication		
Codeine	Morphine	Cimetidine
Thiouracil	Gold salts	Tetracycline
Macrolides	Neomycin	Artovastatin calcium
Adrenal steroids	Antivirals	Cardiovascular/antihypertensives
Menthol	Cocaine	Amphetamine
Medical/surgical interventions		
Total laryngectomy	Rhinoplasty	Thyroidectomy
Chemotherapy	Craniotomy	Adrenalectomy
Hemodialysis	Flu vaccine	Sinus surgery
Radiation therapy	Gastrectomy	Oopherectomy
Neoplasms		
Esthesioneuroblastoma	Nasal adenoCA	Temporal lobe tumor
Frontal lobe glioma	Meningiomas	Aneurysms
Pituitary tumors	Craniopharyngiomas	Corpus callosum tumors

Adapted with permission from Murphy C, Doty RL, Duncan HJ. Clinical disorders of olfaction. In: Doty RL, ed. Handbook of Olfaction and Gustation, 2nd ed. New York, NY: Marcel Dekker; 2003:461–478.

excessive esophageal reflux, which can dry the nose and cause hyposmia. Computed tomographic scanning can be used prudently if there is a suspicion of chronic infection and a possible failure of appropriate medications. The use of magnetic resonance imaging should be limited and coordinated with the internist or neurologist if a workup of Alzheimer disease or other central neurological disorders seems indicated. The likelihood of finding an olfactory tumor is extremely small.

The University of Pennsylvania Smell Identification Test (UPSIT) can be used to identify smell disturbances and to evaluate the efficacy of any therapy. This test includes 40 scratch and sniff odorants. Most of the odorants relate to smell, but there are at least 6 that are trigeminal stimulants to reveal whether the patient is a malingerer or whether the patient has a global neurological problem affecting more than one cranial nerve. Normative data are provided with the test for females and males based on their age. Women have a slightly better sense of smell at all ages, even into old age. The tests can be done with one or both nostrils open but are best done with both nostrils open. If the patient has some nasal congestion, a topical nasal decongestant can be used before the test, since the test is looking for the integrity of the neural organ and not the nature of the nasal airway.

The treatment of smell disturbances is very limited compared with its high prevalence in the elderly. The treatment of anosmia is similar to the treatments for chronic rhinitis. The hallmark of this treatment is topical steroid sprays used morning and night bilaterally to open the nasal airway. In addition, oral steroids maybe an effective treatment because they reduce inflammation in the nose, sinuses, and brain. Their specific effect on the olfactory epithelium is to thin the mucosa. The long-term use of oral steroids may have significant side effects on emotions, psychological status, and the stomach, which can be problematic in the elderly. If there are signs of chronic infection, then antibiotics should be used. Because the sense of smell is important to the sense of taste, the patient should be counseled to use nonsalt additives to enhance the smells and flavors while reducing the side effects of excessive salt intake.

Rhinitis in the Elderly

There are many forms of rhinitis in the elderly. Some of them are normal variations of rhinitis that affect every age group. Some of the common forms of rhinitis vary in their presentations in the elderly. There are also special forms of rhinitis that are more common in the elderly, such as gustatory rhinitis and vasomotor rhinitis. Of all of the common complaints of the elderly, a runny nose is high on the list. Many geriatric patients complain that they walk around all day with a tissue in hand, which interrupts their eating and social activities. The elderly patient may also complain of postnasal drip, chronic cough, and sneezing, which are variations on the rhinorrhea complaint. In addition, many patients have upper respiratory problems in conjunction with their asthma. Some elderly patients have nasal obstruction and shortness of breath, which they may confuse with congestive heart failure or bronchial disease. Some elderly patients have rhinorrhea from prior occupational exposures in factories or from long-term smoking.

The most common form of rhinitis in all age groups is due to allergic rhinitis. Between 15 and 42% of the general population has some form of allergic rhinitis. It has been estimated that ~ 3 to 12% of the geriatric population has allergic rhinitis.[30] Allergies and hay fever are due to type-1 hypersensitivity and are immunoglobulin E (IgE) mediated. External allergens are trapped in the nose by its turbulent airflow and get deposited in the nasal mucosa, which is rich in mast cells. Mast cell mediators include histamines, leukotrienes, bradykinins, serotonin, and prostaglandins, which are then expelled into the nose. There is an early- and late-phase response, which sometimes makes it difficult to determine what causes the allergic response in the nose and upper airways.[31] Although there is an age-related decrease in total serum IgE, the specific IgE levels remain the same in all ages, including the elderly.[30] There are other related immune changes with aging, such as a reduction of IgG4, and with thymic involution the T cell function tends to decline.[32] In addition there may be a decrease in cytokine production associated with old age that affects T helper cells. This may turn on the allergic response as one ages, even though some adults think that they have already outgrown the "allergy years."

The diagnosis of allergic rhinitis needs to be by history and allergy testing—either skin or blood radioallergosorbent tests (RASTs). Many elderly patients live in older homes and are exposed to allergens from collections of books, papers, and old furniture. Many elderly patients have pets, who live and sleep with them and have the potential to cause significant allergies. A good history will include these environmental factors. Some elderly patients will not tolerate normal skin testing because of dermal sensitivity, fear of a skin reaction, inability to stop medications that can affect the test, and the desire to avoid skin itching, which may prevent a good night's sleep. Fortunately blood RASTs or modified blood RASTs can provide a good appraisal if significant IgE-mediated allergies are causing the nasal symptoms. The treatment of allergic rhinitis in the elderly includes antihistamines, antileukotrienes, topical nasal steroid sprays, and antihistamine sprays. The secret for success in treating allergies in the elderly is to use medications only when needed (e.g., during allergy season), to enable patients to avoid known allergens (e.g., by suggesting use of dust mite covers on pillows and mattress), and to advocate prudent use of the topical nasal sprays in conjunction with water-based ointments or nasal saline sprays to limit side effects such as pain or bloody spotting. Immunotherapy is a scientific option but is usually avoided by most elderly who do not have the time, strength, or mobility to go for weekly injections. Oral steroids can be used for allergic crises or complications but must be limited due to their psychiatric, emotional, and gastrointestinal side effects.

The most common type of nonallergic rhinitis is vasomotor, which is an autonomic dysfunction. It is a combined parasympathetic and sympathetic dysfunction, which may cause simultaneous rhinorrhea and nasal congestion. This type of rhinitis is noneosinophilic and may be caused by neurogenic reflex mechanisms. A variation of this is gustatory rhinitis, which is caused by eating or thinking of eating. In younger people, it is caused by the capsaicin in spicy foods, which causes a parasympathetic response. In the elderly patient, temperatures of food, oils, and other stimuli related to eating may turn on the nasal secretions without warning. The best method to treat vasomotor rhinitis is to give ipratropium bromide nasal spray, which is a topical anticholinergic agent freely soluble in water. It can be used several times a day when the patient is eating or uncomfortable, but it should be limited to maintain its fullest effect. It is recommended to start with the lower of two concentrations in most elderly patients. Systemic decongestants can be used but are limited by their α-adrenergic effects on blood pressure, their ability to dessicate the nose causing atrophy, and their negative effect on sleeping.

Medications can also cause rhinitis in the geriatric patient. The elderly patient often takes several medications per day. Many of the medications commonly used by the elderly patient can cause rhinitis, including analgesics, angiotensin-converting enzyme inhibitors, diuretics, and lipid-lowering drugs. Most of the antidepressants and antipsychotics also cause a clear nasal rhinorrhea. The mechanism for medication-induced rhinitis is generally unknown, but in cardiac medications it may be due to changes in the sympathetic and parasympathetic tone. For example, α- and β-blockers inhibit sympathetic tone, which may cause vasodilation and a weepy nasal discharge. The treatment of medication-induced rhinitis is to recognize the side effect and to withdraw the offending medication if possible (**Table 12.3**).[33]

Table 12.3 Drugs associated with medication-induced rhinitis

Type	Drugs
Analgesics	Aspirin and nonsteroidal anti-inflammatory drugs
Antihypertensives	Angiotensin-converting enzyme inhibitors: enalapril, captopril, lisinopril
	Angiotensin II receptor antagonist: eprosartan
	Angiotensin blockers: doxazosin, indoramin, phenoxybenzamine, prazosin, tamsulosin, terazosin, carvedilol, propranolol, pindolol
	Centrally acting antihypertensives: clonidine, methyldopa, reserpine
	Diuretics: amiloride, chlorothiazide, hydrochlorothiazide
	Postganglionic adrenergic blockers: guanethidine
	Vasodilator: hydralazine
Antidepressants	Alprazolam and citalopram
Antipsychotics	Thioridazine, amitriptyline, perphenazine, chlorpromazine, risperidone
Hypnotics	Chlomethiazole
Lipid-lowering drugs	Niacin
Phosphodiesterase type 5 inhibitors	Sildenafil, tadalafil, vardenafil
Miscellaneous	Gabapentin, pergolide, cocaine

Adapted with permission from Nocon CC, Pinto JM. Clinical presentation and management of geriatric rhinitis. Aging Health 2009;5(4):569–583.

Another form of ill-defined rhinitis in the elderly is atrophic rhinitis. It may be due to dryness in the nose, glandular atrophy, loss of turbinate vessels, reduced mucociliary clearance, and direct changes in the respiratory lining of the nose. The combination of dehydration with the foregoing changes could lead to thick mucus in the nose and nasal congestion. A secondary form of atrophic rhinitis can occur after excessive nasal surgery, which results in a removal of the respiratory lining of the nose or turbinates. Radiation therapy, asbestosis, granulomatous disorders, and sarcoidosis can also cause a form of atrophic rhinitis affecting the elderly. The treatment of atrophic rhinitis is to return moisture to the nose by topical water-based gels, topical nasal saline, topical nasal saline gel sprays, humidification, and hydration.

Sinusitis in the Elderly Patient

Sinusitis and infectious rhinitis are as common in the elderly as in any other age group. Their diagnosis is often overlooked because of the high prevalence of other forms of noninfectious rhinitis. They are among the most common forms of chronic complaint in the geriatric age group.[34] Infections in the sinuses result from anatomical changes violating Proetz's principles, bacterial or fungal infections of the sinuses, immunological deficiencies, mucous disorders, and ciliary dyskinesias. Thickened secretions from atrophic rhinitis or other antihypertensive or cardiac medications could also cause stasis in the osteomeatal complex, which could predispose the patient to sinusitis. Maxillary sinusitis may be caused by infected maxillary teeth, failed bone grafts, or misplaced dental implants. The symptoms of sinusitis in the elderly include purulent rhinorrhea, facial pain, headaches, postnasal drip, anosmia, and cough. These symptoms may overlap with the normal rhinitis of aging and go unrecognized by the patient and the primary care physician.

The geriatric patient may suffer from short-term infections, recurrent infections, and chronic infections. The most common viral infections causing sinusitis include rhinovirus and coronavirus, which can affect all age groups. The most common acute bacterial sinusitis is caused by *Streptococcus pneumoniae* and *Haemophilus influenzae* type b. In the future, the use of vaccines against these two bacteria will dramatically reduce their prevalence, but it will take at least another 40 years for the vaccines to reduce them in the elderly, because the vaccines were not introduced until the 1990s. The most common types of nosocomial acquired sinusitis is *Staphylococcus aureus*, *Pseudomonas aeruginosa*, and anaerobes. It is possible that the overuse of antibiotics and contaminated irrigations may be the source of these chronic organisms. The most common types of chronic sinusitis are from coagulase negative staphylococci, pseudomonas, other forms of gram-negative rods, and other forms of *Staphylococcus aureus*. It has been estimated that over 40% of the population is a carrier for some form of *Staphylococcus* in the front of the nose.

Biofilms may contribute to the treatment failures of chronic sinusitis in adults. Bacterial biofilms form when aggregates of bacteria form a matrix, which adheres to a surface such as the sinus or nasal lining. Phenotypic switching of bacterial forms may make the bacteria harder to remove. It is unclear whether the elderly have a greater or lesser chance of developing biofilms. However, the elderly often have been in hospitals more than younger adults and so may have been exposed to nasogastric tubes, nosocomial infections of intensive care units, and intubation tubes. *Staphylococcus* and *Pseudomonas* are common in these settings and can readily form biofilms.[35]

Fungal sinusitis is another common form of chronic sinusitis. There is invasive fungal sinusitis, which is rare, and opportunistic fungal sinusitis, which is more common. The secondary form is caused by *Aspergillus* species and *Alternaria*. Culturing fungus is very difficult and may take up to 6 weeks. Common cultures do not reveal fungus, but silver stains and periodic acid-Schiff stains can show fungus. Occasionally biopsies of the sinus lining may show fungus or fungal balls. Fungal sinusitis can be allergic and nonallergic. Its appearance on computed tomographic (CT) scanning is usually that of an opacified sinus with a central hyperattenuation with possible mucocele formation. Aggressive fungal sinusitis can show erosion of the bony margins of the sinuses and expansion of the lamina papyracea. Any of these aggressive findings in the geriatric patient is an immediate indication for surgery.

Epistaxis in the Elderly Patient

Epistaxis is a very frightening problem for the elderly patient for several reasons. First, most patients do not know how to take care of the bleeding nose. Second, the respiratory mucosa of the nose is more friable in the elderly and may bleed more readily than in the younger adult. Third, the elderly patient may have high blood pressure, which will increase the bleeding. Fourth, the patient may be taking medications such as a daily aspirin or a blood thinner, which will dramatically increase the bleeding. This constellation of issues makes epistaxis a significant worry in the elderly and a challenge for the patient and physician to treat.

Epistaxis is most common during certain times of the year. March, August, and November are the seasonal epicenters for epistaxis. This is due to the extreme weather changes, which may cause the anterior vessels on the septum to expand when going from a warm to a cold environment. If there is any irritation to the anterior septal mucosa or there is hard nose blowing, the vessels may become engorged and bleed. Because allergic rhinitis is common in the elderly, patients on average may be blowing their nose more often, irritating these vessels. Winter may also dessicate the front of the nose and will promote easy bleeding. Any rubbing of the nose due to any form of geriatric rhinitis will also increase the risk of rubbing the anterior mucosa and causing additional bleeding. With the temperature changing early in the morning before sunrise, the nose has naturally to warm and humidify, which increases the chance that the combination of temperature and overnight dehydration of the nose can cause early morning bleeding.

The care of the elderly bloody nose is similar to the care of epistaxis in younger adults, with some small modifications. First, the patient should squeeze the nose at the area of the septum for at least 5 to 8 minutes. The Lee–White bleeding time for the average adult is 5 to 8 minutes. Most elderly patients need to be shown the correct site to squeeze and understand that when the nose is bleeding 5 to 8 minutes seems like a very long time. The patient should be encouraged to sit down so as not to increase the blood pressure and to sit straight upright to avoid the discomfort of swallowing the blood and secretions. Most patients are impatient and run to the bathroom or lie down without touching their nose, which may increase the bleeding and the patient's panic. If the patient is on daily aspirin (81 mg), this may double the normal bleeding time to 10 to 16 minutes, which may seem like an eternity to the elderly, scared patient.

There are several other maneuvers that elderly patients should be encouraged to do if the bleeding continues. First, they should place some ointment on the septum to reduce dryness near the bleeding site. Second, if they do not have a cardiac arrhythmia, they can try a small dose of a vasoconstricting spray in the nose, which may slow bleeding long enough to let local pressure be effective. Third, they can place some tissue in the front of the nose infused with ointment to increase the pressure on the septum if they do not have the strength to do it themselves. This tissue should be left in for over 30 minutes to reduce the risk of removing the new clot and restarting bleeding.

Patients with recurrent bleeding should be sent to the emergency room. In the emergency room, a nasal pack or a preset nasal tampon can be placed into one or both sides of the nose. This will quickly stop the bleeding and give the emergency physician long enough time to check for a coagulation deficiency, anemia, infection, and uncontrolled hypertension. If there is a posterior bleed, then a posterior pack or a double balloon can be inserted. Placing posterior packs is difficult in the younger patient and can be very traumatizing and painful to the elderly patient. Water-based gels on the pack and local anesthetizing sprays should be used. The procedures need to be explained to the patient before they are performed, and the family should be encouraged to help the patient deal with the early discomfort. Every patient with a posterior pack or a balloon in the posterior nasopharynx needs to be admitted and placed in a monitored bed to avoid hypo-oxygenation due to nasopharyngeal reflexes.

If the patient comes into the office, the nose can be easily examined once the bleeding has slowed. If the site of the bleed is identified, then silver nitrate cauterization can be used. In the elderly, the anterior respiratory mucosa can be very thin, and bilateral cauterization should be avoided to prevent a possible septal perforation. If there is a more aggressive bleed, then electric cautery can be used, but topical anesthesia by spray or injection will be required. Every patient with epistaxis should have the posterior nasopharynx checked for tumors or ulcers and the posterior sphenopalatine arteries checked for bleeding. Usually, one can pass a small fiberoptic scope through one side to examine both sphenopalatine arteries and both sides of the nasopharynx. This will reduce the discomfort to an elderly patient who is probably already uncomfortable from the anterior nasal manipulation and the stress of the bleeding.

Although most posterior packs are left in the younger adult patient for 48 to 72 hours, the elderly patient may not tolerate them for that long nor have the cardiac or respiratory reserve to merit it. The elderly are at greater risk for a cardiac event or respiratory arrest due to the lowered oxygenation. Some otolaryngologists would recommend going to the operating room to avoid posterior packs in the elderly. They believe it is easier to control the bleeding with less cardiac stress and risk from the posterior packs. The literature may even agree with this plan for younger patients. Patients must be competent to sign their own consent, or the family should be engaged early in the process so they understand the possible need for surgical control of the bleeding.

Even when the bleeding stops, the elderly patient is at risk of recurrent bleeding. This must be carefully and explicitly reviewed. These patients should use a bedroom humidifier for an extended period of time. They should also use ointment in the nose, preferably a water-based one at night time, so they do not inhale it by mistake and develop either a lipoid pneumonia or chronic unexplained cough. Patients should be examined in 1 to 2 weeks to make sure that they are adhering to the recommendations, to answer questions, and to recauterize if necessary.

Once an elderly patient bleeds, there is a greater risk of rebleeding, which most patients and families need to appreciate.

Examination of the Elderly Nose and Sinuses

All examinations of elderly patients should start with observation of how they breathe. The sound of their voice—whether nasal or clear—will give the observant physician an early sign of major nasal complaints. Sniffling and coughing will also highlight excess mucus in the nose or upper throat. Whether the patient is carrying a handkerchief or tissue will also indicate possible infection or rhinorrhea.

Although aging patients will need the same exam as younger adults, they may need different-sized instruments. If the patient is on blood thinners or long-term aspirin therapy, the nose should be carefully addressed. Most elderly patients will tolerate pediatric-sized specula. Although rigid endoscopes are frequently used in younger adults, the elderly patient may find them irritating and they can induce small amounts of bleeding. A fiberoptic endoscope will give similar information and allow examination of the nose, sinus ostia, nasopharynx, and larynx at the same time. The multiple smaller pediatric and infant fiberoptic endoscopes can be used atraumatically and often without any mucosal irritation. If medication is needed, then small amounts of vasoconstricting agents and local anesthetics can be used. The use of liquid cocaine should be avoided due to drug interactions, cardiac toxicity, and its negative effects on patients with arrhythmias and hypertension, conditions that are common in the elderly. If there has been bleeding in the past, then ointment can be applied to the nasal septum before examination to avoid further complications or pain.

Postoperative examination and nasal–sinus debridements may require a change in methodology to be successful in the elderly patient. After sinus surgery, the sinus ostia need to be kept open and the sinuses cleaned of any retained secretions, clots, or polypoid changes. Elderly patients need to know before surgery that they will need one to four nasal sinus debridements. The surgeon needs to make clear that they will feel some discomfort, and that the procedure may take longer if they need to take several breaks. In addition to vasoconstricting agents and local anesthetics, the surgeon may want to have available nasal saline, antibiotic-infused saline, and other emollients to spray into the nose to reduce any dryness or irritation. If there were positive fungal or bacterial cultures from the sinuses at the time of surgery, then local sprays with antifungal agents and antibiotics should be sprayed at the time of debridement. Any use of irrigations will need to be explained or shown to elderly patients, who may not remember the instructions when they get home. Written instructions with diagrams are essential, depending on the patient's competence, memory, and family involvement.

Cultures of the nose and sinuses may be necessary in the patient with infection. Anterior swabs are easy to do but sinus cultures are a challenge in the elderly patient. Aspiration with a curved sterile suction may be performed atraumatically from the ethmoid and maxillary sinuses. If an endoscopically driven culture needs to be taken, then pediatric 2 mm endoscopes should be employed. This can be performed in the surgically opened sphenoid and frontal sinuses with ample preparation and anesthetic spray. The patient should lie down in a tolerable position, which is often at 30 degrees. Younger adults can be placed supine, but the elderly may have degenerative spine disease or significant reflux, which will limit their optimum positioning.

CT scanning of the nose and sinuses is often necessary. There should be attention to the number of X-rays that patients receive and the rads they have had in the previous year. Many elderly patients have other diseases, such as malignancies, lung disease, or inflammatory bowel disease, which may require frequent CT scanning. Therefore, CT scanning of the sinuses should be reserved for those times when the diagnosis is in question, when there is an impending complication such as blindness or a brain abscess, or when there is a need for presurgical planning and CT guidance. An attempt should be made to have limited-radiation CT scanning, which should be done in conjunction with the radiologist. CT scanning should not replace good medical judgment or be used routinely to document sinusitis that could be clinically documented.

Medical Therapy

Otolaryngologists are known to use many medications and sprays for the treatment of nasal and sinus disease. One of the great challenges for the physician is how to prescribe multiple medications to the elderly without interactions or side effects.[36,37] Therefore, the treatment of sinusitis in the elderly is problematic, because it involves simultaneously prescribing several different medications to reduce sinusitis symptoms. Treatment of sinonasal diseases is divided into five general groups. The first are medications, which dry the nose or reduce allergic symptoms. The second are nasal sprays, which are steroid based, antihistamine, or mucous reducing. The third are antibiotics. The fourth are steroids. The fifth are inhaled medications.

Decongestants are commonly given to dry the nose of excess secretions. Their benefit is that they can be given in small doses and can be long acting. For the geriatric patient, their use is problematic, however, since they elevate blood pressure; increase heart rate, which can induce arrhythmias; and dry the throat, which can cause coughing or preasthma and can cause sleep deprivation. Antihistamines are commonly given for allergic rhinitis but have many side effects. They may cause some dehydration and make the elderly patient overly sedated. Many of the newer antihistamines are 24-hour medications, which makes them difficult to split or reduce. As a rule of thumb, most geriatric patients should not take mixed medications because they may have multiple side effects. It is better to take one medication per pill and only take the minimum required to reduce symptoms. This will also make it easier for the patient to understand which pill will help a specific side effect and when to take it.

The steroid sprays are essential to reduce inflammation from a variety of causes, including allergies, weather changes, and infection. There are different steroids in each of the sprays, with different preservatives and spray formats. Some elderly patients find some of the odors, especially the flowery ones, to be noxious or irritating. Elderly patients need to be shown how to best use the sprays by pointing them away from the septum toward the ears and to lower the face when doing it to get better penetration deep into the lateral nose. Some spray bottles may be easier to use than others based on whether the patient has arthritis in the hands. For example, some spray bottles use a different thumb and finger combination and others use a hand-squeezing technique. The physician should talk to the patient about hand dexterity before ordering multiple sprays, which may be expensive and difficult to introduce into the nose. Trying a sample spray bottle in the office will improve compliance and reduce buying medications that the elderly may find challenging to afford and difficult to manipulate.

Antibiotics are the hallmark of treatment for bacterial infections of the nose and sinuses. Many of the antibiotics have potential drug interactions, as shown in **Table 12.4**.[38] The elderly patient should be given shorter-term and lower-dose antibiotics to avoid complications. If the medications are not working within 72 hours, then one may want to consider changing the antibiotics. The advantage of electronic medical records is that prior successful and failed therapies with antibiotics and their side effects can be more easily identified and retrieved. Some physicians prefer to give long-term antibiotics lasting 3 to 4 weeks to younger adults, a treatment protocol that is usually avoided in the elderly, who may find the long-term medications irritating to their stomach. Also, the stronger medications may place the elderly patient at greater risk of dehydration.

Steroids reduce inflammation and are the basic treatment of fungal infections of the sinuses. They also may cause gastritis and severe reflux. Some elderly patients may also develop steroid psychosis, with either euphoria or depression. These medications should not be avoided but the side-effects should be carefully discussed and understood by the elderly patient before taking them. Systemic antifungal agents can be used if there are cultures showing the type of fungus or the suspicion of fungus is high. Inhaled antibiotics and aerosolized antifungal agents are also available. Many elderly patients find the devices difficult to use and irritating to the nose. Just as with other medications, the single medication format for the aerosolized medications will help the elderly patient avoid medications that irritate them while identifying the drugs that may help them. If combination aerosols are used, the patient may want to stop all of them, which may limit the physician's choice of medical therapy.

The neti pot and saline washes are commonly given for nasal and sinus disease treatment. The elderly patient may have a dry nose from natural reduction in the mucoserous glands and the use of other cardiac and antihypertensive medications. The saline washes help to clear the nose and provide necessary moisture. Showing patients how to use the bottles before they leave the physician's office will improve compliance and proper usage. There are, however, several disadvantages to the saline washes that the patient and physician need to appreciate. First, the bottles need to be kept clean daily and should not be stored in the bathroom, so as to reduce bacterial contamination. Second, the irrigations should be done gently, because ear congestion from reflux up the eustachian tube is common and may reduce the hearing of the elderly patient who may already be wearing a hearing aid. Third, the water used should be distilled, because tap water may have a variety of heavy metals or small amounts of other contaminants. Fourth, the patient should be instructed in the use of the saline packets or how to mix their own combinations of salt and baking soda to provide the proper osmolarity and pH for the irrigating fluid.

■ Surgical Therapy

The indication for sinus surgery in the elderly is the same as in younger adults, with some modifications. The absolute indications include impending complications, such as blindness or brain abscess, severe unremitting headaches from the frontal or

Table 12.4 Antibiotics with interactions with drugs commonly used by the elderly

Antibiotic	Interacting drugs	Effects
Macrolides	Digoxin	Increases effects
	Theophylline	Nausea, seizures, apnea
	Viagra	Increases effects
	Lipitor	Increases effects
	Dilantin	Increases level
	Warfarin	Increases PT and bleeding
	Carbamazepine	Nystagmus, ataxia, nausea
	Steroids	Increases effects
Clindamycin	Erythromycin	Increases effects
	Diazepam	Prolongs paralysis
Ampicillin	Allopurinol	Increases chance of rash
Tetracyclines	Digoxin	Increases level, toxicity for months
	Antacids	Decreases absorption
	Barbiturates	Decreases levels
	Warfarin	Increases chance of bleeding
TMP/SMX	Diuretics	Increases potassium and decreases sodium
	Digoxin	Increases levels
	Cyclosporine	Decreases levels, increases Cr
	Warfarin	Increases chance of bleeding
	Methotrexate	Increases bone marrow
		Suppression
	Phenobarbital	Decreases sulfa absorption
Fluoroquinolones	Insulin	Alteration of blood sugar levels
	Carafate	Decreases absorption
	Antacids and vitamins	Decreases levels
	Nonsteroidal anti-inflammatory drugs	Increases central nervous system and seizures
	Warfarin	Increases chance of bleeding
	Antiarrhythmics	Increases Q-T interval
	Caffeine	Increases levels
	Dilantin	Alters levels
Aminoglycosides	Furosemide	Increases oto- and nephrotoxicity
	Cisplatin	Increases oto- and nephrotoxicity
	Neuromuscular blockers	Apnea
Flagyl	Alcohol	Flushing and diarrhea
	Warfarin	Increases chance of bleeding

Adapted with permission from Fairbanks DNF. Pocket Guide to Antimicrobial Therapy in Otolaryngology-Head and Neck Surgery. 13th ed. AAO-HNS; 2007:77–80.

sphenoid sinuses, severe cough from chronic sphenoiditis, and sinusitis resulting from complex dental problems that may put dental implants at risk. The relative indications are the same as in young adults, and the need for surgery will depend on the ability of the patient to tolerate medical therapy. Some geriatric patients have multiple antibiotic allergies, which limits the options available to treat an infection. Some cannot take sprays with sulfites or with certain preservatives. Others cannot tolerate the symptoms of sinus infections or have had recurrent pneumonia from their infections. The one thing to avoid is thinking that age-related rhinorrhea or anosmia will improve with sinus or nasal surgery.

The approach to geriatric patients is different than that for young adults needing nasal or sinus surgery. First, the indications need to be clearly outlined to patients to overcome fear, which could lead them to avoid necessary treatment. Second, the surgeon should offer to have the same discussion within the scope of Health Insurance Portability and Accountability Act of 1996 (HIPAA) guidelines with any caregivers in order that the caregivers understand and are capable of discussing the situation with patients and helping them with postoperative care. This may entail taking the patients back and forth to the hospital for the surgery and to the doctor's office for the necessary postoperative care. This postoperative "contract" with patients and families should include a reasonable review of the time needs over the first postoperative year when recurrences are prone and need to be avoided. Third, the surgeon needs to triangulate with the primary care doctor to ensure that all of the preoperative testing and treatment protocols are performed. This may include changing the timing of medication and stopping blood thinners for a few days preoperatively or admitting the patient to the hospital for a change in anticoagulation. If there is a pacemaker and cautery is possible, then the electrophysiologist needs to be part of the discussion, or the appropriate bipolar cautery must be available. Fourth, any ophthalmological problems and vision changes need to be documented and a postoperative plan prearranged. The risks of surgery need to be balanced with the benefits of success and recorded in the chart as part of the preoperative risk assessment.

Fifth, do not take the anesthesia for granted. The patient may want to talk with the anesthesiologist in advance, particularly if there have been any prior anesthesia experiences the anesthesiologist should know about and plan for. Because of a weak voice or prior pneumonia or reflux, the choice of intubation or the use of a LMA should be predetermined. Generally, the elderly patient's nasal and sinus surgery can be more safely performed under a light general anesthesia (level 1) than local with sedation. The patients who have local anesthesia may be more uncomfortable, be unable to tolerate their own secretions or minor bleeding, and need the procedure to stop several times due to variations in the blood pressure.

An essential question is whether one can perform nasal and sinus surgery safely in the geriatric patient. The overall answer is yes, with some limitations. Over the past 15 years there have been six papers and presentations that have addressed this question. Jiang and Hsu in 2001 looked at 171 geriatric patients who had surgery for chronic sinusitis. They found that there were good outcomes at all age groups, but a higher share of minor operative complications.[39] Catalano et al in 2004 looked at a group of 100 geriatric patients (average age 74.5) who underwent minimally invasive sinus techniques with 84% reporting a significant increase in quality of life standards. The only complication was epistaxis in 2%.[40] Edelstein and Jackman in 2003 reported on a group of 63 elderly patients between the ages of 65 and 89 who had presented with similar complaints and symptoms as younger adults, all of whom underwent nasal and sinus surgery. Remarkably, most of the patients needed nasal septal correction for access to their sinuses and had a greater prevalence of sphenoid sinus surgery than controls. The complication rate was unchanged, and there were insignificant differences in the younger versus older surgical groups.[41]

Ramadan and VanMetre in 2004 also asked the question whether complication rates were higher in the younger versus the geriatric group. The authors compared 46 patients over the age of 65 with a control group of 522 under 65. The complication rate was higher in the older group with a 22% rate versus 13% for the younger control group. They also found that there were more frontal and sphenoid surgeries due to more chronic infections involving sinuses, which were close to the brain and needed to be opened due to failure of medical therapy. There was a higher prevalence of bleeding in the older group at 6.5% versus the younger group's 3.4%. The older group also had more postoperative periorbital ecchymosis, especially in the revision cases.[42] Colclasure et al in 2004 looked at 56 patients over the age of 61. Their patients had only endoscopic sinus surgery and all had improved Sino-Nasal Outcome Test (SNOT-20) quality of life outcomes. The worst complications were postoperative crusting, and there were no major complications and no revisions within the first postoperative year.[43] Busaba and Hossain in 2004 looked at 40 geriatric patients who had septal and turbinate reduction surgery. Half of the patients had general anesthesia and half underwent the surgery with light sedation without any problems. Using the Short-Form Health Survey (SF-12) scores, the authors found a trend of improvement after the surgery for nasal breathing. They found improvement in postnasal drip, rhinorrhea, and congestion, but not nasal or sinus pain or headaches. They note that there was a significant reduction in nasal medications postoperatively, which was one of the goals of the surgery. The study excluded patients who had chronic sinusitis.[44]

Halmos et al recently published on the comorbidity, complications, and survival of sinonasal malignancies comparing the younger adult under 70 with the elderly patient over the age of 70. As predicted, the comorbidities were greater in the older group, but, surprisingly, there was no significant difference in complications. The only predictor for complications was the length of surgery, which is similar for other surgery in the elderly. The elderly showed no change in survival based on cell type, but this may have been due to lower numbers of patients. The authors highlighted that preoperative evaluation and careful patient selection led to these excellent results in the geriatric patient with nasal tumors.[45]

Newer techniques such as balloon sinuplasty have a place in all sinus care but present special challenges for the elderly patient. Balloon sinuplasty can be done in the operating room as part of the surgical plan; however, it may pose many problems for the elderly patient if performed in the office setting. First, there may be a need for cardiac monitoring. Second, there is a need for larger amounts of anesthetics, which may have adverse cardiac effects and give patients a sense that they cannot swallow. Third, small amounts of bleeding may end the procedure prematurely. However, sinuplasty can open sinuses without significant manipulation and help the surgeon avoid a return to the operating room, which the elderly patient may want to avoid for a variety of reasons. Once the ballooned sinuses are open, focused cultures can be taken and the sinuses can be further examined for other disease.

The surgical treatment of the nose and sinuses requires some small changes in the decision tree and surgical mapping for geriatric patients as compared with young adults. First, the surgery should be carefully mapped out in advance and possible critical areas noted, especially in relation to the orbit and base of the skull. Second, there should be extra attention given to whether the patient had prior trauma near the eye, which would predispose the patient to periorbital ecchymosis or edema. Third, the area near the anterior ethmoid sinuses and anterior inferior turbinate should be carefully touched to prevent lacrimal problems because the elderly already have a slightly higher prevalence of epiphora. Fourth, because the elderly may have a slower healing process, there should be limited removal of any respiratory mucosa, which will also limit crusting and scarring. Fifth, there should be limited removal of any turbinate tissue, because the geriatric nose can be dry from a variety of causes. Radiofrequency reduction will shrink large turbinates without touching the mucosa. Sixth, although there is an urge to avoid septal surgery in the elderly to minimize the time spent under general anesthesia, the septal spurs need to be removed because most geriatric patients will not tolerate the cleaning and care needed for the sinuses if the nose hurts from the use of endoscopes. Seventh, the surgeon needs to appreciate the bony landmarks and the downside risks of violating the cribriform in the elderly patient, who may not recover easily from additional neurosurgery. Eighth, limit the use of vasoconstricting agents and restrict the use of cocaine pledgets if the patient has severe cardiac disease. Ninth, prepare for postoperative complications by following the patient more closely, thinking of using minor packing or pledgets if there is any bleeding, and checking the patient more often in the recovery room until he or she is awake and ready to leave the hospital or surgical center (**Table 12.5**).

Table 12.5 Key points in the surgical decision making in the elderly patient

1. Understand the absolute and relative indications for surgery
2. Discuss the surgery with all of the caregivers
3. Triangulate with the primary care doctor the necessary preoperative assessment and any pre- and postoperative care changes and needs
4. Document any ophthalmological problems preoperatively and involve the ophthalmologist intraoperatively and postop as needed
5. Do not take anesthesia for granted; plan ahead with anesthesiologist
6. Map out the surgery in advance and understand the pitfalls
7. Avoid nasolacrimal ducts, base of skull, and excessive removal of nasal, turbinate, or sinus mucosa
8. Consider septal repair for breathing and to prepare for postop care
9. Limit vasoconstricting agents
10. Prepare for complications and consider patient's tolerance for further surgery or manipulation
11. Outline the postoperative "contract" with patients and caregivers
12. See the patient as often as needed for examination, care, discussion of problems, and to answer questions

Sinus surgery for chronic sinusitis can be done effectively with good results in the geriatric patient. Nasal and sinus surgery can have excellent results so long as Proetz's original principles, upon which all nasal and sinus surgery is based, are followed.[46] Patients must be properly prepared for the surgery and the immediate postoperative period, particularly if they are going home. They must also understand the need for close follow-up and cleaning of the sinuses, including debridement. Each patient needs to understand the surgical "contract" and the need to follow instructions, take postoperative medications, and make plans to return to the office as needed. The expectations of the patient, family, and surgeon need to be aligned. The patient's primary care doctor needs to understand the indications and be on board to help with the preoperative assessment for anesthesia and with any changes in the patient's medication protocols before and after the surgery. This will reduce the anxiety before the surgery, help the patient understand the goals, prepare the caregivers to have time for postoperative care, and be ready for any irregularities in postoperative healing.

Conclusion

As the population ages, the number of patients over the age of 65 with rhinologic complaints will increase dramatically. Physicians need to differentiate development in the fetal period from growth in childhood from the normal adult nose. They also need to appreciate the changes that occur to the nose in senescence. Most otolaryngologists treat the geriatric patient and are well equipped to understand the hearing loss of aging and the dysphonia or dysphagia of the elderly, but they are not equipped to appreciate the problems facing the aging of the nose and sinuses. Our medical treatments and surgical decision trees need to be modified, and our biases when dealing with the elderly changed, to adapt to an expanding pool of geriatric patients.

References

1. U.S. Census Bureau. International database. Table 094. Midyear population, by age and sex, 2003
2. Kinsella K, Velkoff V; U.S. Census Bureau. An Aging World: 2001. Washington, DC: U.S. Government Printing Office; 2001. Series P95
3. U.S. Census Bureau. Briefs. Table 4: Age and Sex Composition. Washington, DC: U.S. Government Printing Office; 2011
4. Pallanch JF, McCaffrey TV, Kern EB. Normal nasal resistance. Otolaryngol Head Neck Surg 1985;93(6):778–785
5. Metson RB, Gliklich RE. Clinical outcomes in patients with chronic sinusitis. Laryngoscope 2000;110(3 Pt 3):24–28
6. Cole P. The Respiratory Role of the Upper Airways. St. Louis, MO: Mosby–Yearbook; 1993:3.
7. Vig PS, Zajac DJ. Age and gender effects on nasal respiratory function in normal subjects. Cleft Palate Craniofac J 1993; 30(3):279–284
8. Friedman O. Changes associated with the aging face. Facial Plast Surg Clin North Am 2005;13(3):371–380
9. Quatela VC, Pearson JM. Management of the aging nose. In: Sclafani AP, ed. Management of the Aging Face Facial Plast Surg 2009 (25):215–221
10. Glanville EV. Nasal shape, prognathism and adaption in man. Am J Phys Anthropol 1969:30(1):29–37
11. Brodie AG. Facial patterns, a theme on variation. Angle Orthod 1946;16:75–87
12. Farkas LG, Posnick JC, Hreczko TM. Growth patterns of the face: a morphometric study. Cleft Palate Craniofac J 1992; 29(4):308–315
13. Enlow DH. A morphogenetic analysis of facial growth. Am J Orthod 1966;52(4):283–299
14. Vetter U, Heit W, Helbing G, Heinze E, Pirsig W. Growth of the human septal cartilage: cell density and colony formation of septal chondrocytes. Laryngoscope 1984;94(9):1226–1229
15. Edelstein DR. Aging of the normal nose in adults. Laryngoscope 1996;106(9 Pt 2, Suppl 81):1–25
16. West MD. The cellular and molecular biology of skin aging. Arch Dermatol 1994;130(1):87–95
17. Cole P. Upper respiratory airflow. In: Proctor DF, Andersen I, eds. The Nose: Upper Airway Physiology and the Atmospheric Environment. Amsterdam, Netherlands: Elsevier Biomedical Press; 1982:171
18. Swift DL. Physical principles of airflow and transport phenomena influencing air modifications. In: Proctor DF, Andersen I, eds. The Nose: Upper Airway Physiology and the Atmospheric Environment. Amsterdam, Netherlands: Elsevier Biomedical Press; 1982:340–341
19. Bosisio E, Scoccimarro A, Rizzi M, Raguso A, Sergi M. Mean transit time, forced expiratory volume and age in healthy male smokers and non-smokers. Respiration 1986;49(1): 23–26
20. Madeo J, Li Z, Frieri M. Asthma in the geriatric population. Allergy Asthma Proc 2013;34(5):427–433
21. Doty RL, Shaman P, Applebaum SL, Giberson R, Siksorski L, Rosenberg L. Smell identification ability: changes with age. Science 1984;226(4681):1441–1443
22. Hoffman HJ, Ishii EK, MacTurk RH. Age-related changes in the prevalence of smell/taste problems among the United States adult population. Results of the 1994 disability supplement to the National Health Interview Survey (NHIS). Ann N Y Acad Sci 1998;855:716–722
23. Murphy C, Schubert CR, Cruickshanks KJ, Klein BE, Klein R, Nondahl DM. Prevalence of olfactory impairment in older adults. JAMA 2002;288(18):2307–2312
24. Spielman AI. Chemosensory function and dysfunction. Crit Rev Oral Biol Med 1998;9(3):267–291
25. Murphy C, Doty RL, Duncan HJ. Clinical disorders of olfaction. In: Doty RL, ed. Handbook of Olfaction and Gustation. 2nd ed. New York, NY: Marcel Dekker; 2003:461–478

26. Smutzer GS, Doty RL, Arnold SE, Trojanowski JQ. Olfactory system neuropathology in Alzheimer's disease, Parkinson's disease and schizophrenia. In: Doty RL, ed. Handbook of Olfaction and Gustation. 2nd ed. New York, NY: Marcel Dekker; 2003:503–525
27. Price JL, Davis PB, Morris JC, White DL. The distribution of tangles, plaques and related immunohistochemical markers in healthy aging and Alzheimer's disease. Neurobiol Aging 1991;12(4):295–312
28. Cerf-Ducastel B, Murphy C. FMRI brain activation in response to odors is reduced in primary olfactory areas of elderly subjects. Brain Res 2003;986(1-2):39–53
29. Serby M, Mohan C, Aryan M, Williams L, Mohs RC, Davis KL. Olfactory identification deficits in relatives of Alzheimer's disease patients. Biol Psychiatry 1996;39(5):375–377
30. Busse PJ, Kilaru K. Complexities of diagnosis and treatment of allergic respiratory disease in the elderly. Drugs Aging 2009;26(1):1–22
31. Pinto JM, Jeswani S. Rhinitis in the geriatric population. Allergy Asthma Clin Immunol 2010;6(1):10
32. Chadwick SJ. Allergic rhinitis in the elderly. In: Calhoun KH, Eibling DE, eds. Geriatric Otolaryngology. New York, NY: Taylor and Francis; 2006:225–238
33. Nocon CC, Pinto JM. Clinical presentation and management of geriatric rhinitis. Aging Health 2009;5(4):569–583
34. Chronic conditions: A challenge for the 21st century. National Academy on an Aging Society 1999;(1):1–6
35. Leibovitz A, Baumoehl Y, Steinberg D, Segal R. Biodynamics of biofilm formation on nasogastric tubes in elderly patients. Isr Med Assoc J 2005;7(7):428–430
36. Beers MH. Explicit criteria for determining potentially inappropriate medication use by the elderly. An update. Arch Intern Med 1997;157(14):1531–1536
37. Budnitz DS, Lovegrove MC, Shehab N, Richards CL. Emergency hospitalizations for adverse drug events in older Americans. N Engl J Med 2011;365(21):2002–2012
38. Fairbanks DNF. Pocket Guide to Antimicrobial Therapy in Otolaryngology–Head and Neck Surgery. 13th ed. Alexandria, VA: AAO-HNS; 2007:77–80
39. Jiang RS, Hsu CY. Endoscopic sinus surgery for the treatment of chronic sinusitis in geriatric patients. Ear Nose Throat J 2001;80(4):230–232
40. Catalano PJ, Setliff RC, Catalano LA. Minimally invasive sinus surgery in the geriatric patient. Operative Techniques in Otolaryngology HNS 2001;12(2):85–90
41. Edelstein DR, Jackman A. Geriatric endoscopic sinus surgery in the geriatric population. Presented at the eastern section of the Triological Society; Boston, MA; January 25, 2003
42. Ramadan HH, VanMetre R. Endoscopic sinus surgery in geriatric population. Am J Rhinol 2004;18(2):125–127
43. Colclasure JC, Gross CW, Kountakis SE. Endoscopic sinus surgery in patients older than sixty. Otolaryngol Head Neck Surg 2004;131(6):946–949
44. Busaba NY, Hossain M. Clinical outcomes of septoplasty and inferior turbinate reduction in the geriatric veterans' population. Am J Rhinol 2004;18(6):343–347
45. Halmos GB, Peters TTA, Roodenburg JLN, van Dijk BA, van der Laan BF. Comorbidity, complications, and survival of sinonasal malignancies in young and elderly treated by surgery. Otolaryngol Head Neck Surg 2013;148(5):860–866
46. Proetz AW. Essays on the Applied Physiology of the Nose. 2nd ed. St. Louis, MO: Annals Publishing; 1953

13 Taste and Smell in the Elderly

Richard L. Doty and Hussam F. Tallab

Introduction

It is well established that taste and smell function decline with age in a large proportion of the population.[1,2] Such decrements are not without consequence. For example, in a study of 750 consecutive patients presenting to our Smell and Taste Center with complaints of chemosensory disturbances, 68% experienced decreased quality of life, 46% reported changes in appetite or body weight, and 56% noted adverse influences on daily living or psychological well-being.[3] In another study of over 400 patients, many of whom were elderly, at least one hazardous event, such as failure to detect fire or leaking natural gas, was reported by 45.2% of those with anosmia, 34.1% of those with severe hyposmia, 32.8% of those with moderate hyposmia, 24.2% of those with mild hyposmia, and 19% of those with normal olfactory function.[4]

This chapter provides an overview of the functional and pathophysiological changes in the senses of taste and smell that are associated with aging. The goal is to provide the clinician with a basic understanding of these changes and information of value in treating and counseling older patients who present with aberrations of these senses. Although smell dysfunction can be an early sign of several age-related diseases, most notably Alzheimer disease and sporadic Parkinson disease, the reader is referred elsewhere for more detailed reviews on these topics.[5,6]

Basic Anatomy of the Taste and Smell Systems

The Oral Taste System

Chemicals that enter the oral cavity are sensed by taste receptors within goblet-shaped taste buds consisting of receptor, supporting, and basal cells (**Fig. 13.1**). Such buds, which number around 8,000 in humans, are embedded within the fungiform, foliate, and circumvallate papillae of the tongue (**Fig. 13.2**), as well as within the mucosa of the soft palate, uvula, epiglottis, rostral esophagus, and laryngeal surface of the epiglottis and spread caudally along the aryepiglottic folds, reaching peak density at the laryngeal side of the arytenoid tubercle. Some taste sensations, such as sweet, bitter, and savory (umami), are dependent upon G-protein-coupled receptor proteins located on receptor cell microvilli within the buds. Interestingly, such proteins are rather ubiquitous throughout the body, being found within the linings of the larynx,

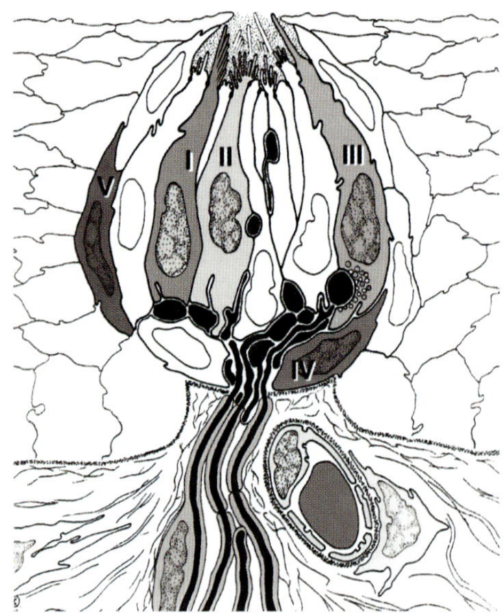

Fig. 13.1 Idealized drawing of longitudinal section of a mammalian taste bud. Cells of types I, II, and III are elongated. These cells have different types of microvilli within the taste pit and may reach the taste pore. Type IV are basal cells and type V are marginal cells. Classically defined synapses occur only between type III cells and nerve fibers. Many of the connecting taste nerves have myelin sheaths. (Reprinted with permission from Witt M, Reutter K, Miller IJ, Jr. Morphology of the peripheral taste system. In: Doty RL, ed. Handbook of Olfaction and Gustation. New York, NY: Marcel Dekker; 2003:651–677.)

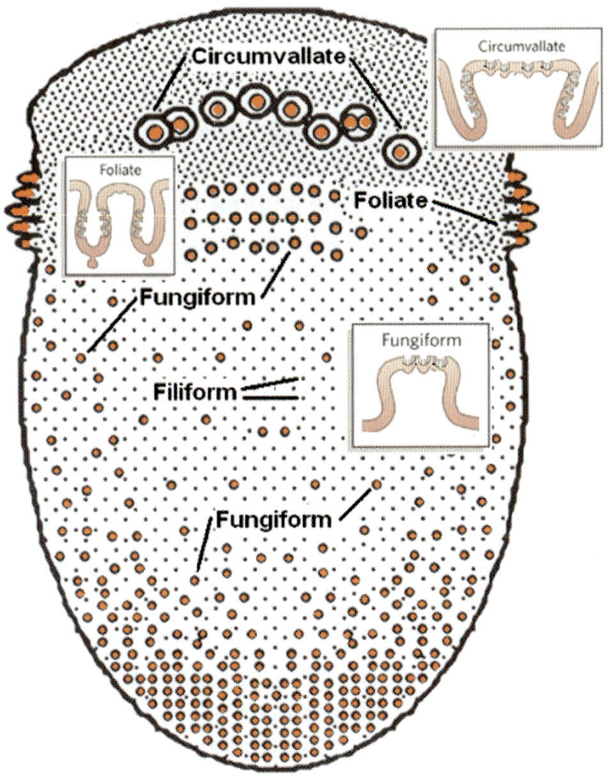

Fig. 13.2 Schematic representation of the tongue demonstrating the relative distribution of the four main classes of lingual papillae, three of which have taste buds (indentations on insets represent taste buds). Taste buds are particularly plentiful on the sides of the foliate and circumvallate papillae. Ebner glands secrete materials into the valleys between the latter papillae. The fungiform papillae can vary considerably in size and are more dense on the anterior lateral regions of the tongue.

epiglottis, stomach, pancreas, and colon. In the gut, they influence chemical absorption, digestion, insulin release, and the metabolism of swallowed foods and beverages.[7]

Several mechanisms are involved in taste transduction, depending on the tastant and its associated qualitative sensations.[8,9] The taste receptors involved in sweet, bitter, and savory sensations fall into distinct G-protein receptor gene families. The gene family associated with sweet and savory sensations comprises three receptor genes (*TAS1R–TAS1R3*), whereas the bitter receptor gene family comprises over 60 receptor genes (*TAS2R1–TAS2R60*), although some are not found in humans or are pseudogenes. In contrast, salty and sour sensations are not mediated by G-protein-related receptors. Salty taste, such as that produced by sodium chloride, requires dissociation of the salt into Na^+ and chloride (Cl^-) ions. The diffusion of the Na^+ ions through specialized membrane pores on the receptor cells induces cell depolarization and transmitter release. Sour taste, such as that induced by hydrochloric acid, is similarly produced via protons (H^+).

The neural projections of the peripheral human taste system are shown in **Fig. 13.3**. The taste buds on the anterior tongue are innervated by the chorda tympani branch of cranial nerve (CN) VII, which merges with fibers of the lingual nerve. The taste buds on the palate are also innervated by CN VII with connections through the geniculate ganglion. The taste buds on the foliate and circumvallate papillae receive their innervation from the glossopharyngeal nerve (CN IX), whereas those on the larynx and esophagus are innervated by the vagus nerve (CN X). In all cases, the afferents from the taste buds enter the brainstem and synapse within the nucleus tractus solitarius (NTS), a structure that extends from the rostrolateral medulla caudally along the ventral border of the vestibular nuclei. The fibers synapse in an orderly rostral to caudal fashion, those from CN VII being rostral to those from CN IX, which in turn are rostral to those from CN X.

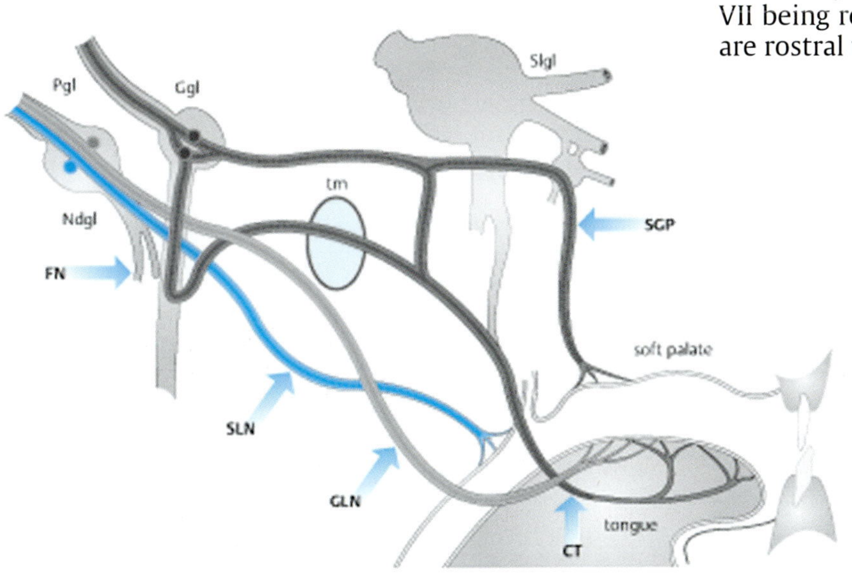

Fig. 13.3 Course of peripheral taste nerves. FN, facial nerve; Ggl, geniculate ganglion; Ndgl, nodosal ganglion; Pgl, petrosal ganglion; SGP, superficial greater petrosal nerve; tm, tympanic membrane; Slgl, semilunar ganglion; SLN, superior laryngeal nerve; GLN, glossopharyngeal nerve; CT, chorda tympani. (Reprinted with permission from Welge-Luessen A. Management of Smell and Taste Disorders. New York, NY: Thieme; 2013.)

The second-order neurons within the NTS ascend ipsilaterally to the parvicellular division of the ventroposteromedial nucleus of the thalamus via the central tegmental tract.[10] From this nucleus, projections are made to the primary taste cortex, a set of structures located at the junction of the anterior insula and the inner operculum. Further projections are then made to other structures, most notably the orbitofrontal cortex, in which interactions occur with neurons from the visual, somatosensory, and olfactory systems.

The Olfactory System

Unlike the taste system, the primary stimuli of this system are vapors. Odorants enter the nose by diffusion or inhalation and dissolve in the mucus that overlies the olfactory neuroepithelium. This pseudostratified columnar epithelium lines the cribriform plate, sectors of the superior septum, and both the superior and middle turbinates. Like the receptors involved in sweet, bitter, and savory taste sensations, the olfactory receptors are G-protein-coupled receptors. They are embedded in the ciliary membranes of 6 to 10 million bipolar receptor cells located in the neuroepithelium (**Fig. 13.4**).[11] Nearly 400 different receptor proteins are expressed in humans. Interestingly, each receptor cell expresses only one type of receptor protein. Unlike the mucus within the nasal epithelium, that of the olfactory region comes from specialized Bowman glands. These secretions are replete with numerous types of enzymes that degrade xenobiotics and odorants.[12] Other cell types found within this specialized epithelium are (1) supporting cells, which, among other things, insulate the olfactory receptor cells from one another; (2) microvillar cells, which likely secrete nitric oxide and play an antibacterial role; and (3) basal stem cells. The latter cells differentiate into the other cell types, replacing them when they sustain damage or death from xenobiotics, aging, or other processes.[13] Unfortunately, receptor cell restoration following damage is often incomplete or nonexistent.

The axons of the olfactory receptor cells coalesce within the lamina propria into multiple bundles, termed the olfactory fila. Each filum contains fascicles ensheathed by glial cells with astrocyte- and Schwann cell mesaxon-like properties.[11] The receptor cell axons course within the fila through the foramina of the cribriform plate to synapse within the olfactory bulb, an outgrowth of the forebrain made up of neurons, nerve fibers, microglia, astrocytes, and blood vessels (**Fig. 13.5**). Considerable neural processing occurs within this structure. The axons of the receptor cells enter into sphere-like structures, termed glomeruli, where they synapse with dendrites of the major projection neurons of the bulb,

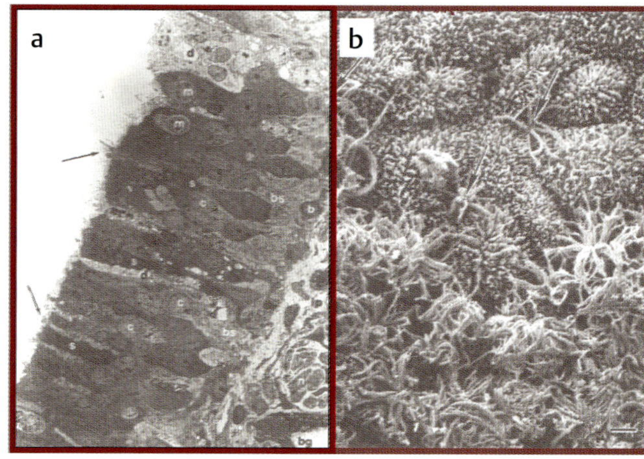

Fig. 13.4 (**a**) Cross-section of the human olfactory epithelium. Four main types of cells can be discerned: bipolar receptor cells (arrows point to largely denuded cilia at dendritic knobs); c, cell body; m, microvillar cell; s, sustentacular cells; b, basal cells. bg, Bowman gland; lp, lamina propria; n, collection of axons within an ensheathing cell; d, degenerating cell; bs, basal cell undergoing mitosis. (Photo courtesy of Dr. David Moran, Longmont, Colorado.) (**b**) A transition zone between the human olfactory epithelium (*bottom*) and the respiratory epithelium (*top*). Arrows signify two examples of olfactory receptor cell dendrites with cilia that have been cut off. Bar = 5 mm. (Used with permission from Menco BPM, Morrison EE. Morphology of the mammalian olfactory epithelium: form, fine structure, function, and pathology. In: Doty RL, ed. Handbook of Olfaction and Gustation. New York, NY: Marcel Dekker; 2003:17–49.)

the mitral and tufted cells. The axons of the receptor cells secrete the excitatory amino acid transmitter glutamate, which activates both N-methyl-D-aspartate (NMDA) and non-NMDA receptors on the dendrites of the mitral, tufted, and other second-order neurons.[14] Some cells intrinsic to the olfactory bulb, termed periglomerular cells, influence neural activity among glomeruli and are largely dopaminergic. These cells serve to modify the incoming signals and, when excessive stimulation occurs, suppress olfactory nerve and mitral/tufted cell activity, in effect decreasing the volume of olfactory bulb output.[15] Cells expressing gamma-aminobutyric acid (GABA), located in the core of the bulb, are termed granule cells and extend processes into more peripheral bulbar layers and modulate olfactory bulb activity, in some cases as a function of bodily needs such as hunger or arousal.[16] Interestingly, these cells, as well as several cells near the glomeruli, termed periglomerular cells, can be repopulated by neuroblasts that migrate from the subventricular zone of the brain through the anterior rostral migratory stream.[17] There is some controversy as to the degree to which this happens in humans.[18]

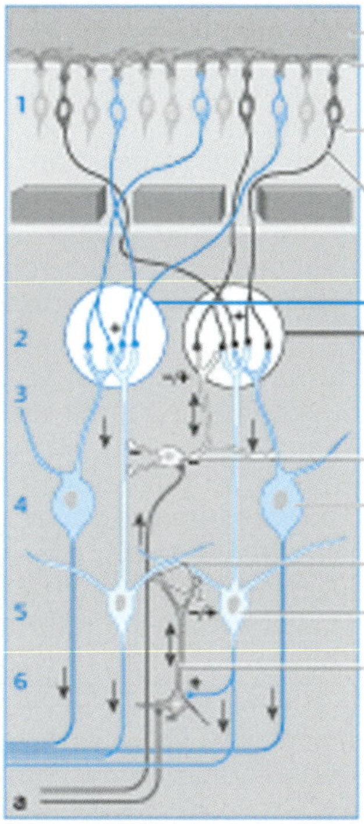

Fig. 13.5 Schematic organization of the olfactory bulb. Arabic numbers indicate the cortical structure: 1, nerve fiber layer; 2, glomerular layer; 3, external plexiform layer; 4, mitral/tufted cell layer; 5, internal plexiform layer; 6, granule cell layer. Glomerular coding: Axons of receptor cell expressing the same olfactory receptor project to only a few analogous glomeruli (e.g., "blue" olfactory receptor neurons converge with "blue" glomeruli). Efferent (bulbofugal, blue) fibers project from mitral/tufted cells to secondary olfactory structures; afferent (centrofugal, gray) fibers project either from contralateral mitral cells or ipsilateral central nuclei and synapse to glomerular or granule cells, respectively. (Reprinted with permission from Welge-Luessen A. Management of Smell and Taste Disorders. New York, NY: Thieme; 2013.)

The mitral and tufted cell axons exit the bulb via the olfactory tract to synapse in the ipsilateral temporal lobe. Major projections include those to the anterior olfactory nucleus (AON), the piriform cortex, the periamygdaloid cortex, and the rostral entorhinal cortex (**Fig. 13.6**). Some tertiary connections to the opposite hemisphere occur via the AON and anterior commissure.

Age-Related Changes in Taste and Smell Perception

Most patients who complain of taste loss have, in fact, altered olfactory function that markedly alters flavors. This is because flavor sensations such as chocolate, mint, pizza, apple, strawberry, and so on are dependent on stimulation of the olfactory receptors via the rear of the nasopharynx (so-called retronasal route). Blocking the nose while eating, for example, greatly decreases or eliminates flavor sensation because active movement of air into the nasopharynx from the oral cavity is significantly impeded.

This section of the chapter specifically addresses age-related deficits observed in taste and smell perception, physiological processes that contribute to such deficits, and medications associated with changes in chemosensation in the elderly.

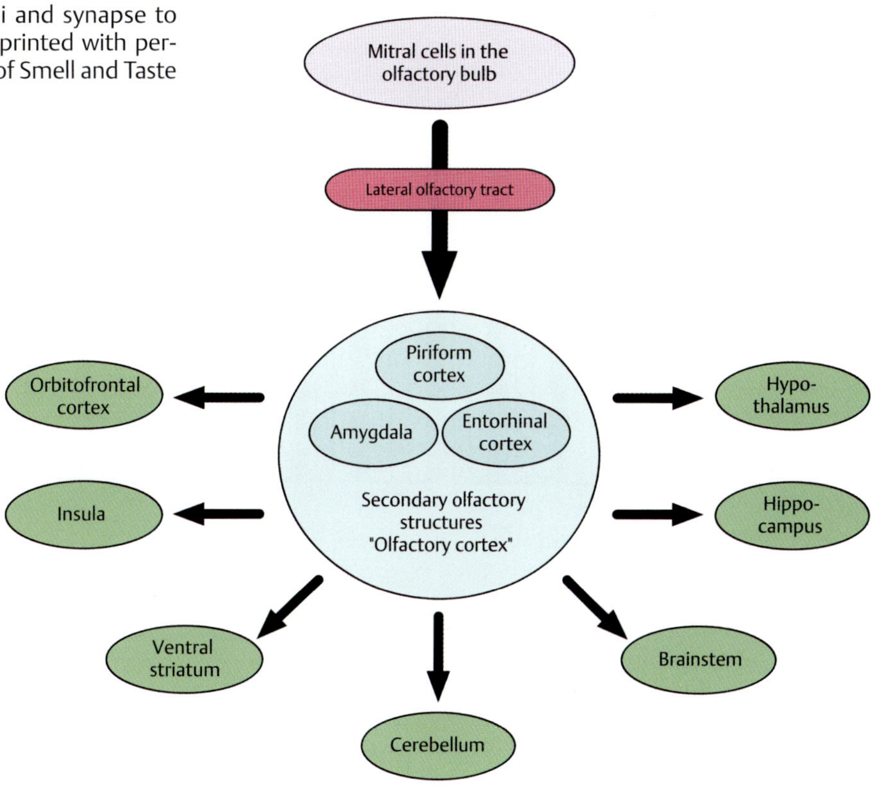

Fig. 13.6 Simplified schematic drawing of the essential bulbofugal olfactory pathways, deriving from mitral cells of the olfactory bulb. The lateral olfactory tract carries direct connections to secondary olfactory structures ("olfactory cortex"), before tertiary olfactory structures are reached. Contralateral projections and other afferents to the olfactory bulb are not indicated. (Reprinted with permission from Welge-Luessen A. Management of Smell and Taste Disorders. New York, NY: Thieme; 2013.)

The Oral Taste System

Age-related decrements in the ability to detect low concentrations of tastants, as measured by taste thresholds, are well documented for both electrical and chemical stimuli. For example, a recent meta-analysis identified 69 studies that have reported age-related declines in taste function, with most reflecting elevated olfactory thresholds.[19] Threshold deficits have been found for all of the major taste qualities and include caffeine, citric acid, hydrochloric acid, magnesium sulfate, phenyl thiocarbamide (PTC), propylthiouracil (PROP), quinine, sodium chloride, sucrose, tartaric acid, and a large number of amino acids.[20–34] However, the magnitude of the effects varies from stimulus to stimulus, and, in general, the effects of age seem to be greater for bitter tastants and the least for sweet tastants.[35–37] Few studies have explored when the age-related progression in dysfunction occurs. An exception is a recent study that obtained electrogustometric thresholds from 461 subjects ranging in age from 15 to 94 years.[22] These investigators concluded that taste loss typically began after the age of 60 years, although in some tongue regions the deficit appeared a decade later.

It should be noted that the detection of age-related deficits depends not only on the oral regions that are assessed but also on the type of testing that is performed. In general, deficits are more marked when testing involves small regions rather than large regions of the tongue. Whole mouth swishing of tastants stimulates multiple nerves and is less sensitive to subtle deficits. An example of the age-related decline in sensitivity of smell regions of the tongue to NaCl is shown in **Fig. 13.7**.[32]

Suprathreshold perception of tastants is also altered by age. Thus, although young people experience a significant increase in the intensity of a taste stimulus as its concentration is increased, some older persons experience a more blunted perception with the increased intensity. In one study, the slope relating intensity magnitude estimates to tastant concentrations was decreased in older adults relative to younger adults by an average factor of 1.76 for bitter-tasting compounds and 2.06 for sweet-tasting compounds.[38] However, in a recent meta-analysis of both threshold and suprathreshold deficits in older cohorts, only 64% (16/25) of the suprathreshold studies evaluated reported a significant age-related deficit, as compared with 87% (20/23) of the threshold studies.[19] Assuming these are accurate proportions,

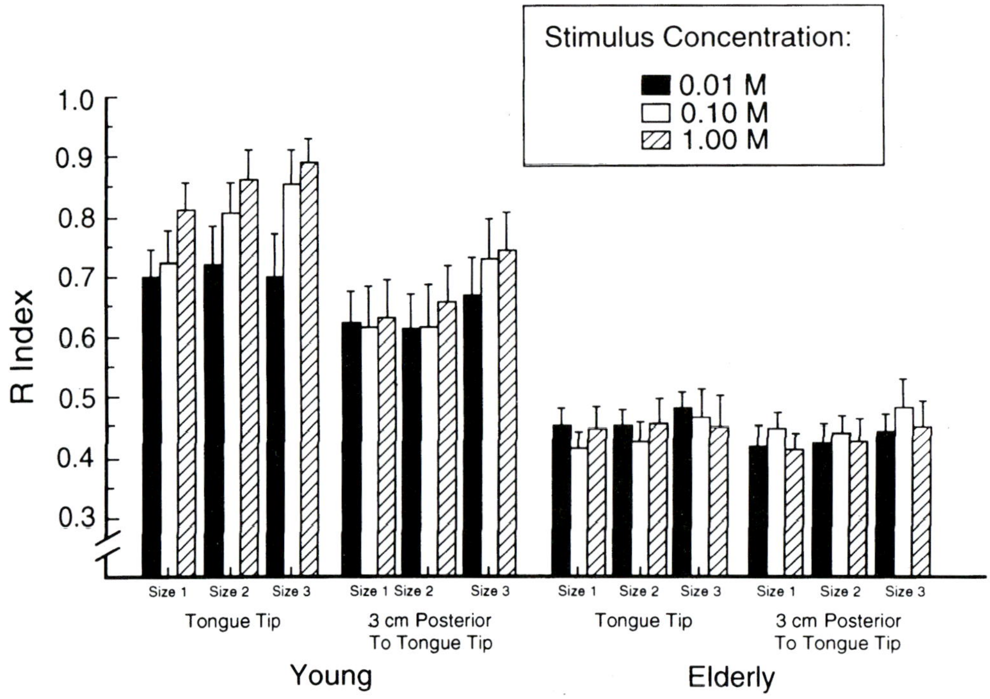

Fig. 13.7 Age markedly depresses regional sensitivity to sodium chloride (NaCl). Mean (± SEM) sensitivity values obtained from 12 young and 12 elderly subjects for NaCl presented to two tongue regions for three stimulation areas (12.5, 25, and 50 mm^2) and three NaCl stimulus concentrations (0.01 M, 0.10 M, and 1 M). Note that the sensitivity of the older subjects was close to chance (0.5) in all tongue regions and for all stimulus areas assessed. Unlike the young subjects, greater sensitivity was not seen on the tongue tip than on a more posterior tongue site. (Reproduced from Matsuda T, Doty RL. Regional taste sensitivity to NaCl: relationship to subject age, tongue locus and area of stimulation. Chem Senses 1995;20:283–290.)

this difference could reflect either more sparing of suprathreshold function or a greater sensitivity of threshold tests to age-related alterations in taste function.

It should be emphasized that, on average, age-related alterations in taste function are not the same for men and women. In general, older women do not exhibit as large a decrease in taste function as older men; as with olfaction, their age-related decline occurs somewhat later in life than that which occurs in men. This phenomenon may reflect a continuance of the sex differences that appear early in life[39]—a sex difference that can be discerned using a range of test procedures, including detection threshold tests,[25,28] recognition threshold tests,[30,40] suprathreshold scaling tests,[41,42] and electrical taste threshold tests.[43]

Although, as described later in this chapter, most of the change in the ability to taste is dependent on changes in the physiology of the taste system, several factors can confound taste measures, including previous smoking history and oral hygiene. As noted by Bartoshuk et al,[44] in some cases age-related decreases in taste sensitivity at low concentrations may reflect a "masking" background taste or mild dysgeusia that results in poor discrimination between the water control and the tastant. This concept is supported by observations that improvement of oral hygiene results in lowering of taste thresholds.[45,46] For example, Langan and Yearick found that elderly persons who received professional oral hygiene therapy three times a week for 5 weeks experienced a lowering of thresholds for sucrose and sodium chloride relative to a control group who were similarly visited by an oral hygienist who only inspected and swabbed the teeth.[46]

The Olfactory System

Major age-related decrements in the ability to smell are well documented.[47–57] An example of the age-related alterations in the ability to identify odors is shown in **Fig. 13.8**.[53] Note that women, on average, outperform men at all ages and that men show an earlier decline in function than women. Importantly, the age-related decline in the sensitivity to odors also occurs for volatiles that enter the olfactory region from the nasopharynx (i.e., vapors from ingested foods and drinks).[58] Because the intensity of retronasal odor perception is influenced by mouth movements that occur during deglutition,[59] some age-related decreases in flavor sensations may reflect fewer molecules reaching the receptor region as a result of decreases in the speed and magnitude of chewing and swallowing. Age-related declines are also present in the responsiveness of the nasal mucosa to chemicals that produce irritation and

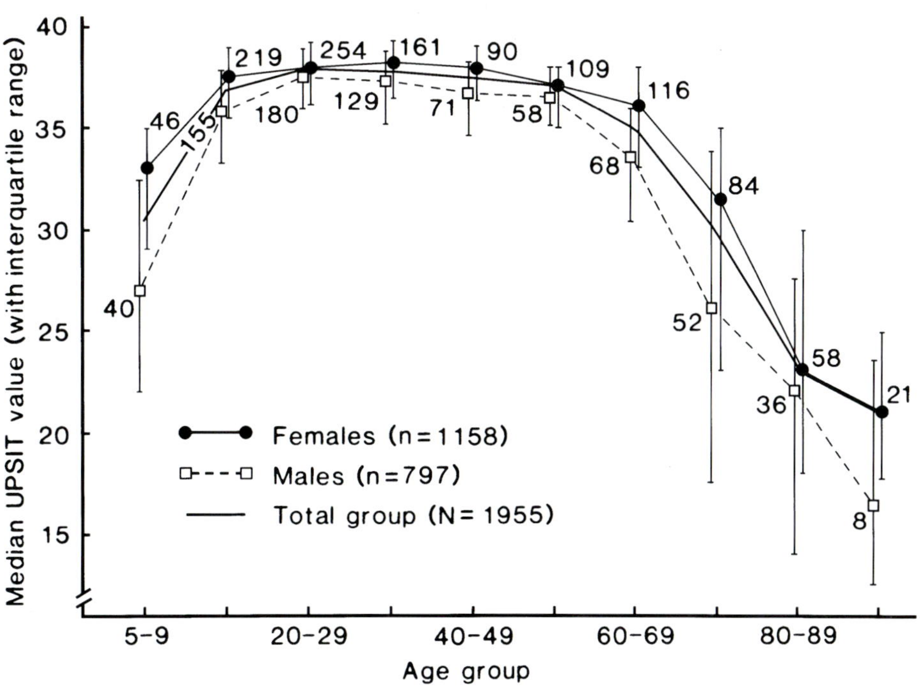

Fig. 13.8 Scores on the University of Pennsylvania Smell Identification Test (UPSIT), a 40-item self-administered smell identification test, as a function of subject age and sex. Numbers by each data point indicate sample sizes. Note that women identify odorants better than men at all ages. (Used with permission from Doty RL, Shaman P, Applebaum SL, Giberson R, Sikorsky L, Rosenberg, L. Smell identification ability: Changes with age. Science 1984;226:1441–1443. Copyright 1984 American Association for the Advancement of Science.)

other skin sensations via the free nerve endings of the trigeminal (CN V) nerve.[60]

In general, individuals who exhibit comparatively low sensitivity to one odorant exhibit low sensitivity to others, whereas those who evidence comparatively high sensitivity to an odorant typically evidence high sensitivity to others. Such observations suggest that a “general olfactory acuity” factor exists, analogous to the general intelligence factor derived from items of intelligence tests.[61,62]

■ The Physiological Basis for Age-Related Chemosensory Deficits

In both the taste and smell systems, age-related changes in the number of functioning receptor elements occur.

The Oral Taste System

Intuitively one would expect an age-related decline in taste function to reflect an age-related decline in the number of taste buds or taste cells. In general, detection thresholds and the perceived intensity of tastants presented to small areas of the anterior tongue are proportional to the number and density of fungiform papillae and taste buds within the stimulated regions.[63–68] The number of stimulus sensations derived from stimulation of individual papillae correlates with the number of taste buds present in the papillae, as determined from autopsy.[69]

Declines in taste bud numbers with age depend on the specific tongue regions evaluated. Age-related declines in taste bud numbers have been reported within the epiglottis and the *circumvallate* papilla.[70] For example, Mochizuki reported the following figures from such papillae: from 0 to 20 years, 242 taste buds; from 21 to 60 years, 196 taste buds; and from 61 to 90 years, 116 taste buds.[71] Such declines are not apparent in taste bud numbers from the anterior and medial regions of the tongues of rodents, monkeys, and humans.[72–75] For example, Arvidson found no age or sex differences in taste bud numbers in 182 *fungiform* papillae collected, at autopsy, from 22 persons ranging in age from 2 to 90 years.[76] Although the number of taste buds in a single papilla varied from 0 to 27, 63% of the papillae had no taste buds at all, 26% had 1 to 3 buds, and the remainder had 4 or more buds. Among individuals, the mean number of taste buds per papillae varied from 0 to 9. Miller found no statistically meaningful relation between age and taste bud densities on either the tip or the midregion of tongues from young adults, although the sample sizes were small for young adults (22–36 years, $n = 5$), middle-aged adults (50–63 years, $n = 7$), and old adults (70–90 years, $n = 6$).[75] Marked variability was observed at all ages—variability that likely obscured any age-related alterations. Mistretta and Oakley found the average percentage of *fungiform* papillae–containing taste buds in Fischer 344 rats aged 4 to 6 months, 20 to 24 months, and 30 to 37 months to be 99.6%, 99.3%, and 94.7%, respectively.[74]

McBride and Mistretta[77] observed decreased neural responses to some salts, acids, and sugars in neurophysiological recordings from the chorda tympani nerves of older rats, even though they found no evidence of a decrease in taste bud numbers.[74] Possible explanations of this phenomenon include changes in the epithelium that might hinder movement of tastants into taste pores, decreases in intrinsic reactivity of taste receptor cells, lowered taste nerve responsiveness, and decreased neural innervation of taste buds by taste fibers. Importantly, taste buds function in a complex milieu in which they are bathed with other secretory products, such as Ebner gland secretions around the foliate papillae, which themselves may undergo age-related changes.

Relatively little is known about changes in central nervous system taste pathways that may be influenced by aging. One functional magnetic resonance imaging (fMRI) study reported that relative to young adults, older adults exhibited, especially when hungry, more frequent and consistent positive activation in brain regions associated with gustatory and reward processing such as the amygdala, caudate nucleus, and orbitofrontal cortex. However, the two groups had equivalent psychophysical detection thresholds for citric acid, sucrose, NaCl, and caffeine.

Taste distortions (dysgeusias) or hallucinations (phantogeusias) are not uncommon in the elderly. Fortunately, most such disorders, which can be quite debilitating, resolve over time, although in some cases such resolution can take years.[78] Several dysgeusias and other taste-related problems of the elderly may be related to their medications, and polypharmacy may be a significant determinant. According to the *Physician's Desk Reference* (PDR), numerous medications commonly prescribed for the elderly are associated with taste-related side effects, as reflected by such terms as *loss of taste, altered taste, ageusia, taste loss, dysgeusia, bad taste, hypogeusia, bitter taste, metallic taste, unpleasant taste,* and *salty taste*.[79] Major offending medications include antimicrobials, antifungals, antihypertensives, antihyperlipidemics, and antidepressants.[80] About 70% of the antihyperlipidemic drugs listed in the PDR are associated with taste side effects, including atorvastatin calcium, fluvastatin, pravastatin, lovastatin, and simvastatin. Over a third of antihypertensives have been reported to have adverse taste side effects, including calcium channel blockers, diuretics (e.g., amiloride), and angiotensin-converting enzyme (ACE) inhibitors. Captopril is more frequently associated than any other ACE inhibitor, with complaints of ageusia, metallic taste, and taste distortion.[81,82] This drug can make sweet-tasting foods taste salty, and can produce chronic bitter or salty sensations, presumably by directly altering ion channels.[83] Drug discontinuance usually reverses the taste disturbance within a few months, although in rare instances dysgeusias fail to resolve even after many months.

The Olfactory System

Age-related changes in the nature and integrity of the human olfactory epithelium are well documented and include a decline in the number of receptor cells, thinning of the epithelium as a whole, and alterations in the zonal distribution of the nuclei of several cell types within the epithelium. Pockets of respiratory epithelium commonly enter into regions previously inhabited by olfactory epithelium, resulting in a spotty, cheesecloth-like appearance of the region.[84–87]

Such changes appear to result from a combination of environmental and physiological factors. In rodents, epithelial damage can be induced by exposures to airborne toxins, such as 3-methyl indole, which mimic to some degree the pathological consequences of aging.[88,89] Interestingly, rats reared in a pathogen-free environment do not show the age-related changes seen in rats reared in a normal laboratory environment.[90] Cumulative induction of olfactory epithelial damage is believed to have occurred in many older persons from exposures to environmental xenobiotics such as viruses, bacteria, and elements of air pollution. It is noteworthy that age-related declines occur in the epithelial expression of phase I and phase II xenobiotic metabolizing enzymes, including glutathione, carnosinase, S-transferases, heat-shock protein 70, and cytochrome P-450 isoforms, potentially predisposing older epithelia to environmental damage.[91–93] There is evidence that environmental factors likely swamp age-related genetic factors in determining the degree of olfactory function in the elderly.[94]

Age-associated changes also occur at the level of the olfactory bulb and in some higher brain structures. Olfactory bulb size declines with age in humans and other animals,[95–97] reflecting to some degree a lack of trophic factors from damaged olfactory epithelia.[98–102] Interestingly, the olfactory bulbs of more than 40% of *nondemented* persons 50 years of age and older exhibit neurofibrillary tangles (NFTs).[103]

In a series of elegant rat studies, Hinds et al provide evidence that much of the age-related change in olfactory bulb volume is probably secondary to the loss of trophic factors from damaged receptor cells. In one study, such volumes were evaluated concurrently with alterations in the olfactory epithelium.[104] A decline in mitral cell body sizes was preceded by a decline in receptor cell numbers on the septal epithelium.

Summary and Conclusions

It is apparent that chemosensory disturbances are very common in the older population and can significantly impact a patient's quality of life, nutrition, safety, and both psychological and physical health. Despite advances in understanding age-related chemosensory disturbances, the structural and functional bases of many such disturbances are multiple, interacting, and complex. Among the disorders that are common in older populations are distortions of taste and smell. Fortunately, many such distortions resolve spontaneously, although resolution can take, in some cases, many months.[78] Although not addressed in this review, it is important for the clinician to be aware that olfactory dysfunction can be an early "preclinical" sign of such age-related diseases as Alzheimer disease and sporadic Parkinson disease.[5,6]

References

1. Doty RL, Kamath V. The influences of age on olfaction: a review. Front Psychol 2014;5:20 doi: 10.3389/fpsyg.2014.00020
2. Methven L, Allen VJ, Withers CA, Gosney MA. Ageing and taste. Proc Nutr Soc 2012;71(4):556–565
3. Deems DA, Doty RL, Settle RG, et al. Smell and taste disorders: a study of 750 patients from the University of Pennsylvania Smell and Taste Center. Arch Otolaryngol Head Neck Surg 1991;117(5):519–528
4. Santos DV, Reiter ER, DiNardo LJ, Costanzo RM. Hazardous events associated with impaired olfactory function. Arch Otolaryngol Head Neck Surg 2004;130(3):317–319
5. Doty RL. Olfaction in Parkinson's disease and related disorders. Neurobiol Dis 2012;46(3):527–552
6. Doty RL. Olfactory dysfunction in Parkinson disease. Nat Rev Neurol 2012;8(6):329–339
7. Breer H, Eberle J, Frick C, Haid D, Widmayer P. Gastrointestinal chemosensation: chemosensory cells in the alimentary tract. Histochem Cell Biol 2012;138(1):13–24
8. Gilbertson TA, Damak S, Margolskee RF. The molecular physiology of taste transduction. Curr Opin Neurobiol 2000; 10(4):519–527
9. Alloway KD, Pritchard TC. Medical Neuroscience. Raleigh, NC: Hayes Barton; 2007
10. Pritchard TC. The primate gustatory system. In: Getchell TV, Doty RL, Bartoshuk LM, Snow JB Jr., eds. Smell and Taste in Health and Disease. New York, NY: Raven; 1991:109–125

11. Menco BP. Ultrastructural aspects of olfactory signaling. Chem Senses 1997;22(3):295–311
12. Ding X, Dahl AR. Olfactory mucosa: composition, enzymatic localization, and metabolism. In: Doty RL, ed. Handbook of Olfaction and Gustation. New York, NY: Marcel Dekker; 2003:51–73
13. Mackay-Sim A. Neurogenesis in the adult olfactory neuroepithelium. In: Doty RL, ed. Handbook of Olfaction and Gustation. New York, NY: Marcel Dekker; 2003:93–113
14. Berkowicz DA, Trombley PQ, Shepherd GM. Evidence for glutamate as the olfactory receptor cell neurotransmitter. J Neurophysiol 1994;71(6):2557–2561
15. Wilson DA, Sullivan RM. Sensory physiology of central olfactory pathways. In: Doty RL, ed. Handbook of Olfaction and Gustation. New York, NY: Marcel Dekker; 2003:181–201
16. Chen WR, Xiong W, Shepherd GM. Analysis of relations between NMDA receptors and GABA release at olfactory bulb reciprocal synapses. Neuron 2000;25(3):625–633
17. Whitman MC, Greer CA. Adult neurogenesis and the olfactory system. Prog Neurobiol 2009;89(2):162–175
18. Wang C, Liu F, Liu YY, et al. Identification and characterization of neuroblasts in the subventricular zone and rostral migratory stream of the adult human brain. Cell Res 2011; 21(11):1534–1550
19. Methven L, Allen VJ, Withers CA, Gosney MA. Ageing and taste. Proc Nutr Soc 2012;71(4):556–565
20. Kleinschmidt EG, Henning L. Threshold for electric stimulation of taste in diabetes mellitus [in German]. Z Gesamte Inn Med 1981;36(12):407–411
21. Le Floch JP, Le Lièvre G, Verroust J, Philippon C, Peynegre R, Perlemuter L. Factors related to the electric taste threshold in type 1 diabetic patients. Diabet Med 1990;7(6):526–531
22. Nakazato M, Endo S, Yoshimura I, Tomita H. Influence of aging on electrogustometry thresholds. Acta Otolaryngol Suppl 2002;122(546):16–26
23. Mavi A, Ceyhan O. Bitter taste thresholds, numbers and diameters of circumvallate papillae and their relation with age in a Turkish population. Gerodontology 1999;16(2):119–122
24. Ahne G, Erras A, Hummel T, Kobal G. Assessment of gustatory function by means of tasting tablets. Laryngoscope 2000; 110(8):1396–1401
25. Baker KA, Didcock EA, Kemm JR, Patrick JM. Effect of age, sex and illness on salt taste detection thresholds. Age Ageing 1983;12(2):159–165
26. Drewnowski A, Henderson SA, Hann CS, Barratt-Fornell A, Ruffin M. Age and food preferences influence dietary intakes of breast care patients. Health Psychol 1999;18(6):570–578
27. Gudziol H, Hummel T. Normative values for the assessment of gustatory function using liquid tastants. Acta Otolaryngol 2007;127(6):658–661
28. Nilsson B. Taste acuity of the human palate. III. Studies with taste solutions on subjects in different age groups. Acta Odontol Scand 1979;37(4):235–252
29. Murphy C, Gilmore MM. Quality-specific effects of aging on the human taste system. Percept Psychophys 1989; 45(2):121–128
30. Fikentscher R, Roseburg B, Spinar H, Bruchmüller W. Loss of taste in the elderly: sex differences. Clin Otolaryngol Allied Sci 1977;2(3):183–189
31. Koertvelyessy TA, Crawford MH, Hutchinson J. PTC taste threshold distributions and age in Mennonite populations. Hum Biol 1982;54(3):635–646
32. Matsuda T, Doty RL. Regional taste sensitivity to NaCl: relationship to subject age, tongue locus and area of stimulation. Chem Senses 1995;20(3):283–290
33. Mojet J, Christ-Hazelhof E, Heidema J. Taste perception with age: generic or specific losses in threshold sensitivity to the five basic tastes? Chem Senses 2001;26(7):845–860
34. Weiffenbach JM. Taste and smell perception in aging. Gerodontology 1984;3(2):137–146
35. Gilmore MM, Murphy C. Aging is associated with increased Weber ratios for caffeine, but not for sucrose. Percept Psychophys 1989;46(6):555–559
36. Cowart BJ. Relationships between taste and smell across the adult life span. Ann N Y Acad Sci 1989;561:39–55
37. Schiffman SS, Gatlin LA, Frey AE, Heiman SA, Stagner WC, Cooper DC. Taste perception of bitter compounds in young and elderly persons: relation to lipophilicity of bitter compounds. Neurobiol Aging 1994;15(6):743–750
38. Schiffman SS, Lindley MG, Clark TB, Makino C. Molecular mechanism of sweet taste: relationship of hydrogen bonding to taste sensitivity for both young and elderly. Neurobiol Aging 1981;2(3):173–185
39. Doty RL. Gender and reproductive state correlates of taste perception in humans. In: McGill TE, Dewsbury DA, Sachs BD, eds. Sex and Behavior: Status and Prospectus. New York, NY: Plenum; 1978:337–362
40. Lassila V, Sointu M, Räihä I, Lehtonen A. Taste thresholds in the elderly. Proc Finn Dent Soc 1988;84(5-6):305–310
41. Weisfuse D, Catalanotto FA, Kamen S. Gender differences in suprathreshold taste scaling ability in an older population. Spec Care Dentist 1986;6(1):25–28
42. Sorter A, Kim J, Jackman AH, Tourbier I, Kahl A, Doty RL. Accuracy of Self-Report in Detecting Taste Dysfunction. Laryngoscope 2008;118:611–617
43. Coats AC. Effects of age, sex, and smoking on electrical taste threshold. Ann Otol Rhinol Laryngol 1974;83(3): 365–369
44. Bartoshuk LM, Rifkin B, Marks LE, Bars P. Taste and aging. J Gerontol 1986;41(1):51–57
45. Hyde RJ, Feller RP. Age and sex effects on taste of sucrose, NaCl, citric acid and caffeine. Neurobiol Aging 1981;2(4): 315–318
46. Langan MJ, Yearick ES. The effects of improved oral hygiene on taste perception and nutrition of the elderly. J Gerontol 1976;31(4):413–418
47. Doty RL. Influence of age and age-related diseases on olfactory function. Ann N Y Acad Sci 1989;561:76–86
48. Yousem DM, Maldjian JA, Hummel T, et al. The effect of age on odor-stimulated functional MR imaging. AJNR Am J Neuroradiol 1999;20(4):600–608
49. Wysocki CJ, Pelchat ML. The effects of aging on the human sense of smell and its relationship to food choice. Crit Rev Food Sci Nutr 1993;33(1):63–82
50. Ship JA, Weiffenbach JM. Age, gender, medical treatment, and medication effects on smell identification. J Gerontol 1993;48(1):M26–M32
51. Murphy C, Schubert CR, Cruickshanks KJ, Klein BE, Klein R, Nondahl DM. Prevalence of olfactory impairment in older adults. JAMA 2002;288(18):2307–2312
52. Choudhury ES, Moberg P, Doty RL. Influences of age and sex on a microencapsulated odor memory test. Chem Senses 2003;28(9):799–805
53. Doty RL, Shaman P, Applebaum SL, Giberson R, Siksorski L, Rosenberg L. Smell identification ability: changes with age. Science 1984;226(4681):1441–1443
54. Schiffman SS. Taste and smell losses with age. Bol Asoc Med P R 1991;83(9):411–414

55. Rawson NE. Olfactory loss in aging. Sci SAGE KE 2006; 2006(5):pe6
56. van Thriel C, Schäper M, Kiesswetter E, et al. From chemosensory thresholds to whole body exposures-experimental approaches evaluating chemosensory effects of chemicals. Int Arch Occup Environ Health 2006;79(4):308–321
57. Deems DA, Doty RL. Age-related changes in the phenyl ethyl alcohol odor detection threshold. Trans Pa Acad Ophthalmol Otolaryngol 1987;39(1):646–650
58. Stevens JC, Cain WS. Aging and the perception of nasal irritation. Physiol Behav 1986;37(2):323–328
59. Burdach KJ, Doty RL. The effects of mouth movements, swallowing, and spitting on retronasal odor perception. Physiol Behav 1987;41(4):353–356
60. Stevens JC, Plantinga A, Cain WS. Reduction of odor and nasal pungency associated with aging. Neurobiol Aging 1982;3(2):125–132
61. Doty RL, Smith R, McKeown DA, Raj J. Tests of human olfactory function: principal components analysis suggests that most measure a common source of variance. Percept Psychophys 1994;56(6):701–707
62. Yoshida M. Correlation analysis of detection threshold data for "standard test" odors. Bull Fac Sci Eng Cho Univ 1984; 27:343–353
63. Smith DV. Taste intensity as a function of area and concentration: differentiation between compounds. J Exp Psychol 1971;87(2):163–171
64. Doty RL, Bagla R, Morgenson M, Mirza N. NaCl thresholds: relationship to anterior tongue locus, area of stimulation, and number of fungiform papillae. Physiol Behav 2001;72(3):373–378
65. Miller SL, Mirza N, Doty RL. Electrogustometric thresholds: relationship to anterior tongue locus, area of stimulation, and number of fungiform papillae. Physiol Behav 2002; 75(5):753–757
66. Zuniga JR, Davis SH, Englehardt RA, Miller IJ Jr, Schiffman SS, Phillips C. Taste performance on the anterior human tongue varies with fungiform taste bud density. Chem Senses 1993; 18:449–460
67. Miller IJJ Jr, Reedy FE Jr. Variations in human taste bud density and taste intensity perception. Physiol Behav 1990; 47(6):1213–1219
68. Segovia C, Hutchinson I, Laing DG, Jinks AL. A quantitative study of fungiform papillae and taste pore density in adults and children. Brain Res Dev Brain Res 2002;138(2):135–146
69. Arvidson K, Friberg U. Human taste: response and taste bud number in fungiform papillae. Science 1980;209(4458): 807–808
70. Arey LB, Tremaine MJ, Monzingo FL. The numerical and topographical relations of taste buds to human circumvallate papillae throughout the life span. Anat Rec 1935;64:9–25
71. Mochizuki Y. Studies on the papilla foliate of Japanese. 2. The number of taste buds. Okajimas Folia Anat Jpn 1939; 18:355–369
72. Mistretta CM, Baum BJ. Quantitative study of taste buds in fungiform and circumvallate papillae of young and aged rats. J Anat 1984;138(Pt 2):323–332
73. Bradley RM, Stedman HM, Mistretta CM. Age does not affect numbers of taste buds and papillae in adult rhesus monkeys. Anat Rec 1985;212(3):246–249
74. Mistretta CM, Oakley IA. Quantitative anatomical study of taste buds in fungiform papillae of young and old Fischer rats. J Gerontol 1986;41(3):315–318
75. Miller IJ Jr. Human taste bud density across adult age groups. J Gerontol 1988;43(1):B26–B30
76. Arvidson K. Location and variation in number of taste buds in human fungiform papillae. Scand J Dent Res 1979;87(6): 435–442
77. McBride MR, Mistretta CM. Taste responses from the chorda tympani nerve in young and old Fischer rats. J Gerontol 1986;41(3):306–314
78. Deems DA, Yen DM, Kreshak A, Doty RL. Spontaneous resolution of dysgeusia. Arch Otolaryngol Head Neck Surg 1996; 122(9):961–963
79. Physician's Desk Reference. Philadelphia, PA: Thomson Reuters; 2009
80. Doty RL, Shah M, Bromley SM. Drug-induced taste disorders. Drug Saf 2008;31(3):199–215
81. Grosskopf I, Rabinovitz M, Garty M, Rosenfeld JB. Persistent captopril-associated taste alteration. Clin Pharm 1984; 3(3):235
82. McNeil JJ, Anderson A, Christophidis N, Jarrott B, Louis WJ. Taste loss associated with captopril treatment. Br Med J 1979;2(6204):1555–1556
83. Zervakis J, Graham BG, Schiffman SS. Taste effects of lingual application of cardiovascular medications. Physiol Behav 2000;68(3):405–413
84. Morrison EE, Costanzo RM. Morphology of the human olfactory epithelium. J Comp Neurol 1990;297(1):1–13
85. Naessen R. An enquiry on the morphological characteristics and possible changes with age in the olfactory region of man. Acta Otolaryngol 1971;71(1):49–62
86. Nakashima T, Kimmelman CP, Snow JB Jr. Structure of human fetal and adult olfactory neuroepithelium. Arch Otolaryngol 1984;110(10):641–646
87. Paik SI, Lehman MN, Seiden AM, Duncan HJ, Smith DV. Human olfactory biopsy. The influence of age and receptor distribution. Arch Otolaryngol Head Neck Surg 1992;118(7): 731–738
88. Peele DB, Allison SD, Bolon B, Prah JD, Jensen KF, Morgan KT. Functional deficits produced by 3-methylindole-induced olfactory mucosal damage revealed by a simple olfactory learning task. Toxicol Appl Pharmacol 1991;107(2):191–202
89. Gaskell BA, Hext PM, Pigott GH, Doe JE, Hodge MC. Olfactory and hepatic changes following a single inhalation exposure of 3-trifluoromethyl pyridine in rats: concentration and temporal aspects. Toxicology 1990;62(1):35–51
90. Loo AT, Youngentob SL, Kent PF, Schwob JE. The aging olfactory epithelium: neurogenesis, response to damage, and odorant-induced activity. Int J Dev Neurosci 1996;14(7-8): 881–900
91. Krishna NS, Getchell TV, Dhooper N, Awasthi YC, Getchell ML. Age- and gender-related trends in the expression of glutathione S-transferases in human nasal mucosa. Ann Otol Rhinol Laryngol 1995;104(10 Pt 1):812–822
92. Kirstein CL, Coopersmith R, Bridges RJ, Leon M. Glutathione levels in olfactory and non-olfactory neural structures of rats. Brain Res 1991;543(2):341–346
93. Getchell TV, Krishna NS, Dhooper N, Sparks DL, Getchell ML. Human olfactory receptor neurons express heat shock protein 70: age-related trends. Ann Otol Rhinol Laryngol 1995; 104(1):47–56
94. Doty RL, Petersen I, Mensah N, Christensen K. Genetic and environmental influences on odor identification ability in the very old. Psychol Aging 2011;26(4):864–871
95. Bhatnagar KP, Kennedy RC, Baron G, Greenberg RA. Number of mitral cells and the bulb volume in the aging human olfactory bulb: a quantitative morphological study. Anat Rec 1987;218(1):73–87

96. Sama-ul-Haq, Tahir M, Lone KP. Age and gender-related differences in mitral cells of olfactory bulb. J Coll Physicians Surg Pak 2008;18(11):669–673

97. Yousem DM, Geckle RJ, Bilker WB, Doty RL. Olfactory bulb and tract and temporal lobe volumes. Normative data across decades. Ann N Y Acad Sci 1998;855:546–555

98. Liss L, Gomez F. The nature of senile changes of the human olfactory bulb and tract. AMA Arch Otolaryngol 1958; 67(2):167–171

99. Meurman OH. Experimental studies of the effect of pathological changes in the nasal mucous membrane on the olfactory bulb. Acta Otolaryngol 1950;38(6):477–483

100. Smith CG. The change in volume of the olfactory and accessory olfactory bulbs of the albino rat during postnatal life. J Comp Neurol 1935;61:477–508

101. Holt CM. Studies on the olfactory bulbs of the albino rat, I: Experiments to determine the effect of a defective diet and of exercise upon the weight of the olfactory bulbs. J Comp Neurol 1917;27:201–234

102. Frühwald V. Die Folgen des einseitigen Nasenverschlusses auf die Riechschleimhaut und auf den Bulbus und Tractus olfactorius. Archiv fur Ohren-, Nasen- und Kehlkopfheilkunde 1935;139:153–173

103. Kishikawa M, Iseki M, Nishimura M, Sekine I, Fujii H. A histopathological study on senile changes in the human olfactory bulb. Acta Pathol Jpn 1990;40(4):255–260

104. Hinds JW, McNelly NA. Aging in the rat olfactory system: correlation of changes in the olfactory epithelium and olfactory bulb. J Comp Neurol 1981;203(3):441–453

14 Inhalant Allergies and Asthma in the Geriatric Population

Karen H. Calhoun

Introduction

Tradition says that older adults are less likely to suffer from allergies, but recent studies show that many elderly people do suffer from allergic diseases and/or asthma.[1] Because there is a general lack of awareness that geriatric atopy occurs, it is often excluded from the differential diagnosis in older patients presenting with nasal congestion, postnasal drip, rhinorrhea, cough, wheezing, or shortness of breath.

In the geriatric patient, there are numerous causes other than atopy that may present with nasal congestion or cough. Some of these include vasomotor or gustatory rhinitis, chronic obstructive pulmonary disease (COPD), and bronchitis, all of which are common in the geriatric population. Add to this the multiple comorbidities often present, and the general lack of knowledge that allergies occur in elderly patients, and it is no surprise that clinicians often fail to consider geriatric atopy. Overlooking this important entity deprives the elderly of appropriate treatment, symptom relief, and, ultimately, improvement in quality of life.[2]

Why Assume Allergies Are Uncommon in the Elderly?

Immunosenescence is defined as aging of the immune system. This affects both the innate and the adaptive immune systems, with a general decrease in immunocompetence. Consequent to this decreased immunocompetence is an increase in chronic and infectious diseases among the elderly.[3,4] There is decreased function of B and T cells, with a reduction in diversity among both populations.[1] With aging, the response to many vaccines is less robust. For example, administering a flu vaccine in young adults causes a response in 70 to 90% of people, whereas a similar vaccination in older patients results in a response of only 17 to 35%.[1,5]

The lower vitamin D levels found in many older patients also hinder a vigorous immune response.[1] Vitamin D promotes the function of antigen-presenting cells (APCs) and T cells. A lack of vitamin D can hinder the induction of T-regulatory (Treg) cells and the development of tolerance, which is a crucial part of the allergy immunotherapy response.

Collective consideration of these facts may help explain why many clinicians assume allergy and asthma are rare in the elderly.

Incidence of Allergies in the Elderly

Allergies affect ~ 20% of the population worldwide. The general assumption is that this is proportionally higher in younger patients, with a slow steady decline as patients age.

Several studies have shown an age-related decrease in total and specific immunoglobulin E (IgE).[1,6] Skin prick testing (SPT) was positive in 28.4% of patients referred to an Italian allergy unit, but this was a selected population of elderly people who had allergy symptoms.[7] Karablut et al looked at geriatric patients with symptoms of allergic rhinosinusitis (AR) compared with a young control group. The rate of SPT positivity was ~ 50% in the older group and ~ 75% in the younger control group.[8]

There are, however, also data suggesting that allergies do not decrease substantially with aging. DiLorenzo et al found no changes in serum IgE or T-helper cell type 2 (Th2) cytokines with aging.[9] A survey of 109 geriatric nursing home patients (mean age 77) tested by interview, SPT, and serum total and specific IgE (sIgE) reported a positive SPT and/or sIgE in ~ 40% of those tested.[10] A large Swiss study using in vitro testing showed the incidence of atopy in men under versus over 60 to be ~ 36% versus 26%, and in women 31% versus 18%.[11] Another researcher noted that severe allergies are worse as the nasal mucociliary clearance time lengthens, which typically happens with aging.[12]

We can accurately conclude that allergies do exist among those over the age of 65 in numbers that are clinically meaningful. If there is, in fact, a lower incidence of inhalant allergies in the elderly compared with the young, this may mean that allergies occur in a greater percentage of the young population and decrease in that same population over time. When today's 70-year-old was age 10, however, the overall incidence of allergies was substantially lower than it is in today's 10-year-olds. Perhaps today's lowered measured incidence of allergy in the older patient represents the constant rate of allergy in an aging cohort, rather than a diminution of allergy over that person's lifetime. Only future longitudinal studies will distinguish between these two possibilities.

Incidence of Asthma

The overall incidence of asthma in individuals over the age of 65 is often quoted as being 6 to 10%.[1] One study in Texas of the elderly reported a 6.3% incidence of asthma, with another 9% having "probable asthma."[13] A Korean study of over 2,000 people noted an incidence of asthma (based on a questionnaire and methacholine challenge) ranging from 2% in those under 40, to 12.7% in those 65 or older.[14] In the aforementioned large Swiss study, a little over 8% of those under 60 had asthma, compared with ~ 7% for those over 60.[11]

Older patients are more likely to have wheezing, shortness of breath (SOB), and cough than younger age groups. These presenting symptoms may be presumed to indicate conditions known to be more common in the older age group (COPD, bronchitis, congestive heart failure) without investigating the possibility of a reversible component. This can lead to major clinical difficulties. It is noteworthy that asthma deaths in younger patients are decreasing, whereas asthma mortality is increasing in older patients. Part of this problem may stem from an inaccurate diagnosis in the elderly to begin with. Hospens et al noted that, among geriatric patients with respiratory problems, the presence of airway hyperreactivity was associated with a more rapid decrease in pulmonary function and significantly worse exacerbations.[15] Spirometry is accurate in the elderly[11] and can be used in the office setting to reliably distinguish reversible from irreversible obstructive pulmonary disease. This useful tool helps prevent the misdiagnosis and consequent inappropriate treatment of a respiratory problem such as COPD when it is actually asthma.

A large significant percentage of asthma in the elderly has allergic triggers.[16] King et al described significantly more inhalant allergies in elderly patients with asthma compared with those without asthma (odds ratio 13).[16] In Baltimore, Huss et al noted that, of 80 asthmatic patients over age 65, 75% had at least one positive SPT.[17] Ariano et al documented that, among patients with asthma, 72% had at least one positive SPT.[18] Jackola et al demonstrated no age-related difference in the incidence of ragweed allergy among asthma patients.[19] Parameswaran et al reported that a history of atopy was a very strong predictor of asthma among the elderly.[20]

How Are Allergy and Asthma Best Diagnosed in the Geriatric Population?

As with most things in medicine, diagnosis begins with a thorough history and physical examination. The history may contain clues such as seasonality (worse symptoms in spring suggests tree pollen allergies), location (symptoms occurring in a musty basement may be due to mold), or proximity (visiting a friend who has a cat always results in wheezing). Daily symptom scores and records of medication use can be used to estimate the severity of allergic disease. On physical examination, there may be "allergic shiners" (dark circles under the eyes due to venous congestion) or an allergic crease on the nose (horizontal wrinkle just above the lower lateral cartilages due to habitual rubbing of the hand upward under the nose), or even frank wheezing. Speculum examination of the nose or endoscopy often reveals edematous mucosa, which is typically pale or faintly bluish in color.

Diagnosis is confirmed with allergy testing, in vitro testing (measuring levels of antigen-specific IgE in the serum), or skin testing (applying small amounts of potential allergen into the skin looking for stimulation of histamine release). Skin testing can be either epicutaneous (SPT) or intradermal dilutional testing (IDT).

SPT is performed with concentrated antigen, usually 1:20 weight to volume (w:v) or equivalent. Because the IDT inserts antigen deeper into the skin where there are more reactive cells, more dilute solutions of antigen are used. Classic IDT uses serial injections of each antigen, ranging from very dilute (dilution no. 6, or 1:312,550) to more concentrated (dilution no. 2, or 1:500). Positive histamine and negative saline controls are used in both types of testing, with a negative glycerine control sometimes also used. There are also methods of combining these two techniques, as in modified quantitative testing.[21]

Other testing used mainly in research includes nasal provocation (insufflation of allergen into the nose while measuring the nasal airway before and after using acoustic rhinometry) and conjunctival challenge (applying allergen directly to the conjunctiva).

A final confounder in the diagnosis of inhalant allergies is local allergic rhinitis (LAR).[22,23] This is a condition where allergic symptoms are present, perhaps even a response to antihistamines, but skin and blood testing are negative. In some of these patients, sIgE is present in nasal secretions, brush biopsy, washings, or tissue biopsy. Rondón et al reported the presence of local nasal sIgE in ~ 40% of patients who had previously been assigned a nonallergic diagnosis.[24,25]

How Does Aging Affect Allergy Testing?

Although the mechanics of in vitro testing are unchanged by age, this investigation is widely regarded as less sensitive than skin testing. Skin changes with aging as skin histamine response declines, with atrophy of the epidermis and dermis and a decrease in collagen and cellularity. Solar damage can cause false-negative skin test results.[26–28] Some suggest that these age-related skin changes generally increase the chance of false-negative testing, and even suggest that we may need different criteria for the interpretation of skin testing in geriatric patients.

One possible alternative is to follow negative SPT with IDT in the elderly patient. An older study by Nelson et al addresses the question of whether negative SPT in older patients with a positive allergic history should be followed by IDT.[29] In this report, patients were divided into four groups based on history, SPT results, and IDT results. Group 1 had a positive history, negative SPT, and positive IDT. Group 2 had a positive history and positive SPT. Group 3 had a positive history and negative SPT and IDT. Group 4 had a negative allergic history and negative SPT. When they defined AR as having a positive response to nasal challenge *and* having current symptoms, the incidence of AR was 46% in group 2 and zero in the other three groups. In other words, in this study, finding a positive IDT after negative SPT did not identify clinical allergic rhinitis.

Who Should Be Tested and How?

Any patient, old or young, with symptomatic asthma, rhinitis, or conjunctivitis should be considered for allergy testing. In addition, patients with sinus disease severe enough to warrant endoscopic sinus surgery (ESS) should be allergy tested if there has been no such testing within the past 5 years. Allergy skin testing is more sensitive and is therefore preferred to in vitro testing when practical and safe. When performing in vitro allergy testing, it is good practice to also obtain a measurement of total serum IgE. In vitro testing is reserved for the specific situations listed in **Table 14.1**.

If in vitro testing is negative and total IgE is elevated, further in vitro testing may be illuminating because clinically significant atopy is likely. If in vitro testing is negative and total IgE is in the normal range, testing can either stop at that point or continue to skin testing, depending on the degree to which the potentially allergic symptoms affect the patient.

Trouble-Shooting Allergy Skin Testing

Antihistaminic medications must be stopped ~ 10 days before allergy skin testing to permit stimulation of an adequate histamine response.

For some patients who have difficulty discontinuing antihistamines, a brief oral steroid burst when the antihistamines are withdrawn may help control severe symptoms before testing. Oral steroids do not interfere with allergy skin testing. Monoamine oxidase inhibitors and tricyclic antidepressants should be stopped ~ 5 days prior to testing.

Beta-blockers are withheld for 2 to 3 days prior to testing, if permitted by the prescribing physician. For a patient on a cardioselective β-blocker that cannot be stopped for 2 to 3 days to permit skin testing, slow, cautious skin testing is generally safe. Because

Table 14.1 Indications for in vitro allergy testing rather than skin testing

Comorbidities that put the patient at high risk for cardiovascular instability—could increase the morbidity/mortality if a systemic reaction occurred
Patient taking a β-blocker, including β-blocker eyedrops—if epinephrine is required for a systemic reaction, the unopposed α-effect could be challenging to manage
Poorly controlled asthma—puts the patient at higher risk for developing a systemic reaction
Antihistamines cannot be stopped (severe urticaria, etc.)—suppresses skin wheal responses
Dermagraphism or other widespread dermatitis—makes accurate interpretation of wheal size difficult
Negative skin testing with high total serum immunoglobulin E (IgE)—suggests that atopy exists
Pregnancy—remote risk of fetal compromise if a severe systemic reaction occurs

the risk of a systemic reaction is related to the total allergic load applied, the tests are applied slowly. If multiple large reactions occur, the remainder of the testing is spread out over one or more additional days. Multiple recent articles suggest that the risk associated with a cardioselective β-blocker is lower than that with one like propranolol, and that the overall risk of a β-blocker and allergy skin testing may have been overestimated.[30]

If SPT is performed and the histamine (positive) control is very small, it is useful to apply the IDT controls. Provided these are satisfactory, IDT is offered to the patient. If the SPT saline (negative) control is positive, IDT may be more accurate. When dermatographism is present, it is worth verifying whether it persists on another day, since it is a response that can vary over time.

What about the patient who has reasonable controls on SPT but no or minimal allergic responses, and yet still has a history strongly suggestive of allergy? It is reasonable to offer these patients IDT. There is controversy about whether positive IDT tests with a no. 2 concentration (~ 1:500 w:v) indicate an allergy of clinical importance. It is this author's view that it does if (1) a no. 2 glycerine control (2% glycerine) remains small, (2) the allergen elicits a wheal of ≥ 7 mm with itching and/or skin erythema surrounding, different from the other test spots, and (3) results coincide with the clinical history such as seasonality, geographic location, similar factors.

How Is Geriatric Allergy Best Treated?

For all allergic patients, there are the three cornerstones of allergy treatment: (1) avoidance of triggers, (2) medications for temporary control, and (3) immunotherapy for long-term tolerance development.

Allergy avoidance is the first choice, particularly with the elderly. Because nothing is ingested, there are no treatment-related risks. Measures like dustmite mattress and pillow covers, carpet removal, and high-efficiency particle arrester (HEPA) filters reduce exposure to perennial allergens. Because homes and furnishings in this age group are also often older, a thorough housecleaning and perhaps replacement of mattresses and other soft furnishings can be very helpful.

Nasal irrigation with saline using a neti pot or other device is another drug-free method of soothing allergic rhinitis and possibly dislodging some allergy-inciting spores/pollens/danders from the nasal mucosa. The only contraindications to this treatment would be surgery or trauma that might cause communication with the intracranial compartment (as with cerebrospinal fluid rhinorrhea) or possibly if a patient requires a very low-sodium diet, although if irrigation is done properly, minimal saltwater is swallowed.

When considering medications for treatment of allergies in older patients, polypharmacy, comorbidities, and general frailty must be considered.[1,8] The package inserts of almost all medications mentioned here include some statement similar to "insufficient numbers of patients over 65 have been tested to know if dose or other adjustments are necessary for patients in this age group." Dosing as will be described here is an extrapolation of information for patients 18 to 64 years old.

Nasal steroid sprays are generally a good choice for the elderly because their primary effects are local rather than systemic, and they have few worrisome interactions with other medications.[31]

There has been concern about the use of nasal steroids in the elderly because of their potential to increase intraocular pressure (IOP) and worsen glaucoma. Two recent studies have failed to show increased IOP after short-term nasal steroid use. One study in which IOP was measured in patients with nasal polyposis before and after 1 month of treatment with intranasal budesonide irrigations found no increase in IOP.[32] In another study, IOP was measured before and showed no change after 6 weeks of nasal beclomethasone spray in patients with known ocular hypertension or controlled glaucoma.[33] Bui et al arrived at different results when they studied IOP in patients with glaucoma who were currently using nasal steroids. IOP was measured before the nasal steroid spray was discontinued, then at 5 weeks and again at 27 weeks following cessation. There was a significant decrease in IOP after cessation, of sufficient magnitude to delay additional glaucoma treatment in many.[34]

This author's recommendation for nasal steroid spray is to use it in patients with no history of increased IOP or glaucoma who have had an ophthalmological examination within the past year. If there has been no recent examination, it is prudent to obtain an ophthalmology assessment documenting IOP prior to starting nasal steroids. When IOP elevation or glaucoma is known to exist, decisions about initiating or continuing nasal steroid sprays are best undertaken in consultation with the patient's ophthalmologist.

Topical nasal antihistamines constitute another localized treatment option, although they are associated with modest systemic absorption. Topical nasal azelastine and olopatadine both carry cautions about use with alcohol or other central nervous system (CNS) depressants.[35,36] In addition, unfortunately, some older patients have dexterity/arthritis/dementia issues, making nasal or oral inhalers more difficult to use than pills.

Oral Antihistamines

The lipophilic nature of first-generation antihistamines facilitates crossing the blood–brain barrier, causing the drowsiness typically associated with these medications. There is also evidence of dose-related cognitive problems when diphenhydramine is used in older hospitalized patients.[37] These first-generation antihistamines should be used with caution in the elderly.

Because second-generation antihistamines do not cross the blood–brain barrier efficiently, they are much less likely to be associated with drowsiness and are generally fairly well tolerated in the elderly.[38] Those currently available in the United States include cetirizine, desloratadine, fexofenadine, levocetirizine, and loratadine.

A summary of the contraindications, cautions, and drug interactions listed on the physicians' package insert of each of these common medications follows.

Cetirizine

Dose adjustment is needed and caution is recommended for patients with renal or hepatic impairment. In 16 geriatric patients (mean age 77) compared with 14 adults (mean age 53), a single 10 mg dose caused 50% prolongation of elimination half-life, and "apparent total body clearance" was 40% lower. The package insert also states that, of the patients in clinical studies, 186 were 65 years and older, and 39 were 75 and older. "No overall differences were observed between these patients and younger patients, but greater sensitivity of some older patients cannot be ruled out."[39]

On the Epocrates Web site, "avoid or use alternative" is suggested for cetirizine with carbinoxamine or doxylamine, and "monitor or modify treatment" for dexmedetomidine because of CNS depression risk.[40]

With a 10 mg dose, somnolence occurred in 14% compared with 6% in placebo.[39] This means use with any other medication that also causes somnolence should be carefully considered. On Epocrates, there is a long list of medications in the "caution advised" category, mostly for risk of CNS depression and psychomotor impairment.[40]

Desloratadine

Dose adjustment is recommended with renal or hepatic impairment. Coadministration with P450 3A4 inhibitors (ketoconazole, erythromycin, or azithromycin) increased plasma concentrations but had no effect on the safety profile. Coadministration with fluoxetine or cimetidine also increased serum levels, again with no effect on the safety profile. Having insufficient numbers of geriatric patients to determine if response was different was mentioned.[41] Epocrates mentions no significant or potentially significant drug interactions.[40]

Fexofenadine

Renal dose adjustment is recommended, but hepatic dose adjustment is usually not needed. It should not be given with fruit juice. Staggering time of dosing by several hours is recommended if antacids containing aluminum or magnesium are also used because these can decrease fexofenadine absorption. Administration with erythromycins or ketoconazole can increase serum levels, but no effect on QT interval was observed. Administration with nevirapine can decrease serum levels.[42]

Levocetirizine

Renal dose adjustment is needed, but no adjustment is required with hepatic impairment. The only medication interactions mentioned in the package insert are with theophylline (small decrease in clearance) and ritonavir (increased half-life and decreased clearance). Somnolence with the 5 mg dose occurred in 6% of subjects, versus 2% with placebo.[43] In normal patients, levocetirizine has no effect on QT interval.[44] Epocrates suggests avoiding combining levocetirizine with carinoxamine or doxylamine because of CNS depression concerns. As with cetirizine, there is a long list of medications under "caution advised," again mainly for sedation concerns.[40]

Loratadine

Renal and hepatic dose adjustments are required. In 12 healthy geriatric patients (age 66–78) the peak plasma level was 50% higher than in young subjects. Erythromycin, ketoconazole, and cimetidine coadministration caused serum level increases but no QT interval changes.[45] On the Epocrates Web site, ranolazine is mentioned as "avoid/use alternative" because the combination could increase serum levels and the related "risk of adverse effects, including QT prolongation, and cardiac arrhythmias." Similarly, use with amiodarone, darunavir, or dasatinib is "caution advised" for the same reasons.[40]

With these caveats considered, second-generation antihistamines are quite useful in the treatment of allergic symptoms in the older population.

Decongestants

These should almost always be avoided in older patients. Contraindications and cautions listed include hypertension arrhythmias, cardiovascular disease, diabetes, glaucoma, hyperthyroidism, prostatic hypertrophy, or renal impairment. Because these conditions are common in the elderly, it is safer to refrain from using this class of medications in most cases.

Leukotriene Modifiers

Montelukast appears generally safe for use in older patients. It should not be administered with grapefruit juice, because this can increase serum levels.[46,47] Dose modification is required in the presence of hepatic impairment but not with renal impairment. Coadministered medications that can decrease montelukast serum levels include barbiturates, carbamazepine, rifampin, or the combination medication of phenobarbital/hyoscyamine/atropine/scopolamine. In treating geriatric asthma, using montelukast, which is a pill, may be easier for some older patients to manage than using inhalers.

Asthma Inhalers

The primary asthma medications used today in the United States are short-acting bronchodilators, inhaled corticosteroids, and combination inhaled corticosteroid/long-acting bronchodilators.

Short-Acting Bronchodilators (2 Agonists) (Rescue Inhalers)

The medications in this class available in the United States include albuterol, metaproterenol, levalbuterol, and pirbuterol. These are used to treat exacerbations of asthma on an as-needed basis. They can increase pulse and blood pressure, making use problematic for older patients with severe cardiopulmonary comorbidities. There is also a potential problem using this class of inhaler when the patient is on a β-blocker medication. Cardioselective β-blockers, which act mainly on heart (β1) receptors may be needed in specific situations (such as after an acute myocardial infarction), where carefully considered benefit outweighs risk. Coadministration with non-potassium-sparing diuretics has the potential for contributing to electrocardiographic changes or hypokalemia. When albuterol and digoxin are used together, serum digoxin levels can increase and should therefore be monitored carefully. Use within 2 weeks of monoamine oxidase inhibitors or tricyclic antidepressants should be avoided.[48]

This class of medications is also used prior to exercise for the prevention of exercise-induced bronchospasm. As more seniors pursue competitive athletics, this has become increasingly relevant.[49]

Inhaled Corticosteroids

These are "controller" medications, used on a regularly scheduled (usually daily or more often) basis to decrease asthma-related pulmonary inflammation. Those available in the United States include beclomethasone, budesonide, ciclesonide, flunisolide, fluticasone, mometasone, and triamcinolone. Contraindications or cautions for many medications in this class include glaucoma, increased intraocular pressure, cataracts, and bone mineral density problems. Inhaled corticosteroids do not appear to increase the rate of diabetes in the elderly, nor do they affect bone density or the risk of fracture.[50–52] Patients using these medications should be encouraged to rinse, gargle, and brush their teeth after using inhaled corticosteroids to decrease the risk of oropharyngeal candidiasis.

Combination inhalers: These combine an inhaled corticosteroid with a long-acting β2 agonist. The three currently available in the United States are fluticasone + salmeterol, budesonide + formoterol, and mometasone + formoterol. The precautions that apply to inhaled corticosteroids and short-acting β-agonists used alone also apply to these combinations.

Can Allergy Immunotherapy Help the Geriatric Allergy/Asthma Patient?

Specific allergy immunotherapy (SIT) is the only treatment of allergy and allergy-triggered asthma that can actually change the natural history of these diseases. However, when we know that the diversity and robustness of the T cell populations decline with aging, is it still worthwhile to consider SIT in older patients? Unfortunately, there are few studies of SIT in this age group.

A Spanish study in 1993 reported using subcutaneous immunotherapy (SCIT) in 22 patients over the age of 60, and noted improved skin reactivity and bronchial hyperreactivity with decreased sIgE.[53] A 2004 Italian study used injection immunotherapy (SCIT) in 37 patients over 54 who were monosensitized to birch or ragweed. This group was compared with 33 younger patients with a median age of 35, also monosensitized to one of these pollens. There was also a group of 37 patients with similar allergies over age 54 who declined immunotherapy and thus served as an additional control group. The two IT groups reported at least 50% improvement in symptoms after 1 to 5 years of IT, with no significant difference between the younger and older groups. Twenty-seven of 37 of the older no-immunotherapy group self-reported unchanged symptoms, and 10 of 37 reported worse symptoms.[54]

Another Italian study published in 2008 used sublingual immunotherapy (SLIT) for patients with persistent rhinitis, mild asthma, and allergy to house-dust mites. When they compared patients aged 18 to 28 ($n = 49$) with patients aged 55 to 65 ($n = 40$), clinical outcome measures improved in all groups. The SLIT patients had fewer new allergies than the non-treated control groups, but there was no age effect.[55]

A crucial part of the competent immune response to allergy immunotherapy is the induction of Treg cells that express CD4, CD25, and foxp3 (forkhead box protein 3). Whereas the percentage of the T cell population that is CD4+ increases with aging, this increase is reflected in an increase in naturally occurring CD4+25+Foxp3+Treg cells. Inducible Tregs, as produced with SIT, decline with aging.[1,3] Interestingly, regular exercise appears to "stimulate greater NK-cell activity, enhance antigen presentation, reduce inflammation, and clear senescent cells in the elderly."[56] Until definitive studies are completed, the current evidence favors the use of SIT in geriatric patients with positive sIgE testing (skin or in vitro) and oculonasal symptoms and/or asthma.

Conclusions

There is a surprising lack of evidence concerning the diagnosis and treatment of allergies and asthma in the geriatric age group. Pending better data in the future, the following are the author's current thoughts and recommendations:

1. Allergies and asthma occur often enough in elderly patients to earn a regular place on the differential diagnosis of patients presenting with oculonasal or respiratory symptoms. Their impact on quality of life is severe enough to make missing this treatable diagnosis unfortunate.
2. In vivo testing (SPT or IDT) is preferred to in vitro testing if it is not medically contraindicated. Whether allergies revealed on IDT following negative SPT are clinically relevant remains unsettled.
3. Geriatric patients with new-onset or worsening apparent COPD, bronchitis, and/or cough should have exhaled fractionated nitric oxide, spirometry (before and after albuterol), or both. Finding a reversible component to a respiratory problem alters the treatment approach, leading to potentially better outcomes for these patients.
4. Avoidance measures, including nasal saline irrigation, are the safest treatment for allergy in all age groups and should be strongly recommended. Many geriatric patients have lived in the same home for decades. Often, the upholstered furnishings and mattresses are older and may harbor mold and dust mites. For smokers, the scent and residue of cigarette smoke may permeate soft furnishings. A thorough cleaning to decrease mold, dust mites, and animal danders is likely to be helpful, even for the nonallergic. Likewise, a HEPA filter, especially in the bedroom, will certainly not hurt, and the resulting improvement in indoor air quality could be helpful to allergic and nonallergic patients alike.
5. The same medications useful in younger groups are useful in the elderly, with the exception of first-generation antihistamines and decongestants. For the available medications, physicians must be familiar with the contraindications, dose modifications, and interactions with other medications. Careful consideration of therapeutic choices is necessary in this age group where comorbidities, polypharmacy, and frailty are common.
6. Pending future age-specific studies, allergy immunotherapy appears to be effective in immune modification and symptom relief in elderly patients. Depending on the physician's treatment philosophy, this means offering allergy immunotherapy early in the course of treatment (the author's preference) or after all environmental changes and possible medications have proven insufficient for reasonable disease control (traditional wisdom).
7. Diagnosis and treatment of inhalant allergies and asthma in the geriatric population become increasingly relevant as the number of older adults in the United States increases. There are a multitude of questions and studies to be performed in this segment of the population, making this a fruitful area of potential research for today's residents and fellows.

References

1. Cardona V, Guilarte M, Luengo O, Labrador-Horrillo M, Sala-Cunill A, Garriga T. Allergic diseases in the elderly. Clin Transl Allergy 2011;1(1):11
2. Wöhrl S, Stingl G. Underestimation of allergies in elderly patients. Lancet 2004;363(9404):249
3. Castelo-Branco C, Soveral I. The immune system and aging: a review. Gynecol Endocrinol 2014;30(1):16–22
4. Jagger A, Shimojima Y, Goronzy JJ, Weyand CM. Regulatory T cells and the immune aging process: a mini-review. Gerontology 2014;60(2):130–137
5. Scichilone N, Augugliaro G, Togias A, Bellia V. Should atopy be assessed in elderly patients with respiratory symptoms suggestive of asthma? Expert Rev Respir Med 2010;4(5):585–591
6. Mediaty A, Neuber K. Total and specific serum IgE decreases with age in patients with allergic rhinitis, asthma and insect allergy but not in patients with atopic dermatitis. Immun Ageing 2005;2(1):9
7. Ventura MT, D'Amato A, Giannini M, Carretta A, Tummolo RA, Buquicchio R. Incidence of allergic diseases in an elderly population. Immunopharmacol Immunotoxicol 2010;32(1):165–170
8. Karabulut H, Baysal S, Acar B, Babademez MA, Karasen RM. Allergic rhinitis (AR) in geriatric patients. Arch Gerontol Geriatr 2011;53(3):270–273
9. Di Lorenzo G, Pacor ML, Esposito Pellitteri M, et al. A study of age-related IgE pathophysiological changes. Mech Ageing Dev 2003;124(4):445–448
10. Bakos N, Schöll I, Szalai K, Kundi M, Untersmayr E, Jensen-Jarolim E. Risk assessment in elderly for sensitization to food and respiratory allergens. Immunol Lett 2006;107(1):15–21
11. Wüthrich B, Schmid-Grendelmeier P, Schindler C, et al. Prevalence of atopy and respiratory allergic disease in the elderly SAPALDIA population. Int Arch Allergy Immunol 2013;162(2):143–148
12. Kirtsreesakul V, Somjareonwattana P, Ruttanaphol S. The correlation between nasal symptom and mucociliary clearance in allergic rhinitis. Laryngoscope 2009;119(8):1458–1462
13. Arif AA, Rohrer JE, Delclos GL. A population-based study of asthma, quality of life, and occupation among elderly Hispanic and non-Hispanic whites: a cross-sectional investigation. BMC Public Health 2005;5:97
14. Kim Y-K, Kim S-H, Tak Y-J, et al. High prevalence of current asthma and active smoking effect among the elderly. Clin Exp Allergy 2002;32(12):1706–1712
15. Hospers JJ, Postma DS, Rijcken B, Weiss ST, Schouten JP. Histamine airway hyper-responsiveness and mortality from chronic obstructive pulmonary disease: a cohort study. Lancet 2000; 356:1313–1317
16. King MJ, Bukantz SC, Phillips S, Mohapatra SS, Tamulis T, Lockey RF. Serum total IgE and specific IgE to Dermatophagoides pteronyssinus, but not eosinophil cationic protein, are more likely to be elevated in elderly asthmatic patients. Allergy Asthma Proc 2004;25(5):321–325
17. Huss K, Naumann PL, Mason PJ, et al. Asthma severity, atopic status, allergen exposure and quality of life in elderly persons. Ann Allergy Asthma Immunol 2001;86(5):524–530
18. Ariano R, Panzani RC, Augeri G. Late onset asthma clinical and immunological data: importance of allergy. J Investig Allergol Clin Immunol 1998;8(1):35–41
19. Jackola DR, Pierson-Mullany LK, Daniels LR, Corazalla E, Rosenberg A, Blumenthal MN. Robustness into advanced age of atopy-specific mechanisms in atopy-prone families. J Gerontol A Biol Sci Med Sci 2003;58(2):99–107
20. Parameswaran K, Hildreth AJ, Taylor IK, Keaney NP, Bansal SK. Predictors of asthma severity in the elderly: results of a community survey in Northeast England. J Asthma 1999;36(7):613–618
21. Krouse JH, Krouse HJ. Modulation of immune mediators with MQT-based immunotherapy. Otolaryngol Head Neck Surg 2006;134(5):746–750
22. Wise SK, Ahn CN, Schlosser RJ. Localized immunoglobulin E expression in allergic rhinitis and nasal polyposis. Curr Opin Otolaryngol Head Neck Surg 2009;17(3):216–222
23. Khan DA. Allergic rhinitis with negative skin tests: does it exist? Allergy Asthma Proc 2009;30(5):465–469
24. Rondón C, Doña I, López S, et al. Seasonal idiopathic rhinitis with local inflammatory response and specific IgE in absence of systemic response. Allergy 2008;63(10):1352–1358
25. Rondón C, Canto G, Blanca M. Local allergic rhinitis: a new entity, characterization and further studies. Curr Opin Allergy Clin Immunol 2010;10(1):1–7
26. Skassa-Brociek W, Manderscheid JC, Michel FB, Bousquet J. Skin test reactivity to histamine from infancy to old age. J Allergy Clin Immunol 1987;80(5):711–716
27. Gilchrest BA, Stoff JS, Soter NA. Chronologic aging alters the response to ultraviolet-induced inflammation in human skin. J Invest Dermatol 1982;79(1):11–15
28. Vocks E, Ständer K, Rakoski J, Ring J. Suppression of immediate-type hypersensitivity elicitation in the skin prick test by ultraviolet B irradiation. Photodermatol Photoimmunol Photomed 1999;15(6):236–240
29. Nelson HS, Oppenheimer J, Buchmeier A, Kordash TR, Freshwater LL. An assessment of the role of intradermal skin testing in the diagnosis of clinically relevant allergy to timothy grass. J Allergy Clin Immunol 1996;97(6):1193–1201
30. Fung IN, Kim HL. Skin prick testing in patients using beta-blockers: a retrospective analysis. Allergy Asthma Clin Immunol 2010;6(1):2
31. Mehle ME. Are nasal steroids safe? Curr Opin Otolaryngol Head Neck Surg 2003;11(3):201–205
32. Seiberling KA, Chang DF, Nyirady J, Park F, Church CA. Effect of intranasal budesonideide irrigations on intraocular pressure. Int Forum Allergy Rhinol 2013;3(9):704–707
33. Yuen D, Buys YM, Jin YP, Alasbali T, Trope GE. Effect of beclomethasone nasal spray on intraocular pressure in ocular hypertension or controlled glaucoma. J Glaucoma 2013;22(2):84–87
34. Bui CM, Chen H, Shyr Y, Joos KM. Discontinuing nasal steroids might lower intraocular pressure in glaucoma. J Allergy Clin Immunol 2005;116(5):1042–1047
35. http://dailymed.nlm.nih.gov/dailymed/lookup.cfm?setid=4b114460-7a1c-11df-8b19-0002a5d5c51b
36. http://dailymed.nlm.nih.gov/dailymed/lookup.cfm?setid=24fb7339-f5a9-4d02-a492-43617729412b
37. Agostini JV, Leo-Summers LS, Inouye SK. Cognitive and other adverse effects of diphenhydramine use in hospitalized older patients. Arch Intern Med 2001;161(17):2091–2097
38. Kaliner MA. H1-antihistamines in the elderly. Clin Allergy Immunol 2002;17:465–481
39. http://www.fda.gov/ohrms/dockets/AC/03/briefing/3999B1_23_Zyrtec.pdf
40. www.epocrates.com
41. https://www.merck.com/product/usa/pi_circulars/c/clarinex/clarinex_pi.pdf
42. http://www.accessdata.fda.gov/drugsatfda_docs/label/2003/20872se8-003,20625se8-010_allegra_lbl.pdf

43. http://products.sanofi.us/xyzal/xyzal.pdf
44. Hulhoven R, Rosillon D, Letiexhe M, Meeus MA, Daoust A, Stockis A. Levocetirizine does not prolong the QT/QTc interval in healthy subjects: results from a thorough QT study. Eur J Clin Pharmacol 2007;63(11):1011–1017
45. http://www.fda.gov/ohrms/dockets/ac/01/briefing/3737b_12_label-claritin.pdf
46. Scichilone N, Battaglia S, Benfante A, Bellia V. Safety and efficacy of montelukast as adjunctive therapy for treatment of asthma in elderly patients. Clin Interv Aging 2013;8:1329–1337
47. Cingi C, Toros SZ, Gürbüz MK, et al. Effect of grapefruit juice on bioavailability of montelukast. Laryngoscope 2013;123(4):816–819
48. http://www.merck.com/product/usa/pi_circulars/p/proventil_hfa/proventil_hfa_pi.pdf
49. http://www.nsga.com/
50. Dendukuri N, Blais L, LeLorier J. Inhaled corticosteroids and the risk of diabetes among the elderly. Br J Clin Pharmacol 2002;54(1):59–64
51. Elmståhl S, Ekström H, Galvard H, Johnell O, Gerhardsson de Verdier M, Norjavaara E. Is there an association between inhaled corticosteroids and bone density in postmenopausal women? J Allergy Clin Immunol 2003;111(1):91–96
52. Hubbard R, Tattersfield A, Smith C, West J, Smeeth L, Fletcher A. Use of inhaled corticosteroids and the risk of fracture. Chest 2006;130(4):1082–1088
53. Armentia A, Fernández A, Tapias JA, et al. Immunotherapy with allergenic extracts in geriatric patients: evaluation of effectiveness and safety. Allergol Immunopathol (Madr) 1993;21(5):193–196
54. Asero R. Efficacy of injection immunotherapy with ragweed and birch pollen in elderly patients. Int Arch Allergy Immunol 2004;135(4):332–335
55. Marogna M, Bruno ME, Massolo A, Falagiani P. Sublingual immunotherapy for allergic respiratory disease in elderly patients: a retrospective study. Eur Ann Allergy Clin Immunol 2008;40(1):22–29
56. Bigley AB, Spielmann G, LaVoy EC, Simpson RJ. Can exercise-related improvements in immunity influence cancer prevention and prognosis in the elderly? Maturitas 2013;76(1):51–56

15 Voice Disorders in the Elderly

Robert T. Sataloff and Karen M. Kost

Introduction

Older adults differ from children and young adults in terms of laryngeal and pulmonary structure and function, hormonal environment and other bodily conditions, aerobic conditioning, susceptibility to injury, intellectual function (including memory) and other factors. Just as physicians must understand functions and limitations of children, so, too, must we become familiar with the special needs, limitations, and challenges of older patients who experience vocal change. Expert diagnosis, medical treatment, voice therapy/training, and occasionally surgery usually can maintain or restore vocal stability and "youth." This is important because voice weakness and instability are interpreted often as reflecting intellectual instability. As a result, presbyphonia can impair the credibility of societies' wisest and most experienced elders. Presbyphonic loss of volume also makes it difficult for patients to talk with their older friends, many of whom are hearing-impaired. This may lead older voice patients to withdraw socially, substantially impairing quality of life.

As the number of individuals aged 65 and older increases, it is not surprising to note an increase in the number of older patients seeking consultations for dysphonia. The reported incidence of vocal complaints in the geriatric population is somewhere between 12% and 35%.[1,2] Twenty to thirty-five percent of patients use their voices for work,[3,4] suggesting that vocal health is a high priority within this subgroup of older patients. In all geriatric patients, dysphonia affects quality of life directly; and it may impair the ability to communicate significantly, particularly with hearing-impaired spouses, family and friends. Indeed, dysphonia and hearing loss frequently coexist in the elderly: those with hearing loss are more likely to have dysphonia than their counterparts without hearing loss.[5] Furthermore, dysphonic seniors suffer from social isolation, anxiety and depression, indicating a need to address both dysphonia and hearing loss when treating these patients.[2,6]

Those over the age of 65 are subject to the same vast array of vocal diagnoses as younger adults, including benign vocal fold lesions (polyps, nodules, cysts, papillomas), chronic inflammatory laryngitis (reflux-related conditions, autoimmune disorders, medication-induced conditions), acute inflammatory laryngitis (viral, fungal and bacterial), muscle tension disorders, neurologic disorders (essential tremor, Parkinson, poststroke, spasmodic dysphonia, amyotrophic lateral sclerosis), vocal fold immobility, vocal malignancies and vocal fold atrophy. Vocal fold atrophy is unusual in younger patients except in the setting of muscle wasting diseases, paresis/paralysis, or extreme weight loss. In all cases, presbylarynx must be a diagnosis of exclusion, after all other possibilities have been considered and eliminated. Despite the high prevalence of dysphonia in the elderly, there are relatively few published studies on the subject. This may be because of the complexity of the subject: the severity of dysphonia in the geriatric patient is a function of not only the primary vocal diagnosis, but also several other factors including the functional status of the patient, co-existing morbidities, pulmonary reserve, medications, and cognitive function.

In a retrospective review of 175 elderly patients seen in a tertiary care laryngology practice in Philadelphia, the most common complaints were hoarseness in 71%, inability to project the voice or decreased volume in 45%, excessive throat clearing/phlegm in 43%, vocal fatigue in 37%, cough in 23%, and breathiness in 22%.[7] Less common complaints included raspiness, pitch breaks, loss of range, globus sensation, tremor and dysphagia. Many patients had more than one complaint. The most commonly identified diagnoses, which frequently co-existed with other conditions such as presbylarynx, included laryngopharyngeal reflux, muscle tension dysphonia, paresis (diagnosed clinically and with EMG in many cases), vocal fold mass, glottic insufficiency, and varicosities/ectasias. As a result of their dysphonia, more than 50% of patients in this study reported a significant impairment in their quality of life, with potentially serious psychosocial implications.[7]

Anatomy and Physiology

Between the periods of young adulthood and older age, the respiratory system undergoes marked anatomic and physiologic changes. Decreased force and rate of contraction of respiratory muscles, stiffening of the thorax and loss of lung tissue elasticity undermine the power source of the voice.[8–11] Lung vital capacity is decreased, and forced expiratory volume and air flow rate decline.[12] These changes and others result not only in decreased power source functions, but also in changes in breathing strategy. Some of these are gender dependent. For example, in men, respiratory changes may be linked with inefficient laryngeal valving that results from the glottal gaps commonly noted with aging. In women, the age-related changes may be more likely to involve valving at the level of the velopharynx, tongue and lips, and women also experience a decline in laryngeal agility.[13,14]

The larynx itself also undergoes extensive anatomic and physiologic change during adulthood,[15] as summarized in previous literature.[16] Cartilages undergo ossification and calcification,[17,18] intrinsic muscles atrophy,[19–21] and joints erode.[22] The nature of age-related changes in the epithelium of the vocal folds has been in dispute. Several investigators report thickening; others have found no evidence of change with aging. In women, the epithelium may progressively increase in thickness with aging, particularly after age 70.[23] A variety of changes in the lamina propria have been documented, including thickening/edema of the superficial layer, degeneration/atrophy of elastic fibers, and a decline in the number of myofibrils.[23,24] In males, it also has been suggested that the epithelium increases in thickness up to age 70 and then decreases with further aging. In elderly men, the mucosa stiffens and increases in viscosity in comparison with women and younger men,[24] resulting in decreased ease of phonation.[24,25] Changes in the larynx from young adulthood to old age are generally more extensive in men than in women, with the possible exception of muscle atrophy about which there is little information on gender differences.[15]

Microscopic changes noted in the superficial layer of the lamina propria in mice include a relative reduction in hyaluronic acid and elastin, with an increase in collagen. In addition, there is an increase in the density and ratio of collagen and reticular fibers which are arranged in thick, disorganized bundles.[26,27] Histologic examination of aged human vocal folds has shown a decrease in the total number of cells, reduction in the intracellular organelles responsible for protein synthesis, and reduced production of extra cellular matrix (ECM) from these cells. The superficial layer of the lamina propria increases in thickness and is more edematous in both men and women, with a change in viscoelastic properties.[28,29] Changes within the cricoarytenoid joint include surface irregularities and disorganization of collagen fibers.[30] Laryngeal cartilages stiffen with progressive calcification and/or ossification.

A great deal of work, summarized by Thomas et al, has revealed changes in the musculature of the aging larynx, which contribute significantly to presbyphonia. Several skeletal muscle changes are known to occur with aging. Although many of these also apply to the thyroarytenoid muscle (TA), there are also notable differences. Sarcopenia refers to the loss in muscle mass, strength and quality often observed with aging. Because the loss in muscle mass is gradual, there is little noticeable loss in function, until the loss extends beyond threshold levels. At this point, functional abilities decline noticeably. Sarcopenia is likely the result of metabolic, neurologic, hormonal and environmental factors.

The TA extends from the thyroid cartilage anteriorly to the vocal process and fovea oblonga of the arytenoid cartilage. It is often thought of as being made up of a medial vocalis and more laterally positioned thyromuscularis. The latter probably plays a role in the rapid shortening of the vocal fold, while the vocalis is likely involved in "fine-tuning" tension along the vocal fold edge and in providing lateral resistance during vocal fold contact. Contraction of the TA results in thickening and stiffening of the vocal fold, and a corresponding "loosening" of the lamina propria. Compared with limb skeletal muscle, the TA differs in several ways including fiber size, contractile protein profiles, mitochondrial content, and aging patterns. Similar differences also have been found in other laryngeal muscles.

The TA in humans contains type I, IIX and IIA fibers, as well as "hybrid fibers." Furthermore, it has been suggested that the fast and slow fibers are arranged along a gradient, with the medial aspect composed of slow fibers and the lateral aspect composed of fast fibers. This unique composition, which results in a rapidly contracting, fatigue-resistant muscle well suited for the TA's role as a muscle of respiration, airway protection, and voice production, is unusual compared with limb skeletal muscle. Elevated levels of mitochondria have been noted in the posterior crycoarytenoid, cricothyroid and thyroarytenoid muscles compared with limb skeletal muscle. This feature may increase resistance to fatigue and facilitate the continuous action required by these muscles for respiration. The TA is richly innervated by the recurrent laryngeal and superior laryngeal branches of the vagus nerve. Motor units are small, with each motor neuron innervating only a few fibers. Laryngeal sensory information is received through mechanoreceptors, chemoreceptors, taste buds, and free nerve endings.

Although loss of muscle mass with aging in the human TA was identified first in 1941, and confirmed in subsequent studies, patterns of fiber loss have not been defined clearly. In older rats, a reduction in force, speed, and endurance has been identified. Changes in the innervation of the TA with age also have been noted. Although there appears to be no net loss of myelinated or unmyelinated fibers with age, there is an increase in myelin-abnormal and myelin-thinning fibers, suggesting an active process of degeneration/regeneration. In the superior laryngeal nerve, there is a reduction in the size and number of myelinated fibers, which correlates with the documented reduction in laryngeal sensitivity with age. Metabolic changes have also been noted in the aging TA. Mitochondrial DNA mutations consisting of the 4977-base pair deletion have been identified, and these are thought to result in the increased production of injurious free radicals. Expression of this mutation appears to increase with age, producing dysfunctional mitochondria which may negatively affect contractile properties of the TA. In addition, laryngeal blood flow decreases by ~ 50% in older rats, with a possible reduction in oxygen, and accumulation of cellular waste products. The influence of hormones on vocal maturation, and in senescence, is recognized widely, and appreciated clinically. The mechanism of action of these hormones, however, remains poorly understood.

Marked anatomic changes in the supraglottic vocal tract have been reported from young adulthood to old age. Facial bones continue to grow during this period[31,32] although the magnitude of that growth (3–5%) is relatively modest. Changes in facial muscles include decreased elasticity, reduced blood supply, atrophy, and collagen fiber breakdown.[33,34] The temporomandibular joints (TMJ) undergo extensive changes with aging including thinning of articular discs, reduced blood supply, and regressive remodeling of the mandibular condyle and glenoid fossa.[35–40] However, age-related changes in the TMJ can be difficult to distinguish histologically from a TMJ that is involved pathologically.[37,39,40] The oral mucosa loses elasticity with aging and thins, with deterioration of attachments of epithelium and connective tissue to bone.[22] However, there is some disagreement as to whether these changes reflect normal aging or result from drugs, disease, or pathological conditions.[40–44] Dental structures also are altered with aging, although tooth loss itself is not an inevitable consequence of aging.[45] Changes in the tongue epithelium include thinning and fissuring of the tongue surface.[46,47] Pharyngeal and palatal muscles also have been reported to undergo age-related degenerative changes.[48–50]

Loss of salivary function can produce symptoms of oral dryness, dysphagia, and oral discomfort in the elderly; susceptibility of oral infection also is reported to increase.[51] The elderly have been reported to experience significant declines in tongue strength, although endurance remains relatively unaffected.[52] Lingual pressure reserves during swallowing decline with aging, although maximum tongue pressures during swallow events remain stable from young adulthood to old age.[53]

Acoustic Changes in the Aging Voice

Mueller opined that "The voice is a mirror of personality and senescence may cloud that image."[54] The aging voice is associated with a change in vocal quality that may be perceived as reduced volume, increased breathiness, a change in pitch, decreased endurance and reduced vocal range. When listening to speech samples, listeners are reasonably accurate in distinguishing between young, middle, and older age groups. Older voices often are associated with a loss of range and described with undesirable adjectives such as "hoarse," "raspy," "breathy," "unsteady," "tremulous," and "shaky." The elderly are a heterogeneous group; and many of these characteristics are not solely the result of aging, but rather from poor physical conditioning that results in weak respiratory and abdominal muscles and ultimately inadequate vocal support. Several studies have shown that listeners can generally differentiate between young and old speakers. Aging affects vocal pitch, loudness, and quality, although the effects are highly variable across the aging population.[55]

Speaking fundamental frequency changes with age, with different patterns of change noted for men and women. In men, the fundamental frequency of speaking drops through about the fifth decade and then rises, perhaps due to vocal fold muscle atrophy or hormonal changes. In women, speaking fundamental frequency remains fairly constant or lowers slightly until menopause, after which additional lowering of fundamental frequency occurs. Interestingly, these changes are less prominent in professional singers, who tend to maintain fairly stable fundamental frequency levels throughout adulthood.[56,57] Speech intensity also changes with age. Men over 70 talk louder than younger men, even after taking hearing loss into account. Elderly women do not have a similar increase in speech intensity. However, both genders experience a decrease in maximum intensity levels with advancing age.[58,59] In addition, women have an elevated minimum intensity level (they cannot phonate as softly as young women).[59]

Although there is variability in vocal intensity with age, most studies agree that in the elderly, vocal intensity of speech and the ability to modulate it are reduced.[60] Notably, these changes are much less apparent in elderly singers compared with non-singers, once again supporting a role for "vocal exercise."

Jitter and shimmer are higher in the elderly when compared with younger people and have been associated with higher Voice Handicap Index scores.[7] Both of these characteristics are related to perceptual qualities of harshness and roughness, which have been identified as characteristics of "old" voices. Singers, as well as other healthy, physically fit older individuals display less jitter and shimmer and sound "younger" compared with their counterparts in poor health.

Examination of patients with an "old voice" using strobovideolaryngoscopy may reveal changes associated with vocal atrophy including variable degrees of bowing, noted as a concavity of the medial edge of the vocal fold during both adduction and abduction, prominent vocal processes, a spindle-shaped glottic chink, and a reduction in amplitude of the mucosal wave.[61,62]

Although some age-related alterations cannot be avoided in specific individuals, not all of them are manifestations of irreversible deterioration. In fact, as our understanding of the aging process improves, it is becoming more and more apparent that many of these changes can be forestalled or even corrected. Woo et al reached similar conclusions recognizing that "presbylarynges is not a common disorder and should be a diagnosis of exclusion made only after careful medical and speech evaluation."[63] As physicians and teachers, we need to look closer before concluding: "I can't help your voice; you're just getting older."

Medical Intervention

Certain aspects of the aging process can be controlled medically through judicious intervention. The decision to intervene much be individualized, carefully weighing the risks against benefits for each intervention. For example, as female singers approach menopause, estrogen deprivation causes substantial changes in the mucous membranes that line the vocal tract, the muscles, and other structures throughout the body. These and other hormonal effects frequently are reflected in the voice, but can be forestalled for many years through the judicious use of hormone replacement therapy in selected patients. Dosage is best determined by checking estrogen levels prior to menopause. Preparations containing androgens should be avoided whenever possible because they can cause permanent masculinization of the voice. However, treating physicians must also be aware of contraindications to hormone replacement, especially if there is a history of other health problems such as breast cancer. Other endocrine problems such as hypothyroidism also are common in the elderly and may cause prolonged dysphonia unless they are recognized and treated.

Systematically attacking the aging process in other areas of the body is also important. The bodily changes characteristic of aging are not unique. In many ways, they are identical to those seen in disease and in disuse such as prolonged bed rest or immobilization of a leg. In particular, muscle disuse causes loss of muscle fibers indistinguishable from that seen with advanced age, as noted above. In skeletal muscle of the limbs, it has long been recognized that muscle disuse/inactivity leads to atrophy that becomes progressively more difficult to reverse with increasing age. Conversely, it is well established that general activity, and in particular exercise programs, positively affect the structure and function of muscle. Resistance training increases muscle mass and strength, while endurance training increases mitochondrial density and may help preserve normal muscle morphology. At a cellular level, exercise positively affects hormonal levels, neuronal input, and enzymatic as well as antioxidant activity. This suggests that decline is not inevitable, and can be minimized or delayed by optimizing health and physical conditioning. Exercise prevents or reverses many of these changes in the young, and it appears to have the same effect when the changes are caused by aging. Appropriate exercise will not only help maintain muscle function and coordination, but it also helps functioning of the cardiovascular system, nervous system, and especially the respiratory system. Respiratory function normally decreases with advancing age. In particular, residual lung volume increases, with a consequent decrease in vital capacity, tending to undermine the primary respiratory improvements resulting from earlier voice training. As a result, as a singer's or speaker's respiratory potential diminishes, it is essential that he or she remain as close as possible to optimum respiratory conditioning. Proper nutrition and weight control also are important. A well-balanced, nutritionally sound diet along with maintaining an optimal weight contributes to a higher quality voice. Oral health includes adequate salivary quality and flow, good dental hygiene, and treatment of any mucosal disorders. Many medications are associated with undesirable effects such as cough, drying effects, and altered cognition, all of which may impact voice negatively. Whenever possible, medications with a deleterious effect on voice should be minimized or changed. Reflux should be identified and treated. Respiratory function, which powers the voice, may decrease with increasing age, as evidenced by an increase in residual volume and a reduction in vital capacity. Good abdominal support is also a crucial component of maintaining a "younger" voice.

The authors find it helpful to think of each individual as having a performance range from his or her poorest performance to his or her optimal performance. Audiences have established a certain level of performance that is acceptable for a professional singer. At the age of 18, a singer with an excellent voice may perform at only 50% of his or her current potential. Yet, he or she may get away with it, because the condition of his or her body is above the acceptable performance standard. However, as a singer ages, physical abilities deteriorate. If the singer still performs at only 50% of his/her new ability, he or she will fall below the acceptable performance standard. However, if, through appropriate training, exercise, medication, and other factors, a singer is able to get to 70, 80, or 90% of potential performance level, professionally acceptable performance may be maintained for many decades. For this reason, in treating age-related dysphonia, a combination of traditional voice therapy, singing training, acting voice techniques, and aerobic conditioning are recommended to optimize neuromuscular performance. In general, rehabilitation is sufficient to restore acceptable voice function and eliminate most of the acoustic information perceived as "old." However, occasionally substantial tissue changes make it impossible for therapy and medical management alone to restore satisfactory voice, and some such patients may benefit from laryngeal surgery. Nevertheless, surgery is unnecessary for the vast majority of patients with age-induced dysphonia.

We are accustomed to thinking of older people as having great latitude in most things by virtue of experience and in deference to their age. When we hear a 70-year-old tenor develop a "wobble," we write it off as "getting old" and are reluctant or embarrassed to challenge him, because, after all, he cannot help aging. We also often do not think of prescribing exercises such as swimming, walking, jogging, or other aerobic exercise for people with gray hair and a little extra weight. However, this reticence is unfair and unproductive. To the contrary, as lungs and thorax lose their elasticity and distensibility and abdominal muscle mass begins to deteriorate, it is all the more important for a professional voice user to be in peak physical condition. A singer whose respiratory and abdominal conditioning is not good enough to allow him or her to walk up a few flights of stairs without becoming winded probably is unable to maintain good abdominal support throughout a recital or opera. When the power source of the voice is undermined in this way, compensatory excessive muscle use in the neck and tongue usually supervenes. Conditioning muscles gradually in a disciplined fashion under medical supervision restores good support. Regular vocal technical training can eliminate the tremolo ("wobble") and improve agility, accuracy, and endurance in the older speaker or singer just as it can in the beginner.

Psychology and Intellect

Other age-related medical changes also may be significant to vocal function in some people. Personality has been most commonly described in terms of five factors: extraversion, emotional stability, agreeableness, conscientiousness, and culture. Peabody and Goldberg described the five replicable factors that emerge from factor analysis of a large number of personality traits.[64] In general, personality traits are quite stable after approximately age 30. It is useful for the physician to understand personality traits and their tendency for stability. These may be helpful in interpreting other psychological changes associated with aging. Certain mental disorders are more common in the elderly, including Alzheimer disease, and disorders of memory and mood. Alzheimer disease is a diagnosis that can only be made with certainty by postmortem examination of the brain, which reveals characteristic neuritic plaques and neurofibrillary tangles. However, clinical observation and decline in cognitive function documented by neuropsychological batteries over time are commonly used to make a presumptive diagnosis. Impairments in cognitive function and other neurological sequelae also are seen in multi-infarct dementia that presents with increasing frequency with advancing age. Mood disorders, including major depression, are not unusual in the elderly and may account for significant decline in cognitive, affective, and behavioral function. In addition, elderly people have a higher incidence of risk factors associated with mental illness, including poverty, bereavement, isolation, sensory deficits, and physical illness. It should also be noted that older people perform differently on some psychodiagnostic tests, and such studies must be interpreted with great caution, especially when attempting to distinguish between dementia and expected mental changes such as benign senescent forgetfulness. In IQ testing of the elderly, age-related decrements on tests such as the WAIS-R are primarily in the speed tests, measuring perceptual-motor skills. There are more often decrements in *fluid* abilities (such as reaction speed) than in *crystallized* abilities (such as fund of knowledge). Verbal ability is retained until very old age. With renorming of the WAIS-R to age-appropriate populations, IQ changes in the elderly are now clearly seen as functions of educational opportunity and health status.[65,66] Alterations in cognition, especially memory, and changes in personality secondary to mood disorders and delusionality may impair a person's ability to concentrate, consistently perform vocal tasks, and cooperate optimally with voice rehabilitation.

Endocrine System

Sexual Dysfunction

Sexual dysfunction is also common among the elderly. It is important to recognize that this is associated with alterations in the hormonal environment that also may affect vocal function. For example, in males, serum levels of testosterone decline along with sexual function. In women, postmenopausal levels of estrogen are low, although their effect on sexual function is less predictable. However, they are associated with changes in mucosal secretions and structure, and in mood. Physicians should be aware that estrogen-androgen medications are prescribed for sexual dysfunction in women. The androgens may cause irreversible masculinization of the voice, and their use should be avoided whenever possible, especially in professional voice users.

In addition to the endocrine problems discussed above, thyroid disease in the elderly deserves special mention. Both hyperthyroidism and hypothyroidism are notoriously difficult to diagnose during advanced age. The elderly patient with hypothyroidism frequently does not display the obvious "typical" features encountered in younger people. These include mental slowing, loss of energy, neurotic behavior, hearing loss, weight gain, musculoskeletal discomfort, dry skin, changes in facial appearance, and other problems. The diagnosis in the elderly is often missed because of many of the symptoms may be inaccurately attributed to age. In addition, elderly patients often have other problems to which their difficulties are ascribed in the absence of clear diagnostic clues to hypothyroidism. Alterations in thyroid function frequently produce substantial changes in vocal quality including loss of range, efficiency, and "muffling" of the voice. These vocal derangements generally resolve when the thyroid abnormality is treated.

Head and Neck

Problems associated with hearing loss are reviewed in greater detail elsewhere and are extremely important in older voice patients. Physicians should determine not only the hearing status of their older voice patients, but also whether they have pitch distortion (diplacusis) and loudness distortion (recruitment).[67] These conditions affect vocal performance, and they may require modifications in rehabilitation strategies. Oral cavity changes associated with aging may be particularly troublesome to singers. Loss of dentition may alter occlusion and articulation causing especially disturbing problems for professional voice users and wind instrumentalists. These difficulties may be avoided to some extent by having impressions made while dentition is still normal. Dentures that are more similar to the person's natural teeth can then be fashioned. Although salivary glands lose up to ~ 30% of their parenchymal tissue over a lifetime, salivary secretion remains adequate in most healthy, nonmedicated people throughout life. Atrophic changes in the oral mucosa render it more susceptible to injury in the elderly. The sensation of xerostomia, when present, may be especially disturbing to singers and other professional voice users. Oral cancers also comprise ~ 5% of all malignancies, and 95% of oral cancers occur in people over 40 years of age. Cancers in the head and neck may result in profound voice dysfunction.

Other Conditions

Many other factors also must be taken into account in diagnosis and treatment of elderly voice patients. These include coronary artery disease, cerebrovascular disease, hypertension, obesity, stroke, diabetes, cancer, diet, osteoporosis, hearing loss, vision loss, swallowing dysfunction, anemia, arthritis, neurological dysfunction including tremor, incontinence, gastrointestinal disorders, memory and concentration ability, and other conditions. All of these may have adverse effects on the voice either through action directly on the larynx or through impairment of the voice-producing mechanism at another anatomical site that affects, for example, the power source or resonators. Some of these maladies have a major impact on ability to respond to and carry over voice retraining and must be considered when planning therapy for elderly patients.

Voice Therapy

Expert voice therapy for presbyphonia can be particularly rewarding. Such therapy is best provided by a team, and therapy must include attention to the entire body, not just the voice. As discussed above, aerobic conditioning is essential. Voice therapy for presbyphonia therefore begins with a general medical evaluation and institution of a medically supervised aerobic conditioning program to restore the power source of the voice, which is essential for speaking, and singing. This is similar to the cardiac rehabilitation programs instituted after myocardial infarction.

In addition to the physician, the voice therapy team approach includes intervention by a speech-language pathologist, singing voice specialist, and frequently an acting voice specialist. The speech pathologist is responsible for identifying and eliminating voice abuse and misuse, teaching vocal hygiene, and developing an exercise program for the spoken voice that emphasizes appropriate breath and abdominal support, relaxation in the muscles of the head and neck, and appropriate use of resonance to optimize audibility.[68]

The Impact of Vocal Exercise

Voice exercise programs such as Vocal Function Exercises and Resonant Voice Therapy have been shown to positively affect laryngeal function and voice. Although direct evidence of the effects on TA muscle structure and morphology is lacking, the well-demonstrated benefits of vocal exercise strongly suggest a beneficial effect on the laryngeal musculature. In a study by Gorman et al, 19 elderly men with a diagnosis of presbylarynx were enrolled in a 12-week program of vocal function exercises.[69] At the end of the program, participants demonstrated improved glottic closure, a decrease in breathiness, an increase in subglottic pressure, and significantly increased maximum phonation time from 22 second to 37 seconds. There is no question that age-related dysphonia impacts quality of life as measured by the validated Voice-Related Quality of Life (VRQOL) survey, a 10-item self-rated questionnaire. Berg et al reported significant improvement in VRQOL scores in 19 elderly patients with dysphonia undergoing voice therapy compared with the 6 controls who chose no treatment.[70] Interestingly, patients who were more compliant with voice therapy had even greater improvements in VRQOLs than those who were less compliant. Although voice therapy is noninvasive, it does require a commitment of time, effort, and resources. It is possible that elderly patients with age-related dysphonia must reach a point at which their voice is sufficiently disabling in order for them to be willing to make the necessary time investment in voice therapy. Voice therapy also requires reasonably good cognition. Elderly patients with impaired memory may have such problems with carry-over that they may not be successful candidates for voice therapy.

In the presence of good physical health, technically good singing, which is symbiotic with physical and voice therapy, reduces the changes associated with the perception of an "old" voice.[60,71] Healthy, fit singers are able to maintain a stable fundamental frequency, intensity range, and vocal quality well into the seventh decade, indicating that physiologic age is more predictive of vocal performance than chronologic age.

The singing voice specialist works symbiotically with the speech-language pathologist, caring for both singers and nonsingers.[72] The purpose of this portion of the therapy program is not to create singers out of every presbyphonic patient. Rather, singing skills are to speaking as running skills are to walking. If we try to rehabilitate a patient who has difficulty walking and if we are able to have that patient jog or run, walking becomes trivial, because it is well within the individual's performance limits. Analogously, singing expands an individual's phonatory limits, increasing breath support and phrase length, increasing frequency and intensity ranges, and strengthening the voice beyond the level necessary for even extended speech. The combination of traditional voice therapy and specialized singing exercises expedites and improves outcomes. This approach is valuable for patients of all ages but is particularly gratifying in older patients.

Since 1995, the value of including an acting voice trainer in the voice team has been recognized.[73] Like singing teachers, acting teachers who choose to work in the medical milieu must acquire additional knowledge and skills that are not an ordinary part of their training. However, the techniques used by actors to develop their speaking voices are different from those used by speech-language pathologists or singing voice specialists, although they are compatible and do not conflict with traditional voice therapy. Acting voice trainers teach techniques not only for development of speaking voice strength and projection, but also for control of face and body function, phonatory expression of emotion, preparation and interpretation of spoken materials, and other communication skills. Learning these techniques improves not only voice quality and vocal authority, but it also gives the patient great confidence in his/her ability to control vocal communication. In some cases, this confidence is almost as therapeutic as measurable acoustic improvements, especially in the elderly.

In our experience, voice therapy is extremely valuable in the geriatric patient. In fact, we even offer programs for "voice cosmesis" for patients whose only concern is the "old" quality of their voices. Such patients have often undergone cosmetic surgery such as rhytidectomy, blepharoplasty, and rhinoplasty to disguise signs of aging, yet their voices "give them away." An expert therapy program can be most helpful in these patients, as well as in those who are even more disabled by presbyphonic changes.

Surgery

In some patients, even the best voice therapy is not sufficient to overcome presbyphonia. When vocal fold thinning or bowing causes failure of glottic closure, hyperfunction (muscular tension dysphonia) develops routinely as the patient tries to compensate in an attempt to eliminate breathiness and improve volume. This muscle hyperfunction is often responsible for voice fatigue, increased hoarseness, and sometimes for vocal nodules, hemorrhages, or other injuries. As voice therapy eliminates the hyperfunction, breathiness becomes audible again, and volume may decrease. If the glottal incompetence is minimal, vocal exercises may increase muscle bulk enough to restore glottic closure. At the same time, improved vocal technique will enhance audibility even if slight breathiness remains. However, when glottal incompetence is too great, surgery should be considered. Appropriate preoperative evaluation and surgical technique are reviewed elsewhere.[74]

In a study by Davids et al, geriatric patients accounted for 21% of referrals.[1] In this older group, the most common diagnoses were vocal fold atrophy in almost 25%, neurological vocal dysfunction in 23%, and vocal fold immobility in 23.1%.[1] Management options offered to patients with vocal fold atrophy consisted of reassurance, voice therapy, injection laryngoplasty, and thyroplasty. Almost 40% of patients were reassured and decided to forgo additional treatment. Fifty-seven percent elected to have voice therapy, with a statistically significant improvement in VRQOL scores post treatment. Similarly, the much smaller proportion of patients who chose injection laryngoplasty also had significant improvement in VRQOL scores following injection. These results indicate that the voice changes associated with vocal fold atrophy in geriatric patients can be treated effectively with the simple interventions of voice therapy, injection laryngoplasty, or a combination of both.

The "Voice Lift"

Voice lift is a term that was developed to describe a multidisciplinary approach to restoring youthfulness to the voice.[73] Voice lift is commonly misunderstood as referring to surgery for voice improvement, analogous to "face lift." Surgery is only one component of the voice lift process, which always begins with a medical evaluation, voice therapy, and retraining of the voice in speech and singing. Surgery is considered only after nonsurgical treatment has been optimized and deemed insufficient by the patient and voice team.

Special Considerations: The Untrained Professional Singer and the Choral Singer

Older, untrained professional singers present special challenges. If they have had successful careers, in many cases they have been singing correctly "naturally," despite the lack of formal training. Most singers who sing abusively with excessive tension and hyperfunction suffer fatigue, injury, and do not build successful, long careers. Even nonclassical singers, such as rock singers, who have survived decades of performance frequently sing technically well much of the time. As such singers age, however, they do not have the knowledge to modify vocal performance techniques to compensate for physiologic changes, or injuries. Consequently, they frequently change from fundamentally good technique to worse technique, resulting in impaired performance ability, and possibly even vocal injury. Helping such singers is relatively easy, once they become convinced that they need help, want help, and that vocal education is not going to damage their vocal style and identity. Training such individuals must begin with medical evaluation, aerobic conditioning, strengthening of the muscles of the back, abdomen, and chest, and vocal re-education. The vocal training should include singing lessons and training for the speaking voice. The singing lessons address basics, as would be taught to a teenager. However, older adults may take longer to respond, particularly when they have to give up habitual hyperfunction, strengthen laryngeal musculature that has not been used effectively, and bring the vocal system "into balance." Since nearly everyone speaks more often than he/she sings, it is helpful to include formal training for the speaking voice (using a speech-language pathologist and/or acting voice specialist) in the retraining process.

The majority of people who sing are choral singers. They are devoted, enthusiastic, and commonly untrained. Unfortunately, a great many choral conductors also are untrained in voice or in vocal technique and vocal health. In fact, many are instrumentalists (often piano or organ) with no knowledge of the fact that instrumental rehearsal technique is not always appropriate for singers.[75] Choral singers, irrespective of age, can be helped through individual singing lessons and must be trained specifically to avoid singing too loudly because of the Lombard effect experienced in noisy choral environments. One guide to the health of a choral rehearsal is the condition of voices at the end of the rehearsal. Singers should not be hoarse following rehearsals. Rather their voices should be clear and, if anything, more "warmed up" following the rehearsal than they were at the beginning. When choirs are well conducted, voices are developed throughout the course of a concert season, not impaired.

Summary

Dysphonia in geriatric patients is common and is expected to increase as demographics continue to shift to an older population. The etiology is often multifactorial, with presbylarynx being a diagnosis of exclusion. Older voices are typically hoarse, weak, breathy, unsteady and tremulous. Examination may reveal prominent vocal processes, atrophic vocal folds, and a spindle-shaped glottic gap. Presbyphonia is associated with depression, anxiety, social isolation, and a reduction in quality of life. Histological changes have been demonstrated in the mucosa, lamina propria, and musculature of aged vocal folds. Similar age-related changes in limb skeletal muscles of elderly patients occur as well. Convincing evidence has shown that many of these changes can be reversed or avoided with maintenance of good general health and conditioning maintained with regular physical exercise. Older singers are perceived to have younger voices compared with elderly nonsingers, presumably because of the benefits of regular vocal exercise. Voice exercise programs in elderly patients with age-related dysphonia provide an effective and noninvasive means of treatment, with a positive impact on quality of life, as well as improvement in acoustic measures, maximum phonation time, and vocal intensity. In selected patients, laryngeal surgery can be beneficial.

Most patients with age-related voice changes can be helped. Intensive management through medical intervention and age-appropriate voice lessons should be encouraged. Because older singers and other professional voice users may have considerably less natural reserve and resilience than youthful performers, we need to be particularly demanding with them. They cannot compensate for or tolerate weakness like teenagers, nor can they recover quickly from vocal injuries. However, with optimal physical and vocal conditioning, proper medical supervision of cardiac and respiratory function, and appropriate medication, weight control, nutrition, and surgery in selected cases, many singers, actors, clergy, politicians, teachers, and others may enjoy extra years or decades of improved voice performance, which are gratifying both to them and to their audiences. Similar results may be even easier to achieve in older voice patients with less taxing vocal demands.

References

1. Davids T, Klein AM, Johns MM III. Current dysphonia trends in patients over the age of 65: is vocal atrophy becoming more prevalent? Laryngoscope 2012;122(2):332–335
2. Roy N, Stemple J, Merrill RM, Thomas L. Epidemiology of voice disorders in the elderly: preliminary findings. Laryngoscope 2007;117(4):628–633
3. Kost K, Yammine N. Dysphonia in the elderly: findings from the McGill Voice Laboratory. Unpublished data
4. Takano S, Kimura M, Nito T, Imagawa H, Sakakibara K, Tayama N. Clinical analysis of presbylarynx—vocal fold atrophy in elderly individuals. Auris Nasus Larynx 2010;37(4):461–464
5. Cohen SM, Turley R. Coprevalence and impact of dysphonia and hearing loss in the elderly. Laryngoscope 2009;119(9): 1870–1873
6. Roy N, Merrill RM, Gray SD, Smith EM. Voice disorders in the general population: prevalence, risk factors, and occupational impact. Laryngoscope 2005;115(11):1988–1995
7. Gregory ND, Chandran S, Lurie D, Sataloff RT. Voice disorders in the elderly. J Voice 2012;26(2):254–258
8. Kahane J. Anatomic and physiologic changes in the aging peripheral speech mechanism. In: Beasley DS, Davis GA, eds. Aging Communication Processes and Disorders. New York, NY: Gune and Stratton; 1981:21–45
9. Dhar S, Shastri SR, Lenora RA. Aging and the respiratory system. Med Clin North Am 1976;60(6):1121–1139
10. McKeown F. Pathology of the Aged. London, UK: Butterworths; 1965
11. Mahler D. Pulmonary aspects of aging. In: Gambert SR, ed. Contemporary Geriatric Medicine. Vol. 1. New York, NY: Plenum Medical Book Company; 1983:45–85
12. Crapo R. The aging lung. In: Mahler DA, eds. Pulmonary Disease in the Elderly Patient. Vol. 63: Lung Biology in Health and Disease. New York, NY: Marcel Dekker; 1993:353–365
13. Hoit JD, Hixon TJ. Age and speech breathing. J Speech Hear Res 1987;30(3):351–366
14. Hoit JD, Hixon TJ, Altman ME, Morgan WJ. Speech breathing in women. J Speech Hear Res 1989;32(2):353–365
15. Linville SE. Vocal Aging. Albany, NY: Delmar Thomson Learning; 2001
16. Sataloff RT, Linville SE. The effects of age on the voice. In: Sataloff RT. Professional Voice: The Science and Art of Clinical Care, 3rd ed. San Diego, CA: Plural Publishing, Inc.; 2005:497–511
17. Malinowski A. [Shape, dimensions and process of calcification of the cartilaginous framework of the larynx in relation to age and sex in the Polish population]. Folia Morphol (Warsz) 1967;26(2):121–132
18. Roncollo P. Researches about ossification and conformation of the thyroid cartilage in sex and certain other factors. Mayo Clin Proc 1949;31:47–52
19. Bach A, Lederer F, Dinolt R. Senile changes in the laryngeal musculature. Arch Otolaryngol 1941;34:47–56
20. Ferreri G. Senescence of the larynx. Italian General Review of Oto-Rhino-Laryngology 1959;1:640–709
21. Rodeño MT, Sánchez-Fernández JM, Rivera-Pomar JM. Histochemical and morphometrical ageing changes in human vocal cord muscles. Acta Otolaryngol 1993;113(3):445–449
22. Kahane J. Age-related changes in the peripheral speech mechanism: Structural and physiological changes. Proceedings of the research symposium on communicative sciences and disorders and aging. ASHA Reports, American Speech Language Hearing Association. Rockville, MD. 1990;19:75–87.
23. Hirano M, Kurita S, Sakaguchi S. Ageing of the vibratory tissue of human vocal folds. Acta Otolaryngol 1989;107(5-6): 428–433

24. Ishii K, Zhai WG, Akita M, Hirose H. Ultrastructure of the lamina propria of the human vocal fold. Acta Otolaryngol 1996;116(5):778–782
25. Chan RW, Titze IR. Viscoelastic shear properties of human vocal fold mucosa: measurement methodology and empirical results. J Acoust Soc Am 1999;106(4 Pt 1):2008–2021
26. Honjo I, Isshiki N. Laryngoscopic and voice characteristics of aged persons. Arch Otolaryngol 1980;106(3):149–150
27. Sato K, Hirano M, Nakashima T. Age-related changes of collagenous fibers in the human vocal fold mucosa. Ann Otol Rhinol Laryngol 2002;111(1):15–20
28. Pontes P, Brasolotto A, Behlau M. Glottic characteristics and voice complaint in the elderly. J Voice 2005;19(1):84–94
29. Hirano MKS, Nakashima T. Growth, development, and aging of human vocal folds. In: Bless DM, Abbs JH, eds. Vocal Fold Physiology. San Diego, CA: College-Hill; 1983:22–43
30. Gorham-Rowan MM, Laures-Gore J. Acoustic-perceptual correlates of voice quality in elderly men and women. J Commun Disord 2006;39(3):171–184
31. Thomas LB, Harrison AL, Stemple JC. Aging thyroarytenoid and limb skeletal muscle: lessons in contrast. J Voice 2008;22:430–450
32. Beiver D, Bless D. Vibratory characteristics of the vocal folds in young adult and geriatric women. J Voice 1989;3:120–131
33. Hooton E, Dupertuis C. Age changes and selective survival in Irish males. In: American Association of Physical Anthropology: Studies in Physical Anthropology, no. 2. New York, NY: Wenner-Gren Foundation; 1951
34. Lasker GW. The age factor in bodily measurements of adult male and female Mexicans. Hum Biol 1953;25(1):50–63
35. Leveque JL, Corcuff P, de Rigal J, Agache P. In vivo studies of the evolution of physical properties of the human skin with age. Int J Dermatol 1984;23(5):322–329
36. Pitanguy I. Ancillary procedures in face-lifting. Clin Plast Surg 1978;5(1):51–69
37. Akerman S, Rohlin M, Kopp S. Bilateral degenerative changes and deviation in form of temporomandibular joints. An autopsy study of elderly individuals. Acta Odontol Scand 1984;42(4):205–214
38. Nannmark U, Sennerby L, Haraldson T. Macroscopic, microscopic and radiologic assessment of the condylar part of the TMJ in elderly subjects. An autopsy study. Swed Dent J 1990; 14(4):163–169
39. Pereira Júnior FJ, Lundh H, Westesson PL. Age-related changes of the retrodiscal tissues in the temporomandibular joint. J Oral Maxillofac Surg 1996;54(1):55–61, discussion 61–62
40. Stratmann U, Schaarschmidt K, Santamaria P. Morphometric investigation of condylar cartilage and disc thickness in the human temporomandibular joint: significance for the definition of osteoarthrotic changes. J Oral Pathol Med 1996;25(5): 200–205
41. de Bont LG, Boering G, Liem RS, Eulderink F, Westesson PL. Osteoarthritis and internal derangement of the temporomandibular joint: a light microscopic study. J Oral Maxillofac Surg 1986;44(8):634–643
42. Scapino RP. Histopathology associated with malposition of the human temporomandibular joint disc. Oral Surg Oral Med Oral Pathol 1983;55(4):382–397
43. Breustedt A. Age-induced changes in the oral mucosa and their therapeutic consequences. Int Dent J 1983;33(3): 272–280
44. Cruchley AT, Williams DM, Farthing PM, Speight PM, Lesch CA, Squier CA. Langerhans cell density in normal human oral mucosa and skin: relationship to age, smoking and alcohol consumption. J Oral Pathol Med 1994;23(2):55–59
45. Ofstehage JC, Magilvy K. Oral health and aging. Geriatr Nurs 1986;7(5):238–241
46. Sonies B. The aging oropharyngeal system. In: Ripich D, ed. Handbook of Geriatric Communication Disorders. Austin, TX: Pro-ed; 1991:187–203
47. Adams D. Age changes in oral structures. Dent Update 1991;18(1):14–17
48. Klein DR. Oral soft tissue changes in geriatric patients. Bull N Y Acad Med 1980;56(8):721–727
49. Sasaki M. Histomorphometric analysis of age-related changes in epithelial thickness and Langerhans cell density of the human tongue. Tohoku J Exp Med 1994;173(3):321–336
50. Kiuchi S, Sasaki J, Arai T, Suzuki T. Functional disorders of the pharynx and esophagus. Acta Otolaryngol Suppl 1969;256: 1–30
51. Tomoda K, Morii S, Yamashita T, Kumazawa T. Histology of human eustachian tube muscles: effect of aging. Ann Otol Rhinol Laryngol 1984;93(1 Pt 1):17–24
52. Zaino C, Benventaon T. Functional, involutional and degenerative disorders. In: Zaino C, Benventano T, ed. Radiographic Examination of the Oropharynx and Esophagus. New York, NY: Springer-Verlag; 1977
53. Vissink A, Spijkervet FK, Van Nieuw Amerongen A. Aging and saliva: a review of the literature. Spec Care Dentist 1996; 16(3):95–103
54. Crow HC, Ship JA. Tongue strength and endurance in different aged individuals. J Gerontol A Biol Sci Med Sci 1996; 51(5):M247–M250
55. Mueller PB. Senescence of the voice. Bulletin. Royal College of Speech and Language Therapists 1991;476:2–5
56. Mueller PB. The aging voice. Semin Speech Lang 1997; 18(2):159–168, quiz 168–169
57. Brown WS Jr, Morris RJ, Hicks DM, Howell E. Phonational profiles of female professional singers and nonsingers. J Voice 1993;7(3):219–226
58. Brown WS Jr, Morris RJ, Hollein H, Howell E. Speaking fundamental frequency characteristics as a function of age and professional singing. J Voice 1991;5:310–315
59. Ptacek PH, Sander EK, Maloney W, Jackson C. Phonatory and related changes with advanced age. J Speech Hear Res 1966;9:353–360
60. Morris R, Brown W. Age-related voice measures among adult women. J Voice 1987;1:38–43
61. Prakup B. Acoustic measures of the voices of older singers and nonsingers. J Voice 2012;26(3):341–350
62. Golub JS, Chen PH, Otto KJ, Hapner E, Johns MM III. Prevalence of perceived dysphonia in a geriatric population. J Am Geriatr Soc 2006;54(11):1736–1739
63. Mirza N, Ruiz C, Baum ED, Staab JP. The prevalence of major psychiatric pathologies in patients with voice disorders. Ear Nose Throat J 2003;82(10):808–810, 812, 814
64. Woo P, Casper J, Colton R, Brewer D. Dysphonia in the aging: physiology versus disease. Laryngoscope 1992;102(2): 139–144
65. Peabody D, Goldberg LR. Some determinants of factor structures from personality-trait descriptors. J Pers Soc Psychol 1989;57(3):552–567
66. Botwinic J. Aging and Behavior. New York, NY: Springer-Verlag; 1978:22–30
67. Anastasi A. Psychological Testing. 6th ed. New York, NY: Macmillan Publishing; 1988:347–351
68. Sataloff RT, Sataloff J, Sokolow CJ. Hearing loss in singers and other musicians. In: Sataloff RT. Professional Voice: The Sci-

ence and Art of Clinical Care. 3rd ed. San Diego, CA: Plural Publishing, Inc.; 2005:513–528

69. Heuer RJ, Rulnick RK, Horman M, Perez KS, Emerich KA, Sataloff RT. Voice therapy. In: Sataloff RT. Professional Voice: The Science and Art of Clinical Care. 3rd ed. San Diego, CA: Plural Publishing, Inc.; 2005:961–986

70. Gorman S, Weinrich B, Lee L, Stemple JC. Aerodynamic changes as a result of vocal function exercises in elderly men. Laryngoscope 2008;118(10):1900–1903

71. Berg EE, Hapner E, Klein A, Johns MM III. Voice therapy improves quality of life in age-related dysphonia: a case-control study. J Voice 2008;22(1):70–74

72. Sataloff RT. Vocal Health and Pedagogy. San Diego, CA: Singular Publishing Group; 1998

73. Sataloff RT, Baroody MM, Emerich KA, Carroll LM. The singing voice specialist. In: Sataloff RT. Professional Voice: The Science and Art of Clinical Care. 3rd ed. San Diego, CA: Plural Publishing, Inc.; 2005:1021–1040

74. Freed SL, Raphael BN, Sataloff RT. The role of the acting-voice trainer in medical care of professional voice users. In: Sataloff RT. Professional Voice: The Science and Art of Clinical Care. 3rd ed. San Diego, CA: Plural Publishing, Inc.; 2005:1051–1060

75. Sataloff RT. Voice surgery. In: Sataloff RT. Professional Voice: The Science and Art of Clinical Care. 3rd ed. San Diego, CA: Plural Publishing, Inc.; 2005:1137–1214

76. Sataloff RT, Smith B. Choral Pedagogy. 2nd ed. San Diego, CA: Plural Publishing, Inc.; 2006

16 Swallowing Disorders in the Elderly

Ozlem E. Tulunay-Ugur

Introduction

According to the U.S. Department of Health and Human Services, persons over the age of 65 currently represent 12.9% of the American population. As the fastest-growing segment of the population, this age group is expected to expand to 30% by the year 2030. Dysphagia is a growing health concern in the aging population. Its prevalence is high in both the unhealthy and the community-dwelling elderly population and is associated with increased risks of malnutrition and aspiration pneumonia.[1] Although the exact incidence of dysphagia across different settings is unclear, conservative estimates suggest that 15% of the geriatric population is affected by dysphagia.[1] The prevalence is much higher in selected populations, such as patients residing in nursing homes, who have reported rates as high as 30 to 40%.[2] Aside from leading to malnutrition, dehydration, and aspiration pneumonia, dysphagia also has major effects on social and psychological well-being.[3] Due to the complex nature of the swallowing system and because the workup and treatment encompasses multiple disciplines, several aspects of the problem remain poorly understood.

Changes in the Physiology of Swallowing with Aging

Age-related changes place older adults at risk for dysphagia for two major reasons: first, natural, healthy aging alters head and neck anatomy as well as the physiological and neural mechanisms that sustain swallowing function. This progressive change contributes to the alterations in swallowing in healthy older adults, and is termed presbyphagia, which is also associated with a diminished functional reserve. Second, disease prevalence increases with age, and dysphagia is a comorbidity of many age-related diseases and/or their treatments.[4]

Swallowing incorporates a complex system of both voluntary and involuntary sensory and motor behaviors. Six cranial nerves and ~ 40 sets of bilaterally innervated muscles coordinate the upper aerodigestive system, which coordinates the main functions of breathing and swallowing. Swallowing occurs in four phases: the oral preparatory, oral phase, pharyngeal phase, and esophageal phase. A large number of muscles and structural movements of bone and cartilage are involved in the following tasks: (1) preparing food in the mouth for swallowing, (2) propelling food through the oral cavity, and (3) propelling food through the pharynx and into the esophagus.[5] To execute swallowing safely, the upper aerodigestive tract reconfigures from a system that valves and moves air for the purposes of breathing and talking to one that interrupts airflow and protects the airway while food, fluid, secretions, and medications are allowed to move into the digestive system for nutrition and hydration.[4] With aging, a reduction in muscle mass and connective tissue elasticity results in loss of strength and range of motion.[1] Aging causes several significant changes in the oropharyngeal swallow, although usually the swallowing mechanism maintains a functional ability to propel food safely and efficiently from the mouth through the pharynx and into the esophagus. The overall effect of aging is to slow deglutition and to mildly but significantly reduce swallowing efficiency.[6]

The oral tongue is the primary propulsive force controlling and forcing the bolus into the pharynx. Todd et al corroborated the findings of Robbins et al and others who reported that isometric tongue strength decreases with age. Furthermore, they demonstrated that, since young and older adults generate similar swallowing tongue strength, swallowing is a submaximal strength activity; yet older adults have less functional reserve.[7–9] The decrease in isometric tongue strength in older adults has been postulated to be due to generalized weakening of skeletal muscle caused by sarcopenia.[10] Nicosia et al showed that patients with oral phase dysphagia had lower isometric tongue strength compared with a control group; and Lazarus et al confirmed similar findings in patients with head and neck cancer.[10,11] The role of tongue strengthening exercises in the treatment of dysphagia is not yet clear and requires further evaluation.

Another significant change in pharyngeal swallow with aging is a slightly delayed triggering of the pharyngeal stage.[5] In those over age 65, the initiation of laryngeal and pharyngeal events, including laryngeal vestibule closure, is significantly longer than in younger adults.[6] Although this may put the elderly at risk for penetration and aspiration, in this population the importance of either one of these consequences is still not thoroughly understood. Using flexible endoscopy and the penetration aspiration scale (PAS), Butler and colleagues reported the prevalence of penetration and aspiration to be 15 and 6.5%, respectively, in *normal* elderly individuals.[12] Alternatively, Allen et al suggested that penetration and aspiration during swallowing represent pathological entities that are not present in people with normal swallowing function. They looked at the prevalence of penetration and aspiration on videofluoroscopic swallowing studies (VFSSs) in normal individuals without dysphagia. One individual aspirated on VFSS, and penetration, which was present in 11.4% of normal adults, was even more common with a liquid bolus.[13] Although the implications of penetration and aspiration continue to be studied, one of the well-known associated risk factors is pooling in the pyriform sinuses and the resultant overflow into the laryngeal vestibule. Upper esophageal sphincter (UES) dysfunction can be a major contributor to postswallow residues. Logemann et al evaluated the biomechanics of the swallowing of eight healthy adults between 21 and 29 years old and eight healthy adults over 80 years old. The study revealed that the movement of the hyoid and larynx to open the UES was identical to the point of the upper sphincter opening for both groups. However, there was a significant difference between the hyoid and laryngeal movements after UES opening. Following the UES opening, the younger men continued the anterior motion of the hyoid bone until they achieved upper sphincter opening and went further by 8 mm. In older subjects, the hyoid anterior movement was just enough to get the UES open and only 1 to 2 mm more. The difference between the amount of hyoid anterior movement needed to open the upper sphincter and the anterior amount of movement actually used in total reflects the functional *reserve* present in any given individual. Logemann and colleagues concluded that, although older men seemed to be more efficient in hyoid anterior movement and achieving UES opening, they in fact exhibited no reserve. Functional reserve is needed to assist in recovery when someone becomes ill and loses muscle strength.[14]

Contributing Factors

Skeletal muscle strength begins to decline at approximately age 45 and is associated with a 30 to 40% decrease in strength by the age of 80.[15] This loss of muscle mass not only causes a reduction in strength, but also may be responsible for as much as a 30% decline in the highest rate of oxygen utilization an individual can achieve while performing an exercise requiring substantial skeletal muscle mass.[16] Loss of skeletal muscle mass below a critical threshold, known as sarcopenia, leads to functional impairment and frailty. Sarcopenia of the lingual muscles correlates with malnutrition, and tongue thickness also correlates with midarm muscle area thickness. It has been suggested that exercises improving tongue thickness and strength could improve oropharyngeal dysphagia.[17]

Xerostomia can hinder bolus flow and results in the retention of material along the upper digestive tract. Functional salivary production has been shown to remain fairly stable throughout the age spectrum, although older adults have some decrease in salivary reserve due to the loss of saliva-producing acinar cells. Consequently, the drying effects of medications are generally more pronounced in older adults.[4] More than 400 drugs are known to cause xerostomia, and the older adult is generally on multiple classes of drugs known to be offenders, such as anticholinergics, antihypertensives, antipsychotics, anti-Parkinson agents, diuretics, and sedatives. Xerostomia can also result from diseases such as Sjögren syndrome and scleroderma.

Neurological and neuromuscular disorders are among the most important causes of dysphagia in older adults. Stroke, Alzheimer disease, dementia, and Parkinson disease are all commonly associated with dysphagia. Dysphagia is highly prevalent following stroke, with estimates ranging from 30 to 65%.[18,19] Complications associated with poststroke dysphagia include pneumonia, malnutrition, dehydration, increased length of hospital stay, increased rehabilitation time, increased mortality, and increased health care costs.[1,4,20] About 25% of stroke patients die of aspiration pneumonia within the first year of rehabilitation.

It has been estimated that up to 45% of patients institutionalized with dementia have some degree of swallowing difficulty.[21] Patients with dementia show slowing of the swallowing process, which may lead to increased time needed to finish meals and, as a result, malnutrition. In addition, cognitive impairment, motor deficits, and loss of appetite lead to further difficulties with feeding. Pneumonia is one of the many dysphagia-related health problems seen in this group, and indeed is one of the common causes of mortality.[1,22]

Clinical Assessment: History

Dysphagia is likely to be underestimated in the older adult. Often perceived as a normal part of aging, it may not be brought up by the patient as a complaint until significant changes in diet have been made to compensate. Therefore, diligence is necessary and mandates a thorough history on all geriatric patients. Most patients will present with the complaint of "food getting stuck" in their throat. The site at which a patient localizes dysphagia is of limited value. Although dysphagia in the retrosternal or epigastric areas frequently corresponds to the site of obstruction, dysphagia localized to the neck may be from either the lower esophagus or the hypopharynx.[23] Nonetheless, a careful history can help differentiate between oropharyngeal and esophageal dysphagia. Patients with oropharyngeal dysphagia will more commonly exhibit symptoms of coughing/choking during meals, especially with liquids. They may also have nasal regurgitation and problems with oral competence.

A clear understanding of the current diet of the patient is important. The types of foods causing difficulty should be determined, as well as the number of meals eaten during a day, aiming to understand whether the patient has an adequate nutritional intake. Unintentional weight loss in the elderly is generally a sign of malnutrition and increases the risk of opportunistic infections such as pneumonia. By leading to malnutrition, dysphagia promotes frailty, which in turn may worsen the dysphagia in older adults.

Aspiration risk should be carefully assessed and may be present at either initial swallow or postswallow due to residue in the hypopharynx. As a result of altered superior laryngeal nerve function in this population, silent aspiration is not rare. A history of aspiration pneumonia and hospitalizations should be sought and noted. In the United States, the prevalence of aspiration pneumonia in nursing homes has been reported to be as high as 8%.[24]

Regurgitation of undigested food, solid food dysphagia, borborygmi in the throat, postprandial or nocturnal coughing, and halitosis are all symptoms that should raise suspicion of the presence of a Zenker diverticulum. These patients are also at risk for malnutrition, dehydration, and aspiration pneumonia. A history of neurological disorders, prior surgeries, or head and neck cancer treatment should alert the clinician to the possibility of dysphagia. The cognitive status of the patient is of importance to understand the inherent difficulties with feeding as well as to plan therapeutic strategies.

Physical Examination

A thorough head and neck examination with special attention to cranial nerve function should be performed. In examining the oral cavity, the presence of xerostomia should be noted. Indirect or direct (flexible) laryngoscopy, an integral part of the examination, may reveal pooling in the vallecula or pyriform sinuses, vocal fold hypo-/immobility, or a glottic gap during phonation (incomplete glottic closure).

The pharyngeal squeeze maneuver (PSM) first described by Bastian is a simple yet very valuable test to evaluate pharyngeal function during flexible laryngoscopy.[25] The patient is asked to make a high-pitched, strained phonation, preferably with increasing effort. This will, in a normal pharynx, result in obvious recruitment of the pharyngeal constrictor musculature.[25,26] This recruitment is reduced or absent in patients with dysphagia. Belafsky and colleagues reported a good correlation between the PSM and the pharyngeal constriction ratio, which is a validated measure of pharyngeal strength.[27]

Diagnostic Evaluation

The clinical examination should aim to accomplish several purposes: (1) to identify possible causes of dysphagia and assess swallowing safety or risk of aspiration, (2) to decide on oral versus alternative feeding routes, (3) to clarify the need for further assessment, and (4) to establish baseline or pretreatment clinical data to be compared with follow-up assessment after intervention or during the course of progressive diseases.[28]

Bedside evaluation techniques have been shown to be of limited value in assessing dysphagia.[29] Numerous methods can be used for bedside evaluation, more commonly in hospitalized patients, aiming to identify those at risk for aspiration. The main advantage of bedside evaluation is that many of the health care providers, such as the nursing staff who generally have initial contact with the patient, can be trained in bedside evaluations, triggering a formal assessment if needed.

Patient self-evaluation can be helpful in determining functional health status and health-related quality of life. Developed by Belafsky et al, the Eating Assessment Tool (EAT-10) is a useful clinical instrument for documenting initial dysphagia severity and the patient's treatment response.[30] The MD Anderson Dysphagia Inventory, developed for head and neck cancer patients, and the Sydney Swallow Questionnaire are some of the other instruments available for patient self-assessment.[31,32]

Methods of Evaluation

Flexible Endoscopic Evaluation of Swallowing and Sensory Testing (FEES and FEESST)

These are convenient and efficient methods of testing that can be performed in the clinic and the in-patient setting. They were introduced by Langmore and colleagues in the late 1980s.[33,34] The principle advantages of flexible endoscopic evaluation of swallowing (FEES) include (1) direct observation of the laryngopharyngeal anatomy, (2) ease of execution in every otolaryngology office, (3) no need for a radiology technician, and (4) no X-ray exposure or administration of barium. Limitations of FEES include (1) it does not allow evaluation of the oral phase, and (2) evaluation of the pharyngeal phase is limited owing to the "whiteout" that occurs during swallowing. However, premature spillage, penetration and aspiration, pooling in the vallecula and pyriform sinuses, and spillage into the larynx due to postswallow residue can all be thoroughly evaluated. Although FEES is limited in showing UES transit, residue in the pyriform sinuses may be an indirect sign of UES dysfunction.

The importance of sensation in swallowing and hence airway protection has been studied extensively. In flexible endoscopic evaluation of swallowing and sensory testing (FEESST), airway protection is assessed by the delivery of a discrete pulse of air to the epithelium innervated by the internal branch of the superior laryngeal nerve to elicit the laryngeal adductor reflex, a brainstem-mediated airway-protective reflex.[35] This enables the clinician to obtain vital information about potential performance before the administration of any food bolus.[36] Setzen et al reported a strong association between motor function deficits and hypopharyngeal sensory deficits. In their study, patients with an absent laryngeal adductor reflex showed significant aspiration with thin liquids and pureed foods.[36]

Videofluoroscopic Swallowing Study (VFSS)

Also known as a modified barium swallow (MBS) study, VFSS is the mainstay of dysphagia evaluation. This is the only study that will show all four phases of swallowing. VFSS is useful in (1) identifying existing oral and pharyngeal motility disorders, (2) ascertaining the presence of penetration or aspiration during swallowing of any food consistency, (3) assessing the speed of the swallow, and (4) evaluating the effects of therapeutic strategies such as postural changes, and swallowing maneuvers.[37] VFSS is also useful in monitoring response to therapy. If esophageal pathology is suspected, VFSS can be ordered to be followed by a formal esophagogram during the same visit. An important advantage to this approach is that aspiration is ruled out during the VFSS. Therefore, the patient can safely be given higher volumes of barium. Not doing a formal esophagogram, but rather using a single esophageal screening swallow, has been reported to have a limited sensitivity (63%).[38]

Transnasal Esophagoscopy (TNE)

With transnasal esophagoscopy (TNE), the entire upper aerodigestive tract from the nasal vestibule to the gastric cardia can be visualized safely.[39] It is easy to perform, well tolerated, safe, and requires only topical anesthesia. Indications include dysphagia, globus sensation, laryngopharyngeal and gastroesophageal reflux, and head and neck cancer screening. The relatively high prevalence of esophageal pathology in this group makes TNE an important addition to the diagnostic armamentarium.[39]

Pharyngeal and Esophageal Manometry

Pharyngeal and upper esophageal sphincter manometry allows for objective measurement of pharyngeal and UES coordination and quantitative pressures. Pharyngeal strength and contraction duration, the completeness of UES relaxation, and coordination between the pharynx and UES during swallowing can also be evaluated.[40]

Esophageal manometry is used to examine upper and lower sphincter function, as well as esophageal peristalsis. Decline of peristaltic amplitude and ineffective peristalsis, polyphasic waves in the esophageal body, incomplete sphincter relaxation, and esophageal dilation have been reported in healthy older adults.[41–43]

Adjunct Testing

Depending on the patient's symptoms 24 hour pH-impedance testing, scintigraphy, ultrasonography, and computed tomography may also be useful in diagnostic testing.

Management

The two principal goals in managing geriatric dysphagia include (1) ensuring that swallowing is safe and the airway is protected and (2) preventing dehydration and malnutrition. Although at times these goals can be achieved through surgical means, the mainstays of treatment consist of swallowing therapy, dietary modifications, and close monitoring of nutritional intake. A multidisciplinary team approach to dysphagia, which includes nurses, dietitians, speech-language pathologists, occupational and physical therapists, as well as primary care physicians, neurologists, otolaryngologists, and gastroenterologists ensures comprehensive and successful management.

Surgical Management

Zenker diverticulum, cricopharyngeal (CP) achalasia and aspiration, all of which are more prevalent in the geriatric population, can be managed successfully with surgery.

With the advancement of endosurgical techniques, endoscopic approaches to Zenker diverticulum and CP achalasia have gained popularity. The apparent advantages of shorter surgical times, shorter or no hospital stay, earlier return to a normal diet, and increased patient comfort have been reinforced by reduced complication rates.[44–46] These are all significant benefits in a patient population usually presenting with a myriad of comorbidities and frailty due to malnutrition. Traditional open approaches, despite the advantage of providing tissue for histopathological analysis in the case of a Zenker diverticulum, are generally associated with longer hospital stays and higher rates of complications that include fistula formation and vocal fold paralysis.[47] In managing a Zenker diverticulum (**Figs. 16.1** and **16.2**), the decision regarding surgery and what approach to employ depends on how symptomatic the patient is, the risk of aspiration pneumonia, surgical risk stratification, the size of the diverticulum, and the anatomy of the patient.

The most important component of successful surgical management is correct patient selection. Unfortunately, there are no well-established guidelines for either a Zenker diverticulum or CP achalasia, and practices vary from institution to institution. There is no gold standard diagnostic test for dysfunction of the CP. Most commonly, diagnosis is based on findings of postcricoid pooling on flexible laryngoscopic examination and abnormalities on videofluoroscopy. The latter, however, is largely subjective, and postcricoid pooling is nonspecific. As a result, clinical suspicion plays an important role in decision making.[48] Improvement in symptoms following botulinum toxin injections into the CP muscle has been used as a diagnostic tool, and further treatment has sometimes been based on the outcomes of therapeutic trial injections. Interestingly, Lawson and Zaninotto et al reported a 72.7% success rate with CP myotomy in patients who did not respond to botulinum toxin injection.[49,50]

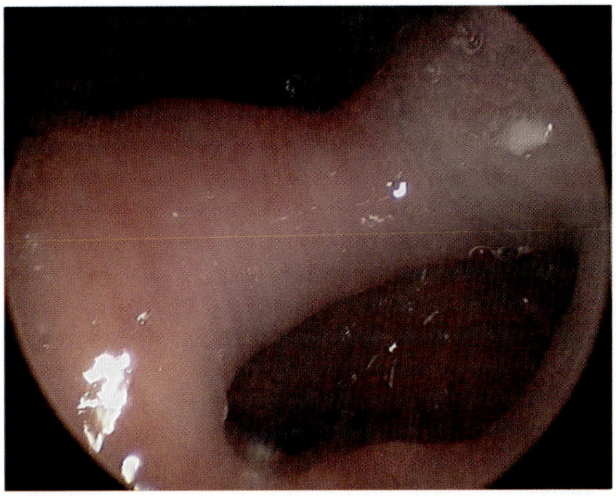

Fig. 16.1 Zenker diverticulum.

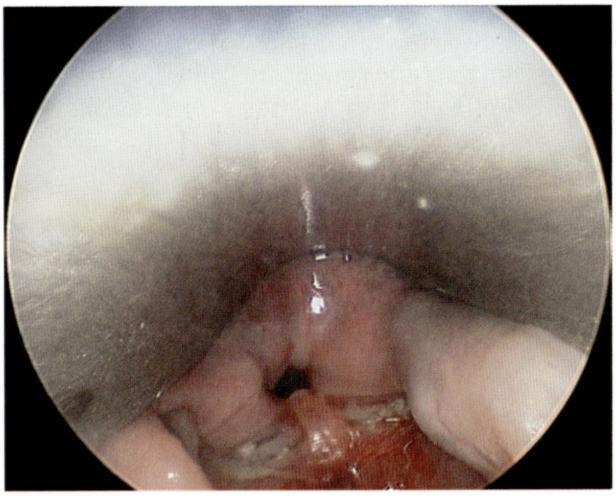

Fig. 16.2 Diverticulotomy performed with stapling.

For dysphagia with intractable aspiration, when all else has failed, surgery may be required. Occasionally, relatively simple procedures that may improve swallowing include augmentation of a paralyzed vocal fold, and cricopharyngeal myotomy or chemodenervation for cricopharyngeal spasm. Often, however, more radical surgery involving definitive separation of the airway and digestive tract is necessary. Options include glottic closure, laryngotracheal separation, and laryngectomy.

Nonsurgical Management

Swallowing therapy plays a central role in the management of dysphagia. Compensatory strategies focus on implementation of techniques to facilitate continued safe oral intake of food and/or liquid, or to provide alternate sources of nutrition to satisfy nutritional needs. They are intended to have an immediate benefit on functional swallowing through simple adjustments that allow patients to continue oral diets safely. Compensatory strategies include, but are not limited to, postural adjustments of the patient, swallowing maneuvers, and dietary modifications.[1] Because of the many conflicting studies on swallowing maneuvers, the role of these strategies without formal therapy has yet to be determined.[1,51,52]

Swallowing rehabilitation, on the other hand, aims to improve physiology through exercises. These exercise-based swallowing interventions have been shown to improve functional swallowing, minimize or prevent dysphagia-related morbidities, and improve impaired swallowing physiology. Although some are directed to comprehensive swallowing function, others focus on strengthening individual swallow subsystems.[1,51,53] Early and vigorous intervention can have a significant positive impact on dysphagia-related complications such as malnutrition and pneumonia.

Enteral Feeding

This is one of the most challenging decisions to be made while caring for an elderly patient with dysphagia. There are many difficult ethical and quality of life considerations involved in the decision-making process. The use of percutaneous endoscopic gastrostomy (PEG) tubes has been increasing, and indications have expanded to include prolonged illness, neurological and psychiatric disorders, anorexia, attempted prevention of aspiration pneumonia, treatment of malnutrition, and the need to provide comfort and improve functional status.[4,54] Within this group, patients with dementia require special attention. Approximately 30% of all PEG tubes have reportedly been placed in patients with dementia, and as many as 10% of institutionalized elderly patients are tube fed.[55] Difficulty eating is common in advanced dementia and is usually an indicator of the terminal phase of the illness. Finucane et al, in reviewing the literature, noted that PEG placement did not prevent aspiration pneumonia, improve survival or function, or reduce the risk of pressure sores or infections.[56] Other studies have also confirmed that nutritional markers such as albumin do not improve with enteral feeding.[55] Feeding tubes do not prevent aspiration, which is a common reason for clinicians to recommend them. Although there is no survival benefit, mortality among tube-fed patients is not insignificant, and among the subgroups of patients requiring tube feeding, patients with dementia have been shown to have the worst prognosis.[4] Therefore, decisions should be individualized after thorough discussion with the family, caregivers, and the responsible primary care physician.

■ Summary

Dysphagia in the older adult is a complex problem due to the nature of the swallowing system and added comorbidities of an aging patient. Effective management of dysphagia depends on early recognition and intervention. This is best accomplished by a multidisciplinary "team" of health care professionals dedicated to dysphagia care. Although the principal goal of the clinician is to improve swallowing safety and to ensure adequate nutrition and hydration, it should be remembered that dysphagia is also a significant quality of life concern. It leads to significant anxiety, social isolation, and depression. A good understanding of the swallowing disorder, relevant ethical considerations, and available medical and surgical management options offers the best opportunity of optimizing care in the elderly patient with dysphagia.

References

1. Sura L, Madhavan A, Carnaby G, Crary MA. Dysphagia in the elderly: management and nutritional considerations. Clin Interv Aging 2012;7:287–298
2. Achem SR, Devault KR. Dysphagia in aging. J Clin Gastroenterol 2005;39(5):357–371
3. McHorney CA, Robbins J, Lomax K, et al. The SWAL-QOL and SWAL-CARE outcomes tool for oropharyngeal dysphagia in adults: III. Documentation of reliability and validity. Dysphagia 2002;17(2):97–114
4. Ney DM, Weiss JM, Kind AJ, Robbins J. Senescent swallowing: impact, strategies, and interventions. Nutr Clin Pract 2009; 24(3):395–413
5. Logemann JA, Curro FA, Pauloski B, Gensler G. Aging effects on oropharyngeal swallow and the role of dental care in oropharyngeal dysphagia. Oral Dis 2013;19(8):733–737
6. Tracy JF, Logemann JA, Kahrilas PJ, Jacob P, Kobara M, Krugler C. Preliminary observations on the effects of age on oropharyngeal deglutition. Dysphagia 1989;4(2):90–94
7. Todd JT, Lintzenich CR, Butler SG. Isometric and swallowing tongue strength in healthy adults. Laryngoscope 2013; 123(10):2469–2473
8. Robbins J, Levine R, Wood J, Roecker EB, Luschei E. Age effects on lingual pressure generation as a risk factor for dysphagia. J Gerontol A Biol Sci Med Sci 1995;50(5):M257–M262
9. Youmans SR, Youmans GL, Stierwalt JAG. Differences in tongue strength across age and gender: is there a diminished strength reserve? Dysphagia 2009;24(1):57–65
10. Nicosia MA, Hind JA, Roecker EB, et al. Age effects on the temporal evolution of isometric and swallowing pressure. J Gerontol A Biol Sci Med Sci 2000;55(11):M634–M640
11. Lazarus CL, Logemann JA, Pauloski BR, et al. Swallowing and tongue function following treatment for oral and oropharyngeal cancer. J Speech Lang Hear Res 2000;43(4):1011–1023
12. Butler SG, Stuart A, Markley L, Rees C. Penetration and aspiration in healthy older adults as assessed during endoscopic evaluation of swallowing. Ann Otol Rhinol Laryngol 2009; 118(3):190–198
13. Allen JE, White CJ, Leonard RJ, Belafsky PC. Prevalence of penetration and aspiration on videofluoroscopy in normal individuals without dysphagia. Otolaryngol Head Neck Surg 2010;142(2):208–213
14. Logemann JA, Pauloski BR, Rademaker AW, Colangelo LA, Kahrilas PJ, Smith CH. Temporal and biomechanical characteristics of oropharyngeal swallow in younger and older men. J Speech Lang Hear Res 2000;43(5):1264–1274
15. Frontera WR, Hughes VA, Lutz KJ, Evans WJ. A cross-sectional study of muscle strength and mass in 45- to 78-yr-old men and women. J Appl Physiol (1985) 1991;71(2):644–650
16. Fleg JL, Lakatta EG. Role of muscle loss in the age-associated reduction in VO2 max. J Appl Physiol (1985) 1988;65(3): 1147–1151
17. Tamura F, Kikutani T, Tohara T, Yoshida M, Yaegaki K. Tongue thickness relates to nutritional status in the elderly. Dysphagia 2012;27(4):556–561
18. Mann G, Hankey GJ, Cameron D. Swallowing function after stroke: prognosis and prognostic factors at 6 months. Stroke 1999;30(4):744–748
19. Smithard DG, O'Neill PA, Parks C, Morris J. Complications and outcome after acute stroke. Does dysphagia matter? Stroke 1996;27(7):1200–1204
20. Martino R, Foley N, Bhogal S, Diamant N, Speechley M, Teasell R. Dysphagia after stroke: incidence, diagnosis, and pulmonary complications. Stroke 2005;36(12):2756–2763
21. Horner J, Alberts MJ, Dawson DV, Cook GM. Swallowing in Alzheimer's disease. Alzheimer Dis Assoc Disord 1994;8(3): 177–189
22. Brunnström HR, Englund EM. Cause of death in patients with dementia disorders. Eur J Neurol 2009;16(4):488–492
23. Edwards D. Discriminatory value of symptoms in the differential diagnosis of dysphagia. Clin Gastroenterol 1976;5:49; Wilcox CM, Alexander LN, Clark WS. Localization of an obstruction esophageal lesion. Is the patient accurate? Dig Dis Sci 1995;40(10):2192–2196
24. Beck-Sague C, Villarino E, Giuliano D, et al. Infectious diseases and death among nursing home residents: results of surveillance in 13 nursing homes. Infect Control Hosp Epidemiol 1994; 15(7):494–496
25. Bastian RW. Videoendoscopic evaluation of patients with dysphagia: an adjunct to the modified barium swallow. Otolaryngol Head Neck Surg 1991;104(3):339–350
26. Merati AL. In-office evaluation of swallowing: FEES, pharyngeal squeeze maneuver, and FEESST. Otolaryngol Clin North Am 2013;46(1):31–39
27. Leonard R, Belafsky PC, Rees CJ. Relationship between fluoroscopic and manometric measures of pharyngeal constriction: the pharyngeal constriction ratio. Ann Otol Rhinol Laryngol 2006;115(12):897–901
28. Speyer R. Oropharyngeal dysphagia: screening and assessment. Otolaryngol Clin North Am 2013;46(6):989–1008
29. Aviv JE, Murry T. Dysphagia evaluation. In: Calhoun KH, Eibling DE, eds. Geriatric Otolaryngology. New York, NY: Informa Healthcare; 2010:293–302
30. Belafsky PC, Mouadeb DA, Rees CJ, et al. Validity and reliability of the Eating Assessment Tool (EAT-10). Ann Otol Rhinol Laryngol 2008;117(12):919–924
31. Chen AY, Frankowski R, Bishop-Leone J, et al. The development and validation of a dysphagia-specific quality-of-life questionnaire for patients with head and neck cancer: the M. D. Anderson dysphagia inventory. Arch Otolaryngol Head Neck Surg 2001;127(7):870–876
32. Wallace KL, Middleton S, Cook IJ. Development and validation of a self-report symptom inventory to assess the severity of oral-pharyngeal dysphagia. Gastroenterology 2000;118(4):678–687
33. Langmore SE, Schatz K, Olsen N. Fiberoptic endoscopic examination of swallowing safety: a new procedure. Dysphagia 1988;2(4):216–219
34. Spiegel JR, Selber JC, Creed J. A functional diagnosis of dysphagia using videoendoscopy. Ear Nose Throat J 1998;77(8): 628–632
35. Aviv JE, Martin JH, Kim T, et al. Laryngopharyngeal sensory discrimination testing and the laryngeal adductor reflex. Ann Otol Rhinol Laryngol 1999;108(8):725–730
36. Setzen M, Cohen MA, Mattucci KF, Perlman PW, Ditkoff MK. Laryngopharyngeal sensory deficits as a predictor of aspiration. Otolaryngol Head Neck Surg 2001;124(6):622–624
37. Logemann JA. Mechanisms of normal and abnormal swallowing. In: Flint PW, Haughey BH, Lund VJ, et al, eds. Cummings Otolaryngology Head and Neck Surgery. 5th ed. Philadelphia, PA: Mosby Elsevier; 2010:1215–1221
38. Allen JE, White C, Leonard R, Belafsky PC. Comparison of esophageal screen findings on videofluoroscopy with full esophagram results. Head Neck 2012;34(2):264–269
39. Postma GN, Cohen JT, Belafsky PC, et al. Transnasal esophagoscopy: revisited (over 700 consecutive cases). Laryngoscope 2005;115(2):321–323

40. Postma GN, Butler SG, Belafsky PC, Halum SL. Normal pharyngeal and upper esophageal sphincter manometry. Ear Nose Throat J 2004;83(12):809
41. Soergel KH, Zboralske FF, Amberg JR. Presbyesophagus: esophageal motility in nonagenarians. J Clin Invest 1964;43:1472–1479
42. Hollis JB, Castell DO. Esophageal function in elderly man. A new look at "presbyesophagus." Ann Intern Med 1974;80(3):371–374
43. Gutschow CA, Leers JM, Schröder W, et al. Effect of aging on esophageal motility in patients with and without GERD. Ger Med Sci 2011;9:Doc22
44. Richtsmeier WJ. Endoscopic management of Zenker diverticulum: the staple-assisted approach. Am J Med 2003;115(Suppl 3A):175S–178S
45. Smith SR, Genden EM, Urken ML. Endoscopic stapling technique for the treatment of Zenker diverticulum vs standard open-neck technique: a direct comparison and charge analysis. Arch Otolaryngol Head Neck Surg 2002;128(2):141–144
46. Stoeckli SJ, Schmid S. Endoscopic stapler-assisted diverticuloesophagostomy for Zenker's diverticulum: patient satisfaction and subjective relief of symptoms. Surgery 2002;131(2):158–162
47. Brigand C, Ferraro P, Martin J, Duranceau A. Risk factors in patients undergoing cricopharyngeal myotomy. Br J Surg 2007;94(8):978–983
48. Pitman M, Weissbrod P. Endoscopic CO2 laser cricopharyngeal myotomy. Laryngoscope 2009;119(1):45–53
49. Lawson G, Remacle M. Endoscopic cricopharyngeal myotomy: indications and technique. Curr Opin Otolaryngol Head Neck Surg 2006;14(6):437–441
50. Zaninotto G, Marchese Ragona R, Briani C, et al. The role of botulinum toxin injection and upper esophageal sphincter myotomy in treating oropharyngeal dysphagia. J Gastrointest Surg 2004;8(8):997–1006
51. Carnaby G, Hankey GJ, Pizzi J. Behavioural intervention for dysphagia in acute stroke: a randomised controlled trial. Lancet Neurol 2006;5(1):31–37
52. Rasley A, Logemann JA, Kahrilas PJ, Rademaker AW, Pauloski BR, Dodds WJ. Prevention of barium aspiration during videofluoroscopic swallowing studies: value of change in posture. AJR Am J Roentgenol 1993;160(5):1005–1009
53. Shaker R, Easterling C, Kern M, et al. Rehabilitation of swallowing by exercise in tube-fed patients with pharyngeal dysphagia secondary to abnormal UES opening. Gastroenterology 2002;122(5):1314–1321
54. Roche V. Percutaneous endoscopic gastrostomy. Clinical care of PEG tubes in older adults. Geriatrics 2003;58(11):22–26, 28–29
55. Cervo FA, Bryan L, Farber S. To PEG or not to PEG: a review of evidence for placing feeding tubes in advanced dementia and the decision-making process. Geriatrics 2006;61(6):30–35
56. Finucane TE, Christmas C, Travis K. Tube feeding in patients with advanced dementia: a review of the evidence. JAMA 1999;282(14):1365–1370

17 Sleep Disturbance in the Geriatric Population

Christopher G. Larsen and M. Boyd Gillespie

Introduction

With an aging population and obesity epidemic, interest in snoring and obstructive sleep apnea has increased substantially over the past 10 to 15 years. Obstructive sleep apnea (OSA) is a prevalent disorder characterized by intermittent cessation of airflow during sleep that results in excessive daytime sleepiness. Sleep disturbance prevalence is ~ 60% in elderly adults and affects nearly 67% of institutionalized elderly adults.[1,2]

The most common presenting symptoms, and the reason many patients seek treatment, are habitual snoring, bed partner/family complaints, and excessive daytime somnolence (EDS). Snoring affects 40% of men and 20% of women[3] and frequently is the first sign of more serious underlying OSA. Geriatric patients also more frequently complain of insomnia and poor sleep quality.

Other associated symptoms that may suggest a sleep disorder include witnessed apnea, nighttime arousal, daytime sleepiness or fatigue, motor vehicle accidents, poor sleep quality, morning headaches, and mood disorders or memory concerns. Due to this wide array of symptoms and manifestations, sleep disorder management requires a multidisciplinary approach. Sleep medicine is the new medical discipline dedicated to treating this condition. Sleep medicine teams frequently involve geriatricians, pulmonologists, otolaryngologists, neurologists, psychiatrists, oral/maxillofacial surgeons, dentists, behavioral psychologists, and nutritionists working together to care for patients with sleep disorders.

This chapter describes the evaluation and management of sleep disorders in elderly patients.

Classification of Obstructive Sleep-Related Breathing Disorders

Sleep-related breathing disorders range in severity from airway narrowing with increased airway effort due to upper airway resistance, to partial (hypopnea) or complete (apnea) airway collapse with respiratory effort (**Tables 17.1** and **17.2**).[4]

Snoring is generated by primarily pharyngeal soft tissue vibration. The sound is typically louder on inspiration when negative pressure and increased tissue collapse are more likely. It can occur without hypopnea or apnea; however, nightly snorers have at least a 50% probability of having sleep apnea on overnight polysomnography (PSG). Therefore testing is recommended in nightly snorers, especially if there is associated daytime sleepiness or fatigue. If testing is performed and the overall apnea-hypopnea index (AHI) is fewer than five events per hour, the diagnosis is primary snoring. Patients with primary snoring rarely have EDS and feel well rested after a full night of sleep. Patients who have fatigue and snoring but PSG testing negative for OSA should be screened for sleep deprivation, restless leg syndrome, hypothyroidism, depression, anemia (especially iron deficiency), Addison disease, collagen vascular diseases, and medication side effects. Polypharmacy is especially prevalent in the geriatric population, and each patients' medication list should be monitored and minimized at every opportunity and clinical encounter.

Upper airway resistance syndrome (UARS) refers to patients who do not meet PSG criteria for OSA

Table 17.1 Respiratory event definitions and types

Respiratory event	Definition
Apnea	A cessation of airflow for at least 10 seconds
Hypopnea	A reduction in airflow (> 30%) at least 10 seconds with > 4% oxyhemoglobin desaturation or electroencephalogram (EEG) arousal
Respiratory effort–related arousal (RERA)	Sequence of breaths for at least 10 seconds with increasing respiratory effort of flattening of the nasal pressure waveform leading to an arousal from sleep when the sequence of breaths does not meet criteria for an apnea or hypopnea
Obstructive	Continued thoracoabdominal effort in the setting of partial or complete airflow cessation
Central	The lack of thoracoabdominal effort in the setting of partial or complete airflow cessation
Mixed	A respiratory event with both obstructive and central features; generally begin as central events and end with thoracoabdominal effort without airflow

Used with permission from Kushida CA, Littner MR, Morgenthaler T, et al. Practice parameters for the indications for polysomnography and related procedures: an update for 2005. Sleep 2005;28(4):499–521.

but have daytime somnolence or other debilitating somatic complaints.[5] In this condition, the PSG demonstrates progressively increased respiratory effort (abnormally negative intrathoracic pressure, with snoring and increased diaphragmatic electromyographic [EMG] activity) terminating in an arousal, commonly referred to as respiratory effort–related arousals (RERAs).[6]

The diagnosis of OSA is established if the patient has both an AHI of ≥ 5 with evidence of excessive daytime sleepiness or fatigue. Each episode must last a minimum of 10 seconds and be associated with reduction in oxygen saturation of 3 to 4% and terminated by brief, often unconscious, arousals from sleep. The United States Medicare guidelines diagnose OSA if the AHI is > 15 or an AHI of 5 with two medical comorbidities and/or excessive daytime sleepiness. The American Academy of Sleep Medicine defines mild OSA as AHI between 5 and 15, moderate between 15 and 30, and severe if > 30.[7] Practitioners should be cognizant that variations in published standards of hypopnea definition may result in differences in AHI.[8]

Epidemiology of OSA in Older Adults

Population-based studies estimate that 2 to 3% of female adults and 4 to 5% of male adults have OSA.[9,10] OSA, however, is even more prevalent in elderly

Table 17.2 Indices of sleep disordered breathing

Indices	Definition
Apnea index	Number of apneas per hour of total sleep time
Hypopnea index	Number of hypopneas per hour of total sleep time
Apnea-hypopnea index (AHI)	Number of apneas and hypopneas per hour of total sleep time
Respiratory effort–related arousals (RERAs) index	Number of RERAs per hour of sleep time
Respiratory disturbance index (RDI)	Number of apneas, hypopneas, and RERAs per hour of total sleep time
Central apnea index	Number of central apneas per hour of total sleep time
Mixed apnea index	Number of mixed apneas per hour of total sleep time

Used with permission from Kushida CA, Littner MR, Morgenthaler T, et al. Practice parameters for the indications for polysomnography and related procedures: an update for 2005. Sleep 2005;28(4):499–521.

patients. In a large study of randomly selected community-dwelling elderly, 65 to 95 years of age, Ancoli-Israel et al reported prevalence rates of 62% for an AHI > 10, 44% for an AHI > 20, and 24% for an AHI > 40.[2] She found that with 18 year follow-up in this population, the AHI remained relatively stable and changed only with associated changes in body mass index (BMI).[11] The Sleep Heart Health Study showed similar findings of increased prevalence of OSA in elderly patients compared with the general population.[12] Patients age 60 to 69 had 51% prevalence of mild to moderate OSA, with increases minimally (54% age 70–79; 56% age 80–89) in prevalence with increasing age. Disease severity was not observed to increase significantly with age.

Other studies estimate that the rate of mild OSA is 50 to 60% in older men and 30 to 40% in older women.[13] This may be due to loss of muscle tone associated with physiological aging.[14] Additional theories include decreased hormone levels[15] and changes in the ratio of fat to lean body mass.[13] Menopausal status appears to be a major determinant in the rate of OSA in females. In the large population-based Wisconsin Sleep Cohort Study, postmenopausal women were found to be 3.5 times more likely than premenopausal women to have AHI > 15.[15] OSA may be underdiagnosed in women due to a lower index of suspicion in practitioners, and atypical symptoms reported by female patients. Insomnia, heart palpitations, and ankle edema were more common complaints in women with OSA.[16]

Although the prevalence of OSA appears to increase steadily with age (and weight), the overall prevalence of the disorder appears to level off after the age of 65.[17] The reason for this may be explained in one of three ways: (1) the incidence of new cases decreases after age 65, (2) the mortality rate of OSA increases after age 65, or (3) OSA remits with older age. Because there is little evidence to support death caused directly by OSA (except in extreme cases) or spontaneous remission, a reduction in incidence after age 65 is the currently favored explanation[13]; however, further investigation is needed to clarify this issue.

Sleep Patterns in Older Adults

Changes in sleep duration and architecture occur as a normal part of the aging process.[18] The duration and need for sleep appear to lessen with age. The average 70-year-old sleeps only 6 hours per night but may make up for loss of nocturnal sleep with daytime naps of 1 to 2 hours.[19] In addition, many older adults have increased difficulty falling asleep once in bed (increased sleep latency), and have greater difficulty staying asleep (decreased sleep efficiency).[20] The number of comorbid medical conditions that have an impact on sleep increases with age and includes depression, arthritis, gastroesophageal reflux, prostate hypertrophy, and renal and pulmonary disorders.[21] In addition, older adults are more likely to take medications such as diuretics that cause nocturia. As a result, up to 40% of older individuals complain of sleep disturbance and undesired daytime fatigue.[22] Additionally, the increased sleep latency, decreased sleep efficiency, and lack of awareness regarding the need for less sleep all combine to create greater complaints of insomnia in this population.

The challenge for the physician presented with complaints of sleep disturbance in older individuals is to determine the degree to which symptoms are related to normal age-related changes in sleep pattern versus an underlying medical disorder or primary sleep disorder. A thorough review of the patient's past medical history, medications, and alcohol and stimulant (caffeine, nicotine) use is required. Improving the management of comorbid conditions (i.e., BPH, arthritis, gastroesophageal reflux disease [GERD], depression) will often result in sleep improvement. A sleep diary to determine times of sleep can also be helpful because many older adults may suffer from advanced sleep phase circadian disorder (early evening sleep; early morning awakening). Advanced sleep phase disorder can often be effectively managed by encouraging more sunlight exposure and walks in the late afternoon as well as melatonin therapy during early morning hours.

Sleep is divided into rapid eye movement (REM) and non–rapid eye movement (NREM) stages. About 80% of normal sleep is spent in NREM and is staged according to electroencephalographic measures. Stage N1, formerly stage 1, is a transition from wakefulness to sleep with a mixed voltage pattern with waves of 3 to 7 cycles per second. Most patients feel as though they are awake during this stage. Stage N2, formerly stage 2, is identified by spindles and K complexes and marks the onset of true sleep. Stage N3, formerly stage 3 and 4, is also referred to as slow wave sleep and is distinguished by delta waves. Stage R is characterized by low-frequency mixed amplitude waves and rapid eye movements. REM typically alternates with NREM periods in 90 minute cycles and increases in length as the night goes on. Early-onset REM (< 8 min) is a marker of narcolepsy, which is formally diagnosed with multiple sleep latency testing (MSLT).

Time spent in REM sleep decreases with age.[23] A large meta-analysis of 65 overnight studies representing 3,577 subjects across the entire age spectrum reported that with age, the percentage time in REM sleep decreased, whereas the percentages of light sleep (N1 and N2) increased.[24] Muscle tone is also decreased during REM sleep, so many patients with OSA have worsening of their upper airway collapse and AHI during REM. This fact may also help explain why elderly patients show no progression or worsening in their OSA with time. Bixler et al studied over 4,000 patients age 22 to 100 and found that the prevalence of OSA increases with age but the severity decreases.[25] For this reason, OSA severity based on AHI is often adjusted in elderly populations such that sleep-disordered breathing is considered present when AHI is > 10 to 15 in patients older than 60.

Pathophysiology

OSA is caused by physical obstruction of the pharyngeal airway during sleep. Most patients with OSA have worsening of symptoms during REM sleep, when muscle paralysis is physiological. Obesity, soft tissue (soft palate, tonsil, tongue base) hypertrophy, and craniofacial structure (retrognathia) contribute to one's propensity to collapse by increasing the extraluminal tissue pressure surrounding the upper airway. Obstruction occurs when the pharyngeal dilator muscles are unable to overcome the negative pressure in the upper airway. The four primary sites of obstruction are the nasal airway, palate, tongue base, and hypopharynx.

Nasal obstruction may worsen OSA or contribute to poor continuous positive airway pressure (CPAP) tolerance, but it is rarely the sole cause of OSA. Patients often report more restful sleep and improved symptoms of snoring and fatigue after surgery to improve nasal airflow, but objective measures of OSA severity (i.e., AHI and lowest oxygen saturation) rarely change.[26] This may be due to lessened open-mouth breathing during sleep, which increases upper airway collapsibility and may decrease the efficacy of pharyngeal dilator muscles.[27]

Obesity is a major risk factor for OSA. Increased fat deposition in the soft tissues of the neck narrows the upper airway and may offset the ability of the pharyngeal dilators to maintain airway patency.[28]

Neuromuscular tone can decrease with age and certainly contributes to the patency of the upper airway. The genioglossus muscle is considered the most important muscle in maintaining pharyngeal airway patency in OSA. Klawe and Tafil-Klawe showed that genioglossus muscle activity increases in response to hypoxia, but there is a decreased genioglossus muscle response to hypoxia in older cohorts.[29] Surgery to address tone and tension in this region has been developed,[30,31] and clinical trials are ongoing for hypoglossal nerve stimulation therapy.[32]

Clinical Sequelae of Untreated OSA

Untreated OSA has been associated with reduced quality of life and serious health conditions. In a retrospective review, He et al found that untreated OSA patients with an apnea index (AI) > 20 had a statistically significant increase in mortality compared with patients whose AI was < 20.[33] The authors also found that untreated patients with moderate to severe OSA had a 63% probability of surviving 8 years, compared with 96% in people with mild or absent OSA. Fatal and nonfatal motor vehicle accidents increase 2.5-fold in patients with untreated OSA.[34]

Reduced Quality of Life

Daytime sleepiness caused by OSA often results in decreased energy, loss of concentration, poor job performance, and reduced social interaction. Executive function, attention, and working memory have all been shown to improve with CPAP treatment.[35] In addition, the loud snoring that often accompanies OSA may result in poor sleep for the sufferer's bed partner. Quality of life has been shown to be improved in both the treated individuals and their bed partners.[36]

An AHI > 5 is associated with concentration difficulty but not memory tasks on self-assessment exams.[37] OSA patients demonstrated significant improvement in daytime sleepiness[38] and in numerous quality of life parameters, including physical functioning, social functioning, vitality, and general health perception after treatment.[39] The relationship between sleepiness (defined by the Epworth Sleepiness Scale [ESS]) and severity of OSA (defined by AHI) is not well defined, especially in older populations. Many elderly people have an AHI > 5 but report minimal or no daytime sleepiness.[40] Unless the AHI is > 15 or there is significant oxygen desaturations (< 90%) and hypertension or coronary artery disease, most would not argue for invasive treatment in this subset of nonsleepy elderly patients.

Cardiovascular Morbidity and Mortality

Evidence supports an increase in cardiovascular mortality 5 years after diagnosis in untreated patients with severe OSA compared with treated patients.[33,41] Another study found that men under age 60 with snoring and EDS were twice as likely to die over a 10-year study period compared with subjects without snoring or snoring without sleepiness.[42] Two large prospective studies suggest that untreated, loud, habitual snorers have a 30 to 40% greater risk of myocardial infarction or stroke relative to non-snorers.[43,44] The risk of sudden cardiac death is significantly increased in patients with OSA and nocturnal hypoxemia, with increased risk in patients with more severe disease.[45]

The foregoing information is contradicted by a recent study by Johansson et al.[46] In community-dwelling elderly age 71 to 87, OSA does not appear to be associated with cardiovascular disease (CVD) or mortality, but central sleep apnea might be a pathological marker of CVD and impaired systolic function associated with higher mortality. One limitation of this study was use of in-home sleep studies and a limited sample size (331 patients).

Hypertension

It has been hypothesized that systemic arterial hypertension is the cause of the increased cardiovascular morbidity and mortality observed in patients with sleep-disordered breathing.[47] Laboratory evidence has demonstrated that sustained arterial hypertension can be induced in animal models subjected to intermittent airway occlusion during sleep.[48] The current epidemiological evidence shows a strong and consistent association between OSA and hypertension. Four large population-based cross-sectional studies found that the odds of hypertension were 1.4 to 2.5 times greater in patients with an AHI > 5 compared with controls.[49–51] Finally, prospective analysis of the Wisconsin Sleep Cohort study found that even minimal elevation in AHI scores was associated with a 42% increased risk of developing hypertension over a 4 year period.[52]

Level I evidence shows that treatment of OSA with CPAP has been reported to lower blood pressure (mean, systolic and diastolic) by ~ 10 mm Hg.[53] In this study, 60 consecutive patients with moderate to severe OSA were randomized to either effective or subtherapeutic nasal CPAP for 9 weeks. Apneas and hypopneas were reduced by 95% in the treatment group and 50% in the subtherapeutic group. The blood pressure reduction demonstrated in the therapeutic CPAP-treated group would be predicted to reduce coronary heart disease event risk by 37% and stroke risk by 56%.

Motor Vehicle Accidents

Epidemiological and laboratory evidence both suggest that patients with OSA are at greater risk for motor vehicle accidents (MVAs). Patients with an AHI > 15 were 7.3 times more likely to have had multiple MVAs in the 5 years before their study, compared with those with lower or no apnea.[54] Hospitalized MVA victims were found to be 6.3 times more likely to have an AHI > 5 compared with community controls.[9,54,55] In addition, patients with severe OSA performed significantly worse on a driving simulator than controls without OSA.[56]

Insulin Resistance

Untreated OSA has been shown to be an independent risk factor for insulin resistance.[57] Thus OSA may contribute to the development of diabetes and metabolic syndrome (the term used to describe concomitant obesity, insulin resistance, hypertension, and dislipidemia). Assoumou et al reviewed a cohort of 806 elderly healthy patients (age 68) and found that 9.8% had metabolic syndrome, and 55.9% had OSA (diagnosed on home sleep study, positive for AHI > 15).[58] Of the subset with OSA, 12.5% had metabolic syndrome. The oxygen desaturation levels and AHI were found to be significantly higher in the subset of patients with metabolic syndrome. Hypoxia and the oxyhemoglobin desaturation index appeared to be the most important factors explaining the association between metabolic syndrome (specifically hyperglycemia and hypertension) and OSA.

Diagnosis of Sleep Disorders in Elderly Patients

A high index of suspicion should accompany evaluation of geriatric patients with obesity (BMI > 30), loud nightly snoring, restless sleep, and daytime fatigue or somnolence. In a large review by Young et al, 70% of adult patients with OSA were found to be obese.[59] Patients who have symptoms without obesity and patients with a positive family history of OSA should also warrant investigation with a detailed sleep history and physical examination. The ESS is an easy to administer, widely used scale to risk stratify patients with daytime sleepiness at risk for OSA (**Fig. 17.1**). OSA is much more likely in patients with an ESS > 10.[60]

A thorough sleep history (**Table 17.3**) helps identify patients at risk for primary sleep disorders seen most commonly in older adults: OSA, restless leg syndrome, insomnia, and sleep maintenance insomnia. Sleep maintenance insomnia is characterized by early morning awakening and is highly associated with alcohol abuse or depression in older individuals.[61] Patients suspected of a primary sleep disorder should undergo overnight PSG to establish the presence and severity of a sleep disorder.

Please answer the following questions based on this scale:

0: would never fall asleep

1: slight chance of dozing

2: moderate chance of dozing

3: high chance of dozing

Situation	Chance of Dozing
Reading	________
Watching TV	________
Sitting in a public place (i.e. theater or meeting)	________
Driving a car, stopped at a traffic light	________
As a passenger in a car for an hour, no break	________
During quiet time after lunch without alcohol	________
Lying down to rest when circumstances permit	________

Fig. 17.1 Epworth Sleepiness Scale.

Table 17.3 Elements of sleep history

Time in bed
Time to sleep
Number of awakenings
Time awake
Food consumption and timing of meals
Amount and time of alcohol consumption
Presence of snoring, witnessed apnea, gasps, or choking spells
Presence of involuntary leg motion or jerking
Level of daytime sleepiness or fatigue (Epworth Sleepiness Scale score)
Time, duration, and number of daytime naps
Medications, including over the counter and herbal
Waking with a headache

Three screening questions are helpful in determining the likelihood of sleep disorder in elderly patients[1]:

1. Is your sleep restorative, or restful?
2. Does lack of sleep or fatigue intrude in your daily activities?
3. Does your bed partner or caregiver report any unusual sleep behavior such as breathing pauses, snoring, gasping, or abnormal movements?

Medication review is especially important in the geriatric patient due to more pronounced side effects in this population. Hypnotic medications may diminish in effectiveness with time, and medications prescribed for insomnia, such as benzodiazepines, often worsen OSA. Don't forget to ask about over-the-counter medications and herbal supplements! Melatonin is used by many to promote sleep, but it should be used with caution in patients on anticoagulant medications such as warfarin. Chamomile tea is also a "relaxing" supplement, but it should not be used in patients with ragweed allergy, because the plants are related. Valerian is reportedly helpful in anxiety and helping patients fall asleep, but it should not be used with other sleep aides or alcohol. One final herbal sleep aide is kava. It is metabolized in the liver and should not be used in patients who are on medications such as statin drugs. Kava use has been tied to severe liver failure, especially when taken with alcohol or other medications metabolized in the liver.

OSA is more prevalent in patients with hypertension, coronary artery disease, congestive heart failure, history of prior stroke, or diabetes as well as in those who are obese or postmenopausal. Screening via PSG is encouraged in this subset of patients with signs or symptoms of sleep disturbance.[4]

Physical exam findings such as BMI, blood pressure measurement, and neck circumference should be recorded. Collar size > 17 inches in men and 15 in women is associated with OSA.[12] Unfortunately, the Sleep Heart Health Study showed that SDB is poorly predicted by obesity, neck circumference, and reports of witnessed apnea in elderly patients.[12] This finding may be due to the high prevalence of disease in elderly patients. Maxilla and mandibular position, nasal deformity (septal deviation or valve collapse), turbinate size and response to decongestant spray, nasal polyps, tongue position, tonsil size, palate length/shape, and hyoid position should be evaluated. Patients with Angle class II malocclusion may benefit most from dental devices or maxillomandibular advancement (MMA) surgery.

Fujita developed a classification system for patterns of obstruction by anatomical location as follows: type I, collapse in the retropalatal region only; type II, collapse in the retropalatal and retrolingual regions; type III, collapse in the retrolingual region only.[62] Classically described surgery to address retropalatal collapse (i.e., uvulopalatopharyngoplasty [UPPP]) often fails in poorly selected patients due to multilevel airway obstruction in most patients with moderate or severe OSA.[63]

Otolaryngologists frequently use flexible fiberoptic nasopharyngoscopy (preferably with supine positioning) with or without sedation or sleep simulation to evaluate for upper airway collapse (**Fig. 17.2**). The Müller maneuver was described to simulate upper airway collapse in an office setting by inhaling against a closed glottis with the nose and mouth closed. This results in negative pharyngeal pressure and allows the physician to identify the site(s) of collapse. Aboussouan et al found that using the Müller maneuver to guide the decision on UPPP resulted in an AHI reduction by 50% in 78% of patients who had retropalatal collapse, compared with only 36% who had multilevel obstruction.[64] The biggest limitation with the Müller maneuver is it fails to demonstrate lower levels of airway obstruction (retrolingual, hypopharyngeal), and it is performed on awake and alert patients with normal muscle tone. It may be more difficult to obtain reliable results with this maneuver in elderly patients with early cognitive impairment.

Office-based supine airway evaluation with fiberoptic scopes may provide more insight into the level of airway collapse than seated erect patient position.[65] Sleep MRI has also been used with some success in predicting level of airway obstruction in snoring patients.[66]

Drug-induced sleep videoendoscopy has been described to guide more effective surgical intervention.[67] Sleep is induced in a monitored setting via pharmacological means, and fiberoptic nasopharyngoscopy is performed to better identify the site(s) of airway collapse. This idea seems to hold the most promise for surgical planning, but the downside is the expense and risk associated with sedation. The levels of obstruction can be treated with surgery to relieve obstruction in each area for patients that can't tolerate or refuse CPAP. The modified Mallampati score (i.e., I–IV without tongue extrusion) (**Fig. 17.3**) has been shown to correlate poorly with airway level obstruction on sleep endoscopy in patients with OSA.[68] It does predict difficult intubation and surgical success (along with tonsil hypertrophy) using UPPP alone to treat OSA (more success with palate position I or II and tonsil hypertrophy).

Nocturnal PSG is the gold standard for diagnosis of OSA, but more and more patients are being screened with home studies. Home studies are most appropriate in patients with suspected mild disease or without complex medical comorbidities. Home sleep studies may miss other causes of excessive daytime sleepiness such as UARS or periodic leg movement during sleep disorder (PLMD). A full diagnostic study includes electroencephalogram, electro-oculogram, submental electromyogram, electrocardiogram, nasal and oral airflow monitors, thoracoabdominal effort, anterior tibial electromyogram, body position monitors, tracheal microphone, and pulse oximetry. Optional additions (14 channel) are end-tidal carbon dioxide monitor, esophageal pressure monitor, and nasal CPAP or BiPAP. These studies are attended by and analyzed by a trained technologist and interpreted by a physician. Split night studies, in which patients demonstrate OSA early in the evening, allow for pressure titration of CPAP or BiPAP for home use.

The anesthesia perioperative assessment literature has popularized the mnemonic questionnaire "STOP-Bang" as a screen for OSA in previously undiagnosed patients. Patients and/or significant others are asked if the patient has: loud Snoring, daytime Tiredness, Observed apneas, high blood Pressure, elevated BMI > 35, Age > 50, Neck circumference > 40 cm, and male Gender. Patients are high risk for OSA if 3 or more are positive and low risk if fewer than 3.[8] The sensitivity of this test was found to be 93% for AHI 15 and 100% for AHI 30. The Society of Ambulatory

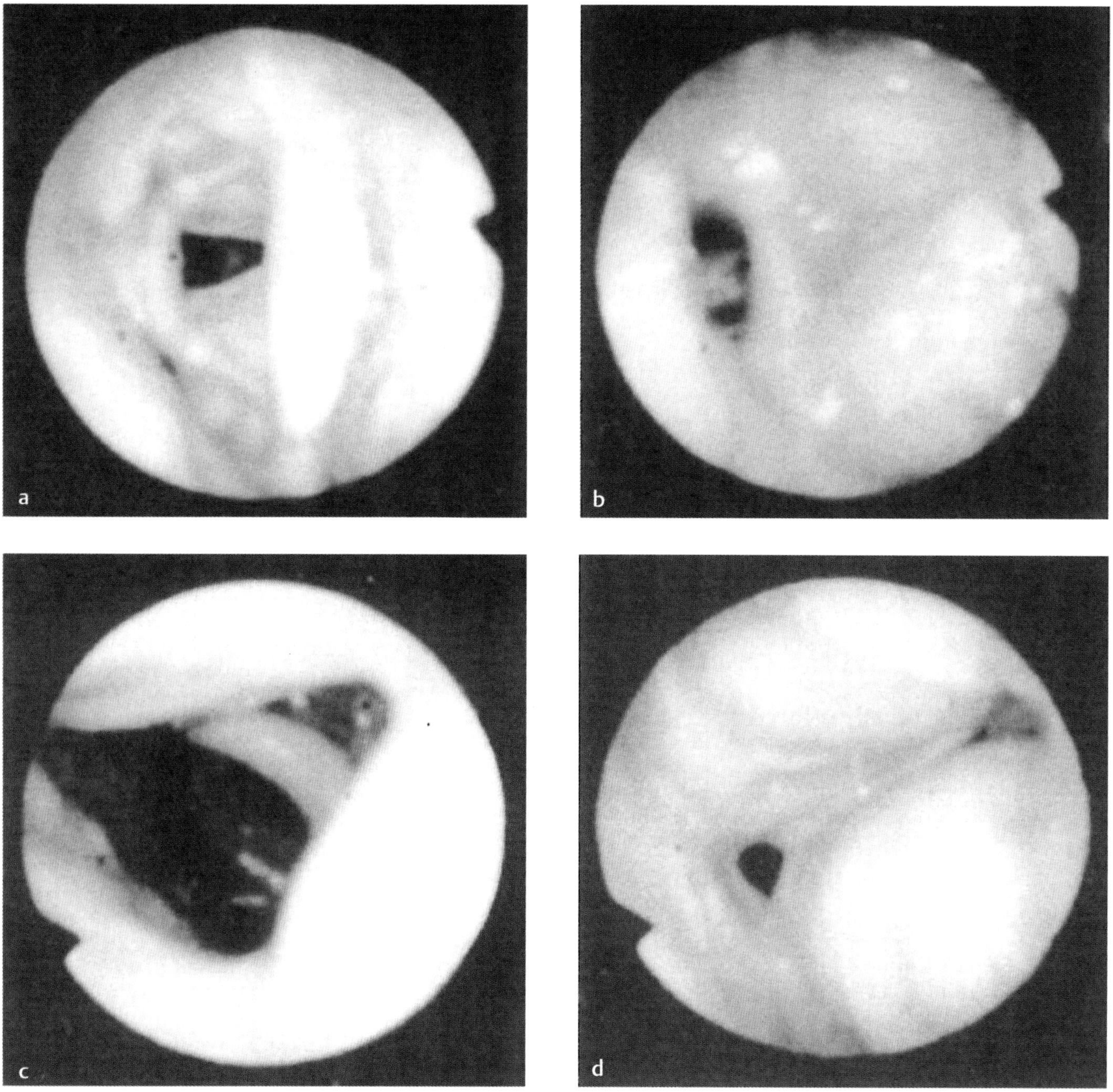

Fig. 17.2 (**a**) Flexible fiberoptic view of normal hypopharyngeal airway. (**b**) Fiberoptic view of base of tongue obstruction. (**c**) Fiberoptic view of the hypopharyngeal airway before the Müller maneuver. (**d**) Fiberoptic view of hypopharyngeal collapse during the Müller maneuver. (Used with permission from Cummings CW. Cummings Otolaryngology Head & Neck Surgery. 4th ed. Philadelphia, PA: Elsevier Mosby; 2005.)

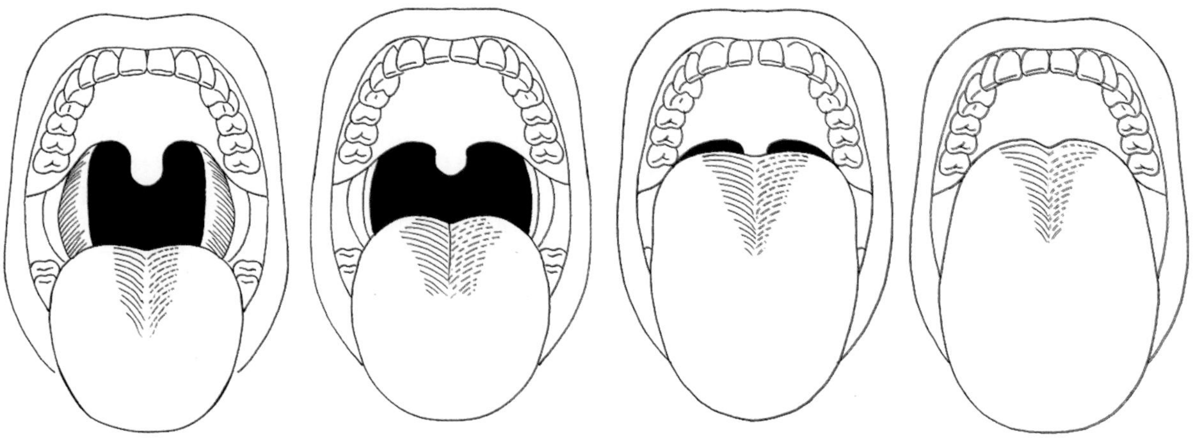

Fig. 17.3 Depiction of the modified Mallampati classification. (Reprinted with permission from Fedok F, Carniol P. Minimally Invasive and Office-Based Procedures in Facial Plastic Surgery. New York, NY: Thieme; 2013.)

Anesthesia recommends screening all adult patients with this questionnaire prior to ambulatory surgery.[69]

Restless legs syndrome (RLS) is characterized by a feeling of restlessness in the legs and sensations such as muscle twitching, aches, or the urge to move. The sensation often occurs in the evening and when awake lying in bed. The discomfort is worsened by inactivity. Typically, the feeling is relieved by pacing or the act of leg motion. It is estimated that 20% of adults over age 80 experience RLS.[70] This disease is in the same spectrum as periodic limb movement disorder (PLMD), which can also be diagnosed with PSG (tibial EMG). PLMD patients, in contrast to RLS patients, are often unaware of their leg movements or their nightly microarousals related to the leg motion. The prevalence of PLMD is estimated at 4 to 11% and increases with age.[71]

Research into the pathophysiology of RLS and PLMD has implicated low iron levels and the nigrostriatal dopaminergic system. For this reason, elderly patients often respond to low doses of carbidopa/levodopa or dopaminergic medications.[72] Elderly patients should also be screened for iron deficiency with ferritin and transferrin saturation levels. Treatment is encouraged for ferritin levels below 18 g/L or transferrin saturation percentage < 16%.[73]

Insomnia is an extremely common complaint in elderly populations. Insomnia is defined as recurrent difficulty with sleep initiation, maintenance, consolidation, or quality that causes daytime dysfunction despite adequate opportunity for sleep.[74] Daytime symptoms may include fatigue or malaise, cognitive impairment, social/vocational difficulty, poor school performance, daytime sleepiness, mood impairment, or reduced motivation. Increased sleep latency may be due to decreased sleep needs or anxiety. Decreased sleep efficiency, with difficulty staying asleep, may be due to an increased percentage of time in lighter stages of sleep that occurs as part of the normal aging process. It may also be due to alcohol abuse or depression. Multiple medical conditions can also adversely affect sleep (chronic pain, nocturia, and concomitant psychiatric illness). Often, the best cure for insomnia is recommending sleep hygiene (**Table 17.4**).[61]

Many elderly patients report spending ~ 10 hours in bed but only sleep ~ 6, thus feeling like they only slept half of the night. This can often be treated with "sleep consolidation or restriction therapy."[61] With this approach, patients are only allowed to stay in bed for the amount of time they claim to sleep. After 2 to 3 days of relative sleep deprivation, they will sleep through that time allotment and feel as though they are sleeping through the night. The allowed time in bed is then extended 15 to 30 minutes per week until complaints subside.

Table 17.4 Sleep hygiene

Be aware of how much sleep you actually need: the average 70-year-old needs only 6 hours/day, total, including naps
Get up at about the same time every day—weekends and weekdays
Go to bed only when sleepy; reserve bed for sleep and sex only
Establish a relaxing presleep routine, such as reading a book or listening to relaxing music
Avoid heavy meals or caffeinated beverages within 5–6 hours of bedtime
Avoid smoking/nicotine products close to bedtime
Avoid sleeping pills for periods longer than a few weeks; don't drink alcohol when taking sleeping pills
Maintain a regular daily schedule that includes exercise, down time, and regular meal times; avoid strenuous exercise within 6 hours of bedtime
Early afternoon naps can prevent early evening dozing
If necessary, restrict caffeine intake, including coffee, tea, caffeinated soda, and chocolate

Used with permission from Barthlen GM. Obstructive sleep apnea syndrome, restless legs syndrome, and insomnia in geriatric patients. Geriatrics 2002;57:34–39.

Treatment

Geriatric patients with OSA should proceed in a stepwise manner from conservative medical measures, to procedural or surgical options if conservative measures fail. Weight loss should be recommended in all overweight patients with OSA. Unfortunately, sustained weight reduction is difficult due to decreased energy associated with the disease, medical comorbidities (i.e., osteoarthritis) and dietary choices in the 21st century (cheap, high calorie, processed foods).

CPAP is the gold standard treatment for obstructive sleep apnea. The positive pressure acts as a pneumatic splint to prevent upper airway collapse. Ballester et al compared two cohorts with moderate to severe OSA.[38] One group was treated with sleep hygiene and weight loss recommendations, whereas the other was treated with CPAP in addition to weight loss and sleep hygiene recommendations. After 3 months of treatment, sleepiness, quality of life, and perceived health were improved in the CPAP treatment group.

A large prospective cohort study of 939 elderly patients (> 65 years old) found that patients with severe OSA (AHI > 30) were at reduced risk for cardiovascular death when treated with CPAP.[75] CPAP treatment was defined as use > 4 hours per night. Patients with mild OSA (AHI < 15) served as the control group.

The evidence regarding CPAP use in OSA patients without daytime somnolence is less convincing. Barbé et al showed that CPAP failed to prevent hypertension and cardiac events in 725 prospective, randomized patients with AHI > 20 but ESS < 10.[76]

Bilevel positive airway pressure (BiPAP) and auto-adjusting positive airway pressure (APAP) have been developed to improve pressure titration and treat patients with underlying neuromuscular disease or chronic lung disease. BiPAP delivers a separately adjustable lower expiratory positive pressure and higher inspiratory pressure. It has not been shown to improve adherence versus CPAP in a randomized, controlled pilot study.[77] APAP devices may eliminate the need for formal PSG CPAP pressure titration in selected patients by autotitrating positive airway pressure to select an effective level of pressure and prevent airway collapse.[78]

The biggest limitation to CPAP is tolerance and compliance. For patients who travel regularly, packing the machine may be a burden. When adherence is defined as > 4 hours of use per night, 46 to 83% of patients have been reported to be nonadherent.[63] The decision to embrace CPAP occurs during the first few days of treatment. Disease severity, as measured by AHI, has been shown to have a weak relationship with CPAP adherence.[66] Not surprisingly, symptom severity influences adherence. Self-reported EDS (ESS > 10) has been shown to be associated with long-term CPAP use.[65] Low CPAP usage was shown in patients with severe OSA but little sleepiness. Most new CPAP machines have "smart cards" that monitor use time per night, and close follow-up should be encouraged in patients with OSA who are treated with CPAP to ensure compliance.

Oral appliances are an option, especially in patients with mild to moderate OSA, relative retrognathia. or overbite (Angle class II occlusion), and poor CPAP tolerance or refusal. Oral appliances are another conservative option in elderly patients who may have medical comorbidities or be poor candidates for general anesthesia. A systematic review of oral appliances showed that AHI was reduced to < 10 in 52% of patients. Compliance in this study was better than with CPAP, with median use 77% of nights.[79] The most often reported complications from oral appliance therapy are tooth, jaw, and temporomandibular joint (TMJ) discomfort. Although oral appliance therapy has higher rates of patient adherence, CPAP has proven to be more effective in reducing AHI.[80]

Soft palate "pillar" implants made of porous polyethylene have been shown to improve AHI and EDS by stiffening the soft palate. Primary benefits are minimal morbidity and outpatient surgery with local/topical anesthesia. Nordgård et al prospectively studied 26 patients with BMI < 30 who had mild to moderate OSA (AHI 10–30).[81] They showed that these implants resulted in improvement in AHI in 81% of patients. The majority of patients (57%) had their AHI reduced to < 10. This benefit appeared to last longer than 1 year. More than 80% of bed partners reported significant improvement in snoring. A large meta-analysis showed soft palate implants to provide benefit for snoring and mild to moderate OSA.[72] The end points measured were reduced snoring, AHI, and ESS improvement. The most common complication was implant extrusion at 9.3%. Patients with hyperactive gag reflex, severe OSA, and/or obesity (BMI > 30) are generally poor candidates for this treatment option.

Upper airway surgery for obstructive sleep apnea can be considered in one of two ways, depending on the goal of surgery: (1) improve CPAP tolerance, or (2) eliminate the need for CPAP.

If the goal is to improve CPAP tolerance, nasal septoplasty, septorhinoplasty, nasal valve repair, and/or inferior turbinate reduction surgery may play an important role. By reducing nasal resistance, often the pressure of CPAP can be reduced and patients feel as if they are no longer sleeping "in a wind tunnel." A good way to determine the probability of success is a three-night trial with oxymetazoline nasal spray prior to CPAP use. This topical decongestant will decrease nasal congestion/obstruction, lasts for 12 hours, and may simulate nasal airway outcomes with nasal surgery. Unfortunately, this medication is associated with rebound congestion when used for more than 3 days consecutively.

For patients with seasonal allergy or reactive nasal congestion, topical nasal corticosteroid (i.e., fluticasone) therapy may provide similar benefits. Systemic absorption has not been found to be problematic, and long-term use is common in patients suffering from perennial allergic rhinitis and rhinosinusitis with nasal polyps. Primary side effects include epistaxis and risk for nasal septal perforation.

Both complications can be minimized or eliminated by teaching patients to use these medications appropriately. Patients should aim the bottle at the ipsilateral medial canthus, away from the nasal septum, bilaterally. Kiely and colleagues reported that the AHI was lower in 24 patients given intranasal fluticasone compared with those given placebo (23 vs. 30).[82]

A recent literature review on the topic of nasal obstruction and OSA came to the following conclusion: nasal obstruction plays a modulation, but not a causative, role in SDB. Nasal interventions may improve subjective aspects of snoring and daytime somnolence but do not improve objective indicators of disease.[26] McLean and colleagues found that treating nasal obstruction with oxymetazoline and nasal valve dilator strips reduced mouth breathing during sleep and the severity of OSA, but did not effectively alleviate the disease.[83]

When patients refuse CPAP or cannot tolerate it, pharyngeal surgery is frequently the next step. Friedman et al popularized a staging system (**Table 17.5**) for predicting which patients were likely to benefit from UPPP and those that may benefit from multilevel (pharynx/palate, and hypopharyngeal) surgery.[84] Friedman palate position was based on the modified Mallampati palate position (I–IV; **Fig. 17.3**) and tonsil size was graded 1 to 4+ (within pillars = 1+; extending to pillars = 2+; extending beyond pillars but not midline = 3+; and "kissing" in midline = 4+). In this study, patients with modified Mallampati palate position I or II, tonsil hypertrophy (3–4+), and BMI < 40 were much more likely to benefit from UPPP alone. Stage I patients had 80% success with UPPP

Table 17.5 Friedman staging to predict treatment success (apnea-hypopnea index reduction by 50% and < 20) with uvulopalatopharyngoplasty alone

	Friedman palate position	Tonsil size	Body mass index (kg/m^2)
Stage I	1	3, 4	< 40
	2	3, 4	< 40
Stage II	1, 2	0, 1, 2	< 40
	3, 4	3, 4	< 40
Stage III	3	0, 1, 2	Any
	4	0, 1, 2	Any
	Any	Any	> 40

Used with permission from Friedman M, Ibrahim H, Joseph NJ. Staging of obstructive sleep apnea/hypopnea syndrome: a guide to appropriate treatment. Laryngoscope 2004;114(3):454–459.

alone, versus only 40% if stage II and 8% if stage III. Surgical success was defined as reduction in RDI to < 50% preop value and < 20.

Critical to the decision for surgery is determining the site(s) of airway obstruction. Steinhart and colleagues evaluated 117 OSA patients and found that 100% had retropalatal obstruction, and 77% had retroglossal obstruction, emphasizing the fact that most patients have multiple levels of obstruction and may require a series of surgeries to adequately treat their condition.[85] More recently, den Herder et al evaluated 127 patients with sleep endoscopy and found that 88% of patients had retropalatal obstruction and 49% had retroglossal obstruction. Of these patients, 51% had exclusive retropalatal obstruction, whereas only 12% had exclusive obstruction at the base of tongue.[69]

UPPP was first described by Fujita in 1981.[86] UPPP is used to treat redundant soft palate tissue and tonsillar obstruction. It is the most commonly performed surgical procedure for OSA regardless of coexisting patient factors such as morbid obesity, tongue position, and retrognathia. For this reason, it is often unsuccessful in treating OSA in poorly selected patients. UPPP is associated with significant morbidity. Kezirian et al reported that this surgery is associated with serious nonfatal complications in 1.5% of patients and mortality in 0.2%.[87] Risks include severe bleeding (1–5%),[71] velopharyngeal insufficiency (hypernasal voice or incompetence when swallowing liquids), taste alteration, dry mouth, foreign body/globus sensation, and inability to wear nasal CPAP if persistent disease exists due to inability to maintain upper airway seal. Fairbanks reported that temporary nasal reflux occurs in 12 to 15% of patients after UPPP.[71]

Modified UPPP with Z-plasty or expansion sphincter palatoplasty, as described by Friedman,[88] Cahil,[89] and Woodson,[74] reduces some of these risks and results in less circumferential scar formation. All three studies showed results superior to traditional UPPP. The suture suspending the palatopharyngeus muscle to the periosteum of the hamulus expands the retropalatal region superiorly and ventrally (**Fig. 17.4**).

Woodson advocates transpalatal advancement pharyngoplasty to decrease retropalatal obstruction by removing a 1 cm portion of the posterior bony maxilla (**Fig. 17.5**).[90] This surgery is often offered to patients who have persistent retropalatal obstruction after UPPP or have small tonsils without characteristic long, thick, soft palate.

Multiple surgical options have been developed to address the tongue base and hypopharyngeal airway collapse.[31] Among the options are hyoid myotomy with suspension, lingual tonsillectomy, midline glossectomy, and genioglossal advancement.

Friedman et al showed that multilevel surgery, including Z-palatoplasty and transoral robotic surgery (TORS) midline glossectomy could safely be performed without tracheostomy tube placement.[75] This study also showed superior results in patients who had Z-palatoplasty with TORS glossectomy compared with matched cohorts who had Z-palatoplasty and radiofrequency ablation in the tongue base or Z-palatoplasty and submucosal minimally invasive lingual excision (SMILE). The goal of midline glossec-

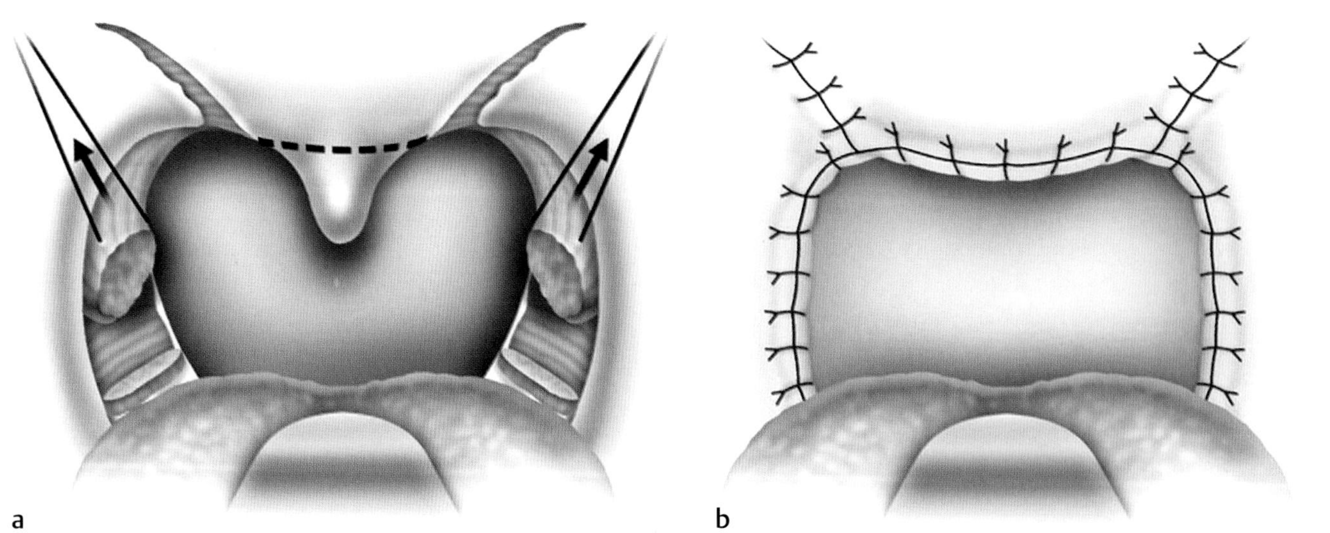

Fig. 17.4 (**a, b**) Modified uvulopalatopharyngoplasty (UPPP), expansion sphincter pharyngoplasty. Note the anterolateral direction of pull (arrows) that widens the retropharyngeal space. (Used with permission from Pang KP, Woodson BT. Expansion sphincter pharyngoplasty: a new technique for the treatment of obstructive sleep apnea. Otolaryng Head Neck Surg 2007;137(1):110–114.)

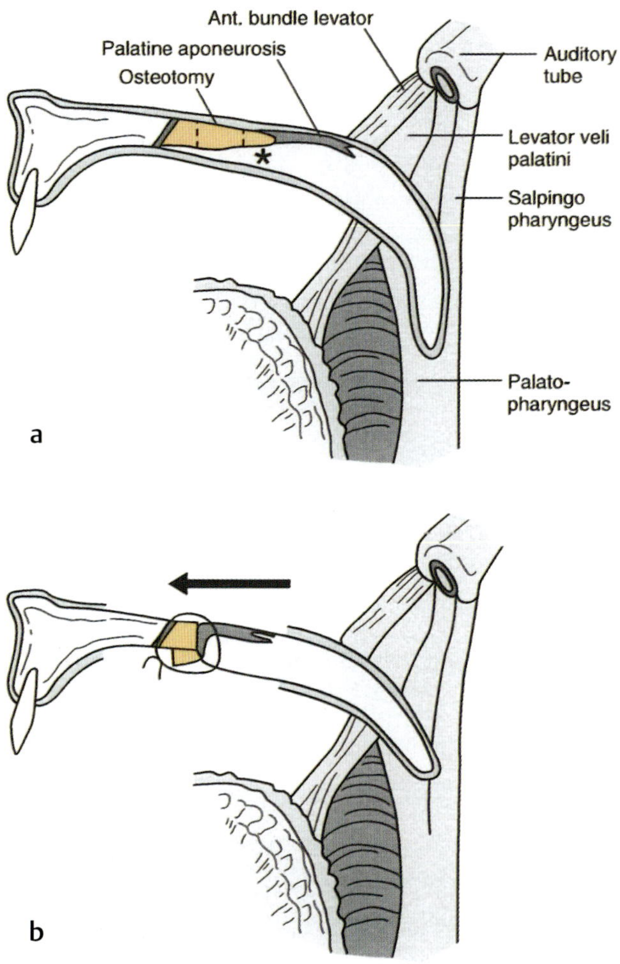

Fig. 17.5 Sagittal illustration of palate showing advancement. (Used with permission from Cummings CW. Cummings Otolaryngology Head & Neck Surgery. 4th ed. Philadelphia, PA: Elsevier Mosby; 2005.)

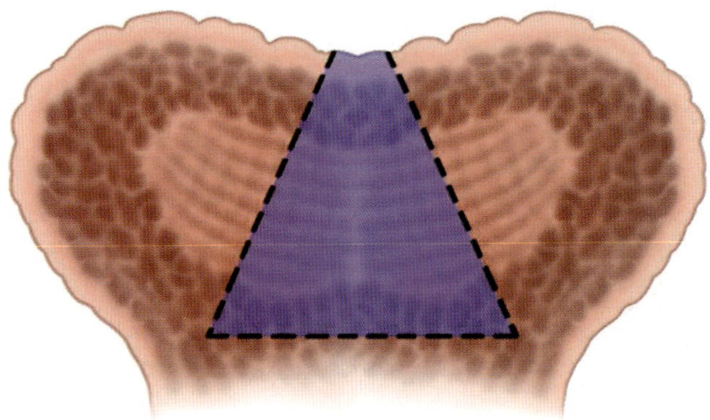

Fig. 17.6 Transoral robotic surgery (TORS) midline glossectomy tissue removal after exposure with a Jennings retractor. (Used with permission from Friedman M, Hamilton C, Samuelson CG, et al. Transoral robotic gossectomy for the treatment of obstructive sleep apnea-hypoapnea syndrome. Otolaryngol Head Neck Surg 2012;146(5):854–862.)

tomy is to remove an inverted triangle of mucosa and muscle (**Fig. 17.6**). The surgical robot is not a necessity,[73] but it helps facilitate visualization and aggressive soft tissue reduction in this difficult-to-expose site. TORS midline glossectomy has been found to result in greater AHI reduction and improvement in LSAT versus the other referenced techniques, but with increased dysphagia and pain.

An alternative, less invasive, option to address hypopharyngeal and retrolingual collapse involves the Repose (Medtronic, Jacksonville, FL) system. This bone-anchored suture suspension system can be used to accomplish results similar to genioglossal advancement (without an osteotomy) and hyoid myotomy (HM) with suspension. Via transcervical (or intraoral for tongue base suspension) incisions, a titanium screw is placed at the lingual cortex of the genial tubercle of the mandible. A permanent suture attached to the screw is passed through the paramedian tongue musculature, submucosally across the tongue base, and then back through the length of the tongue, and anchored to pull the tongue base anteriorly. Through the same incision, two additional screws can be anchored to the mandible laterally and used to suspend the hyoid bone anteriorly and superiorly after freeing the inferior muscular attachments. Success rates for HM after UPPP range from 52 to 78% in patients with BMI less than 30.[31,91]

Although aggressive options, especially in geriatric populations, one should not forget about MMA, surgical tracheostomy, or bariatric surgery in patients with severe, refractory OSA and/or morbid obesity. Varela et al showed that weight loss surgery significantly improves obesity-related OSA with improvement as early as 1 month postop.[92] MMA surgical success rate approaches 90%[93] but complications include dental malocclusion, nerve paresthesia, prolonged maxillomandibular fixation, and bony malunion.

Nonsurgical treatment for sleep disorders should begin by encouraging patients to lose weight (if indicated), and avoid alcohol and sedating medications before bedtime. Patients should also be heavily cautioned against driving and instructed to avoid activities requiring sustained vigilance until the sleep disorder is successfully treated. Long-term treatment with hypnotic medications is not advised because they often lose efficacy within a few weeks, have side effects of respiratory depression, and may worsen OSA (**Table 17.6**).

Conclusion

Sleep disturbance in the elderly population is extremely common. The differential diagnosis includes primary snoring, upper airway resistance

Table 17.6 Selected pharmacotherapies for insomnia and restless legs syndrome in older adults

Agent	Dose/timing	Comments
Nonbenzodiazepine	**Hypnotics**	**For insomnia**
Zolpidem tartrate (Ambien)	5 mg at bedtime	Drug of choice for treatment of sleep-onset and sleep maintenance insomnia, duration 2–3 wk
Zaleplon (Sonata)	5 mg at bedtime	Shown to cause daytime drowsiness, duration 2–3 wk
Benzodiazepine	**For insomnia**	**If obstructive sleep apnea (OSA) ruled out**
Temazepam (Restoril)	7.5 mg at bedtime	Rule out OSA first
Hormone replacement	**Menopausal insomnia**	
Conjugated estrogens	0.3–1.25 mg in the AM	Shown to improve sleep and reduce OSA
Antidepressants	**For insomnia**	**and depression**
Sertraline HCl (Zoloft)	50 mg in the AM	Well tolerated
Fluoxetine HCL (Saralem)	20 mg in the AM	Well tolerated
Mirtazapine (Remeron)	15 mg at bedtime	In cases of depression associated with severe insomnia and anxiety, shown to be superior to above SSRIs
Dopaine agonists for	**Restless legs syndrome**	
Carbidopa/levadopa (Sinemet)	25/100 mg at bedtime	May cause shift of symptoms to daytime
Pramipexole (Mirapex)	0.125 mg at bedtime	Newer dopamine agonist, may cause excessive sleepiness

Used with permission from Barthlen GM. Sleep disorders. Obstructive sleep apnea syndrome, restless legs syndrome, and insomnia in geriatric patients. Geriatrics 2002;57(11):34–39; quiz 40.

syndrome, sleep apnea, restless leg syndrome, sleep manifestation of systemic disease (diabetes, congestive heart failure, BPH, depression, alcoholism, etc.), periodic limb movement disorder, physiological aging, poor sleep hygiene, and insomnia. Diagnosis and treatment by a multidisciplinary sleep medicine team is likely to improve outcomes and patient quality of life.

All geriatric patients (> 65 years old) should be screened by history and physical examination for sleep-disordered breathing given the extensive prevalence of at least mild OSA (AHI > 5 but < 15) in this age group and the severe potential health and quality of life consequences of undiagnosed sleep apnea. Evidence supports treatment of OSA in individuals with the following findings:

- AHI > 5 with excessive daytime sleepiness
- AHI > 5 with cardiovascular comorbidities
- AHI > 15 with or without excessive daytime sleepiness
- Oxyhemoglobin desaturation < 90%

Patients with an AHI between 5 and 15 who do not have excessive daytime sleepiness are likely to be at low risk for cardiovascular sequelae and unlikely to be compliant with therapy because they have no self-perceived sleepiness. Multiple medical and surgical treatment options exist based on the diagnosis and underlying cause of the sleep disturbance. Treatment selection depends largely on the level of obstruction, severity, presence of medical comorbidities, presence of anatomical deformities, and patient preference.

CPAP is the gold standard treatment for OSA, but compliance can be problematic. Untreated OSA can lead to increased mortality, increased cardiovascular disease, and neurocognitive difficulty. It has also been demonstrated to be an independent risk factor for insulin resistance, GERD, MVAs, and decreased attention, working memory, and executive function. When CPAP is not tolerated or is refused by the patient, alternative surgical and procedural options should be considered. General anesthesia can be avoided with pillar soft palate implants or dental prosthesis creation and should be considered in CPAP-intolerant patients with mild to moderate disease.

UPPP is the most commonly performed surgical procedure for OSA and is often misused as the first line of surgical therapy regardless of coexisting patient factors (retrognathia, obesity, multilevel obstruction). As a result, it is often unsuccessful in treating OSA in poorly selected patients. Expansion Z-palatoplasty, midline glossectomy, and tongue base/hyoid suspension procedures have shown improved outcomes for CPAP-intolerant patients with moderate and severe OSA.

■ Acknowledgment

The authors would like to thank Josh Mark, MS IV, and Kevin Sykes, MPH, for their assistance.

■ References

1. Barthlen GM. Sleep disorders: obstructive sleep apnea syndrome, restless legs syndrome, and insomnia in geriatric patients. Geriatrics 2002;57(11):34–39, quiz 40
2. Ancoli-Israel S, Kripke DF, Klauber MR, Mason WJ, Fell R, Kaplan O. Sleep-disordered breathing in community-dwelling elderly. Sleep 1991;14(6):486–495
3. Norton PGDE, Dunn EV, Haight JS. Snoring in adults: some epidemiologic aspects. Can Med Assoc J 1983;128(6):674–675
4. Kushida CA, Littner MR, Morgenthaler T, et al. Practice parameters for the indications for polysomnography and related procedures: an update for 2005. Sleep 2005;28(4):499–521
5. Guilleminault C Sr, Stoohs R, Clerk A, Cetel M, Maistros P. A cause of excessive daytime sleepiness. The upper airway resistance syndrome. Chest 1993;104(3):781–787
6. Ayappa I, Norman RG, Krieger AC, Rosen A, O'Malley RL, Rapoport DM. Non-Invasive detection of respiratory effort-related arousals (REras) by a nasal cannula/pressure transducer system. Sleep 2000;23(6):763–771
7. Seet E, Chung F. Obstructive sleep apnea: preoperative assessment. Anesthesiol Clin 2010;28(2):199–215
8. Chung F, Yegneswaran B, Liao P, et al. STOP questionnaire: a tool to screen patients for obstructive sleep apnea. Anesthesiology 2008;108(5):812–821
9. Davies RJ, Stradling JR. The epidemiology of sleep apnoea. Thorax 1996;51(Suppl 2):S65–S70
10. CJ D. Prevalence of obstructive sleep apnea-hypopnea and related clinical features in the elderly: a population-based study in the general population aged 71–100. Presented at the World Conference 2001 Sleep Odyssey. Montevideo, Uruguay; 2001
11. Ancoli-Israel S, Gehrman P, Kripke DF, et al. Long-term follow-up of sleep disordered breathing in older adults. Sleep Med 2001;2(6):511–516
12. Young T, Shahar E, Nieto FJ, et al; Sleep Heart Health Study Research Group. Predictors of sleep-disordered breathing in community-dwelling adults: the Sleep Heart Health Study. Arch Intern Med 2002;162(8):893–900
13. Young T, Peppard PE, Gottlieb DJ. Epidemiology of obstructive sleep apnea: a population health perspective. Am J Respir Crit Care Med 2002;165(9):1217–1239
14. Klawe JJT-KM, Tafil-Klawe M. Age-related response of the genioglossus muscle EMG-activity to hypoxia in humans. J Physiol Pharmacol 2003;54(Suppl 1):14–19
15. Young T, Finn L, Austin D, Peterson A. Menopausal status and sleep-disordered breathing in the Wisconsin Sleep Cohort Study. Am J Respir Crit Care Med 2003;167(9):1181–1185
16. Shepertycky MRBK, Banno K, Kryger MH. Differences between men and women in the clinical presentation of patients diagnosed with obstructive sleep apnea syndrome. Sleep 2005;28(3):309–314
17. Young T, Shahar E, Nieto FJ, et al; Sleep Heart Health Study Research Group. Predictors of sleep-disordered breathing in community-dwelling adults: the Sleep Heart Health Study. Arch Intern Med 2002;162(8):893–900
18. Piani A, Brotini S, Dolso P, Budai R, Gigli GL. Sleep disturbances in elderly: a subjective evaluation over 65. Arch Gerontol Geriatr Suppl 2004;9(9):325–331
19. Van Cauter E, Leproult R, Plat L. Age-related changes in slow wave sleep and REM sleep and relationship with growth hormone and cortisol levels in healthy men. JAMA 2000;284(7):861–868
20. Boselli M, Parrino L, Smerieri A, Terzano MG. Effect of age on EEG arousals in normal sleep. Sleep 1998;21(4):351–357
21. Foley D, Ancoli-Israel S, Britz P, Walsh J. Sleep disturbances and chronic disease in older adults: results of the 2003 National Sleep Foundation Sleep in America Survey. J Psychosom Res 2004;56(5):497–502
22. Bliwise DL. Sleep in normal aging and dementia. Sleep 1993;16(1):40–81
23. Van Cauter E, Leproult R, Plat L. Age-related changes in slow wave sleep and REM sleep and relationship with growth hormone and cortisol levels in healthy men. JAMA 2000;284(7):861–868
24. Ohayon MMCM, Carskadon MA, Guilleminault C, Vitiello MV. Meta-analysis of quantitative sleep parameters from childhood to old age in healthy individuals: developing normative sleep values across the human lifespan. Sleep 2004;27(7):1255–1273
25. Bixler EO, Vgontzas AN, Ten Have T, Tyson K, Kales A. Effects of age on sleep apnea in men: I. Prevalence and severity. Am J Respir Crit Care Med 1998;157(1):144–148
26. Meen EK, Chandra RK. The role of the nose in sleep-disordered breathing. Am J Rhinol Allergy 2013;27(3):213–220
27. Meurice JCMI, Marc I, Carrier G, Sériès F. Effects of mouth opening on upper airway collapsibility in normal sleeping subjects. Am J Respir Crit Care Med 1996;153(1):255–259
28. Patil SPSH, Schneider H, Schwartz AR, Smith PL. Adult obstructive sleep apnea: pathophysiology and diagnosis. Chest 2007;132(1):325–337
29. Klawe JJ, Tafil-Klawe M. Age-related response of the genioglossus muscle EMG-activity to hypoxia in humans. J Physiol Pharmacol 2003;54(Suppl 1):14–19
30. Practice parameters for the treatment of obstructive sleep apnea in adults: the efficacy of surgical modifications of the upper airway. Report of the American Sleep Disorders Association. Sleep 1996;19(2):152–155
31. Kezirian EJ, Goldberg AN. Hypopharyngeal surgery in obstructive sleep apnea: an evidence-based medicine review. Arch Otolaryngol Head Neck Surg 2006;132(2):206–213

32. Van de Heyning PH, Badr MS, Baskin JZ, et al. Implanted upper airway stimulation device for obstructive sleep apnea. Laryngoscope 2012;122(7):1626–1633
33. He J, Kryger MH, Zorick FJ, Conway W, Roth T. Mortality and apnea index in obstructive sleep apnea. Experience in 385 male patients. Chest 1988;94(1):9–14
34. Sassani A, Findley LJ, Kryger M, Goldlust E, George C, Davidson TM. Reducing motor-vehicle collisions, costs, and fatalities by treating obstructive sleep apnea syndrome. Sleep 2004;27(3):453–458
35. Quan SFWR, Wright R, Baldwin CM, et al. Obstructive sleep apnea-hypopnea and neurocognitive functioning in the Sleep Heart Health Study. Sleep Med 2006;7(6):498–507
36. Parish JMLP, Lyng PJ. Quality of life in bed partners of patients with obstructive sleep apnea or hypopnea after treatment with continuous positive airway pressure. Chest 2003; 124(3):942–947
37. Jennum P, Sjøl A. Self-assessed cognitive function in snorers and sleep apneics. An epidemiological study of 1,504 females and males aged 30-60 years: the Dan-MONICA II Study. Eur Neurol 1994;34(4):204–208
38. Ballester E, Badia JR, Hernández L, et al. Evidence of the effectiveness of continuous positive airway pressure in the treatment of sleep apnea/hypopnea syndrome. Am J Respir Crit Care Med 1999;159(2):495–501
39. Pichel F, Zamarrón C, Magán F, del Campo F, Alvarez-Sala R, Suarez JR. Health-related quality of life in patients with obstructive sleep apnea: effects of long-term positive airway pressure treatment. Respir Med 2004;98(10):968–976
40. Young T, Peppard PE, Gottlieb DJ. Epidemiology of obstructive sleep apnea: a population health perspective. Am J Respir Crit Care Med 2002;165(9):1217–1239
41. Partinen M, Jamieson A, Guilleminault C. Long-term outcome for obstructive sleep apnea syndrome patients. Mortality. Chest 1988;94(6):1200–1204
42. Lindberg E, Janson C, Svärdsudd K, Gislason T, Hetta J, Boman G. Increased mortality among sleepy snorers: a prospective population based study. Thorax 1998;53(8):631–637
43. Hu FB, Willett WC, Manson JE, et al. Snoring and risk of cardiovascular disease in women. J Am Coll Cardiol 2000;35(2): 308–313
44. Koskenvuo M, Kaprio J, Telakivi T, Partinen M, Heikkilä K, Sarna S. Snoring as a risk factor for ischaemic heart disease and stroke in men. Br Med J (Clin Res Ed) 1987;294(6563):16–19
45. Gami AS, Olson EJ, Shen WK, et al. Obstructive sleep apnea and the risk of sudden cardiac death: a longitudinal study of 10,701 adults. J Am Coll Cardiol 2013;62(7):610–616
46. Johansson P, Alehagen U, Svanborg E, Dahlström U, Broström A. Clinical characteristics and mortality risk in relation to obstructive and central sleep apnoea in community-dwelling elderly individuals: a 7-year follow-up. Age Ageing 2012; 41(4):468–474
47. Lavie P, Herer P, Peled R, et al. Mortality in sleep apnea patients: a multivariate analysis of risk factors. Sleep 1995;18(3): 149–157
48. Tilkian AG, Guilleminault C, Schroeder JS, Lehrman KL, Simmons FB, Dement WC. Hemodynamics in sleep-induced apnea. Studies during wakefulness and sleep. Ann Intern Med 1976;85(6):714–719
49. Nieto FJ, Young TB, Lind BK, et al. Association of sleep-disordered breathing, sleep apnea, and hypertension in a large community-based study. Sleep Heart Health Study. JAMA 2000;283(14):1829–1836
50. Bixler EO, Vgontzas AN, Lin HM, et al. Association of hypertension and sleep-disordered breathing. Arch Intern Med 2000;160(15):2289–2295
51. Young T, Peppard P, Palta M, et al. Population-based study of sleep-disordered breathing as a risk factor for hypertension. Arch Intern Med 1997;157(15):1746–1752
52. Peppard PE, Young T, Palta M, Skatrud J. Prospective study of the association between sleep-disordered breathing and hypertension. N Engl J Med 2000;342(19):1378–1384
53. Becker HF, Jerrentrup A, Ploch T, et al. Effect of nasal continuous positive airway pressure treatment on blood pressure in patients with obstructive sleep apnea. Circulation 2003; 107(1):68–73
54. Young T, Blustein J, Finn L, Palta M. Sleep-disordered breathing and motor vehicle accidents in a population-based sample of employed adults. Sleep 1997;20(8):608–613
55. Terán-Santos J, Jiménez-Gómez A, Cordero-Guevara J; Cooperative Group Burgos-Santander. The association between sleep apnea and the risk of traffic accidents. N Engl J Med 1999;340(11):847–851
56. Findley LJ, Fabrizio MJ, Knight H, Norcross BB, LaForte AJ, Suratt PM. Driving simulator performance in patients with sleep apnea. Am Rev Respir Dis 1989;140(2):529–530
57. Ip MSLB, Lam B, Ng MM, Lam WK, Tsang KW, Lam KS. Obstructive sleep apnea is independently associated with insulin resistance. Am J Respir Crit Care Med 2002;165(5): 670–676
58. Assoumou HG, Gaspoz JM, Sforza E, et al. Obstructive sleep apnea and the metabolic syndrome in an elderly healthy population: the SYNAPSE cohort. Sleep Breath 2012;16(3): 895–902
59. Young T, Palta M, Dempsey J, Skatrud J, Weber S, Badr S. The occurrence of sleep-disordered breathing among middle-aged adults. N Engl J Med 1993;328(17):1230–1235
60. Johns MW; MW J. A new method for measuring daytime sleepiness: the Epworth sleepiness scale. Sleep 1991;14(6): 540–545
61. Barthlen GM. Sleep disorders: obstructive sleep apnea syndrome, restless legs syndrome, and insomnia in geriatric patients. Geriatrics 2002;57(11):34–39, quiz 40
62. Fairbanks MD, David NF, Mickelson SA, et al, eds. Snoring and Obstructive Sleep Apnea. 3rd ed. New York, NY: Raven; 2002:101–128
63. Weaver TEGR, Grunstein RR. Adherence to continuous positive airway pressure therapy: the challenge to effective treatment. Proc Am Thorac Soc 2008;5(2):173–178
64. Aboussouan LS, Golish JA, Wood BG, Mehta AC, Wood DE, Dinner DS. Dynamic pharyngoscopy in predicting outcome of uvulopalatopharyngoplasty for moderate and severe obstructive sleep apnea. Chest 1995;107(4):946–951
65. McArdle N, Devereux G, Heidarnejad H, Engleman HM, Mackay TW, Douglas NJ. Long-term use of CPAP therapy for sleep apnea/hypopnea syndrome. Am J Respir Crit Care Med 1999;159(4 Pt 1):1108–1114
66. Budhiraja R, Parthasarathy S, Drake CL, et al. Early CPAP use identifies subsequent adherence to CPAP therapy. Sleep 2007;30(3):320–324
67. Barbé F, Mayoralas LR, Duran J, et al. Treatment with continuous positive airway pressure is not effective in patients with sleep apnea but no daytime sleepiness: a randomized, controlled trial. Ann Intern Med 2001;134(11):1015–1023
68. den Herder C, van Tinteren H, de Vries N. Sleep endoscopy versus modified Mallampati score in sleep apnea and snoring. Laryngoscope 2005;115(4):735–739
69. Joshi GP, Ankichetty SP, Gan TJ, Chung F. Society for Ambulatory Anesthesia consensus statement on preoperative selection of adult patients with obstructive sleep apnea scheduled for ambulatory surgery. Anesth Analg 2012;115(5):1060–1068

70. Phillips B, Young T, Finn L, Asher K, Hening WA, Purvis C. Epidemiology of restless legs symptoms in adults. Arch Intern Med 2000;160(14):2137–2141
71. Hornyak M, Feige B, Riemann D, Voderholzer U. Periodic leg movements in sleep and periodic limb movement disorder: prevalence, clinical significance and treatment. Sleep Med Rev 2006;10(3):169–177
72. Grewal M, Hawa R, Shapiro C. Treatment of periodic limb movements in sleep with selegiline HCl. Mov Disord 2002; 17(2):398–401
73. Gamaldo CEEC, Earley CJ. Restless legs syndrome: a clinical update. Chest 2006;130(5):1596–1604
74. Roth T. Insomnia: definition, prevalence, etiology, and consequences. J Clin Sleep Med 2007;3(5, Suppl):S7–S10
75. Martínez-García MA, Campos-Rodríguez F, Catalán-Serra P, et al. Cardiovascular mortality in obstructive sleep apnea in the elderly: role of long-term continuous positive airway pressure treatment: a prospective observational study. Am J Respir Crit Care Med 2012;186(9):909–916
76. Barbé F, Durán-Cantolla J, Sánchez-de-la-Torre M, et al; Spanish Sleep and Breathing Network. Effect of continuous positive airway pressure on the incidence of hypertension and cardiovascular events in nonsleepy patients with obstructive sleep apnea: a randomized controlled trial. JAMA 2012;307(20):2161–2168
77. Powell ED, Gay PC, Ojile JM, Litinski M, Malhotra A. A pilot study assessing adherence to auto-bilevel following a poor initial encounter with CPAP. J Clin Sleep Med 2012;8(1): 43–47
78. Littner M, Hirshkowitz M, Davila D, et al; Standards of Practice Committee of the American Academy of Sleep Medicine. Practice parameters for the use of auto-titrating continuous positive airway pressure devices for titrating pressures and treating adult patients with obstructive sleep apnea syndrome. An American Academy of Sleep Medicine report. Sleep 2002;25(2):143–147
79. Ferguson KA, Cartwright R, Rogers R, Schmidt-Nowara W. Oral appliances for snoring and obstructive sleep apnea: a review. Sleep 2006;29(2):244–262
80. Engleman HMMJ, McDonald JP, Graham D, et al. Randomized crossover trial of two treatments for sleep apnea/hypopnea syndrome: continuous positive airway pressure and mandibular repositioning splint. Am J Respir Crit Care Med 2002;166(6):855–859
81. Nordgård S, Hein G, Stene BK, Skjøstad KW, Maurer JT. One-year results: palatal implants for the treatment of obstructive sleep apnea. Otolaryngol Head Neck Surg 2007;136(5): 818–822
82. Kiely JLNP, Nolan P, McNicholas WT. Intranasal corticosteroid therapy for obstructive sleep apnoea in patients with co-existing rhinitis. Thorax 2004;59(1):50–55
83. McLean HAUA, Urton AM, Driver HS, et al. Effect of treating severe nasal obstruction on the severity of obstructive sleep apnoea. Eur Respir J 2005;25(3):521–527
84. Friedman M, Ibrahim H, Joseph NJ. Staging of obstructive sleep apnea/hypopnea syndrome: a guide to appropriate treatment. Laryngoscope 2004;114(3):454–459
85. Steinhart H, Kuhn-Lohmann J, Gewalt K, Constantinidis J, Mertzlufft F, Iro H. Upper airway collapsibility in habitual snorers and sleep apneics: evaluation with drug-induced sleep endoscopy. Acta Otolaryngol 2000;120(8):990–994
86. Fujita S, Conway W, Zorick F, Roth T. Surgical correction of anatomic abnormalities in obstructive sleep apnea syndrome: uvulopalatopharyngoplasty. Otolaryngol Head Neck Surg 1981;89(6):923–934
87. Kezirian EJ, Weaver EM, Yueh B, et al. Incidence of serious complications after uvulopalatopharyngoplasty. Laryngoscope 2004;114(3):450–453
88. Friedman M. Z-palatoplasty. Oper Tech Otolaryngol 2007; 18:2–6
89. Cahali MB, Formigoni GG, Gebrim EM, Miziara ID. Lateral pharyngoplasty versus uvulopalatopharyngoplasty: a clinical, polysomnographic and computed tomography measurement comparison. Sleep 2004;27(5):942–950
90. Woodson BT, Robinson S, Lim HJ. Transpalatal advancement pharyngoplasty outcomes compared with uvulopalatopharyngoplasty. Otolaryngol Head Neck Surg 2005;133(2): 211–217
91. Vicente E, Marín JM, Carrizo S, Naya MJ. Tongue-base suspension in conjunction with uvulopalatopharyngoplasty for treatment of severe obstructive sleep apnea: long-term follow-up results. Laryngoscope 2006;116(7):1223–1227
92. Varela JEHM, Hinojosa MW, Nguyen NT. Resolution of obstructive sleep apnea after laparoscopic gastric bypass. Obes Surg 2007;17(10):1279–1282
93. Troell RJRR, Riley RW, Powell NB, Li K. Surgical management of the hypopharyngeal airway in sleep disordered breathing. Otolaryngol Clin North Am 1998;31(6):979–1012

18 Facial Plastic Surgery in Geriatric Patients

J. Regan Thomas

Introduction

Several predictable changes and alterations are typical and normal sequelae of the neck and facial aging process. Unlike other components of the body's predictable aging changes, aging in the face and neck region carries other significant implications, including those that impact cultural, social, and personal perceptions. Historically there has been an evolution of facial rejuvenation procedures in response to those perceptions. The procedures have gained significant public acceptance and desirability. In the not too distant past facial procedures were often felt to be within the realm of wealthy celebrities or others in the entertainment business. Today these procedures are widely accepted and actively explored by a wide spectrum of social, economic, and ethnic backgrounds. The goal is to achieve an enhanced self-perception of greater fitness and youth coupled with a response to cultural pressures to maintain a youthful appearance related to work, economic, and various social interactions.[1,2]

Although the geriatric population requires facial plastic surgery for facial trauma and fractures, facial neoplasms, and occasionally persistent congenital defects, the focus of facial plastic surgery in the geriatric population more frequently addresses facial aging processes. An individual's age is usually judged according to appearance of the skin.[3] Although much attention is focused on cutaneous gerontology, the appearance of cutaneous senescence is actually based on a combination of skeletal structure, soft tissue, and skin (**Fig. 18.1**). The primary changes in a person's three-dimensional skeletal contour contribute to secondary changes in the overlying soft tissue and skin. It has been said that a youthful face represents that period in time when a particular set of skeletal proportions are ideal for their soft tissue envelope.

What is generally termed facial aging is in reality a combination of the aforementioned factors. Facial wrinkles or rhytids are related to changes in the skin secondary to a variety of factors, including chronological skin aging, ultraviolet (UV) and other environmental factors leading to photoaging, hyperdynamic facial expressions, and skin folding secondary to loss of soft tissue support and skeletal changes. Reversal or techniques to counteract these changes create the foundation for facial plastic surgery in the geriatric patient (**Fig. 18.2**).

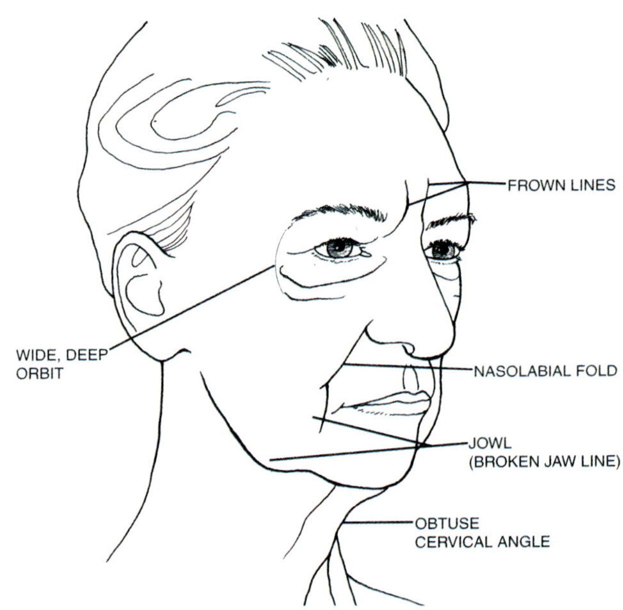

Fig. 18.1 Typical aging changes. (Used with permission from Facial Plast Surg Clin North Am 2001;9(2):179–187.)

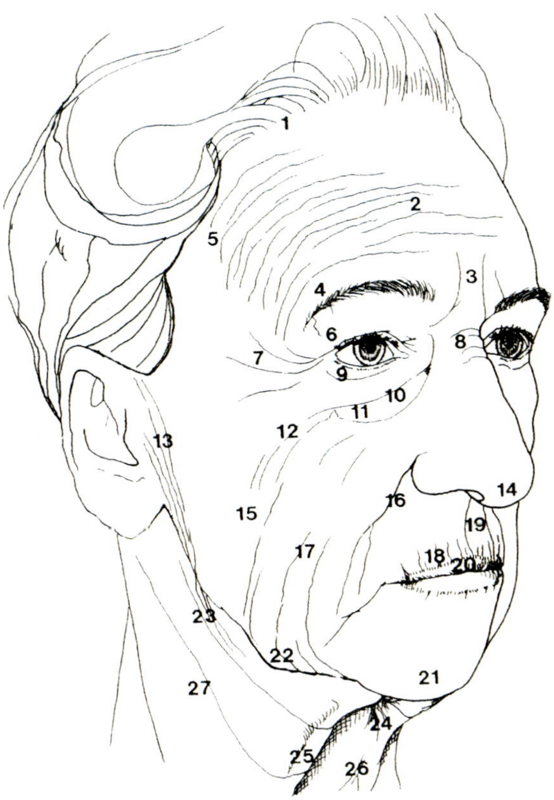

Fig. 18.2 Topographic geriatric facial changes. (Used with permission from Facial Plast Surg Clin North Am 2001;9(2): 179–187.)

Analysis and Pathophysiology of Facial Aging

Geriatric skin changes are a product of two basic processes. First is chronological aging, sometimes referred to as intrinsic aging, the changes of which are primarily genetic. Second is environmental or extrinsic aging, particularly from such stressors as sun exposure or smoking. Skin changes often seen in the geriatric patient include dyschromia, roughness, and multiple rhytids followed by persistently deeper folds. Structurally this occurs due to dermal atrophy, decreased collagen, and loss of cutaneous fat coupled with loss of inherent elasticity and increased melanogenesis[4]

The structural changes in soft tissue already noted are variable but can be significant as part of the aging process, two major forces impact these changes. First is chronological aging of the skin related to intrinsic passage of time and second, photoaging related to chronic ultraviolet light exposure. Other components may impact this as well, such as smoking and certain dietetic aspects.[5] The skin of geriatric patients shows declining changes with age, which ae further accelerated in UV exposed photoaged skin. Photoaging is responsible for many of the age-associated cosmetic concerns, including dispigmentation, laxity, changes of pores, telangiectasia, a leathery appearance, and wrinkling. Vascular changes increase during this period, creating the tendency for bruising during activities of daily life as well as medical procedures. Loss as well as shifting and redistribution of subcutaneous tissue further contribute to folds and drooping skin. Because of these changes, dealing with soft tissue in the geriatric patient carries additional considerations as compared with more youthful patients:

- Cell replacement
- Immune response
- Injury response
- Barrier function
- Sensory perception
- Sweat production
- Sebum production
- Vitamin D production

The facial changes typically associated with the geriatric patient are a result of a combination of forces related to facial aging including gravity, soft tissue maturation, skeletal remodeling, facial muscular changes, and solar changes to the skin. The aging process comprises a complex and diverse set of elements, each of which leaves a specific and distinctive result on the aging face. The anatomical and tissue changes already noted are intimately interconnected, each having an impact on the other components. Skin, soft tissue, muscle, and skeleton, although affected individually by the aging process, present themselves as an interactive aging process acting in concert to result in the facial appearance typically seen in the geriatric patient.

Geriatric Skin Changes

The geriatric patient displays several predictable changes related to ongoing aging affect. These changes include secondary results of gravity acting on skin that is becoming progressively thinner, dryer, and less elastic. There are genetic factors also influencing the location of facial wrinkles, and these progress as a result of cutaneous senescence combined with cumulative environmental insults.

Chronic solar exposure and UV interaction constitute the major environmental component contributing to the clinical changes that are typical of aging skin. This is accurately termed photoaging and is distinct from intrinsic or chronological aging.

The relationship of inherent aging changes in the geriatric patient's skin can be contrasted with those changes that are compounded by photoaging and chronic solar exposure. More photologic changes and sun-protected skin consist primarily of fine wrinkling and laxity with occasional benign neoplasm development. Those who leave their skin exposed to chronic solar damage demonstrate changes of texture, color, and functional capacity. Color changes include dyschromia, often a yellow pallor, lentigines, and the gradual appearance of telangiectasia. Textural changes likewise accompany these variations and include a loss of palpable smoothness, keratosis, and increasing rhytids ending in persistent deep folds and creases. Histological changes associated with aging skin begin with a thinning of the viable epidermis and flattening of the dermal–epidermal junction. This is in contrast to photoaged skin in which the epidermis becomes increasingly thicker with a flattening of the dermal–epidermal junction.

Of the dermal structural elements, elastic fibers are prominently affected by the sequelae of both chronologically damaged and photodamaged skin. Chronically aged skin reveals elastic fibers that are slightly increased in thickness. Photodamaged skin shows striking histological changes with the presence of massive quantities of thickened bundles of degraded elastic fibers or dermal elastosis. The result of these various histological reactions and changes in aging skin is that the skin itself is less stretchable and less resilient. The loss of inheritant elasticity results in skin that is more lax with dependent draping that is prone to wrinkling from gravitational effects. There is also an increase in mechanical fragility and a susceptibility to lateral sheer stress combined with an increase in dryness and skin irritability.[6]

Geriatric Facial Musculature

Contractions and sphincteric actions of the facial musculature are responsible for facial expressions exhibiting emotion as well as functional actions including eye closing, lip movement, and numerous others. However, over time and combined with aging skin changes facial rhytids and folds are accentuated by this normal muscular action and begin to contribute to changes in facial appearance associated with aging in the geriatric patient. For example, continued contraction of the orbicularis component of the orbicularis oculi creates concentric folds emanating from the lateral canthus resulting in lines referred to as crow's feet. The corrugator supercilii lies deep to the frontalis muscle and has it origin on the frontal bone medial to the eyebrows near the superior medial orbital rim. The corrugator acts as a brow abductor drawing the brows inferiorly and medially and thus ultimately producing vertical frown lines. In the same anatomical region, the procerus muscle originates on the lower part of the nasal bone and inserts in the skin overlying the nasion. This likewise pulls the medial brow inferiorly, creating transverse wrinkles over the nasal bridge. The antagonist of the brow depressors is the frontalis muscle, which is ultimately responsible for horizontal forehead creases. All of these actions, which are normal facial movements, ultimately contribute to an aging facial appearance and are key areas addressed, particularly by Botox (Allergan, Irvine, CA), as a treatment modality. Similarly, the normal muscle actions of the lower facial mimetic muscles and the perioral muscles all contribute to rhytids and skin folds related to aging changes in the lower face. Although it is a normal process for these hyperdynamic facial lines, crow's feet, and glabellar furrows to reflect underlined muscular anatomy, the ultimate result is reflective of what are typically thought of as unaesthetic changes in the face related to aging.

The Aging Nose

Often overlooked in terms of facial anatomical changes that are recognized as aging in the face are the progressive changes to nasal appearance and its impact on facial aesthetics. The nose at a central location is a key component of facial aesthetics and facial relationships, and the aging changes that affect the nose affect the rest of the facial appearance. Aging alters the nasal skeleton, cartilaginous framework, and soft tissue covering.[7] Progressive descent of the nasal tip is often associated with loss of support from changes and attachment of the upper and lower level cartilages, which then lengthen and weaken the nasal tip support, thus lengthening and enlarging the nose. The nasal labia angle becomes increasingly acute in relationship to this loss of tip structure. The relative appearance of a nasal dorsal hump is exaggerated as the tip decreases in its projection. Pyriform remodeling affects the alar base, and, in combination with upper maxillary resorption, it results in superior repositioning and thus further narrowing of the nasal labial angle and accentuation of the tip ptosis. Chin pad ptosis secondary to bony resorption further contributes to the illusion of increased nasal length (**Fig. 18.3**).

Rhinoplasty of the geriatric patient often not only contributes to a more youthful appearance based on repositioning of the nasal anatomy but also frequently contributes to airway improvement. Aging changes to the nose that impact nasal function include loss of the internal nasal valve support, external valve collapse, and changes of narrow airway openings related to loss of tip support. Rhinoplasty is a frequent requirement in the aging patient because of these functional and airway difficulties

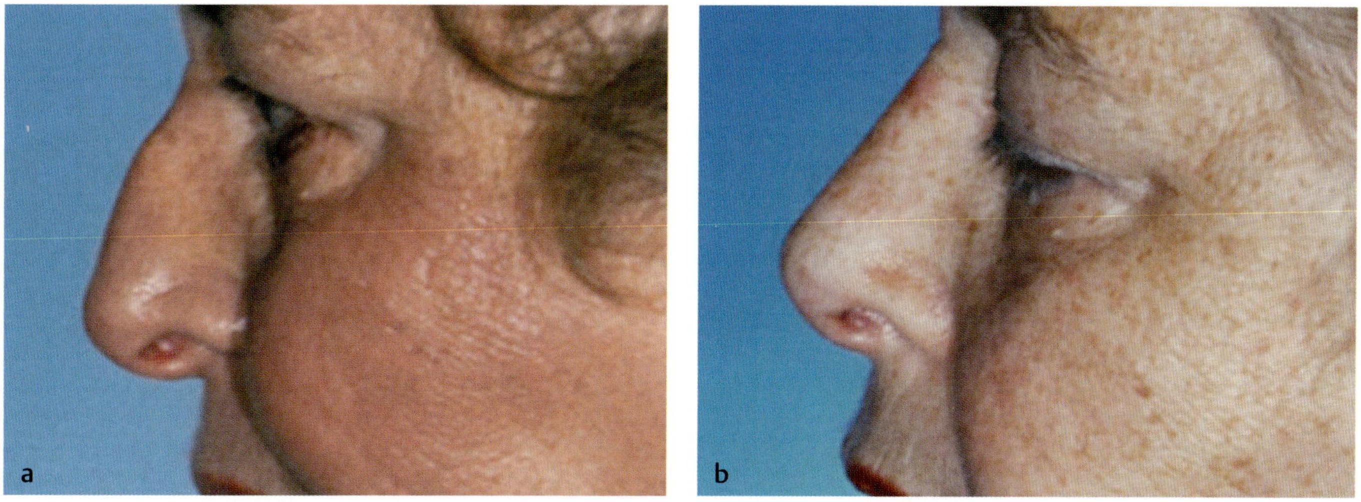

Fig. 18.3 (**a**) Typical findings in the geriatric nose include soft tissue thickening, loss of tip support, and narrowing of the nasolabial angle. (**b**) Postoperative improvements following rhinoplasty in the geriatric patient.

in addition to aesthetic goals of attaining greater youthfulness and enhanced aesthetic facial appearance in the geriatric patient.

Eyebrows and Eyelids in the Geriatric Patient

The combination of gravity, loss of tissue elasticity, a loss of subcutaneous tissue, and at times bony resorption lead to inferior displacement of the brow. With aging, typically the eyebrow position descends from above the supraorbital rim to point of some portion below it. This contributes to excess accumulation of upper lid skin that accentuates ongoing skin changes of dermatochalasis with loss of eyelid creases and additional folds of skin over the upper lid. Excess sliding of skin and a weakened orbital septum allow interorbital fat to herniate, creating eyelid bags and protruding adipose tissue. The periorbital soft tissue in the more youthful patient is often shallow and described as an unbroken convex line from the lower eyelid to the cheek. With progressive aging those relationships change the dimensions and become wider and deeper as time progresses. Ptotic cheek fat may descend inferiorly, contributing to a melolabial fold leaving a cheek depression that can be accentuated by buccal fat attenuation. The orbicularis muscle becomes increasingly ptotic; with aging its inferior border becomes increasingly apparent. This creates the malar decent of the zygomatic eminence laterally resulting in deepening of the nasojugal fold, which continues to deepen with aging. Multiple surgical procedures in the aging patient are designed to correct and reverse these predictable changes. Procedures used individually or in combination include upper and lower blepharoplasty, brow lift, and forehead lift. These surgical procedures may be used independently or in combination with other facial aesthetic procedures depending on the severity of the aging changes in the geriatric patient as well as the patient's aesthetic goals.

Jowl and Neck in the Aging Patient

The typical changes of the aging neck arise from a combination of changes, including changes in the skin, fat distribution, the platysmal muscle, and the underlying bony cartilaginous framework. The continual downward pull of the platysma creates jowls with the loss of definition of chin and jowl line. The jowl region along the margin of the mandible as created by ptosis of the facial portion of the platysmal muscle skin accordingly can also become lax over the platysma, developing horizontal rhytids. Typically in the aging patient anterior edges of the platysma separate and lose tone, creating the interior neck banding and, particularly in the male patient, the so-called turkey neck deformity. The common entity is development of a large submental fat pad deep to the platysmal bands as well as a similar fat pad in the subcutaneous area above the platysma. These fat accumulations contribute to the double chin appearance in those patients in addition to the sagging skin and loss of muscular support. In many patients the hyoid bone and larynx will gradually descend with age, making the larynx appear more prominent and blunting the cervicomental angle.

A variety of techniques to correct these predictable changes of aging have been described and are frequently used. These include an array of essentially facelift procedures that entail tightening of the skin and subcutaneous tissue, correction of the loosening and displaced musculature support, and elevation of the connective tissue of the face with redraping of redundant skin. These are often combined with soft tissue and facial skin surface modalities of treatment to further smooth the skin surface, which improve the appearance of cutaneous skin rhytides and act as adjuncts to surgical correction of these redundant sagging tissues of the geriatric patient facial anatomy.

Nonsurgical Treatment in the Geriatric Face

Botulinum Toxin

Injectable botulinum toxin can be of help in correcting certain nonaesthetic anatomical changes in the aging face. Botulinum toxin is available in various types; however, type A (Botox) has become the most frequently used agent. Botox does not offer a permanent solution; however, the relative ease of treatment on an outpatient basis has added to its popularity. Although it may be more useful in the younger patient without additional soft tissue aging changes there are certainly applications for the patient in the geriatric age group, and it is frequently used in this fashion. The toxin disrupts the nerve cells' ability to release acetylcholine. Facial rhytides or wrinkles that occur naturally over time secondary to repetitive contraction of underlying facial musculature are often felt to be nonaesthetic and a sign of aging. Temporarily weakening or paralyzing the musculature of the face in the area of rhytid formation allows the skin to settle and conform to the face without the dominate influence of muscle contraction. In most cases this will alleviate the appearance of rhytides and thus enhance facial appearance.[8]

Although there are a variety of types of botulinum toxin available, botulinum toxin type A is the most common neurotoxin used clinically for facial aesthetic treatment. The most common treatment indications are in the area of the upper third of the face and include forehead rhytides, thytids, and brow elevation. The periocular region, particularly in the lateral crow's feet areas, can also be safely helped in our frequent area of indication. Areas of required facial animation in the lower face, such as the lips, must be approached with great care. Facial animation is vital to expressing human emotions, and lack of activity or emotion in those areas can have a negative effect in terms of interaction and aesthetic result.

There are certain contraindications to the use of botulinum toxins. The materials are certainly contraindicated in those with a known allergic response to any component of the product or with a general history of anaphylaxis. Additionally patients with neuromuscular conditions or peripheral motor neuropathies such as myasthenia gravis, amyotrophic lateral sclerosis, or similar syndromes are not perfect candidates. In the geriatric patient group many of the individuals are on a variety medications for treatments, and this should be explored in depth. The use of botulinum toxin should be avoided in patients using medications that may create difficulties. These would include depolarizing blockers, anticholinesterases and lincosamides, and aminoglycosides. The use of botulinum toxin is also contraindicated in those individuals with autoimmune, dermatologic, or other systemic disorders that predispose to poor wound healing or exuberant inflammatory response. Blood thinners can be considered a relative contraindication due to ecchymosis or potential hematoma formation.

The older geriatric patient should be approached in a very conservative fashion. The treating physician should remember that although the goal with botulinum toxin is to smooth some facial rhytides related to muscle contraction, this may be counterproductive in the geriatric patient. Those patients with significantly loose soft tissues and lax skin may find that, for example, smoothing the forehead rhytides creates a lowering of the upper brow to an unacceptable degree. Injection should generally be avoided within 1 cm of the margin of the ridge of the supraorbital rim and most importantly at the midpupillary line where diffusion can affect the upper eyelid levator. Treatment should be adjusted and individualized for the patient and customized based on the soft tissue anatomy and patient needs. Treatment in the lower half of the face, particularly in the perioral region, although described, should be approached very conservatively. Often at best it can offer only modest relief in specific areas and can lead to both functional and aesthetic negative appearance. Areas of inappropriate muscle weakness can potentially be a result of the injections.

Treatment in the neck area and of the platysmal muscle should likewise be approached very conservatively in the geriatric patient. Although this is described in the literature and used effectively in certain patient categories, senior or geriatric patients may have increased laxity of soft tissue of the neck that is unaesthetic and counteracts any potential improvement in the platysmal bands themselves.

Facial Peels in the Geriatric Patient

Laser resurfacing has become increasingly popular as technical advances of new modalities have been developed. Chemical peels continue to be a potential adjunct for many patients and are actively used by some treating physicians in the aging patient with specific aging skin issues. These problems for the patient include photoaging, rhytides, keratosis, pigmentary dyschromias, and some level of superficial scarring such as from acne. There may be some improved elastic and tensile strength to the skin with some tightening of the skin. Because of this peels may be beneficial to some geriatric patients but as with all the treatments it should be individualized for the patient. There is a wide array of chemical peel modalities available, and these should be individualized according to the patients' needs.

Skin texture and skin type can be assessed using the Glogau classification for photoaging as well as the Fitzpatrick classification of sun reactivity type. These are useful when determining which treatment agent to use (**Table 18.1**).

Most individuals classify chemical peels based on histological depths of reaction and treatment. The knowledge of this reaction of the peeling agent is useful in determining the appropriate selection of the correct peeling method. Superficial light peels exfoliate with fresh skin at the level of the epidermis, whereas medium-depth and deep peels can work in the papillary and the reticular dermis, respectively.

Superficial peels would include the α-hydroxyl acids such as glycolic acid 30 to 70% and Jessner solution or trichloroacetic acid (TCA) peels 10 to 20%. Medium peels, which are used for the papillary upper reticular dermis, will include Jessner solution with TCA, and deep peels would typically use a version of the Baker–Gordon phenol peel. The key ingredients are 88% phenol and croton oil.

It should be recognized that there are indeed complications with the peels, particularly in the medium and deeper depth peel solutions. The postoperative complications can include prolonged erythema, acne and milia, infection, skin dyschromia, and scarring.

As noted earlier, in the geriatric patient, it is important to determine preoperatively any medical conditions or possible interactions with other medications. Likewise, although the peels may be helpful in terms of surface improvement they will not correct significantly redundant flaccid skin, which is often associated with the older patient age group.

Laser Skin Resurfacing in the Geriatric Patient

The goal of laser resurfacing is to give aging skin a more youthful appearance by improving dispigmentation, wrinkles, and potentially other lesions. Two different types of laser resurfacing have been developed: nonablative and ablative. Generally nonablative resurfacing is used where the surface texture has minimal wrinkling and surface change, and the treatment is usually able to spare the epidermis through adjunctive surface cooling. Ablative laser resurfacing is the more aggressive treatment for skin tightening and textural enhancement, because it removes the entire epidermis and parts of the dermis in an attempt to regenerate smoother-appearing skin in place of photodamaged skin. The treatment effect is much like the ultimate effect from dermabrasion or chemical peels. In general nonablative techniques are used in younger patients with mild and fine rhytides and perhaps early melasma. Ablative laser resurfacing is often more useful in the older patient age group where moderate to severe facial rhytides and wrinkling are present on the facial skin surface.[9]

Nonablative laser therapy uses a wide array of alternatives for this treatment modality, including

Table 18.1 Glogau classification of aging skin

Severity	Typical age	Features
Mild		Smooth skin, minimal keratosis
Moderate	35–50	Early rhytides, wrinkling, early actinic keratosis
Advanced	50–65	Persistent rhytids and wrinkles, discoloration with telangiectasia and actinic keratosis
Severe	60–75	Marked wrinkling and photoaging with dynamic rhytides, active actinic keratosis difficult to cover with makeup

light-emitting diode (LED), potassium-titanyl-phosphate (KTP), pulsed dye, neodymium:yttrium-aluminum-garnet (Nd:YAG), and intense pulsed light (IPL), among others. Each wavelength choice tends to offer certain advantages at the expense of some disadvantages, and the physician must balance those aspects when selecting the treatment modality. In general the nonablative skin rejuvenation treatments treat earlier photodamage and wrinkling and offer the advantage in appropriate patients of reducing patient downtime and recovery.

Ablative laser resurfacing should give results similar to dermabrasion or chemical peels. Its proponents argue that there is greater control over depth of injury with the adjunctive additional benefit of thermocoagulation of the dermis, and that that effect is helpful in collagen tightening and dermal remodeling. The two major laser wavelengths employed in recent years for ablative laser resurfacing include pulsed carbon dioxide (CO_2), and erbium:YAG (Er:YAG). Er:YAG laser resurfacing is typically reserved for patients with less severe and more superficial photodamage, whereas pulsed CO_2 is more appropriate for those with deep, severe rhytidosis who are willing to accept the associated prolonged downtime. Some systems combine the Er:YAG and subablative CO_2 systems to get the best of both techniques.

Complications related to laser resurfacing include prolonged erythema that may persist up to several months or longer. Infection should be rare but can happen and can be of bacterial, viral, or even fungal etiology. Acne and milia are relatively common early on but more minor for most patients in terms of their issues. Hyperpigmentation can occur 3 to 4 weeks after resurfacing and may persist for several months if treatment is not begun. Often exposure to sunlight during the healing period can stimulate melanocyte activity. Sun avoidance and sun screens are key in the postresurfacing period. More severe complications from laser treatment include hypertrophic scarring and unintended soft tissue changes such as lower lid ectropion.

Blepharoplasty in the Geriatric Patient

The eyes play a key role in expression as well as facial identity and contribute significantly to the overall appearance of the face. The eyes are one of the first areas of the face to demonstrate aging changes and thus are a frequent component of patients' self-evaluation and request for treatment. Actual changes are first manifest as smile lines or crow's feet in the lateral canthus region and progress to excess skin (dermatochalasis) and fat pseudoherniation. Both the upper and lower lids typically present with changes effected by these aging sequelae. These changes combined with brow ptosis can contribute to a "tired" as well an aging look.

Upper Eyelid Blepharoplasty

Upper blepharoplasty is performed to address aging changes of the upper eyelid. The steps typically include excision of excess skin from the upper lid and removal of pseudoherniating fat as needed; most often this in the medial fat compartment. The procedure may be done in conjunction with lower lid blepharoplasty and other facial aesthetic procedures.[10]

The preoperative eyelid evaluation consists of examining for effective skin and fat pseudoherniation of the medial and central compartments. The eyelid crease should be approximately 9 to 10 mm above the lash line for the skin in the female. This crease in the male can be slightly shallower, in the 8 to 10 mm region. The technique begins with preoperative marking, typically done in the preoperative area with the patient in the upright animated position. The inferior level of the incision falls along the tarsal crease and typically extends superiorly as one approaches the orbital rim. Determination of the appropriate amount of redundant skin is then marked on the patient. It is helpful to use forceps to gently pinch the excess skin to determine the appropriate amount.

Once marking has been completed the skin is infiltrated with 1% lidocaine to 1:100,000 epinephrine, typically using 1 to 2 mL per side. The face is prepped and the skin incision performed. A helpful technique is to combine a small amount of hyaluronidase with the injection to allow the skin to be pinched according to the preoperative planning lines that will remain in that pinched state and facilitate excision. In some patients where greater definition is required for the upper lid, a small strip of orbicularis oculi muscle can be resected just above the sulcus. Ophthalmic cautery or bipolar cautery is used throughout to maintain hemostasis. The fat compartment can be opened and gently teased out with cotton-tipped applicator dissection, the base cauterized and excised. The wound is then closed with placement of key 6–0 polypropylene sutures followed by a running 6–0 polypropylene suture (**Fig. 18.4**).

Lower Lid Blepharoplasty

Lower lid blepharoplasty begins with appropriate marking with the patient in the preoperative holding area in the upright animated position, noting areas with redundant skin as well as possible pseudoherniation of fat pads. A variety of procedures are used depending on the patient's preoperative status. Those patients with appropriate skin and muscle tightness in the lower lid but with fat protrusion can be approached through a transconjunctival approach. For the patients where it is appropriate to tighten the dermatochalasis of the lower lid, a subciliary incision can be used. Various fat preservation techniques have been described from fat repositioning to camouflaging of the orbital rim and filling the so-called tear trough or nasojugal depression. A variety of fat injections are also appropriate at times.

Typically for lower lid procedures general anesthesia or sedation may be used. For the transconjunctival approach with fat excisions local anesthesia is infiltrated in the conjunctival side of the lid with the lid retracted. An incision is made typically just below the inferior tarsal plate as the lid is retracted appropriately inferiorly. A conjunctival flap is then developed and retracted superiorly with a 5–0 silk suture exposing the lower lid fat compartments. The orbital septum is opened to each fat compartment and the appropriate amount of fat is dissected away with a cotton-tipped applicator, the base cauterized or excised. At this point the flap is released and typically no closure is required. Ophthalmic antibiotic ointment is applied within the sulcus. An iced sterile oval eye pad is then placed as the opposite side is done, and a light cold dressing is maintained postoperatively. In certain patients a transconjunctival approach can be used with fat preservation. In this situation the medial and at times middle fat compartment can be maneuvered into a subperiosteal pocket created at the orbital rim. This fat can be further held in place with a transcutaneous absorbable suture that is left in place for several days postoperatively.

The transcutaneous approach to blepharoplasty follows local injection of the lower lid, and a subciliary incision is made easily leaving several millimeters below the lash line. A submuscular flap is developed and a "skin-muscle" flap is developed and typically extended down to the orbital rim. The medial and lateral fat pads can be identified, the periosteum opened, and fat removed as needed. If orbital fat is preserved the arcus marginalis is identified and the periosteum elevated and the subperiosteal pocket is created as is described in the transconjunctival flap. The excess skin-muscle flap is then redraped and the excess skin excised. It is important to leave edge to edge apposition of the flap so that the excision can be closed without tension so as to prevent ectropion. A lateral muscle suspensory suture is often helpful suturing the orbicularis muscle component of the flap to the lateral orbital rim periosteal tissue near the lateral tarsus. Typically a polydioxanone suture is used for this. The skin is closed with interrupted or running subciliary absorbable sutures using 6–0 fast-absorbing gut, and the lateral component is typically reinforced with several 6–0 polypropylene sutures, which are removed 1 week afterward.

■ Facelift in the Geriatric Patient

As in most aesthetic facial procedures, the patient in whom the aging process has been less severe tends to present the best postoperative appearance and most successful facelift procedure. Those patients who are minimally obese and have what is most often described as good bone structure tend to make the best candidates. As in all aesthetic procedures, the patient must have realistic expectations regarding surgery. Psychological evaluation of the patient along with the physical facial findings is an important part of the patient evaluation. The geriatric patient must be counseled that severely aged skin with loss of elasticity and changes in collagen as well as elastic fibers will minimize the amount of correction and longevity of the procedure. The more obese a patient is, the less likely the patient is a favorable candidate. Patients with minimal adipose content and a high cervical angle with high positioning of the hyoid and thyroid complex allows for superior results in the lower face and neck region.

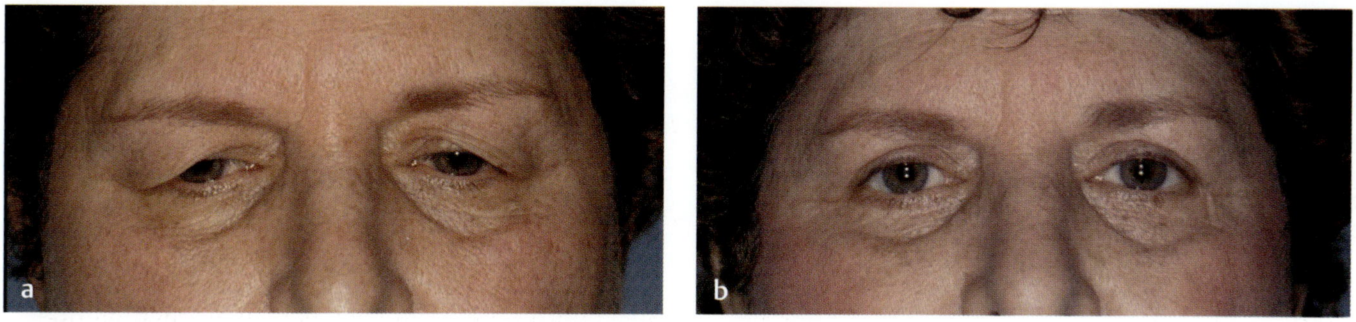

Fig.18.4 (**a**) Geriatric eyelid appearance prior to blepharoplasty demonstrating both aesthetic and functional changes of the upper lids. (**b**) Postoperative appearance following upper lid blepharoplasty in the geriatric patient.

Obese patients should be counseled that their results will be limited, and their expectations should be lowered. It may be wise to counsel the patient on a realistic weight loss program prior to pursuing surgery. Due to the elective nature of this procedure geriatric patients should ideally have no systemic or complicating factors related to their ability to safely undergo surgery and avoid postoperative complications. Medications that have any anticoagulant effect, including aspirin and other nonsteroidal anti-inflammatory drugs, should be stopped. An appropriate evaluation of prescription medications should be coordinated with the patient's personal physician, and cardiac issues should be cleared by their physician appropriately before anesthesia and surgery. Smoking is a significant issue for facelift patients, and the surgeon should insist that the patient stop smoking completely and abstain for at least 3 to 6 months prior to surgery.

An extremely wide array of procedures within the facelift category have been described and are used. These range from relatively minimal incisional "mini lifts," which can be done under local anesthesia on an outpatient basis, to very extensive open procedures performed under general anesthesia to correct multiple layers of facial anatomy. Often, ancillary procedures, particularly in the submental area, are used for submental correction including some form of submental liposuction and platysmal plication.

A wide variety of approaches are described and used. The majority of surgeons at this point in time are using a variation of periauricular incisions starting in the temple area going either pre- or posttragal, extended beneath and behind the ear, and then frequently extended into the postauricular occipital hairline. The two most frequently described flaps would include skin elevation and the subcutaneous level to a varying degree followed by elevation and lifting in support of the superficial musculoaponeurotic system (SMAS) layer. At this point the skin flap would be redraped and redundant skin excised. It is best to have closure with minimal tension to enhance the postoperative appearance of these incisional scars.

Another frequently used alternative procedure would incorporate elevation of a short subcutaneous skin flap followed by a so-called sub-SMAS or deep plane facelift elevation keeping the facial and SMAS attachments distally intact. Closure then is similar with elevation and resupporting of the SMAS layer with absorbable sutures followed by excision of redundant excess skin with an edge-to-edge apposition closure. Depending on technique and surgeon preference a drain may or may not be used following the procedure (**Fig. 18.5**).

A variety of authoritative technique texts and articles are available to the surgeon through the literature. Appropriate selection of technique is based not only on surgeon preference but also on the goals and physical state of anatomy of the patient.[1]

Complications from facelift should be infrequent, but the possibility should be discussed with the patient preoperatively. As already noted external factors, including smoking, use of aspirin or nonsteroidal anti-inflammatory drugs, and other systemic disorders can greatly increase the risk of postoperative complications.

Hematoma is reported as the most common complication following facelift.[11] A hematoma within the first several hours of facelift is a surgical emergency and should be treated quickly to avoid the possibility of postoperative healing difficulty. Infection is reported but is a rare complication in facelift. Wound drainage and antibiotic therapy should be initiated with continued antibiotics guided by culture.

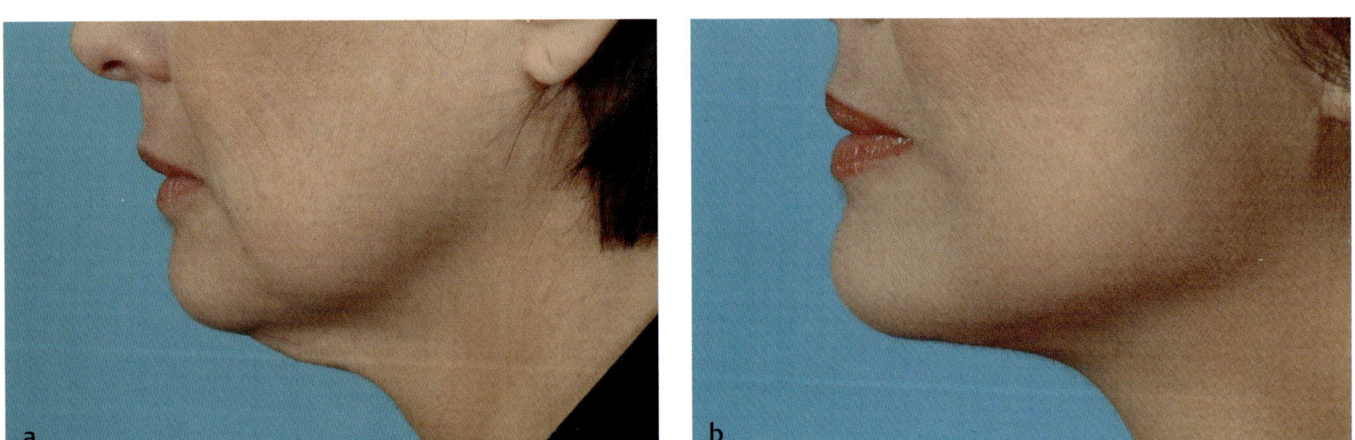

Fig. 18.5 (**a**) Typical aging changes seen in the face, submental, and neck regions. (**b**) Appearance following facelift procedure.

Patients should be warned that nearly all individuals will have hypoesthesia for 4 to 12 weeks following facelift surgery, and this is expected. However, motor weakness from damage to the facial nerve branches or more is a more significant injury.

Incisional scars that are widened or even hypertrophic are possible after facelift. Often this is related to excessive tension on the closure, and tension should be avoided, with edge to edge position of the skin closure as part of the technique. Similarly, earlobe deformity or pulling of the inferior portion of the ear may be related to scar contracture or too much tension in this area. This can be treated by release of the earlobe and advancement of the incision. It is best avoided through the initial surgical technique.

Conclusion

In addition to the key treatment areas to reverse facial aging, including resurfacing, blepharoplasty, and facelift, there are multiple other additional techniques and surgical procedures that may be used based on the surgeon's experience and preference and the patient's desires and needs. Some patients may benefit from variations of brow and forehead lift, including direct browlift, open or variations of coronal browlifts, and endoscopic approaches to lifting. Likewise, often the neckline can be enhanced by chin implantation as well as other facial enhancement with various facial implants such as cheek implants and submalar implants. With so many modalities available it is obvious that, in addition to the experience of the surgeon, preoperative evaluation and facial analysis are key to a satisfactory result.

Geriatric patients find the aging process has affected them in a variety of ways. Changes to the skin, muscle, muscle fat, and connective tissue all contribute to the characteristics that we recognize as aging in the geriatric patient's face. These changes result in poor skin tone, poor surface appearance of the skin itself, ptosis of the muscles of facial expression, and drooping of the fat compartments combined with the appearance of facial rhytides. The treating surgeon should understand that geriatric patients continue to have a level of self-image and self-recognition goals that they wish to achieve. Significant evaluation and discussion preoperatively should encompass these goals to achieve appropriate and satisfactory results for both the patient and the surgeon.

As noted, changes in the skin may be the earliest and most obvious characteristic of the aging process in the geriatric patient. The loss of elasticity is progressive and continues to increase and can be exacerbated based on ultraviolet light exposure and other external factors. Photoaging in the geriatric patient also results in lentigines, keratosis, loss of elasticity, and telangiectasias in addition to the usual rhytides. Accompanying this loss of skin elasticity and in addition to the skin aging we see the loss and change of position of subcutaneous fat, ptosis of muscles, and lengthening of fibrous attachments. Gravitational forces in addition to facial animation all tend to give the characteristic eyelid bags, cheek and jowl laxity, submental laxity, and platysmal banding.

Ultimately aesthetic facial procedures in the geriatric patient must be evaluated as elective in nature. Safety as well as potential improvement should be a key factor in the geriatric patient. That being said, however, it should not be forgotten how important facial appearance typically is to everyone, regardless of age, and how self-image and self-perception impacts all of our patients as they enter the geriatric age group. Perhaps the ideal quote is from Mark Twain who said, "Age is an issue of mind over matter. If you don't mind, it doesn't matter."

References

1. Thomas JR, Humphrey CD. Thomas Procedures in Facial Plastic Surgery: Facelift. Shelton, CT: PMPH Publisher; 2011
2. Tardy ME, Thomas JR. Facial Aesthetic Surgery. St. Louis, MO: Mosby Yearbook, Hank; 1995
3. Zimbler MS, Kokoska MS, Thomas JR. Anatomy and pathophysiology of facial aging. Facial Plast Surg Clin North Am 2001;9(2):179–187, vii
4. Thomas JR, Dixon TK, Bhattacharyya TK. Effects of topicals on the aging skin process. Facial Plast Surg Clin North Am 2013;21(1):55–60
5. Barkenpern N, Glaser DA. Anatomy and Physiology of the Skin: Advanced Therapy in Facial Plastic and Reconstructive Surgery. 1st ed. Shelton, CT: PMPH Publishers; 2010
6. Bhawan J, Andersen W, Lee J, Labadie R, Solares G. Photoaging versus intrinsic aging: a morphologic assessment of facial skin. J Cutan Pathol 1995;22(2):154–159
7. Guyuron B. The aging nose. Dermatol Clin 1997;15(4): 659–664
8. Pollard JD, Moulthrop HM, Jonhson CM. Botulinum Toxin. Thomas Procedures in Facial Plastic Surgery; Non-Invasive Procedures. Shelton, CT: PMPH Publishers; 2012:17–31
9. Banthia V, Hantash BM, Koch RJ. Laser Skin Resurfacing. Thomas Procedures in Facial Plastic Surgery; Non-Invasive Procedures. Shelton, CT: PMPH Publishers; 2012:33–44
10. Earnest LA, Papel ID. Upper Lid Blepharoplasty. Thomas Procedures in Facial Plastic Surgery; Blepharoplasty. Shelton, CT: PMPH Publishers; 2012:19–22
11. Jones BM, Grover R. Avoiding hematoma and cervical facial rhytidectomy: a personal eight year quest. Plast Reconstr Surg 2004;113:381–387

19 Oral Cavity Disorders in Geriatric Patients

Elliot Regenbogen and Denise A. Trochesset

Introduction

In 1900, there were 3.1 million people aged 65 and over in the United States. As the population 65 years and over steadily increased throughout the 20th century, the older population reached 40.3 million in 2010. Although there was an increase in overall population of ~ 10% between 2000 and 2010, those 65 years and over increased by 15%.[1]

As people live longer, there will be an increase in chronic conditions and illnesses that will affect both systemic and oral health.[2,3] Arthritis, hypertension, heart disease, sinus diseases, and diabetes are some of the most common chronic diseases in the elderly. All of these conditions, and in many instances their treatments, can have oral consequences.

The effects of oral diseases are not necessarily limited to the oral cavity. Oral pathogens can cause immediate systemic complications (e.g., aspiration pneumonia, bacteremia) or, by complex immunologic pathways, may be associated with long-term problems (e.g., coronary heart disease and cerebrovascular disorders).[4–7]

This chapter reviews age-related changes in oral tissues and common oral conditions in the geriatric population, as well as the influence of systemic diseases and their treatments.

Oral Mucosa

Age-Related Changes

The clinical appearance of the oral mucosa is most commonly the result of recurrent mild trauma from cheek biting, chronic mucosal disease such as lichen planus, tobacco use, and increased friction as a result of salivary hypofunction. Histological changes may include epithelial thinning, loss of submucosal elastin and fat, and increased fibrotic connective tissues with degenerative alteration in collagen.[8] The resulting clinical appearance may be one of dry, thin, smooth tissue, which is prone to further trauma and infection, particularly with denture use in the face of salivary hypofunction. Although oral mucosal immunity is believed to undergo some age-related changes, wound healing and regeneration of the oral mucosa are generally not affected (**Fig. 19.1**).[9,10]

Conditions

Many lesions are attributable to poorly fitting dentures. The persistent low-grade irritation caused by the prostheses moving and rubbing against tissue, or by patients wearing dentures 24/7 without cleaning or removing them regularly, can induce chronic inflammation, causing denture stomatitis, papillary hyperplasia, and even atrophy of the bone of the alveolar ridges. Hyperplastic reactions can also occur leading to the formation of redundant soft tissue (epulis fissuratum) or alteration of the mucosa such as frictional hyperkeratosis. Other conditions may be grouped as follows.

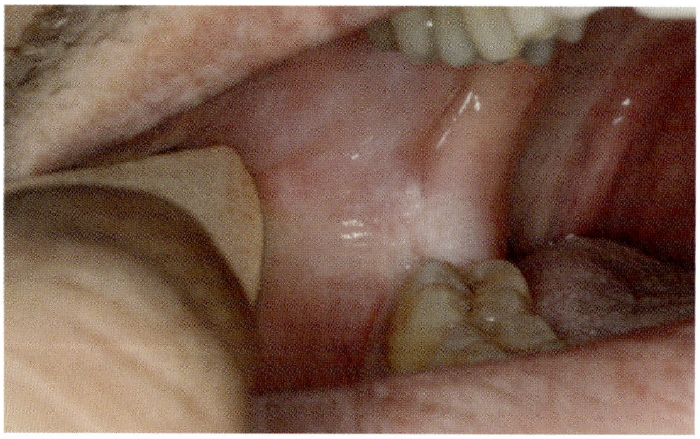

Fig. 19.1 Hyperkeratosis of the retromolar pad.

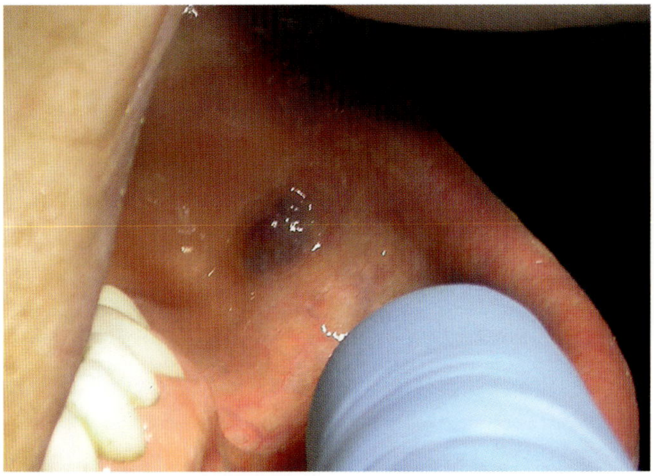

Fig. 19.2 Mucosal varix of the labial mucosa.

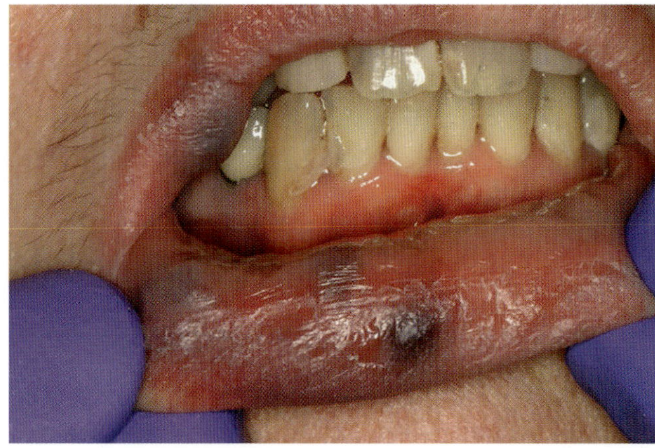

Fig. 19.3 Varices of the lip.

Benign Pigmented Mucosal Lesions

Conditions demonstrating change in mucosal color can include mucosal varices (venous lake) (**Figs. 19.2** and **19.3**), lingual varicosities, amalgam tattoos, melanosis from medications (e.g., Plaquenil), and melanotic macules.

Benign Soft Tissue Growths

Various benign soft tissue lesion may present in the oral cavity. Some common lesions that present as submucosal swellings include reactive lesions like pyogenic granuloma, epulis fissuratum, and fibromas. Other benign growths include lipoma, neuroma, papilloma, and granular cell tumor. Benign bone growths include tori and exostoses. Ectopic sebaceous glands are seen as submucosal creamy or white dots on the lips, buccal, and labial mucosa.

Vesiculobullous Diseases

Lichen planus, pemphigus vulgaris, and cicatricial pemphigoid are some of the oral vesiculobullous diseases that can be found more frequently in the geriatric population. The most common of these is lichen planus, which is a recurrent, chronic, inflammatory, and immune-regulated mucocutaneous disorder that affects ~ 1% of the population, of which ~ 35% are aged 50 years or older (**Fig. 19.4**).[11] In the oral cavity, there are two major forms of lichen planus, reticular and erosive. Only the erosive type needs to be treated, but all patients with oral lichen planus should be monitored at regular intervals due to a slightly increased risk of developing squamous cell carcinoma.

Lichenoid mucositis can be caused by a variety of medications commonly prescribed in older patients (e.g., acyclovir, gold salts, methyldopa, and thiazide diuretics) as well as over-the-counter products such as mouth rinses or chewing gum (**Fig. 19.5**).

Pemphigus vulgaris is a potentially serious autoimmune disorder that usually affects individuals in their fifth and sixth decades (**Fig. 19.6**). Cicatricial pemphigoid is another immunologically mediated disorder; it affects primarily older women (**Fig. 19.7**).

The use of tissue-supported complete or partial dentures in any of these conditions can cause exacerbation of disease leading to vesicle formation, then rupture and formation of ulcers.

Recurrent Aphthous Stomatitis

This condition is less common in elderly people than in younger people; however, nutritional and hematologic deficiencies that are common in older adults

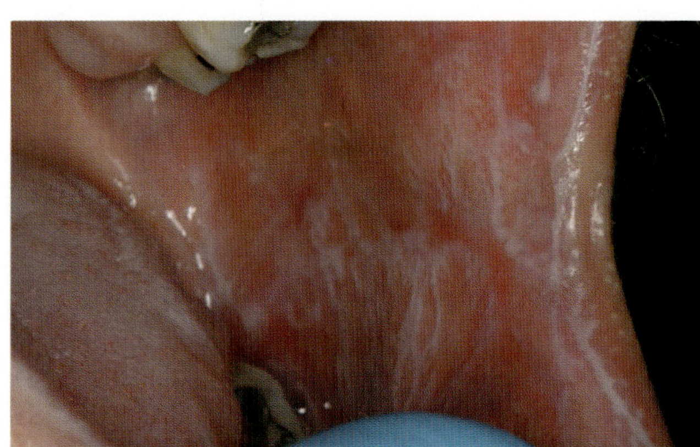

Fig. 19.4 A 63-year-old man with reticular lichen planus.

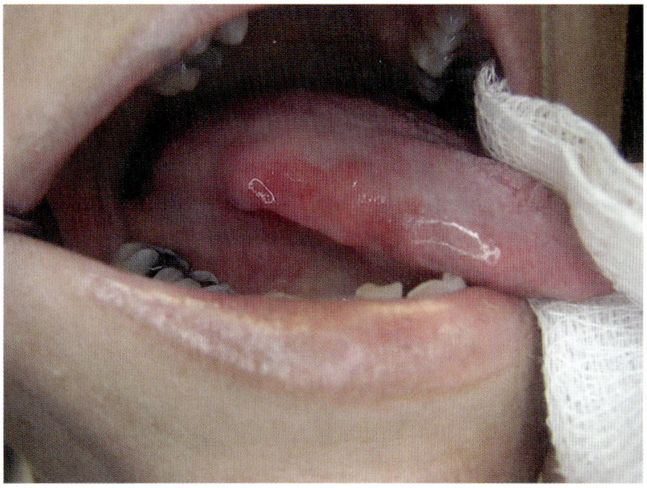

Fig. 19.5 Lichenoid mucositis. Erythema and erosion of the ventral lateral tongue in a patient with hepatitis C.

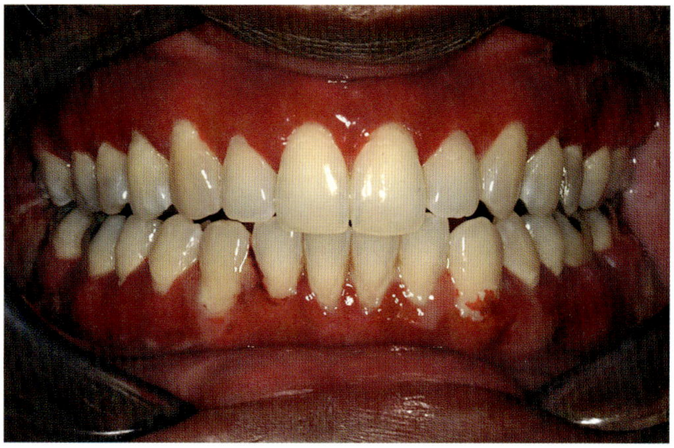

Fig. 19.6 Pemphigus vulgaris. Severe gingival erosion and ulceration.

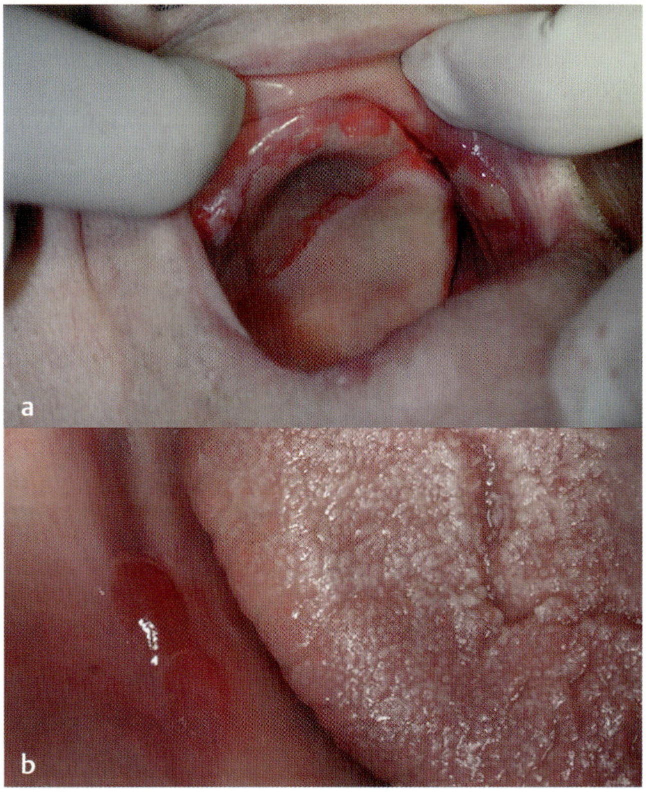

Fig. 19.7 An 83-year-old man with mucous membrane pemphigoid. (**a**) Ulceration of the anterior hard palate associated with the use of a full upper denture. (**b**) Vesicle formation on the lateral aspect of the mandibular alveolar ridge in the same patient

can predispose to recurrent ulcers,[12] as can gastrointestinal (GI) diseases such as Crohn disease, celiac disease, and *Helicobacter pylori* infection, which have been associated with aphthous stomatitis.

Oral Cancer

The incidence increases with age, with over 90% of all cases occurring in individuals 45 and older.[13] Although there is a trend in recent years toward younger individuals, the American Cancer Society's 2013 estimate for the average age of most people diagnosed with these cancers is 62. The most common risk factors are increased age and the use of tobacco and alcohol. In general, ~ 80% of oral cavity and pharynx cancers are squamous cell carcinoma.[14] These lesions can appear as exophytic, poorly demarcated, and ulcerated, erythroplakic, and/or leukoplakic (**Fig. 19.8**). The most common premalignant oral lesion is leukoplakia, and the incidence of leukoplakic lesions undergoing malignant transformation rises sharply with age. Mortality rates for oral cancer also increase with age.[15]

Infections

The oral cavity of older adults is more likely to be susceptible to opportunistic infections due to age and disease-related changes in the oral and systemic immune system. The older patient is more likely to suffer systemic infection from viral, fungal, and bacterial organisms that invade, infect, and become latent in the hard and soft tissues of the oropharyngeal region.[16]

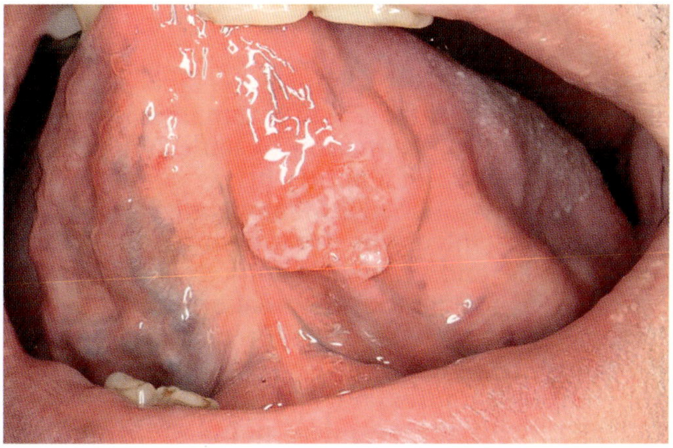

Fig. 19.8 Squamous cell carcinoma in a 67-year-old man.

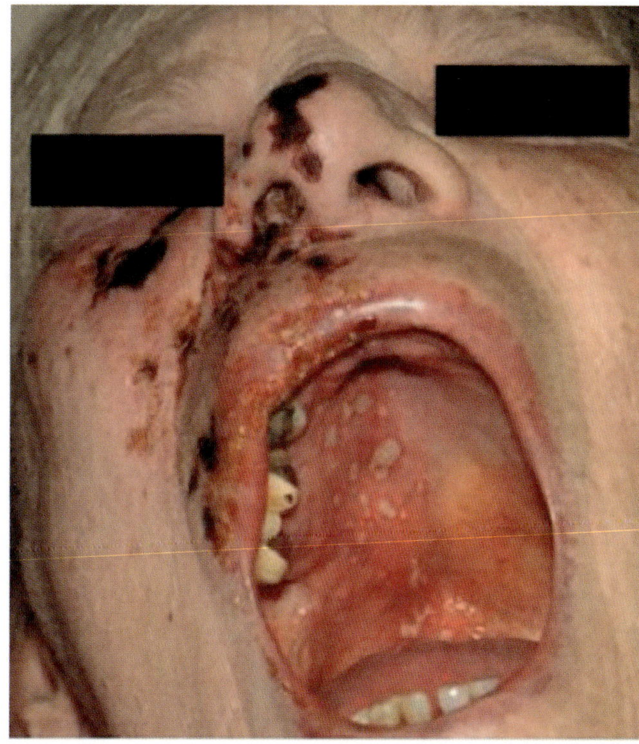

Fig. 19.9 Patient with herpes zoster. (Picture courtesy of Dr. Charles Consky.)

Herpes

Of the viral infections, the most common come from the herpes family. Herpes zoster (HZ) is a neurocutaneous disease that is caused by the reactivation of varicella-zoster virus (VZV) from a latent infection of dorsal sensory or cranial nerve ganglia. Although the initial infection typically occurs in childhood, reactivation of the latent virus may be secondary to immunosuppression, trauma, stress, or concurrent infections. Shingles, the result, is an acute condition with very painful and frequently incapacitating oral-facial vesicular lesions on the skin and mucous membranes in the areas that follow the unilateral distribution of ophthalmic, maxillary, or mandibular divisions of trigeminal sensory nerves (**Fig. 19.9**). The clinical presentation in an older adult will be similar to that in a younger person, but lesions may persist longer. The incidence of HZ increases sharply among patients aged ~ 50 to 60 years and continues an upward course in the decades > 60 years. In the Duke Established Populations for Epidemiological Studies of the Elderly,[17] the lifetime risk of having HZ increased significantly with age even among elderly patients (odds ratio, 1.20 for every 5 year interval in patients > 65 years old; 95% confidence interval, 1.10–1.31). Extrapolating from HZ epidemiological studies, experts calculate the lifetime incidence rate of HZ to be 10 to 20% in the general population and as high as 50% of a cohort surviving to age 85 years. Not only is HZ considerably more common among elderly people, but so too is chronic HZ pain. This increased incidence of HZ and postherpetic neuralgia with age correlates with the simultaneous age-related decrease in VZV-specific cell- mediated immunity.[18]

In addition, recurrent infections from herpes simplex virus (HSV) may continue into old age. Although most commonly occurring on the lip, recurrent lesions may be seen on the skin of the face, the nose, and the ear. Intraoral recurrent lesions are restricted to the keratinized mucosa of the gingiva and hard palate and tend to present in crops of vesicles, which rupture into ulcerations and often will coalesce into one large ulcer. HSV 1 has historically been seen in the oral cavity, but increasingly HSV 2 infections are seen as well.

Candida Infections

Oral candidiasis, a common opportunistic infection of the oral cavity caused by an overgrowth of *Candida*, can result in difficulty eating as well as systemic infections. The most frequently identified risk factors for the development of oral candidiasis are the wearing of dentures, the degree of *Candida* colonization, a lack of oral hygiene, tobacco use, xerostomia, a deterioration in the general state of health, steroid use, and antibiotic therapy (**Fig. 19.10**).[19]

The bacteria that cause the most common oral mucosal infections are those associated with new and recurrent dental caries (*Streptococcus mutans, Lactobacillus*), periodontal diseases (*Porphyromonas gingivalis, Treponema denticola*), and acute and chronic salivary infections (*Staphylococcus aureus, Streptococcus viridans*).[20]

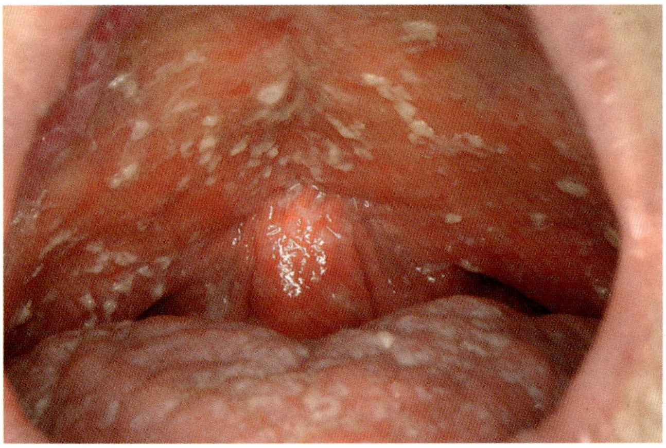

Fig. 19.10 Pseudomembranous candidiasis (thrush).

Treatments

Risk factors and treatment are summarized in **Table 19.1**. The treatment of traumatic oral lesions begins with the elimination of underlying factors such as the repair of a poorly fitting denture. Topical analgesics can be helpful along with antibiotics for secondary infections. Treatment of vesiculobullous disease and erosive lesions depends on the severity of the condition. Topical oral steroids may be mixed with oral adhesives like Orabase (Colgate-Palmolive Co., New York, NY). Systemic steroids and immunosuppressant agents may need to be considered. In the geriatric population, particular care must be exercised with such medications in the face of common concurrent medical issues such as heart disease, diabetes, osteoporosis, and depression.

Prevention of oral cancer begins with the elimination of established risk factors (e.g., the use of tobacco and alcohol). Early detection is a key component of successful treatment. Older edentulous individuals are four times less likely to see a dentist than are dentate individuals and should therefore be targeted for regular annual examinations for head and neck cancer.[21,22] Dental management before, during,

Table 19.1 Risk factors and treatment of oral mucosa disease

Disease	Risk factors	Treatment
Oral cancer	Tobacco, alcohol, human papilloma virus, human immunodeficiency virus, radiation, immunosuppression, leukoplakia, erythroplakia, family history, asbestos, printers (polycyclic aromatic hydrocarbons), betel quid	Surgery Radiation therapy Chemotherapy
Traumatic lesions	Poorly fitting denture, chronic lip chewing, traumatic ulcers, secondary infection	Oral rinses Viscous lidocaine Diphenhydramine elixir Dyclonine Sucralfate Systemic medications Penicillin Amoxicillin Erythromycin
Vesiculobullous and erosive disease	Drug reaction, trauma, allergy	Topical medications Fluocinonide gel Triamcinolone acetonide gel Clobetasol propionate gel Oral rinses Dexamethasone elixir Diphenhydramine elixir Dyclonine Sucralfate Systemic medications Prednisone Immunosuppressant Nutritional supplements Fluid intake

and after treatment of oral cancer is essential to prevent complications. Oral cancer is treated by surgery, chemotherapy, and radiotherapy. Common sequelae include stomatitis, dysphagia, pain, paresthesias, oral motor dysfunction, salivary hypofunction, and an increased risk of developing osteoradionecrosis.

Prevention of the spread of viral lesions in elderly patients can be accomplished by avoidance of individuals who have active infections. Although the lesions are usually self-limited, supportive measures are necessary to maintain adequate nutritional and fluid intake and to diminish pain. However, early diagnosis can diminish morbidity in older patients. In particular, immunocompromised adults are susceptible to recurrent herpes infections and require immediate and aggressive antiviral treatment. Acyclovir, valacyclovir, and famciclovir are common antiviral medications that can, in general, be used safely in older patients and are well tolerated. The drugs are excreted by the kidneys and should be dosed appropriately for patients with renal insufficiency. Randomized, controlled trials indicate that orally administered acyclovir (800 mg 5 times a day for 7 days), famciclovir (500 mg every 8 h for 7 days), and valacyclovir (1 g three times a day for 7 days) reduce acute pain and the duration of chronic pain in elderly patients with HZ who are treated within 72 hours of the onset of rash.[23] Unfortunately, 20 to 30% of treated patients in antiviral trials had pain 6 months from HZ onset, indicating that patients who have been treated can develop postherpetic neuralgia. In the most recent trial of acyclovir and prednisone, time to uninterrupted sleep, return to daily activity, and cessation of analgesic therapy was significantly accelerated in patients who received corticosteroids.[24] The patients in the trial had an average age of 60 years and no relative contraindications to corticosteroids such as hypertension, diabetes mellitus, or osteoporosis. Therefore, some experts advocate orally administered corticosteroids for otherwise healthy older adults with moderate to severe pain and no contraindications to corticosteroids.

Prevention of bacterial infections and candidiasis involves good oral and denture hygiene, the judicious use of antibiotics and immunosuppressants, and the elimination of underlying local and systemic etiologic factors such as salivary hypofunction, diabetes, or immunodeficiency. The use of antifungal creams, rinses, and lozenges is usually successful, but persistent infections require systemic antifungal agents. If a patient has a denture or other prosthesis, both the oral cavity (rinse, troches, etc.) and the prosthesis (antifungal denture bath) should be treated to limit fungal burden. Concurrent use of an antifungal (often needed only once or twice per day) is prudent when potent topical corticosteroids are used in patients with diabetes or severe salivary hypofunction or in immunocompromised patients to decrease the chance of developing thrush. Systemic antifungal agents will have limited effectiveness in patients with decreased or no salivary flow.

■ Periodontium

Age-Related Changes

With the increasing retention of the natural dentition, the number of teeth in older adults at risk of developing periodontal disease is growing.[25] Gingival recession and loss of periodontal attachment and alveolar bone are nearly universal age-related changes. Several systemic conditions and medications that are more prevalent among older adults have been linked with periodontal disorders.

Conditions and Treatments

Gingivitis is much more likely to develop in older patients because of oral and systemic factors. Dental plaque, gingival bleeding, and calculus accumulations develop as a result of softer diets, reduced oral motor activity, and salivary gland hypofunction. Advanced periodontal diseases have been associated with nonoral diseases such as pneumonia, bacteremia, infective endocarditis, coronary heart disease, and brain abscesses, and they may interfere with the treatment of systemic diseases.

There is some evidence that severe osteoporosis significantly reduces the bone mineral content of the jaws and that it may be associated with greater periodontal attachment loss and tooth loss.[26] Studies have been conducted to evaluate the effect of hormone replacement therapy in modifying the periodontal conditions in postmenopausal women. The clinical significance of hormone replacement therapy in periodontal health is not well established.[27]

Medications and medical problems that are common among older adults have an adverse effect on periodontal health. Calcium channel blockers, phenytoin, and cyclosporine, which are prescribed frequently for older persons, have been associated with gingival overgrowth or hyperplasia.[28] Diabetes, even when well controlled, is associated with increased risk of periodontal disease.[29] The prevalence of diabetes among adults age 65 and older increased by more than 50% between 1997 and 2006.[30] Oral mucocutaneous diseases such as erosive lichen planus and cicatricial pemphigoid can demonstrate the clinical appearance of desquamative gingivitis (**Fig. 19.11**).

If the periodontal disease is believed to arise from the patient's medical conditions and their treatment, then a systemic approach to oral health management is required. Drug-induced gingival hyperplasia fre-

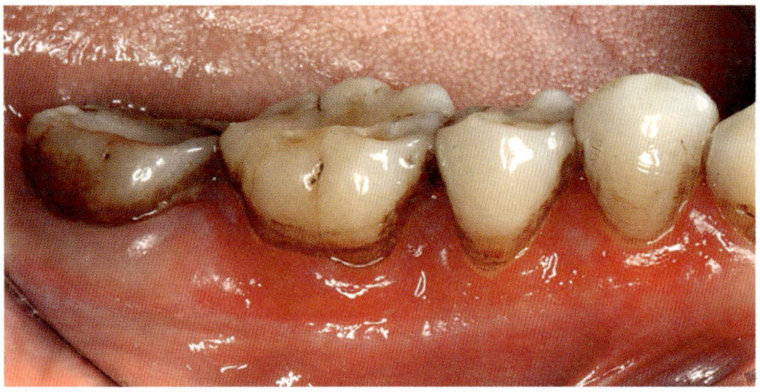

Fig. 19.11 Desquamative gingivitis. (Picture courtesy of Dr. Albert Yoo.)

quently requires surgical reduction along with plaque control and the consideration of alternative medication. Other dental issues commonly found in older patients, such as restoration problems, poorly fitting dentures, and caries need to be addressed as well.

Finally, there are oral and sociobehavioral factors that influence the progression of periodontal disease in elderly people. Irregular dental visits, smoking, psychosocial stress, and poor socioeconomic status all are predictors of periodontal attachment loss in older patients.[31,32] Periodontal maintenance and prevention regimens are similar for all age groups but may require additional time, equipment, and recall visits to dental professionals depending on the functional and mental capacity of the individual. Periodontal health can be maintained with tooth brushing and flossing after each meal and with regularly scheduled professional dental examinations and cleanings. In older adults who are homebound, institutionalized, or physically and/or behaviorally compromised, all additional caregivers need to be made part of this routine. Dental professionals must be actively involved and must instruct caregivers on the proper use of oral and denture hygiene techniques for their patients.

Dentition

Age-Related Changes

With improvement in oral care, prevention, tooth preservation, and restoration major epidemiological changes have occurred over the past several decades in regard to retention of dentition. Only ~ 30% of adults aged ≥ 65 years are completely edentulous.[33] Age-related changes are attributable to normal physiological processes and to pathological changes in response to functional and environmental stresses. Discoloration, loss of enamel, abrasion, and erosion are seen commonly.

Conditions and Treatments

Increases in caries in the elderly are influenced by two trends: a greater retention of teeth among elderly persons, and a decline in caries among younger people.[34] Dental plaque is the primary source of microorganisms, which contribute to caries in the elderly. With diminished salivary gland function, disturbances in oral motor function, and difficulty in performing oral hygiene older patients are more susceptible to new and recurrent tooth decay. When detected early, caries can be restored with a variety of dental materials. In addition to pain and tooth loss, untreated caries can progress to cellulitis, abscess, and bacteremia.

Rigorous oral hygiene, including brushing and flossing after each meal, is the most important part of preventive care. The use of fluoride-containing rinses, gels, and varnishes can help in the remineralization of existing decay and the prevention of new caries.[35] Regular dental visits for prophylaxis, examination, and early treatment of dental caries are also required. The treatment of coronal and root surface dental caries has been facilitated by the improvement in restorative materials. Cosmetic and implant dentistry has also made considerable advances that have implications for older adults.

Patients affected with medical conditions that are known to cause salivary hypofunction (e.g., Sjögren syndrome, diabetes, head and neck irradiation, Alzheimer disease) must be monitored more closely. Similarly, patients who are taking medications associated with salivary hypofunction (e.g., antidepressants, antihypertensives, antipsychotics) should be recalled more frequently than other patients to dental professionals. The older patient with salivary hypofunction requires rigorous oral hygiene practices with the addition of supplemental fluoride gels and rinses.

Salivary Glands

Age-Related Changes

It was previously thought that changes in qualitative and quantitative salivary production were associated with normal aging. This may have been partly due to the common complaint of xerostomia (mouth dryness) in older people. Published work presents a conflicting picture of the effects of age on salivary flow. The different results are likely to be due primarily to the varying methodologies, including the age of the individuals, the number of individuals, the exclusion and inclusion criteria, cross-sectional rather than longitudinal design, method of stimulation (mechanical or chemical), and duration of collection period, all of which make comparisons between the studies difficult; but the age-old mantra of decreased salivation with increased age is not supported by the literature. Changes in anatomy and physiology, including sensation, with age can account for changes in salivary flow.[36] In addition, no age-related decreases in the secretion of certain salivary constituents (e.g., total proteins, proline-rich proteins, lactoferrin, sodium, and potassium) are seen in a healthy elderly population. The loss of fluid-producing acinar cells increases the susceptibility of an older individual to salivary perturbations such as those caused by medications with anticholinergic side effects.[37]

Conditions and Treatments

The most common pathogens associated with acute salivary gland infections are *Staphylococcus aureus* and anaerobic bacteria. The predominant anaerobes include gram-negative bacilli (i.e., *Prevotella* spp, *Porphyromonas* spp, *Fusobacterium* spp) and *Peptostreptococcus* spp. Additionally, *Streptococcus* spp (including *S. pneumoniae* and *S. pyogenes*) and aerobic and facultative gram-negative bacilli (including *Escherichia coli*) have been reported. Aerobic and facultative gram-negative organisms are often seen in hospitalized patients. Organisms less frequently found are *Haemophilus influenzae*, *Klebsiella pneumoniae*, *Salmonella* spp, *Pseudomonas aeruginosa*, *Treponema pallidum*, *Bartonella henselae*, and *Eikenella corrodens*. *Mycobacterium tuberculosis* and atypical mycobacteria are rare causes of parotitis.[38]

Appropriate antibiotic therapy for salivary gland infections should be based on diagnostic culture and sensitivity testing, when possible. Hydration, the use of a sialogogue, massage of the infected gland, and the use of an amoxicillin and clavulanic acid (clindamycin if the patient is allergic to penicillin) can be started immediately. Diagnosis and treatment of salivary gland obstructions may require imaging tests (radiography, ultrasonography, sialography) and subsequent removal of the obstruction.

Tongue

Age-Related Changes

The tongue is a frequent site of oral soft tissue changes. Changes may range from varying forms of glossitis to mass formation. This section discusses various lingual changes that may be recognized in the elderly patient and, where appropriate, their associated treatments.

Conditions and Treatments

Median Rhomboid Glossitis

Median rhomboid glossitis is characterized by a rhomboid-shaped smooth atrophic erythematous mucosa with missing filiform papillae, located at the dorsal midline or paramedian of the tongue, just anterior to the circumvallate papillae on the dorsal midline of the tongue (**Fig. 19.12**). The area usually produces little symptoms other than occasional burning or itching. Men are affected three times more often than women. This lesion has traditionally been thought to be the result of a lack of fusion of the two lateral processes (lingual tubercles) resulting in a lack of coverage of the central structure formed from the first and second branchial arches, the tuberculum impar.[39,40] However, there is also an association with candidal infections and a response to antifungals (e.g., nystatin, fluconazole, clotrimazole) given as a suspension or oral troche. *Candida* can be confirmed with a scraping or culture. More frequent *Candida* infections may be the cause of the higher incidence of median rhomboid glossitis in those with diabetes. Other surfaces of the mouth are characteristically spared. A possible premalignant or malignant phenomenon should be ruled out when the clinical aspects contradict those expected.

Atrophic Glossitis

The smooth, glossy appearance associated with atrophic glossitis is due to atrophy of the filiform papillae. In most cases atrophic glossitis is a manifestation of an underlying condition, many of which are summarized in the **Table 19.2**. Treatment can include nutrient replacement or treatment of the underlying condition.

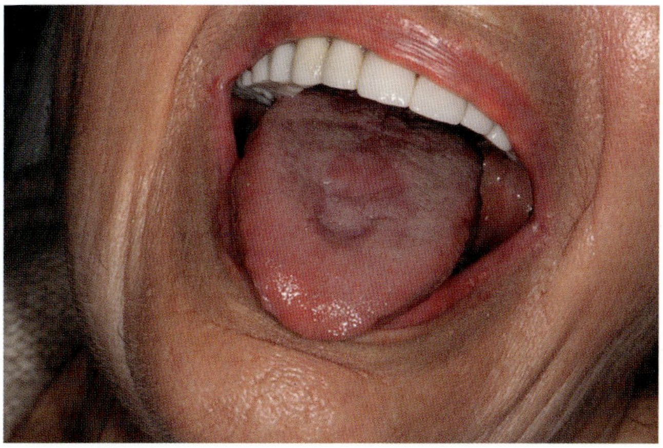

Fig. 19.12 Patient with median rhomboid glossitis.

Table 19.2 Conditions associated with atrophic glossitis

Amyloidosis
Celiac disease
Chemical irritants
Drug reactions
Local infections (candidiasis)
Nutritional deficiencies (iron, folic acid, B12, riboflavin, niacin)
Vesiculoerosive diseases (pemphigoid, pemphigus vulgaris, erythema multiforme, Stevens–Johnson syndrome)
Pernicious anemia
Protein-calorie malnutrition
Sarcoidosis
Sjögren syndrome
Systemic infections (syphilis)

Fissured Tongue

The deep grooves of a fissured tongue are deepening of normal tongue fissures (**Fig. 19.13**). These typically occur with aging and require no treatment unless trapped food and bacteria cause inflammation. Gentle brushing can alleviate most symptoms. Fissured tongue has also been associated with Down syndrome, acromegaly, psoriasis, and Sjögren syndrome. Melkersson-Rosenthal syndrome is accompanied by severe tongue fissuring, relapsing orofacial edema, and facial nerve palsy.

Geographic Tongue

The prevalence of geographic tongue, also known as benign migratory glossitis or erythema migrans, has been reported to vary between 0.28% and 14.4%, but most surveys show a range between 1 and 2.5%. Differences in sampling, diagnosis, type of examination, and ethnic group studied may explain the wide range in reported rates.[41,42] The cause of the disease remains unknown. It has been associated with several conditions, such as pustular psoriasis, allergy, hormonal disturbances, juvenile diabetes, Reiter syndrome, Down syndrome, nutritional deficiencies (vitamin B complex in particular), psychological upsets, fissured tongue, lichen planus, and lithium treatment. A geographic tongue in an otherwise healthy person may indicate a tendency to develop generalized pustular psoriasis. Geographic tongue is not related to infection with human immunodeficiency virus or use of tobacco. A family history of geographic tongue is reported in most patients, suggesting the presence of hereditary factors.

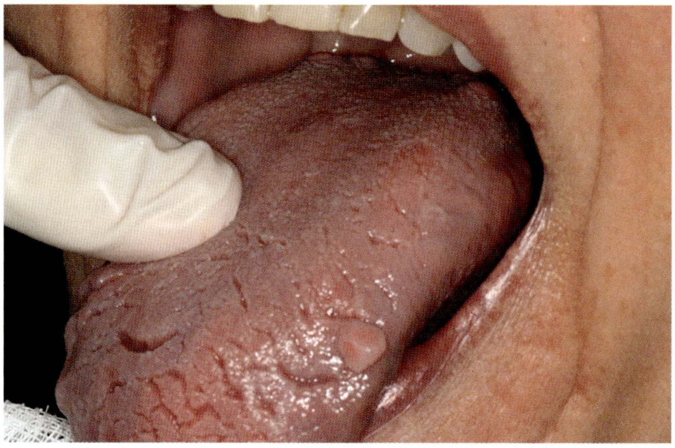

Fig. 19.13 Patient with geographic tongue, fissure tongue, and fibroma.

With geographic tongue, the dorsal tongue develops areas of papillary atrophy that appear smooth and are surrounded by raised, serpiginous borders (see **Fig. 19.13**). With resolution and recurrence of atrophy the areas appear to migrate. The condition is benign and localized, generally requiring no treatment except reassurance. Some patients may have sensitivity to hot or spicy foods. Topical steroid gels (e.g., triamcinolone dental paste) and antihistamine mouth rinses (e.g., diphenhydramine elixir, 12.5 mg per 5 mL diluted in a 1:4 ratio with water) can reduce tongue sensitivity.[43]

Hairy Tongue

The morphology of hairy tongue is due to excess keratin accumulation on the filiform papillae of the dorsal surface. The color can range from white or tan to black (**Fig. 19.14**). It occurs most commonly in smokers and in persons with poor oral hygiene and has been associated with use of certain antibiotics (i.e., tetracycline, olanzapine, and bismuth).[44]

Most patients are asymptomatic, but some have halitosis or abnormal taste. No treatment is required, but gentle daily debridement with a tongue scraper or soft toothbrush can remove keratinized tissue. Keeping well hydrated and eating raw fruit and vegetables to provide roughage on the tongue can also help. Although medications are rarely required, the use of clotrimazole, nystatin, retinoids, triamcinolone, gentian violet, salicylic acid, vitamin B complex, and urea solution has been reported. The use of yogurt or other acidophilus-containing products may also be helpful.[45]

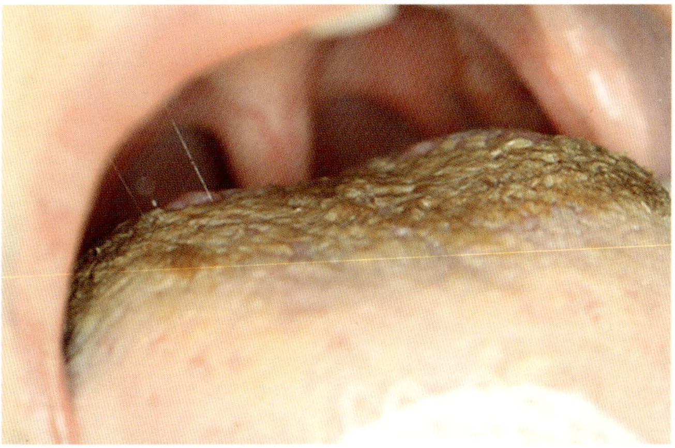

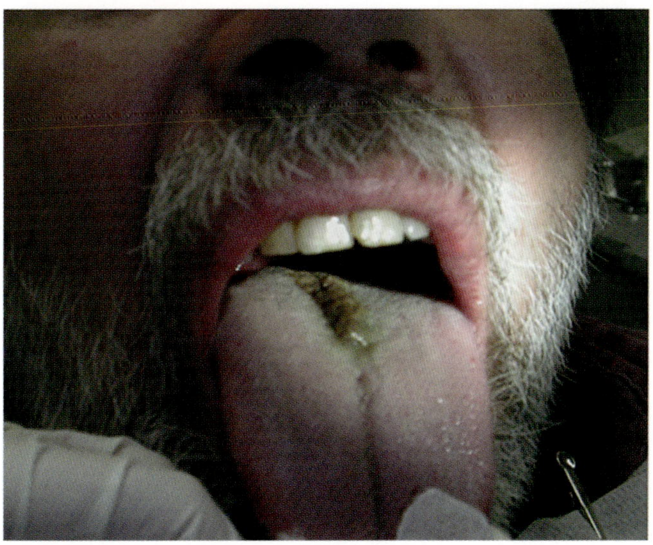

Fig. 19.14 Patient with hairy tongue.

Oral hairy leukoplakia appears on the lateral margins of the tongue and may be unilateral or bilateral. It is associated with immunosuppression and is caused by the Epstein-Bar virus. In the absence of a known immunocompromising condition, human immunodeficiency virus (HIV) testing should be considered. Antiviral medications such as acyclovir may be used for 1 to 3 weeks, although recurrence is common.[41]

Other Lesions

Granular Cell Tumors

Granular cell tumors are small, solitary, painless tumors that can involve the dorsal surface of the tongue. The tumors typically have a smooth surface and are more common after age 30 and in women. Biopsy is necessary to confirm the diagnosis, and malignant transformation is rare.[46]

Traumatic Fibromas

Traumatic fibromas are common, typically appearing along the bite line. The lesion is usually dome-shaped, pink, and smooth (see **Fig. 19.13**). It is caused by the accumulation of dense connective tissue at the site of chronic irritation. Diagnosis and treatment should be made with biopsy if another diagnosis is suspected.[47]

Leukoplakic and Erythroplakic Lesions

Leukoplakic and erythroplakic lesions appear as adherent patches of red or white coloration (**Fig. 19.15**). They both have premalignant potential, more so with erythroplakia. Strong consideration should be given for biopsy and close follow-up. The most common associated factor is tobacco use.

Lingual Thyroid

This condition appears as a smooth, nodular mass in the midline, posterior, dorsal surface of the tongue. Its presence usually represents a lack of descent of thyroid tissue, and up to 70% of patients are hypothyroid.[48]

Lymphoepithelial Cysts

The lesions are yellow nodules located on the ventral surface of the tongue, tonsil regions, or floor of the mouth. They are benign and thought to represent minor salivary or mucosal tissue entrapped during development. Biopsy is necessary to confirm diagnosis.

Macroglossia

This entity is an abnormal enlargement of the tongue relative to the morphology of the mouth and jaws. A scalloped lateral margin due to crowding against

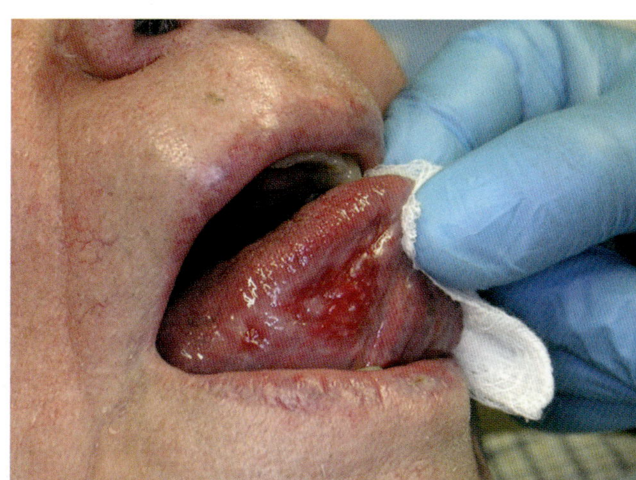

Fig. 19.15 Erythroplakia on the ventral tongue in a 90-year-old man.

the teeth is common. Associated conditions include Down syndrome, hypothyroidism, tuberculosis, sarcoidosis, amyloidosis, multiple myeloma, neurofibromatosis, infection (e.g., syphilis), vascular malformations (**Fig. 19.16**), and angioedema or allergic reaction. Diagnosis and treatment should be directed at the underlying disorder.

Squamous Papilloma

These common lesions are present in up to 1% of adults. The disorder is usually associated with papillomavirus type 6 or 11.[49] They may present as a single pedunculate lesion or involve a more diffuse area. Diagnosis and treatment involve surgical excision.

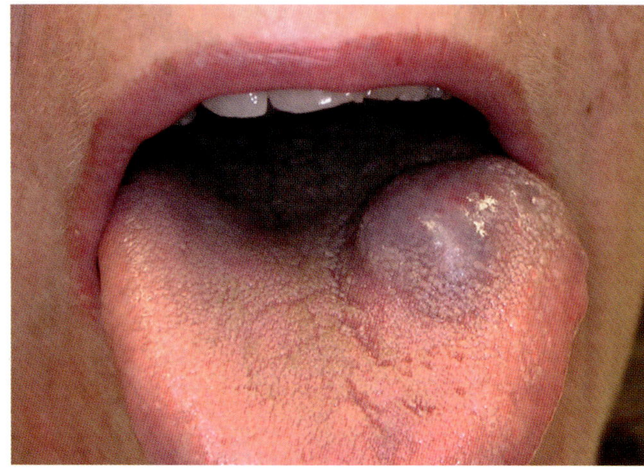

Fig. 19.16 Hemangioma/arteriovenous malformation macroglossia in a 65-year-old woman.

Specific Conditions

Xerostomia and Salivary Hypofunction

A sensation of oral dryness (xerostomia) is a frequent complaint among the elderly.[48] This may occur despite normal salivary gland activity because saliva does not necessarily wet the whole mouth uniformly and localized areas of dryness can trigger the sensation of dry mouth.[50] Nevertheless, whatever the original salivary flow rate, sensation of oral dryness occurs when the flow rate is diminished by 50%.[51]

Possible causes of dry mouth are summarized in **Table 19.3**. Common habits such as tobacco smoking, alcohol use (including in mouthwashes), and use of beverages containing caffeine (coffee, tea, some soft drinks) can cause some oral dryness.

A wide range of drugs can cause reduced salivation (**Table 19.4**). The drugs most commonly implicated in dry mouth are the tricyclic antidepressants, antipsychotics, atropinics, β-blockers, and antihistamines. Dry mouth is a common complaint in the elderly, mainly as a consequence of the large number of drugs used and the high frequency of polypharmacy.[52,53] Even in elderly patients with advanced cancer, dry mouth was the fourth most common symptom (78% of patients), but the usual cause was drug treatment, and there was an association with the number of drugs prescribed.[54]

Systemic diseases (e.g., Sjögren syndrome) should be identified, managed, and controlled. Tests to be considered in the evaluation of xerostomia are summarized in **Table 19.5**. In medication-associated xerostomia, elimination, substitution, or reduction of the causative drug, in collaboration with the patient's physicians, is the ideal solution. For patients receiving head and neck radiation therapy for oropharyngeal cancers, contralateral parotid gland preservation techniques can help diminish postirradiation xerostomia.[55]

Treatments of xerostomia are summarized in **Table 19.6**. Patients with xerostomia who have some remaining viable salivary parenchymal tissue will respond to salivary stimulants; these include sugarless candies, mints, and gums; and nonsugared, nonacidic beverages, used frequently. A combination of alcohol-free mouthwash and sugarless chewing gum, although the effect is short-lived, has been shown to improve xerostomia secondary to radiotherapy.[56] Vitamin C has been shown to be subjectively more effective than artificial saliva but less effective than other salivary stimulants.[57] Malic acid, found in fruits

Table 19.3 Etiology of xerostomia

Cystic fibrosis
Dehydration
Drugs
Graft vs. host disease
Infections
Human immunodeficiency virus
Hepatitis C
Human T lymphotropic virus 1
Irradiation
Primary biliary cirrhosis
Psychogenic
Sarcoidosis
Sjögren syndrome

Table 19.4 Examples of drugs associated with xerostomia

Drug class / examples
Antihistamines
Cyclizine, chlorpheniramine, diphenhydramine
Antihypertensive medication
Beta-blockers, clonidine, methyldopa
Antipsychotics
Clozapine, chlorpromazine
Bronchodilators
Ipratropium, tiotropium
Decongestants
Pseudoephedrine
Diuretics
Furosemide, hydrochlorothiazide, spironolactone
Eyedrops
Atropine, tropicamide
Gastroesophageal reflux medication
H2 antagonists and proton pump inhibitors
Pain medications
Opioids
Parkinson disease medication
Procyclidine, benzatropine
Tricyclic antidepressants
Amitryptyline, imipramine
Urinary incontinence medication
Oxybutynin, tolterodine tartrate

Table 19.5 Tests to be considered for xerostomia evaluation

Complete blood count
Anemia may indicate chronic disease
White cell count abnormal in immunodeficiency, Sjögren syndrome (SS) or systemic lupus erythematosis (SLE)
Thyrombocytopenia in SS or SLE
Blood chemistry
Increased urea and creatinine in dehydration
Increased alkaline phosphatase in primary biliary cirrhosis (PBC)
Serum angiotensin-converting enzyme elevated in sarcoidosis
Immunology
SSA/Ro and SSB/La antibody for Sjögren syndrome
Rheumatoid factor for SS, rheumatoid arthritis, SLE
Antinuclear antibody for SLE (anti-double stranded DNA) and SS
Antimitochondrial antibody for primary biliary cirrhosis
Histopathology minor salivary gland
Sjögren syndrome: focal lymphocytic infiltrate
Sarcoidosis: noncaseating granuloma
Other
Sialometry, sialography, sialoendoscopy, salivary flow analysis

such as pears and apples, can also be effective in the treatment of xerostomia, but both vitamin C and malic acid's main disadvantage is their acidic pH and detrimental effect on tooth enamel.

Pilocarpine is a muscarinic receptor agonist and has been shown to improve symptoms of radiation-induced xerostomia. The effects of pilocarpine are usually immediate; however, in radiation-induced xerostomia, they can take up to 12 weeks. The increase in saliva production generally lasts for 4 hours. Its undesirable side effects include perspiration, flushing, lacrimation, urinary frequency, and gastrointestinal disturbances. As a result of its cholinergic effect, it is contraindicated in patients with asthma, chronic obstructive airway disease, heart diseases, narrow-angle glaucoma, epilepsy, hyperthyroidism, and Parkinson disease. Other muscarinic agents include cevimeline, bethanechol, carbachol, and pyridostigmine.[58–60]

Finally, it is vital that precautions be taken to prevent the deleterious consequences of diminished salivary production. These precautions include frequent dental recall, daily use of fluorides, brushing and flossing after meals, and excellent prosthesis hygiene.

Burning Mouth

Many elderly patients present with a complaint of oral burning of the tongue or other location in the oral cavity. If the sensation of oral burning is a symptom of other local, systemic, or psychogenic diseases, then this is referred to as oral burning disorder; oth-

Table 19.6 Treatments of xerostomia

Treatments of xerostomia
Mechanical and gustatory (sugarless)
Chewing gum
Sucking ointment
Menthol
Sweet
Acid
Vitamin C
Ice chips
Pharmaceutical
Pilocarpine
Bethanechol
Carbachol
Cevimeline
Physostigmine
Anethole trithione
Bromhexine
Palliative measures
Homemade mouthwash
– Saline, sodium bicarbonate, glycerol, mint or lemon
Commercial mouthwash (alcohol free)
Saliva substitutes
Fluoride rinse, gel, and varnishes (in dentate only)

erwise the term *burning mouth syndrome* (BMS) is used, making it a diagnosis of exclusion.[61] Historically, BMS has been referred to by many names based on the quality or location of pain: glossodynia, glossopyrosis, glossalgia, sore tongue, burning tongue, scalded mouth syndrome, oral dysesthesia, and burning mouth condition. The use of these multiple terms reflects the confusion and uncertainty that exists in the scientific literature and in clinical practice. The International Classification of Diseases (version 9) has assigned the term *glossodynia*, which includes the adjunctive terms *glossopyrosis* and *painful tongue*, and a specific identity code number (529.6).[62] Several definitions have been proposed, but most often the patient presents with sensations of burning pain in the mouth without any obvious clinical signs. The physician is unable to definitively diagnose the cause even with the use of diagnostic testing or imaging.

The prevalence of burning mouth symptoms reported from international studies ranges from 0.6 to 15%.[63] BMS seems to increase with age in both males and females, mainly affecting females in the fifth to seventh decade.[64,65]

Possible etiologies of oral burning are summarized in **Table 19.7**. Up to a third of patients associate the onset of symptoms with a previous illness such as an upper respiratory infection, dental procedure, or use of a medication. Other individuals claim the onset of symptoms relates to traumatic life stressors. Typically, the symptoms occur continuously for months or years without periods of cessation or remission. There have been reports of complete/partial remission (with or without intervention) in ~ 50% of patients and of complete spontaneous remission in ~ 20% of patients within 6 to 7 years of onset.[66–68]

Although anxiety and depression have been consistently demonstrated among patients with BMS, suggesting a psychogenic etiology, it is unclear whether psychological dysfunction is present just in association with chronic pain. The reported success of biobehavioral techniques in the treatment of BMS may be related more to an improvement in pain-coping strategies than to cure of the disorder.[69,70]

Vitamin deficiencies such as B1, B2, B6, and zinc deficiencies, as well as diabetes, have not shown a consistent link to BMS.[71,72] Mucosal ulcerative lesions, periodontitis, geographic tongue, and changes in intraoral soft or hard tissues have not been found to have a significant relationship with BMS. Likewise, chemical irritation and allergic reaction to dental materials have not been found to be important causative factors.[73–75]

Because the majority of women in BMS studies are postmenopausal, hormonal changes are considered to be an important factor. However, only one controlled clinical trial has examined the role of hormone replacement therapy in postmenopausal women with BMS. The diagnostic criteria and outcome measures were unclear. There were fewer than 10 participants in each treatment arm, and comparability of groups at baseline was not discussed. Due to methodological flaws, there are insufficient data to draw any reliable conclusions on the effectiveness of hormone replacement therapy for postmenopausal women with BMS.[76]

Patients with BMS have a higher incidence of perceived mouth dryness. However, salivary flow rate studies have not offered supporting evidence of this. Alterations in levels of mucin, immunoglobulin A (IgA), phosphates, and pH have been found, but the relationship of these to symptomatology remains unknown.[69,71]

A possible relationship may exist between disturbance in taste and BMS. There are an increased number of persons with enhanced abilities to detect taste, "supertasters," among patients with BMS. Supertasters have a higher density of taste buds, each surrounded by pain neurons of the trigeminal

Table 19.7 Possible causes of oral burning

Allergy
Dental restorations
Denture material
Foods
Preservatives, additives, flavorings
Autoimmune
Elevated antinuclear antibody
Elevated rheumatoid factor
Cranial nerve injury/neuropathy/neoplasm
Dry mouth
Sjögren syndrome
Radiation therapy
Chemotherapy
Altered saliva content
Endocrine
Diabetes
Thyroid disease
Menopause
Hormonal deficiencies
Medication
Angiotensin-converting enzyme inhibitors
Mucosal disease
Candidiasis
Fissured tongue
Lichen planus
Migratory glossitis (geographic tongue)
Viral
Nutritional deficiency
Vitamin B complex, iron, zinc
Mechanical
Bruxism
Clenching
Dental/denture
Neurological
Psychological
Anxiety
Depression
Phobia

nerve.[77,78] The ability to detect bitter taste has been found to decrease with menopause. Reduction in bitter taste at the level of the chorda tympani, cranial nerve VII, is associated with increased taste sensations from the area of the glossopharyngeal nerve (cranial nerve IX) and the production of taste phantoms.[79] These are frequently evaluated in the process of establishing the diagnosis of BMS.

BMS is a diagnosis of exclusion. A thorough history and physical examination are critical. Most patients report increased pain intensity during the course of the day, decreased pain with eating, pain that does not wake them in the night, xerostomia that has varying intensity with burning, and taste disturbance. If symptoms persist after other problems have been excluded and treated, BMS may be considered and treatment offered. Clinical tests are summarized in **Table 19.8**.

Epidemiological surveys suggest that both acute pain and chronic oral-facial pain are significant problems among elderly people and that they require a thorough multidisciplinary approach to diagnosis and management.[80,81] Oral, systemic, psychological, and behavioral problems are more likely to be major contributors to oral-facial pain. No clear evidence indicates that age per se is a factor in treatment outcome for an older patient with pain.[82] Although it was once assumed that there is a decline in sensitiv-

Table 19.8 Clinical tests considered for burning mouth syndrome

Allergy testing
Change of medications
Angiotensin-converting enzyme inhibitors
Cultures
Fungal, viral, bacterial
Gastroesophageal reflux studies
Hematologic
Autoimmune panel
Chemistry including glucose, iron, vitamin B, zinc
Complete blood count with differential
Endocrine including thyroid
Imaging
Magnetic resonance imaging, computed tomography (if indicated)
Salivary flow rates
Salivary uptake scans
If low salivary flow rates and Sjögren syndrome suspected
Psychometric tests

ity to painful stimulation with aging, more studies have not found this to be the case, and differences in the clinical presentation of disease may account for altered pain association.[83,84] Aging and the incremental effects of dental wear, previous restorative treatments, oral diseases, and oral hygiene practices can induce structural changes in teeth and periodontal tissues that can affect the perception of pain in elderly individuals. There is little research evidence to provide clear recommendations for management of patients who have BMS.[74] Initially, the clinician must determine if the patient is suffering from primary (essential/idiopathic) BMS or oral burning in which symptoms are attributable to underlying local or systemic conditions (secondary BMS). Treatments are summarized in **Table 19.9**.

Halitosis

Although the majority of causes of halitosis in otherwise healthy people is localized to the oral cavity, halitosis can also signal serious systemic illnesses, including diabetes, gastroesophageal reflux disease, or liver or kidney failure. Considering the older adult who may have several medical problems treated with multiple medications, a multifactorial etiology of the malodor is not unexpected. Halitosis may also provide a helpful clue leading to the diagnosis of a previously undetected condition.[85] Causative and management strategies are summarized in **Tables 19.10, 19.11, 19.12, 19.13**.[86]

Table 19.9 Treatments for burning mouth syndrome

Treatment
Behavioral/cognitive therapy
Topical therapy
Clonazepam[a]
Lidocaine
Topical capsaicin
Topical doxepin
Systemic therapy
Tricyclic antidepressants
Nortriptyline[a]
Amitriptyline[a]
Selective serotonin reuptake inhibitor
Paroxetine[a]
Sertraline[a]
Atypical antipsychotic agents
Amisulpride[b]
Levosulpiride[b]
Benzodiazepine
Clonazepam[a]
Anticonvulsant
Gabapentin[a]
Antioxidant
Alpha-lipoic acid
Atypical analgesic
Capsaicin[b]

[a]Off-label use.
[b]Not available in the United States.

Table 19.10 Potential causes of halitosis

Cause
Oral
Poor oral hygiene: dental caries, gingivitis, candidiasis, denture colonization, retained debris
Aphthous and other ulcers
Tonsillitis, tonsillith, pharyngeal abscess
Xerostomia, hyposalivation, Sjögren syndrome
Carcinoma
Nasal
Sinusitis, abscess, atrophic rhinitis, foreign body
Carcinoma
Lower respiratory
Infection
Carcinoma
Gastrointestinal
Reflux, pyloric stenosis, malabsorption syndrome, infection, carcinoma
Hepatic
Liver failure (dimethyl sulfide and ketones in expired air)
Renal
Uremia
Systemic
Starvation, dehydration
Vitamin deficiencies
Leukemia
Blood dyscrasia
Psychogenic

Table 19.11 Drugs associated with halitosis

Amphetamines
Chloral hydrate
Cytotoxic agents
Dimethyl sulphoxide (DMSO)
Disulfiram
Nitrates and nitrites
Phenothiazines
Solvent abuse

Table 19.12 Bacteria and by-products associated with halitosis

Porphyromonas gingivalis
Prevotella intermedia
Fusobacterium nucleatum
Bacteroides forsythus
Treponema denticola
Volatile sulfur compounds (VSCs)
Methyl mercaptam, hydrogen sulphide, dimethyl sulphide
Volatile aromatic compounds
Indole, skatole
Polyamines
Putrescine and cadaverine
Short-chain fatty acids: butyric, valeric, acetic, and propionic acids

Table 19.13 Management of halitosis

Patient education
Treat underlying cause: oral and systemic
Avoiding smoking and certain foods (i.e., onions, garlic, cauliflower, radish)
Eating regular meals including fibrous fruits, vegetables
Good oral hygiene: brushing, flossing, tongue cleaning
Denture cleaning: leave them out at night and in chlorhexidine
or dilute hypochlorite solution
Use of oral care products: toothpastes and mouthwashes containing: chlorhexidine, triclosan, amine fluoride/ stannous fluoride, metal ions
Oral deodorants: sugar-free chewing gum, parsley, mint, cloves, or fennel seeds
Recalcitrant cases: metronidazole 200 mg three times a day for 7 days

Summary

Recognizing that older adults are the most rapidly growing segment of the population, health care providers will need to address the unique issues regarding this age group on a more routine basis. With regard to oral health, primary and systemic disease can interact to produce a wide range of symptoms and pathologies. The prevention and treatment of these problems can have a dramatic impact on the quality of life of this population, making it imperative for the practitioner to have a broad fund of knowledge to meet the needs of elderly patients.

References

1. Werner CA. The older population: 2010. 2010 Census Briefs. https://www.census.gov/prod/cen2010/briefs/c2010br-09.pdf
2. Ghezzi EM, Ship JA. Systemic diseases and their treatments in the elderly: impact on oral health. J Public Health Dent 2000;60(4):289–296
3. Chávez EM, Ship JA. Sensory and motor deficits in the elderly: impact on oral health. J Public Health Dent 2000;60(4): 297–303
4. Loesche WJ, Schork A, Terpenning MS, Chen YM, Kerr C, Dominguez BL. The relationship between dental disease and cerebral vascular accident in elderly United States veterans. Ann Periodontol 1998;3(1):161–174
5. Garcia RI, Krall EA, Vokonas PS. Periodontal disease and mortality from all causes in the VA Dental Longitudinal Study. Ann Periodontol 1998;3(1):339–349
6. Fourrier F, Duvivier B, Boutigny H, Roussel-Delvallez M, Chopin C. Colonization of dental plaque: a source of nosocomial infections in intensive care unit patients. Crit Care Med 1998;26(2):301–308
7. Wu T, Trevisan M, Genco RJ, Falkner KL, Dorn JP, Sempos CT. Examination of the relation between periodontal health status and cardiovascular risk factors: serum total and high density lipoprotein cholesterol, C-reactive protein, and plasma fibrinogen. Am J Epidemiol 2000;151(3):273–282
8. Williams DM, Cruchley AT. Structural aspects of aging in the oral mucosa. In: Squier CA, Hill MW, eds. The Effect of Aging in Oral Mucosa and Skin. Boca Raton, FL: CRC Press; 1994:65–74
9. Farthing PM, Walton LJ. Changes in immune function with age. In: Squier CA, Hill MW, eds. The Effect of Aging in Oral Mucosa and Skin. Boca Raton, FL: CRC Press; 1994:113–120
10. Hill MW, Karthigasan J, Berg JH, Squier CA. Influence of age on the response of oral mucosa to injury. In: Squier CA, Hill MW,

eds. The Effect of Aging in Oral Mucosa and Skin. Boca Raton, FL: CRC Press; 1994:129–142

11. Scully C, Beyli M, Ferreiro MC, et al. Update on oral lichen planus: etiopathogenesis and management. Crit Rev Oral Biol Med 1998;9(1):86–122
12. Ship JA, Chavez EM, Doerr PA, Henson BS, Sarmadi M. Recurrent aphthous stomatitis. Quintessence Int 2000;31(2): 95–112
13. Howlader N, Noone AM, Krapcho M, et al. SEER Cancer Statistics Review, 1975-2010, National Cancer Institute. Bethesda, MD, http://seer.cancer.gov/csr/1975_2010/results_merged/topic_age_dist.pdf, based on November 2012 SEER data submission, posted to the SEER web site, April 2013
14. Howlader N, Noone AM, Krapcho M, et al. SEER Cancer Statistics Review, 1975-2010, National Cancer Institute. Bethesda, MD, http://seer.cancer.gov/csr/1975_2010/results_merged/topic_histologic_tabs.pdf, based on November 2012 SEER data submission, posted to the SEER web site, April 2013
15. U.S. Cancer Statistics Working Group. United States Cancer Statistics: 1999–2011 Incidence and Mortality Web-based Report. Atlanta: U.S. Department of Health and Human Services, Centers for Disease Control and Prevention and National Cancer Institute; 2014. Available at: http://apps.nccd.cdc.gov/uscs/cancersbyraceandethnicity.aspx
16. Shay K, Ship JA. The importance of oral health in the older patient. J Am Geriatr Soc 1995;43(12):1414–1422
17. Schmader K, George LK, Burchett BM, Pieper CF, Hamilton JD. Racial differences in the occurrence of herpes zoster. J Infect Dis 1995;171(3):701–704
18. Schmader K. Herpes zoster in older adults. Clin Infect Dis 2001;32(10):1481–1486
19. Chiappelli F, Bauer J, Spackman S, et al. Dental needs of the elderly in the 21st century. Gen Dent 2002;50(4):358–363
20. Guiglia R, Musciotto A, Compilato D, et al. Aging and oral health: effects in hard and soft tissues. Curr Pharm Des 2010; 16(6):619–630
21. Gift HC, Newman JF. How older adults use oral health care services: results of a National Health Interview Survey. J Am Dent Assoc 1993;124(1):89–93
22. Guggenheimer J, Hoffman RD. The importance of screening edentulous patients for oral cancer. J Prosthet Dent 1994;72(2):141–143
23. Kost RG, Straus SE. Postherpetic neuralgia—pathogenesis, treatment, and prevention. N Engl J Med 1996;335(1): 32–42
24. Whitley RJ, Weiss H, Gnann JW Jr, et al; The National Institute of Allergy and Infectious Diseases Collaborative Antiviral Study Group. Acyclovir with and without prednisone for the treatment of herpes zoster. A randomized, placebo-controlled trial. Ann Intern Med 1996;125(5):376–383
25. Huttner EA, Machado DC, de Oliveira RB, Antunes AG, Hebling E. Effects of human aging on periodontal tissues. Spec Care Dentist 2009;29(4):149–155
26. Wactawski-Wende J. Periodontal diseases and osteoporosis: association and mechanisms. Ann Periodontol 2001;6(1): 197–208
27. Pizzo G, Guiglia R, Licata ME, Pizzo I, Davis JM, Giuliana G. Effect of hormone replacement therapy (HRT) on periodontal status of postmenopausal women. Med Sci Monit 2011;17(4): PH23–PH27
28. Nakib N, Ashrafi SS. Drug-induced gingival overgrowth. Dis Mon 2011;57(4):225–230
29. Mealey BL, Oates TW; American Academy of Periodontology. Diabetes mellitus and periodontal diseases. J Periodontol 2006;77(8):1289–1303
30. AARP Public Policy Institute. Chronic Care: A Call to Action for Health Care Reform, Part 1: Chronic Conditions Among Older Americans. 2009; http://assets.aarp.org/rgcenter/health/beyond_50_hcr_conditions.pdf. Accessed August 19, 2010
31. Genco RJ, Ho AW, Kopman J, Grossi SG, Dunford RG, Tedesco LA. Models to evaluate the role of stress in periodontal disease. Ann Periodontol 1998;3(1):288–302
32. Peruzzo DC, Benatti BB, Ambrosano GM, et al. A systematic review of stress and psychological factors as possible risk factors for periodontal disease. J Periodontol 2007;78(8): 1491–1504
33. Kramarow E, Lentzner H, Rooks R, et al. Health and Aging Chartbook. Health, United States, 1999. Hyattsville, MD: National Center for Health Statistics; 1999
34. Burt BA. Epidemiology of dental diseases in the elderly. Clin Geriatr Med 1992;8(3):447–459
35. Davies RM. The rational use of oral care products in the elderly. Clin Oral Investig 2004;8(1):2–5
36. Smith CH, Boland B, Daureeawoo Y, Donaldson E, Small K, Tuomainen J. Effect of aging on stimulated salivary flow in adults. J Am Geriatr Soc 2013;61(5):805–808
37. Wu AJ, Atkinson JC, Fox PC, Baum BJ, Ship JA. Cross-sectional and longitudinal analyses of stimulated parotid salivary constituents in healthy, different-aged subjects. J Gerontol 1993;48(5):M219–M224
38. Brook I. The bacteriology of salivary gland infections. Oral Maxillofac Surg Clin North Am 2009;21(3):269–274
39. Lee JJ, Hung HC, Cheng SJ, et al. Carcinoma and dysplasia in oral leukoplakias in Taiwan: prevalence and risk factors. Oral Surg Oral Med Oral Pathol Oral Radiol Endod 2006;101(4): 472–480
40. Llewellyn CD, Johnson NW, Warnakulasuriya KA. Risk factors for squamous cell carcinoma of the oral cavity in young people—a comprehensive literature review. Oral Oncol 2001;37(5):401–418
41. Assimakopoulos D, Patrikakos G, Fotika C, Elisaf M. Benign migratory glossitis or geographic tongue: an enigmatic oral lesion. Am J Med 2002;113(9):751–755
42. Yarom N, Cantony U, Gorsky M. Prevalence of fissured tongue, geographic tongue and median rhomboid glossitis among Israeli adults of different ethnic origins. Dermatology 2004;209(2):88–94
43. Reamy BV, Derby R, Bunt CW. Common tongue conditions in primary care. Am Fam Physician 2010;81(5):627–634
44. Refaat M, Hyle E, Malhotra R, Seidman D, Dey B. Linezolid-induced lingua villosa nigra. Am J Med 2008;121(6):e1 doi: 10.1016/j.amjmed.2008.02.023
45. Tamam L, Annagur BB. Black hairy tongue associated with olanzapine treatment: a case report. Mt Sinai J Med 2006; 73(6):891–894
46. Gardner ES, Goldberg LH. Granular cell tumor treated with Mohs micrographic surgery: report of a case and review of the literature. Dermatol Surg 2001;27(8):772–774
47. Kornbrot A, Tatoian JA Jr. Benign soft tissue tumors of the oral cavity. Int J Dermatol 1983;22(4):207–214
48. Närhi TO. Prevalence of subjective feelings of dry mouth in the elderly. J Dent Res 1994;73(1):20–25
49. Syrjänen S. Human papillomavirus infections and oral tumors. Med Microbiol Immunol (Berl) 2003;192(3):123–128
50. Fox PC, Busch KA, Baum BJ. Subjective reports of xerostomia and objective measures of salivary gland performance. J Am Dent Assoc 1987;115(4):581–584
51. Dawes C. How much saliva is enough for avoidance of xerostomia? Caries Res 2004;38(3):236–240

52. Närhi TO, Meurman JH, Ainamo A. Xerostomia and hyposalivation: causes, consequences and treatment in the elderly. Drugs Aging 1999;15(2):103–116
53. Loesche WJ, Bromberg J, Terpenning MS, et al. Xerostomia, xerogenic medications and food avoidances in selected geriatric groups. J Am Geriatr Soc 1995;43(4):401–407
54. Davies AN, Broadley K, Beighton D. Xerostomia in patients with advanced cancer. J Pain Symptom Manage 2001;22(4): 820–825
55. Henson BS, Eisbruch A, D'Hondt E, Ship JA. Two-year longitudinal study of parotid salivary flow rates in head and neck cancer patients receiving unilateral neck parotid-sparing radiotherapy treatment. Oral Oncol 1999;35(3):234–241
56. Nieuw Amerongen AV, Veerman EC. Current therapies for xerostomia and salivary gland hypofunction associated with cancer therapies. Support Care Cancer 2003;11(4): 226–231
57. Björnström M, Axéll T, Birkhed D. Comparison between saliva stimulants and saliva substitutes in patients with symptoms related to dry mouth. A multi-centre study. Swed Dent J 1990;14(4):153–161
58. Rieke JW, Hafermann MD, Johnson JT, et al. Oral pilocarpine for radiation-induced xerostomia: integrated efficacy and safety results from two prospective randomized clinical trials. Int J Radiat Oncol Biol Phys 1995;31(3):661–669
59. LeVeque FG, Montgomery M, Potter D, et al. A multicenter, randomized, double-blind, placebo-controlled, dose-titration study of oral pilocarpine for treatment of radiation-induced xerostomia in head and neck cancer patients. J Clin Oncol 1993;11(6):1124–1131
60. Fox PC, van der Ven PF, Baum BJ, Mandel ID. Pilocarpine for the treatment of xerostomia associated with salivary gland dysfunction. Oral Surg Oral Med Oral Pathol 1986;61(3):243–248
61. Klasser GD, Fischer DJ, Epstein JB. Burning mouth syndrome: recognition, understanding, and management. Oral Maxillofac Surg Clin North Am 2008;20(2):255–271, vii
62. International Classification of Diseases–9–CM, (1979). Wonder.cdc.gov
63. Zakrzewska JM, Hamlyn PJ. Facial pain. In: Crombie IK, ed. Epidemiology of Pain. Seattle, WA: IASP Press; 1999:175–182
64. Bergdahl M, Bergdahl J. Burning mouth syndrome: prevalence and associated factors. J Oral Pathol Med 1999;28(8): 350–354
65. Ferguson MM, Carter J, Boyle P, Hart DM, Lindsay R. Oral complaints related to climacteric symptoms in oöphorectomized women. J R Soc Med 1981;74(7):492–498
66. Sardella A, Lodi G, Demarosi F, Bez C, Cassano S, Carrassi A. Burning mouth syndrome: a retrospective study investigating spontaneous remission and response to treatments. Oral Dis 2006;12(2):152–155
67. Hammarén M, Hugoson A. Clinical psychiatric assessment of patients with burning mouth syndrome resisting oral treatment. Swed Dent J 1989;13(3):77–88
68. Tammiala-Salonen T, Hiidenkari T, Parvinen T. Burning mouth in a Finnish adult population. Community Dent Oral Epidemiol 1993;21(2):67–71
69. Browning S, Hislop S, Scully C, Shirlaw P. The association between burning mouth syndrome and psychosocial disorders. Oral Surg Oral Med Oral Pathol 1987;64(2):171–174
70. Rojo L, Silvestre FJ, Bagan JV, De Vicente T. Prevalence of psychopathology in burning mouth syndrome. A comparative study among patients with and without psychiatric disorders and controls. Oral Surg Oral Med Oral Pathol 1994;78(3): 312–316
71. Ship JA, Grushka M, Lipton JA, Mott AE, Sessle BJ, Dionne RA. Burning mouth syndrome: an update. J Am Dent Assoc 1995;126(7):842–853
72. Basker RM, Sturdee DW, Davenport JC. Patients with burning mouths. A clinical investigation of causative factors, including the climacteric and diabetes. Br Dent J 1978;145(1): 9–16
73. Grushka M. Clinical features of burning mouth syndrome. Oral Surg Oral Med Oral Pathol 1987;63(1):30–36
74. Svensson P, Kaaber S. General health factors and denture function in patients with burning mouth syndrome and matched control subjects. J Oral Rehabil 1995;22(12):887–895
75. Grushka M, Epstein JB, Gorsky M. Burning mouth syndrome. Am Fam Physician 2002;65(4):615–620
76. Zakrzewska JM, Forssell H, Glenny AM. Interventions for the treatment of burning mouth syndrome. Cochrane Database Syst Rev 2005; (1):CD002779
77. Bartoshuk LM, Duffy VB, Miller IJ. PTC/PROP tasting: anatomy, psychophysics, and sex effects. Physiol Behav 1994; 56(6):1165–1171
78. Whitehead MC, Beeman CS, Kinsella BA. Distribution of taste and general sensory nerve endings in fungiform papillae of the hamster. Am J Anat 1985;173(3):185–201
79. Yanagisawa K, Bartoshuk LM, Catalanotto FA, Karrer TA, Kveton JF. Anesthesia of the chorda tympani nerve and taste phantoms. Physiol Behav 1998;63(3):329–335
80. Riley JL III, Gilbert GH, Heft MW. Health care utilization by older adults in response to painful orofacial symptoms. Pain 1999;81(1-2):67–75
81. Lipton JA, Ship JA, Larach-Robinson D. Estimated prevalence and distribution of reported orofacial pain in the United States. J Am Dent Assoc 1993;124(10):115–121
82. Sorkin BA, Rudy TE, Hanlon RB, Turk DC, Stieg RL. Chronic pain in old and young patients: differences appear less important than similarities. J Gerontol 1990;45(2):64–68
83. Heft MW, Cooper BY, O'Brien KK, Hemp E, O'Brien R. Aging effects on the perception of noxious and non-noxious thermal stimuli applied to the face. Aging (Milano) 1996;8(1):35–41
84. Ship JA, Heft M, Harkins S. Oral facial pain in the elderly. In: Lomranz J, Mostofsky DI, eds. Handbook of Pain and Aging. New York, NY: Plenum; 1997:321–346
85. Durham TM, Malloy T, Hodges ED. Halitosis: knowing when 'bad breath' signals systemic disease. Geriatrics 1993; 48(8):55–59
86. Scully C. Halitosis (oral malodour). In: Scully C, ed. Oral and Macillovacial Medicine: The Basis of Diagnosis and Treatment UK: Churchill Livingstone/Elsevier; 2013:98–102

20 Advanced Cutaneous Malignancies in the Elderly

Kelly Michele Malloy and Chaz L. Stucken

Introduction and Epidemiology

Skin cancer is the most commonly diagnosed malignancy in the United States.[1] The term *cutaneous malignancy* represents a diverse group of epithelial and nonepithelial cancers, but, generally speaking, the majority tend to be the result of *cumulative* sun exposure. As a person ages, the amount of ultraviolet (UV) light exposure accumulates, thus making age and cumulative UV exposure difficult to distinguish as independent risk factors. In a 2003 study by Godar et al, Americans were estimated to receive 22.73% of their lifetime UV exposure by the age of 18, 46.53% by the age of 40, and 73.71% by age 59; this study assumed a lifespan of 78 years, at which point it is assumed one would have received 100% UV dose. With current life expectancies of over 80 for men and women, sun exposure likely exceeds well beyond the maximum "dose."[2] This also argues for vigilant sun protection precautions regardless of age.

Age alone is recognized as a risk factor for developing certain cutaneous malignancies, particularly with regard to melanoma. The National Cancer Institute (NCI) Surveillance, Epidemiology and End Results (SEER) Program reports that 44.5% of newly diagnosed melanomas occur in individuals aged 65 years or older, with an additional 22% of new cases occurring in those 55 to 64 years.[3] Although accurate epidemiological data on nonmelanoma skin cancers are not available, it is generally felt that this pattern of increasing incidence with age is also true for other cutaneous malignancies, such as squamous cell carcinoma (SCC) and basal cell carcinoma (BCC). It is worth making special mention of Merkel cell carcinoma (MCC) given its increasing incidence and association with advancing age. The incidence of MCC tripled from 1986 to 2001, and quadrupled by 2006[4,5]; SEER data indicate an incidence of 0.6 per 100,000 annually in the United States. The majority of MCCs occur in the elderly, with a mean age of 72 years at diagnosis; only 5% of MCCs occur in patients younger than 50 years.[6] Although sun exposure has been associated with MCC, more recently the Merkel cell polyomavirus has been implicated in the majority of MCCs. Although exposure to this virus tends to occur earlier in life, it is postulated that failure of immune surveillance with increasing age predisposes to the development of this malignancy.

Cutaneous malignancies tend to be readily curable when diagnosed early and treated with definitive surgery; the vast majority of these early cases are treated by dermatologists, never entering the purview of the otolaryngologist. More advanced skin cancers of the head and neck do require the expertise of head and neck surgeons for both resection and reconstructive surgery. Surgery remains the mainstay of treatment for most cutaneous malignancies and can range in extent from simple wide local excision to sentinel lymph node biopsy (SLNB), to parotidectomy and neck dissection. Reconstructive options may include skin grafts, local flaps, regional flaps, and free tissue transfer. Adjuvant radiation or chemotherapy may be considered, depending on final tumor stage and comorbidities.

This chapter focuses first on the management of the geriatric patient with an advanced cutaneous malignancy, reviewing the available literature to provide practical guidelines for perioperative care. This is followed by a brief review of the specifics of the major subtypes of skin cancer, including staging and treatment considerations.

Preoperative Concerns

Many surgeons may experience reticence when evaluating an elderly patient for major surgery. Although a nonagenarian on the preoperative clinic schedule may inspire some trepidation, it is important to remember that chronological age is not as important as functional age. An 80-year-old retired professor who still walks the golf course is a different surgical candidate compared with a 70-year-old who is wheelchair-bound following a cerebral vascular accident. There are several tools for assessing surgical risk reasonably well in geriatric patients, and these would also apply to surgical risk for cutaneous malignancy: activities of daily living, instrumental activities of daily living, gait speed, exercise tolerance, frailty, and the comprehensive geriatric assessment. With respect to the specific risk advanced age poses to the surgical care of patients with advanced cutaneous malignancy, it is possible to draw some conclusions and make recommendations based on recent investigations for head and neck surgical care in the elderly.

Genther and Gourin recently investigated the outcomes of major head and neck surgery in the elderly, particularly with respect to the effect of comorbidity.[7] Their retrospective analysis of a large sample of elderly head and neck cancer patients in the Nationwide Inpatient Sample sought to evaluate the impact of frailty in the surgical care of this group of patients. They accurately point out that age alone is not a good marker for health status and therefore sought to investigate the impact of "frail elderly" status on both short-term outcomes and cost of health care. *Frail elderly* is defined by the U.S. Census Bureau as "people 65 years or older with significant physical and cognitive health problems."[8] Genther and Gourin adapted this to be defined as patients 65 or older with a comorbidity score of 2 or higher using the Romano adaptation of the Charlson comorbidity index. In their sample of 61,740 patients, patients 80 years and older were more likely to have advanced comorbidity (most commonly cardiovascular and chronic pulmonary diseases); however, postsurgical complications did not differ significantly by comorbidity score and were reported at an overall rate of 11%. This includes no significant difference in wound complications or postoperative infections based on comorbid status alone. Frail elderly patients are indeed at an increased risk of acute medical complications as evidenced by the finding that these occur in only 18% of elderly patients without comorbidity, in 32% of patients with a comorbid score of 1, in 49% of those with a score of 2, and in 63% of those with a score of 3 or more ($p < 0.01$). Frail elderly patients were noted to be at significantly greater risk of acute cardiac and pulmonary events, acute renal failure, stroke, sepsis, pneumonia, and urinary tract infection. On multiple logistic regression analyses, risk of in-hospital death was associated with both age over 75 years and frail elderly status, as well as weight loss, major ablative procedures, and the use of pedicled or free flap reconstruction. Interestingly postoperative surgical complications were not associated with frail elderly status, although acute medical complications were. Finally, frail elderly status was significantly associated with greater length of stay (LOS) and increased hospital-related costs and need for advanced care following discharge, among other variables.[7]

Extrapolating this information to the treatment of advanced head and neck cutaneous malignancy in the elderly is not perfect for obvious reasons, but it may help define some guidelines when counseling patients for surgery. The Genther and Gourin study defined neck dissection alone as a "minor procedure."[7] If it is assumed that parotidectomy is not more complicated than neck dissection alone in terms of overall operative risk, then it follows that most surgery performed for head and neck cutaneous malignancy is indeed on the more "minor" end of the head and neck surgery spectrum in terms of overall operative risk and complications. This study noted that both in-hospital mortality and postsurgical complications were significantly associated with major ablative procedures and with cases requiring major flap reconstruction (both regional and free tissue transfer) in this elderly study group. This does not appear to be the case with more "minor" ablative surgery, such as neck dissection or parotidectomy, let alone SLNB and wide local excision. Thus there does not appear to be a robust reason to recommend against "minor" ablative surgery in the elderly based on procedure alone. That said, frail elderly status was associated with in-hospital death and acute postoperative medical complications; as always, functional age and comorbidity remain important considerations in assessing surgical risk.[9,10]

Generally speaking, it is recommended that healthy older patients with little to no comorbidity be treated no differently than younger patients who present with the same clinical stage and prognosis, because the literature does not support that age alone impacts outcome. For frail elderly patients however, standard of care treatment recommendations may bring risks that are not in line with the patient and family's goals for treatment and quality of life. The literature cited earlier, while not specifically studying advanced cutaneous malignancies, gives surgeons a rough framework to begin the discussion of risks of perioperative death, acute medical complications, and need for advanced aftercare that many elderly patients are concerned about as they consider surgery for their advanced cutaneous malignancy. A frank discussion of prognosis, with respect to both the malignancy and any comorbidity, is imperative. Geriatric medicine consultation can be invaluable to help assess for coexisting geriatric syndromes and assist with advising the patient and family in decision making. A more palliative approach to treatment may be very appropriate in some frail elderly patients, but these alternative treatment strategies are best developed under the auspices of a multidisciplinary cutaneous malignancy team, which includes dermatologists, head and neck surgical oncologists, radiation oncologists, and medical oncologists.

Operative Considerations

Although the various operative procedures for advanced cutaneous malignancy are not necessarily technically different when performed in the elderly, the operative management of these diseases is particularly well suited to the older patient. BCC and SCC are easily resected under local anesthesia as an office procedure in many cases. Mohs micrographic surgery is a well-established, safe operative technique for these malignancies as well. Although the dermatology literature is similar to the head and neck literature in its lack of prospective assessment of elderly patients, there are some early efforts to establish safety in Mohs for older patients.[11,12] In many cases, wide local excision with margin analysis is all that is needed for treatment and, with same-day or staged reconstruction, can be performed under local anesthesia with or without conscious sedation, and entirely on an outpatient basis.

For the patients with melanoma and MCC, SLNB at the time of wide local excision may be indicated to assess for early regional metastases. Again, this is in many ways a procedure ideally suited to the elderly patient because it requires only a brief general anesthetic event and is routinely performed on an outpatient basis. The primary defect is reconstructed secondarily once final margins are cleared, and this can often be performed under local anesthesia, with or without sedation, as an outpatient, or at the time of completion lymphadenectomy should the sentinel node(s) be positive for metastasis.

If a patient requires parotidectomy and/or neck dissection for known regional metastasis, this is of course performed under general anesthesia and most often involves a short inpatient or observation stay. Working efficiently to minimize general anesthesia time is important in reducing operative risk, particularly in frail elderly patients.

Occasionally, patients with advanced cutaneous malignancy will require major head and neck reconstruction to address their ablative defect; in many institutions these are addressed with microvascular free tissue transfer. The literature for both ablative and free tissue transfer surgery in the elderly cutaneous malignancy patient is limited. The few cohort studies of free tissue use in elderly head and neck mucosal surgery patients are limited by low patient numbers and retrospective design, and only conclude that elderly patients are at higher risk for postoperative morbidity and require a thorough preoperative work up of any comorbid conditions.[13] The need for free tissue transplant indicates an advanced primary malignancy requiring a lengthy surgical procedure. Involving geriatric medicine consultants in these cases is important in optimizing medical comorbidities prior to a major surgical event.

Postoperative Care and Other Considerations

As with the preoperative management of elderly advanced cutaneous malignancy patients, postoperative care must look beyond simple wound issues. The stress of surgery may unveil previously well-compensated issues, be they hearing loss, early dementia, or depression. Awareness of well-described geriatric syndromes (see Chapter 3) assists in safely managing patients through the perioperative period. Early consultation of geriatric medicine provides for effective multidisciplinary care. Occupational therapy and physical therapy are also excellent resources for patients who may experience temporary or permanent disability in the aftermath of their surgery.

Finally, thoughtful postoperative consideration of reconstruction and donor site choices in this patient population is very important. No two older patients will be quite alike; thus attention to the details of their overall functional status is critical to their quality of life and safety. For example, older patients tend to require glasses. Most of us would be unable to complete simple activities of daily living without being able to see, but in the elderly, this can be a safety issue as well. A patient who has had a paramedian forehead flap for nasal reconstruction may ultimately be pleased with her cosmetic result but will suffer if she cannot put on glasses for the weeks during which inosculation is taking place. The patient who requires a partial auriculectomy might have a similar issue not being able to wear a long-standing hearing aid while bolster dressings are in place and wound healing is ongoing. Optometrists and audiologists can offer adjustments to help patients get through the perioperative period of time safely and mitigate impact on quality of life.

Disease-Specific Considerations

With the risk of cutaneous malignancy increasing with advancing age, a general review of diagnosis, staging, and treatment recommendations is helpful when approaching any patient with these cancers. There are many types of cutaneous malignancy; this chapter focuses on BCC, SCC, Merkel cell carcinoma, and melanoma.

Nonmelanoma Skin Cancer (NMSC)

Nonmelanoma skin cancer (NMSC) is the most common cancer in the United States, accounting for more malignancies than all other cancers combined. In 2006, ~ 2.1 million people were diagnosed with NMSC, compared with 1.4 million people with all other cancer types. Despite the high incidence of NMSC, these cancers are responsible for less than 0.1% of all cancer deaths.[14,15]

Basal Cell Carcinoma (BCC)

Basal cell carcinoma (BCC) is the most common cutaneous malignancy, accounting for ~ 80% of NMSCs. These lesions are of particular importance to the otolaryngologist because 80% of all BCC occurs in the sun-exposed head and neck region.[16] The most important risk factor associated with the development of BCC is sun exposure in fair-skinned patients. In contrast to squamous cell carcinoma, which is related to cumulative sun exposure, basal cell carcinoma is more strongly related to intense intermittent UV exposure during childhood and adolescence. Other known risk factors include male gender, red or blond hair, light eye color, and immunosuppression. A personal history of BCC increases the risk of developing another BCC by a factor of 10.[17]

The most common form of BCC is nodular, which accounts for over 75% of all cases. These classic lesions present as a pearly papule or nodule with overlying telangiectasia and a rolled border with or without central crusting or ulceration. Superficial BCC is the second most common type, but it is usually seen on the trunk and extremities. The morpheaform type is rare, but almost all cases are found in the head and neck. It is characterized by invasion deeper into the dermis and is more aggressive than the nodular and superficial types. Other rare types include micronodular, infiltrative, and basosquamous, all of which are more aggressive variants associated with higher rates of local recurrence.

The American Joint Committee on Cancer (AJCC) staging of BCC is the same as for NMSC and is reviewed in **Tables 20.1** and **20.2**.[17] The National Comprehensive Cancer Network (NCCN) stratified BCC into low-risk and high-risk groups based on their possibility for local recurrence—these risk factors are reviewed in **Table 20.3**.[18] The risk of regional metastasis is quite low, ranging from 0.0028 to 0.55%.[19]

Table 20.1 TNM classification of non-eyelid nonmelanoma skin cancer

Tumor classification (T)	Characteristics
T1	≤ 2 cm and < 2 high-risk features
T2	> 2 cm or ≥ 2 high-risk features
T3	Invasion of maxilla, mandible, orbit, or temporal bone
T4	Invasion of skeleton or perineural invasion of skull base
Nodal classification (N0)	
N0	No lymph node metastases
N1	Metastasis to single ipsilateral node ≤ 3 cm in greatest dimension
N2a	Metastasis to a single ipsilateral node, 3–6 cm in greatest dimension
N2b	Metastasis to multiple ipsilateral nodes, ≤ 6 cm in greatest dimension
N2c	Metastasis to bilateral or contralateral nodes, ≤ 6 cm in greatest dimension
N3	Metastasis to a lymph node > 6 cm in greatest dimension
Metastasis classification (M)	
M0	No distant metastases
M1	Distant metastases

Used with permission from Edge SE, Byrd DR, Compton CC, et al, eds. AJCC Cancer Staging Manual. 7th ed. New York, NY: Springer; 2010.

Note: High risk features include > 2 mm thickness, Clark level ≥ IV, perineural invasion, primary site on the ear, primary site on non-hair-bearing lip, and poorly differentiated or undifferentiated.

Table 20.2 Anatomical stage and prognostic groups of non-eyelid nonmelanoma skin cancer

Pathological stage	Tumor classification	Nodal classification	Metastasis classification
I	T1	N0	M0
II	T2	N0	M0
III	T3	N0	M0
	T1	N1	M0
	T2	N1	M0
	T3	N1	M0
IV	T1	N2	M0
	T2	N2	M0
	T3	N2	M0
	Any T	N3	M0
	T4	Any N	M0
	Any T	Any N	M1

Used with permission from Edge SE, Byrd DR, Compton CC, et al, eds. AJCC Cancer Staging Manual. 7th ed. New York, NY: Springer; 2010.

Table 20.3 Risk factors for recurrence of basal cell carcinoma

H&P	Low risk	High risk
Location/size	Area L < 20 mm Area M < 10 mm Area H < 6 mm[1]	Area L ≥ 20 mm Area M ≥ 10 mm Area H ≥ 6 mm[1]
Borders	Well defined	Poorly defined
Primary versus recurrent	Primary	Recurrent
Immunosuppression	No	Yes
Site of prior radiation therapy	No	Yes
Pathology		
Subtype	Nodular,[2] superficial	Agressive growth pattern[3]
Perineural invasion	No	Yes

Adapted with permission from the NCCN Clinical Practice Guidelines in Oncology (NCCN Guidelines®) for Basal Cell Skin Cancer V.1.2015. © 2015 National Comprehensive Cancer Network, Inc. All rights reserved. The NCCN Guidelines® and illustrations herein may not be reproduced in any form for any purpose without the express written permission of the NCCN. To view the most recent and complete version of the NCCN Guidelines, go online to NCCN.org. NATIONAL COMPREHENSIVE CANCER NETWORK®, NCCN®, NCCN GUIDELINES®, and all other NCCN Content are trademarks owned by the National Comprehensive Cancer Network, Inc.

Area L: trunk and extremities (excluding pretibia, hands, feet, nail units, and ankles).

Area M: cheeks, forehead, scalp, neck, and pretibia.

Area H: "mask areas" of face (central face, eyelid, eyebrow, periorbital, nose, lips [cutaneous and vermilion], chin, mandible, preauricular and postauricular skin/sulci, temple, and ear, genitalia, hands, and feet).

[1]Location independent of size may constitute high risk in certain clinical settings.

[2]Low risk histologic subtypes include nodular, superficial and other non-aggressive growth patterns such as keratotic, infundibulocystic, and fibroepithelioma of Pinkus.

[3]Having morpheaform, basosquamous (metatypical), sclerosing, mixed infiltrative, or micronodular features in any portion of the tumor.

Early and small tumors may be treated with simple excision or curettage and electrodissection. Because it is a common, slow-growing malignancy, the majority of BCC is treated by family physicians and dermatologists. However, locally aggressive tumors that are in proximity to functionally important and cosmetically sensitive anatomical structures are frequently referred to otolaryngologists. Surgical resection is the mainstay of treatment for lesions that are not amenable to curettage and electrodissection. Low-risk BCC should be excised with 4 mm margins. High-risk BCC may be treated with excision with wider margins and comprehensive intraoperative margin control. Mohs surgery remains the preferred treatment of high-risk BCC, because it allows intraoperative assessment of all margins and a 5-year disease-free survival rate of 99%. As is the case with all of the cutaneous malignancies discussed in this chapter, surgical margins should be discussed, because individual patient preferences may guide the treatment goals. In some cases, patients will accept closer margins to preserve function or cosmesis. In other cases, patients will decline surgery altogether and opt for radiation or targeted agents. Radiation therapy is usually reserved for patients with uncontrollable margins or for those who are poor surgical candidates.[18]

Patients with metastatic, multiply recurrent, or locally advanced BCCs now have another potential treatment modality in the form of a drug called vismodegib. Almost all BCCs have a loss of inhibition of the smoothened homologue (SMO) protein in the hedgehog signaling pathway, leading to uncontrolled proliferation of basal cells. Vismodegib is a novel targeted agent inhibitor of SMO that recently obtained Food and Drug Administration (FDA) approval based on the results of a phase 2 trial in patients with advanced BCC who had been previously treated with surgery, radiotherapy, and/or other systemic therapies. The metastatic disease response rate was 30%, and the locally advanced disease response rate was 43%. Both groups responded for a mean duration of 7.6 months, and 21% had complete responses. This hedgehog pathway inhibitor has been studied only in advanced, recurrent, and metastatic disease, and further study will elucidate its role, if any, in less advanced BCCs.[20]

Squamous Cell Carcinoma (SCC)

SCC is less common than BCC, representing ~ 10% of cutaneous malignancies. The risk of SCC is related to chronic, cumulative UV radiation exposure and is more commonly found in patients of northern European descent with fair skin (Fitzpatrick 1 and 2 skin types), light eye color, and a history of multiple sunburns.[21] SCC incidence is increased in sunny climates close to the equator, and increased risk of SCC is noted in the elderly, in those with a history of previous cutaneous malignancy or premalignant lesion, and in male patients. Risk of SCC is also higher in patients with a history of previous radiation treatment or occupational radiation exposure[22]; elderly patients may have a history of radiation treatment to the skin for treatment of acne because this was a common approach to acne treatment between 1920 and 1960. Arsenic exposure is associated with an increased risk of both SCC and BCC; although not commonly seen as an etiologic agent, some geriatric patients may have been exposed to Fowler's solution (potassium arsenic) in their youth, because this was a popular general tonic through the 1930s. SCC may also arise in the context of previous trauma, particularly burns and scars (e.g., Marjolin ulcer). Immunosuppression is widely recognized as a risk factor for SCC and portends more aggressive behavior of the cancer with increased rates of recurrence and metastasis.[23] Human papilloma virus (HPV) has also been associated with the development of SCC, particularly in immunosuppressed populations.

Clinically, SCC typically presents as an ulcerated, crusting lesion, often with a surrounding area of raised induration (**Fig. 20.1**). Staging of SCC is identical to that of BCC and is reviewed in **Tables 20.1** and **20.2**. SCC has a higher risk of both regional and distant metastasis compared with BCC, with a 10% occult metastasis rate[24]; nonetheless over 95% of nonmelanoma cutaneous malignancy will present as local disease only. The National Comprehensive Cancer Network (NCCN) has sought to define risk factors for aggressive behavior in SCC to help guide management. Most SCCs are low-risk and are diagnosed and treated at an early stage and under the auspices of dermatologists. Treatment of low-risk lesions would include definitive wide local excision, as well as judicious use of cryotherapy, electrotherapy, or photodynamic therapy in patients with early or in situ disease. High-risk SCC in the head and neck includes tumors that are 1 cm or larger on the cheeks, forehead, scalp, and neck, and tumors that are 6 mm or larger on the mask areas of the face, the chin/jawline region, and the periauricular region (**Fig. 20.2**). High-risk SCC parameters recognized by the NCCN also include the following: recurrent tumors; those with diffuse, poorly defined clinical borders; immunosuppression; previous radiation; rapid tumor growth; neurological symptoms or pathological perineural or perivascular invasion; and depth of tumor ≥ 2 mm. Poorly differentiated tumors and those of the adenoid, adenosquamous,

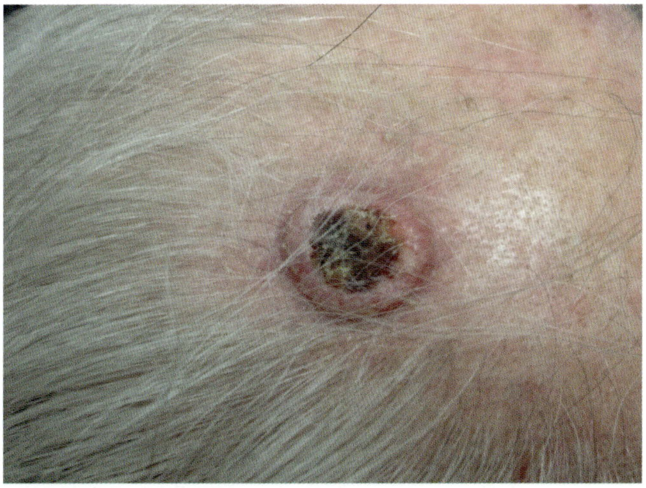

Fig. 20.1 Classic presentation of a squamous cell carcinoma of the scalp in an elderly, fair-skinned man. (Photo courtesy of Dr. Karen Kost.)

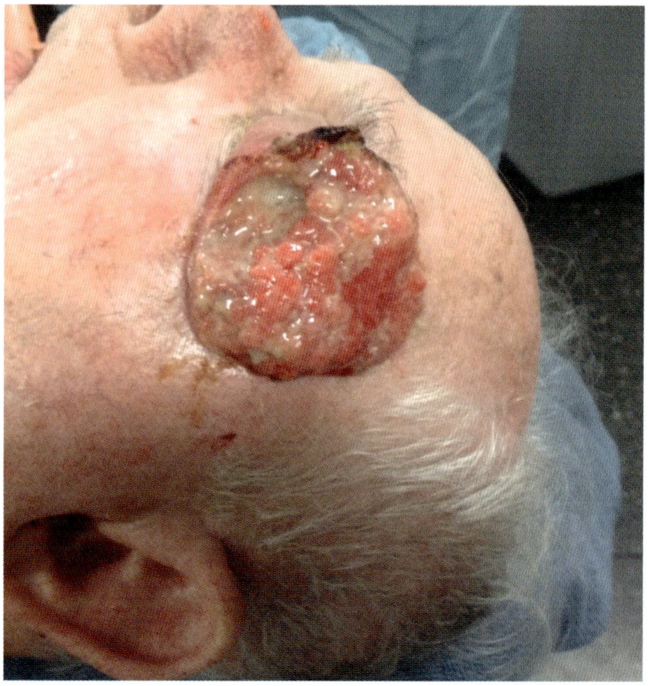

Fig. 20.2 Large squamous cell carcinoma of the left temple and upper eyelid. This is a high-risk lesion given its location and large size. (Photo courtesy of Dr. Karen Kost.)

and desmoplastic subtypes are also considered as potentially more aggressive.[23,25]

Treatment of high-risk SCC is primarily surgical. The primary lesion may be addressed with either Mohs surgery or wide local excision with intraoperative margin assessment. Concern for neck or parotid lymph node involvement on exam should prompt fine needle biopsy of the node(s); lymphadenectomy, including parotidectomy if appropriate, is recommended for regional metastasis. Interestingly, parotid lymph node metastasis portends a poor prognosis.[26,27] The use of SLNB in cutaneous SCC is an area of active investigation, and SLNB does appear to be a reliable method for staging early regional metastasis in SCC.[28,29] Adjuvant radiation is recommended for tumors with perineural invasion, close or positive tumor margins, and positive metastatic lymph nodes, particularly with evidence of extracapsular spread (ECS). Recommendations for chemoradiation (typically platinum based) are based on data from head and neck mucosal SCC; chemoradiation is recommended for cases with ECS and microscopically involved primary tumor margins.[23]

Merkel Cell Carcinoma (MCC)

While a relatively rare malignancy, MCC deserves special mention because it is primarily a disease of the elderly. It is an aggressive neuroendocrine tumor with high rates of local recurrence (25–30%), regional metastasis (52–59%), and distant metastasis (34–36%); its mortality rate surpasses that of melanoma, with 5 year overall survival rates between 30 and 64%.[30] Risk factors for MCC include fair skin types, age 65 years or older, and a history of extensive sun exposure. As with other cutaneous malignancies, MCC is more likely to occur in immunosuppressed patients, for example, those with allogeneic organ transplants, human immunodeficiency virus (HIV) infection, or lymphoproliferative disease. MCC appears to be related to infection by a polyomavirus, since named Merkel cell polyomavirus (MCV). MCV is ubiquitous, even a part of normal flora for humans, and infection is both common and typically asymptomatic. MCV infection typically occurs in childhood and results in viral integration into the host genome with subsequent quiescent chronic infection. Although still an area of active investigation, it is hypothesized that failure of cellular immune surveillance is responsible for tumor development; host immunity may be compromised by immunosuppressive therapy, HIV infection, lymphoproliferative disease, or possibly by aging itself; hence the association of MCC with these patient populations.[31]

MCC most commonly presents as a painless, indurated, pink to bluish-red colored intracutaneous nodule. Patients often describe it as initially looking like a blemish, but one that undergoes rapid growth. Over a third of MCC occurs on the face, scalp, or neck, making the head and neck the most common body region for MCC (36%), followed by upper limbs and shoulders (22%).[32] MCC is diagnosed by biopsy of the primary lesion, and immunohistochemistry is needed to differentiate this malignancy from other "small blue tumors"; MCC stains positive for cytokeratin 20 and thyroid transcription factor-1, and negative for S100, high molecular weight cytokeratins, and leukocyte common antigens, which helps differentiate it from metastatic small cell lung cancer.[33–35] Assessment of the patient for regional metastasis should be performed clinically; palpable lymph nodes may indicate nodal metastasis, whereas a clinically negative neck indicates that the patient may be eligible for SLNB for further staging.

MCC is such an uncommon malignancy that there is a paucity of prospective clinical trials to guide the development of guidelines for evaluation and treatment. The NCCN recently updated its guidelines based on available lower-level evidence, and its consensus is that overall, tumor stage and primary tumor size > 2 cm appear to portend a poor prognosis.[30] The AJCC staging for MCC is provided in **Table 20.4**.[17]Generally speaking the NCCN guidelines advocate for MCC patients to be evaluated and treated by a multidisciplinary cutaneous malignancy group given the rarity and complexity of this disease.[30,36] Surgery remains the cornerstone of

Table 20.4 TNM Staging of Merkel cell carcinoma

Tumor classification (T)	Characteristics
T1	≤ 2 cm
T2	> 2 cm and ≤ 5 cm
T3	> 5 cm
T4	Primary tumor invades bone, muscle, fascia, or cartilage
Nodal classification (N0)	
N0	No lymph node metastases
N1	Metastasis in regional lymph node(s)
N1a	Micrometastasis[a]
N1b	Macrometastasis[b]
N2	In transit metastasis[c]
Metastasis classification (M)	
M0	No distant metastases
M1a	Metastasis to skin, subcutaneous tissues or distant lymph nodes
M1b	Metastasis to lung
M1c	Metastasis to all other visceral sites

Used with permission from Edge SB, Byrd DR, Compton CC, eds. AJCC Cancer Staging Manual. 7th ed. New York, NY: Springer, 2010.
[a] Micrometastases are diagnosed after sentinel or elective lymphadenectomy.
[b] Macrometastases are clinically detectable nodal metastases verified by therapeutic lymphadenectomy or needle biopsy.
[c] In transit metastasis is tumor distinct from primary and located either between primary lesion and draining regional lymph nodes or distal to the primary lesion.

MCC treatment. Wide local excision of the primary cancer with 1 to 2 cm margins, coupled with SLNB for the clinically N0 neck is the standard primary approach; if the neck is clinically suspicious, needle biopsy should be performed, and plans for appropriate lymphadenectomy made should the needle biopsy be positive for metastatic MCC. Small postresection defects may be closed primarily; however, large primary defect reconstruction should be delayed if adjacent tissue rearrangement, extensive skin grafting, or free tissue transfer is expected to be required.

There is increasing evidence that adjuvant radiation may be beneficial in both locoregional control and overall survival.[37–39] There is significant heterogeneity in the design and patient populations of this limited literature; therefore the NCCN recommends a broad approach to adjuvant radiation in this rare, aggressive disease. Although observation may be considered for small primary lesions without lymphovascular invasion or nodal disease, adjuvant radiation should be considered in those cases with tumors ≥ 2 cm, perineural or lymphovascular spread, and nodal metastasis. It is also recommended for immunosuppressed patients and may be substituted for lymphadenectomy in patients who are high-risk surgical candidates.[30]

Melanoma

Melanoma is one of the fastest-growing cancers in the United States, with the incidence rising 5% per year over the past 2 decades. In 2007, the lifetime risk of developing a cutaneous melanoma was 1 in 52, compared with 1 in 1,500 in 1935. Melanoma is most commonly a malignancy found in adults and the elderly, with a median age of diagnosis at 63 years old for men and 56 years old for women.[40] The early detection of thin melanomas prior to the development of metastatic disease is paramount. The 5-year survival rates for individuals with localized, regional, and distant stage disease are 98.2%, 61.7%, and 15.2%, respectively.[41]

As previously discussed, the most important environmental risk factor is sun exposure, which varies depending on geographic latitude, occupation, outdoor leisure activities, and tanning. Other factors that contribute to the risk of melanoma include increasing age, male gender, fair skin, immunosuppression, and the presence of > 20 pigmented nevi. Men are 1.5 times more likely to develop melanoma,[40] and older men are at a particularly increased risk of developing melanomas that are ≥ 3 mm in thickness or of the nodular subtype.[42] Dysplastic nevi are not considered a precursor lesion—the annual risk for a dysplastic nevus to transform into melanoma is < 1 in 30,000 moles. However, dysplastic nevi are a marker for patients who are at increased risk of developing melanoma. Indeed, patients with one dysplastic nevus are 1.6 times more likely to develop melanoma, and patients with five or more dysplastic nevi are 10.5 times more likely to develop melanoma.[43]

In the geriatric population, it is not uncommon for patients to develop multiple cutaneous malignancies. In patients who have a personal history of NMSC, the relative risk of developing a melanoma is 4.28.[44] In patients with a personal history of melanoma, 11% will develop a second primary tumor within 5 years.[45] Patients with a family history of melanoma are 1.74 times more likely to develop a melanoma than the general population[44]; familial atypical multiple moles and melanoma (FAMMM) syndrome is an autosomal dominant disorder caused by a mutation of the *INK4a* antioncogene that encodes p16 on the 9p21 chromosome.[46]

There are multiple types of melanoma, of which the most common subtype is superficial spreading melanoma (**Fig. 20.3**). Superficial spreading melanoma is characterized by a radial growth phase followed by a vertical growth phase. In comparison, nodular melanoma is characterized by a rapid vertically invasive growth phase that leads to thicker lesions with a worse prognosis (**Fig. 20.4**). There are two subtypes that appear to have a particular propensity to occur in the elderly population—lentigo maligna melanoma and desmoplastic melanoma. Lentigo maligna melanoma is an invasive, slow-growing subtype with a relatively favorable prognosis that arises from the lentigo maligna precursor lesions. Desmoplastic melanoma is an aggressive subtype that frequently presents as an amelanotic lesion with a tumor thickness of ≥ 2 mm and has a propensity to have perineural invasion. Because desmoplastic melanoma tends to present with a more advanced stage and perineural invasion, there is a high rate of local recurrence, and many patients undergo adjuvant radiation therapy after surgery. Other less common melanoma subtypes include acral lentiginous, malignant blue nevus, and mucosal melanoma. Of note, up to 50% of mucosal melanomas occur in the head and neck, and this subtype is very aggressive, with 5-year survival rates ranging between 10 and 30%.

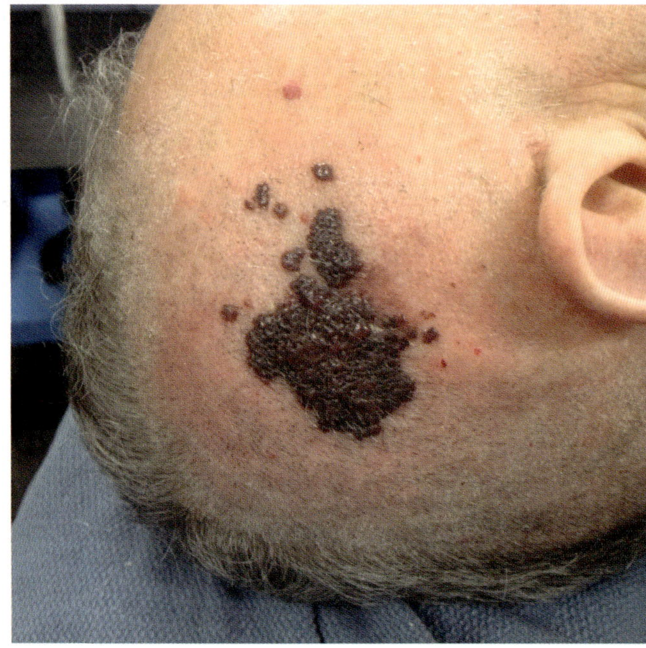

Fig. 20.3 Classic appearance of a scalp melanoma; note the presence of satellite lesions. (Photo courtesy of Dr. Karen Kost.)

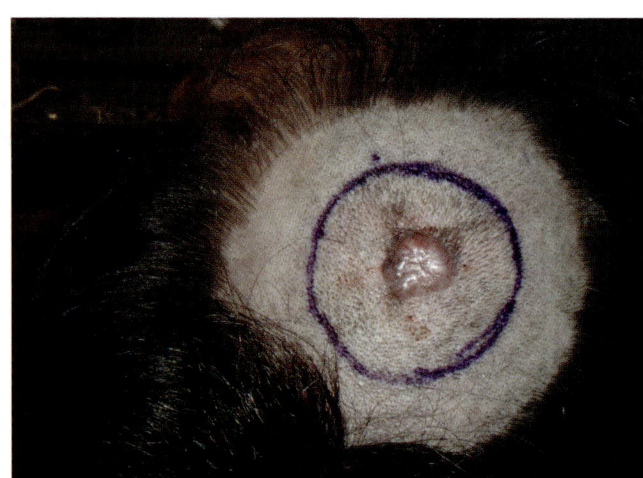

Fig. 20.4 Nodular melanoma. (Photo courtesy of Dr. Karen Kost.)

Staging of melanoma is based on the 2010 AJCC staging system; a summary of the staging system can be viewed in **Tables 20.5** and **20.6**. The factors of the primary tumor that most affect survival are tumor thickness, ulceration, and mitotic rate. The 10-year survival rate is 92% for patients with T1 lesions (≤ 1 mm thickness), 80% for T2 lesions (1.01–2 mm), 63% for T3 lesions (2.01–4 mm), and 50% for T4 lesions (> 4 mm). Mitotic rate was introduced into the newest staging system, replacing the Clark level of invasion, which was not a statistically significant prognostic factor when both mitotic rate and ulceration were taken into account.[47]

The treatment of melanoma is generally surgical, consisting of complete excision of the primary tumor with adequate margins, followed by adjuvant therapy based on the stage of disease. Based on the NCCN guidelines, recommended surgical margins for wide local excision are 0.5 to 1 cm for melanoma in situ, 1 cm for T1 tumors, 1 to 2 cm for T2 tumors, and 2 cm for T3 and T4 tumors.[48] A 1 to 2 cm margin in the complex head and neck region can result in

Table 20.5 TNM staging of melanoma

Tumor classification (T)	Thickness (mm)	Ulceration/mitoses
T1	≤ 1	a: without ulceration AND mitosis < 1/mm² b: with ulceration OR mitosis ≥ 1/mm²
T2	1.01–2	a: without ulceration b: with ulceration
T3	2.01–4	a: without ulceration b: with ulceration
T4	> 4	a: without ulceration b: with ulceration
Nodal classification (N)	Number of metastatic nodes	Nodal metastatic burden
N0	0	N/A
N1	1	a: micrometastasis b: macrometastasis
N2	2–3	a: micrometastasis b: macrometastasis c: in transit metastases/satellites without metastatic nodes
N3	4+ metastatic nodes, or matted nodes, or in transit metastases/satellites with metastatic nodes	
Metastasis classification (M)	Site	Serum LDH
M0	No distant metastases	Not applicable
M1a	Distant skin, subcutaneous, or nodal metastases	Normal
M1b	Lung metastases	Normal
M1c	All other visceral metastases Any distant metastasis	Normal Elevated

Used with permission from Edge SB, Byrd DR, Compton CC, eds. AJCC Cancer Staging Manual. 7th ed. New York, NY: Springer, 2010.

Note: Micrometastases are diagnosed after sentinel lymph node biopsy and completion lymphadenectomy (if performed).

Note: Macrometastases are defined as clinically detectable nodal metastases confirmed by therapeutic lymphadenectomy or when nodal metastasis exhibits gross extracapsular extension.

Table 20.6 Anatomical stage and prognostic groups of melanoma

Pathological stage	Tumor classification	Nodal classification	Metastasis classification
IA	T1a	N0	M0
IB	T1b T2b	N0 N0	M0 M0
IIA	T2b T3a	N0 N0	M0 M0
IIB	T3b T4a	N0 N0	M0 M0
IIC	T4b	N0	M0
IIIA	T1–4a T1–4a	N1a N2a	M0 M0
IIIB	T1–4b T1–4b T1–4a T1–4a T1–4a	N1a N2a N1b N2b N2c	M0 M0 M0 M0 M0
IIIC	T1–4b T1–4b T1–4b Any T	N1b N2b N2c N3	M0 M0 M0 M0
IV	Any T	Any N	M1

Used with permission from Edge SB, Byrd DR, Compton CC, eds. AJCC Cancer Staging Manual. 7th ed. New York, NY: Springer, 2010.

a significant functional disability or aesthetic deformity. It is important to discuss the implications of adequate surgical margins with elderly patients so that patients may provide their input in balancing both oncological and functional concerns. Adjuvant radiation may improve local control when adequate margins are not obtained due to functional concerns.

In patients with clinical evidence of regional spread, neck dissection is indicated. Patients with a clinically N0 neck have been the subject of controversy over the past few decades, but recent studies have clarified the treatment recommendations. In 2012, the American Society of Clinical Oncology and Society of Surgical Oncology released clinical practice guidelines on the use of lymphatic mapping and SLNB in patients with melanoma.[49] According to these guidelines, SLNB is recommended for patients with intermediate-thickness melanomas (1–4 mm) and thick melanomas (> 4 mm) for staging purposes and regional disease control. SLNB may be considered in selected patients with thin melanomas (< 1 mm) with high-risk features when staging outweighs the risks of the procedure. The final report of the phase 3 Multicenter Selective Lymphadenectomy Trial (MSLT-I) confirmed that SLNB for intermediate-thickness melanomas significantly improves 10-year disease-free and melanoma-specific survival.[50] Completion lymph node dissection is indicated for patients with a positive SLNB.

Adjuvant radiation therapy for primary disease is considered for patients with desmoplastic melanoma with narrow margins, locally recurrent disease, or extensive perineural invasion. Radiation therapy is also considered for regional disease that has gross extracapsular extension, more than one node within the parotid gland, more than two nodes in the neck, or nodal size ≥ 3 cm. Palliative radiation may be considered in unresectable nodal, satellite, or in-transit disease.[48]

Patients with stage III melanoma are at increased risk of developing distant metastases. Pegylated interferon-a-2b (IFNa2b) administered over a 5-year course has been shown to improve relapse-free survival from 38.9% to 45.6% in a randomized trial of 1,256 patients with completely resected stage III disease.[51] IFNa2b therapy has significant toxicity and side effects, including fatigue and nausea, which may limit its use in the elderly population.

The prognosis of patients with metastatic melanoma is dismal, but novel immunotherapy agents have shown promising results in recent years. Ipilimumab is a monoclonal antibody that stimulates T cells to promote antimelanoma immunity, and it was FDA approved for the treatment of metastatic melanoma in 2011. In two different phase 3 trials, ipilimumab lengthened survival from 6.4 to 10.1 months compared with treatment with glycoprotein 100 peptide vaccine, and it lengthened survival from 9.1 to 11.2 months compared with treatment with dacarbazine.[52,53]

Between 40 and 60% of patients with metastatic melanoma have a *BRAF* mutation in which glutamic acid is substituted for valine at codon 600 (V600E), which activates signaling of the mitogen-activated protein kinase (MAPK) pathway. Vemurafenib, dabrafenib, and trametinib are immunotherapy agents that inhibit *BRAF* and are increasingly being used in unresectable and metastatic melanoma patients with *BRAF* mutations. In a phase 3 trial comparing vemurafenib to dacarbazine, vemurafenib significantly improved 6-month overall survival from 64 to 84%. One important side effect of *BRAF* inhibitor therapy is the development of cutaneous SCC, which may occur in up to 18% of patients.[54]

As with all malignancies, clinical surveillance is necessary after treatment. General recommendations include skin and regional node examination at least yearly for 5 years and annually thereafter. Elderly patients who were offered SLNB but declined, or those with a positive SLNB who declined completion neck dissection, may be followed by cervical ultrasonography. High-risk patients may require surveillance imaging depending on their stage, but there is little reliable data to guide the use of laboratory or radiographic testing.[48]

Conclusion

Advanced cutaneous malignancies occur most commonly in elderly patients. Accordingly, adherence to sound geriatric principles of patient management is vital to the safe and effective treatment of the older patient with advanced skin cancer. Early involvement of the patient's geriatric specialist and/or consultation of geriatric medicine when needed will greatly enhance the care and outcomes for these patients. Finally, a patient- and caregiver-centered approach to treatment decisions, under the auspices of a multidisciplinary team, is important to the comprehensive care of these complex patients.

References

1. www.cdc.gov/cancer/skin/statistics
2. Godar DE, Urbach F, Gasparro FP, van der Leun JC. UV doses of young adults. Photochem Photobiol 2003;77(4):453–457
3. National Cancer Institute. Stat Fact Sheets SEER: Melanoma of the Skin. 2011. seer.cancer.gov/statfacts/html/melan.html
4. Hodgson NC. Merkel cell carcinoma: changing incidence trends. J Surg Oncol 2005;89(1):1–4
5. Albores-Saavedra J, Batich K, Chable-Montero F, Sagy N, Schwartz AM, Henson DE. Merkel cell carcinoma demographics, morphology, and survival based on 3870 cases: a population based study. J Cutan Pathol 2010;37(1):20–27
6. Agelli M, Clegg LX. Epidemiology of primary Merkel cell carcinoma in the United States. J Am Acad Dermatol 2003; 49(5):832–841
7. Genther DJ, Gourin CG. Effect of comorbidity on short-term outcomes and cost of care after head and neck cancer surgery in the elderly. Head Neck 2014. doi: 10.1002/hed.23651
8. Kinsella K, Velkoff VA. An Aging World: 2001. U.S. Census Bureau, Series P95/01-1. Washington, DC: U.S. Government Printing Office; 2001
9. Sanabria A, Carvalho AL, Vartanian JG, Magrin J, Ikeda MK, Kowalski LP. Comorbidity is a prognostic factor in elderly patients with head and neck cancer. Ann Surg Oncol 2007;14(4): 1449–1457
10. Piccirillo JF. Importance of comorbidity in head and neck cancer. Laryngoscope 2000;110(4):593–602
11. Delaney A, Shimizu I, Goldberg LH, MacFarlane DF. Life expectancy after Mohs micrographic surgery in patients aged 90 years and older. J Am Acad Dermatol 2013;68(2):296–300
12. Pascual JC, Belinchon I, Ramos JM. Mortality after dermatologic surgery for nonmelanoma skin cancer in patients aged 80 years and older. J Am Acad Dermatol 2013;69(6): 1051–1052
13. Tsai CH, Chang KP, Hung SY, Chen WF, Cheng MH, Kao HK. Postoperative morbidity in head and neck cancer ablative surgery followed by microsurgical free tissue transfer in the elderly. Oral Oncol 2012;48(9):811–816
14. Rogers HW, Weinstock MA, Harris AR, et al. Incidence estimate of nonmelanoma skin cancer in the United States, 2006. Arch Dermatol 2010;146(3):283–287
15. American Cancer Society. Cancer Facts and Figures 2006. Atlanta, GA: American Cancer Society; 2006
16. Kim RH, Armstrong AW. Nonmelanoma skin cancer. Dermatol Clin 2012;30(1):125–139, ix
17. Edge SE, Byrd DR, Compton CC, et al, eds. AJCC Cancer Staging Manual. 7th ed. New York, NY: Springer; 2010
18. National Comprehensive Cancer Network. NCCN clinical practice guidelines in oncology: basal cell and squamous cell skin

cancers (version 2.2014). http://www.nccn.org/professionals/physician_gls/pdf/nmsc.pdf

19. Rubin AI, Chen EH, Ratner D. Basal-cell carcinoma. N Engl J Med 2005;353(21):2262–2269
20. Sekulic A, Migden MR, Oro AE, et al. Efficacy and safety of vismodegib in advanced basal-cell carcinoma. N Engl J Med 2012;366(23):2171–2179
21. Weinstock MA. Epidemiology of ultraviolet radiation. In: Miller SJ, Maloney ME, eds. Cutaneous Oncology: Pathophysiology, Diagnosis, and Management. Malden, MA: Blackwell Science; 1998:121–128
22. Perkins JL, Liu Y, Mitby PA, et al. Nonmelanoma skin cancer in survivors of childhood and adolescent cancer: a report from the childhood cancer survivor study. J Clin Oncol 2005; 23(16):3733–3741
23. Miller SJ, Alam M, Andersen J, et al. Basal cell and squamous cell skin cancers. J Natl Compr Canc Netw 2010;8(8): 836–864
24. Martinez JC, Cook JL. High-risk cutaneous squamous cell carcinoma without palpable lymphadenopathy: is there a therapeutic role for elective neck dissection? Dermatol Surg 2007;33(4):410–420
25. Bichakjian CK, Alam M, Andersen J, et al. NCCN Clinical Practice Guidelines in Oncology (NCCN Guidelines): Basal Cell and Squamous Cell Skin Cancers, Version I.2013. Fort Washington, PA: National Comprehensive Cancer Network; 2013
26. Palme CE, O'Brien CJ, Veness MJ, McNeil EB, Bron LP, Morgan GJ. Extent of parotid disease influences outcome in patients with metastatic cutaneous squamous cell carcinoma. Arch Otolaryngol Head Neck Surg 2003;129(7):750–753
27. Ch'ng S, Maitra A, Allison RS, et al. Parotid and cervical nodal status predict prognosis for patients with head and neck metastatic cutaneous squamous cell carcinoma. J Surg Oncol 2008;98(2):101–105
28. Ahmed MM, Moore BA, Schmalbach CE. Utility of head and neck cutaneous squamous cell carcinoma sentinel node biopsy: a systematic review. Otolaryngol Head Neck Surg 2014;150(2):180–187
29. Schmitt AR, Brewer JD, Bordeaux JS, Baum CL. Staging for cutaneous squamous cell carcinoma as a predictor of sentinel lymph node biopsy results: meta-analysis of American Joint Committee on Cancer criteria and a proposed alternative system. JAMA Dermatol 2014;150(1):19–24
30. Bichakjian CK, Olencki T, Alam M, et al. Merkel cell carcinoma, version 1.2014. J Natl Compr Canc Netw 2014;12(3): 410–424
31. Amber K, McLeod MP, Nouri K. The Merkel cell polyomavirus and its involvement in Merkel cell carcinoma. Dermatol Surg 2013;39(2):232–238
32. Albores-Saavedra J, Batich K, Chable-Montero F, Sagy N, Schwartz AM, Henson DE. Merkel cell carcinoma demographics, morphology, and survival based on 3870 cases: a population based study. J Cutan Pathol 2010;37(1):20–27
33. Ratner D, Nelson BR, Brown MD, Johnson TM. Merkel cell carcinoma. J Am Acad Dermatol 1993;29(2 Pt 1):143–156
34. Leech SN, Kolar AJ, Barrett PD, Sinclair SA, Leonard N. Merkel cell carcinoma can be distinguished from metastatic small cell carcinoma using antibodies to cytokeratin 20 and thyroid transcription factor 1. J Clin Pathol 2001;54(9):727–729
35. Chan JK, Suster S, Wenig BM, Tsang WY, Chan JB, Lau AL. Cytokeratin 20 immunoreactivity distinguishes Merkel cell (primary cutaneous neuroendocrine) carcinomas and salivary gland small cell carcinomas from small cell carcinomas of various sites. Am J Surg Pathol 1997;21(2):226–234
36. Schwartz JL, Wong SL, McLean SA, et al. NCCN Guidelines implementation in the multidisciplinary Merkel Cell Carcinoma Program at the University of Michigan. J Natl Compr Canc Netw 2014;12(3):434–441
37. Lewis KG, Weinstock MA, Weaver AL, Otley CC. Adjuvant local irradiation for Merkel cell carcinoma. Arch Dermatol 2006; 142(6):693–700
38. Jouary T, Leyral C, Dreno B, et al; Groupe de Cancérologie Cutanée of the Société Française de Dermatologie. Adjuvant prophylactic regional radiotherapy versus observation in stage I Merkel cell carcinoma: a multicentric prospective randomized study. Ann Oncol 2012;23(4):1074–1080
39. Mojica P, Smith D, Ellenhorn JD. Adjuvant radiation therapy is associated with improved survival in Merkel cell carcinoma of the skin. J Clin Oncol 2007;25(9):1043–1047
40. Little EG, Eide MJ. Update on the current state of melanoma incidence. Dermatol Clin 2012;30(3):355–361
41. Siegel R, DeSantis C, Virgo K, et al. Cancer treatment and survivorship statistics, 2012. CA Cancer J Clin 2012;62(4): 220–241
42. Chamberlain AJ, Fritschi L, Giles GG, Dowling JP, Kelly JW. Nodular type and older age as the most significant associations of thick melanoma in Victoria, Australia. Arch Dermatol 2002;138(5):609–614
43. Goldstein AM, Tucker MA. Dysplastic nevi and melanoma. Cancer Epidemiol Biomarkers Prev 2013;22(4):528–532
44. Gandini S, Sera F, Cattaruzza MS, et al. Meta-analysis of risk factors for cutaneous melanoma: III. Family history, actinic damage and phenotypic factors. Eur J Cancer 2005;41(14): 2040–2059
45. Ferrone CR, Ben Porat L, Panageas KS, et al. Clinicopathological features of and risk factors for multiple primary melanomas. JAMA 2005;294(13):1647–1654
46. Czajkowski R, Placek W, Drewa G, Czajkowska A, Uchańska G. FAMMM syndrome: pathogenesis and management. Dermatol Surg 2004;30(2 Pt 2):291–296
47. Balch CM, Gershenwald JE, Soong SJ, et al. Final version of 2009 AJCC melanoma staging and classification. J Clin Oncol 2009;27(36):6199–6206
48. National Comprehensive Cancer Network. NCCN Clinical Practice Guidelines: Melanoma (version 2.2014). http://www.nccn.org/professionals/physician_gls/pdf/melanoma.pdf
49. Wong SL, Balch CM, Hurley P, et al; American Society of Clinical Oncology; Society of Surgical Oncology. Sentinel lymph node biopsy for melanoma: American Society of Clinical Oncology and Society of Surgical Oncology joint clinical practice guideline. J Clin Oncol 2012;30(23):2912–2918
50. Morton DL, Thompson JF, Cochran AJ, et al; MSLT Group. Final trial report of sentinel-node biopsy versus nodal observation in melanoma. N Engl J Med 2014;370(7):599–609
51. Eggermont AM, Suciu S, Santinami M, et al; EORTC Melanoma Group. Adjuvant therapy with pegylated interferon alfa-2b versus observation alone in resected stage III melanoma: final results of EORTC 18991, a randomised phase III trial. Lancet 2008;372(9633):117–126
52. Hodi FS, O'Day SJ, McDermott DF, et al. Improved survival with ipilimumab in patients with metastatic melanoma. N Engl J Med 2010;363(8):711–723
53. Robert C, Thomas L, Bondarenko I, et al. Ipilimumab plus dacarbazine for previously untreated metastatic melanoma. N Engl J Med 2011;364(26):2517–2526
54. Chapman PB, Hauschild A, Robert C, et al; BRIM-3 Study Group. Improved survival with vemurafenib in melanoma with BRAF V600E mutation. N Engl J Med 2011;364(26):2507–2516

21 Head and Neck Cancer in the Elderly

Mihir R. Patel, Raymond Chai, and Ara A. Chalian

■ Prevalence of Head and Neck Cancer among the Elderly

The definition of *elderly* continues to evolve as human lifespans increase. The National Institute of Aging and the National Institutes of Health use three categories to define aged patients: 65 to 74 years as young old, 75 to 84 years as older old, and 85 and over as oldest old.[1] A chronological landmark is considered the age of 70, because an increased incidence of age-related physiological changes becomes present at this age, resulting in pharmacokinetic changes that may lead to increased treatment-related toxicity.[2] Although aging is associated with a variety of declining physiological functions, due to the fact that biological age may differ greatly from chronological age, thorough evaluation and risk assessment are needed for decision making in the setting of head and neck cancers. It is imperative for the treating physicians to consider the factors that might affect a patient's ability to withstand cancer treatment. In addition, it is important to estimate the life expectancy of a patient when treatment strategies are planned. In Western societies, age-adjusted life expectancy is ~ 13.6 years for a 70-year-old man and 16.4 years for a 70-year-old woman.[2]

Head and neck cancers occur within the paranasal sinuses, nasal cavity, oral cavity, pharynx, and larynx. In 2014, there were an estimated 55,070 new cases of head and neck cancers, with 12,000 head and neck cancer-related deaths in the United States.[3] Worldwide, head and neck cancer is the sixth most common cancer, with roughly 650,000 new cases reported annually. Despite the increasing prevalence of cancer related to the human papillomavirus, which primarily affects younger patients,[4,5] head and neck cancer remains principally a cancer of an older population. According to the Surveillance, Epidemiology, and End Results database, ~ 47% of all patients diagnosed with head and neck cancer in the United States between 1973 and 2008 were age 65 and older.[6] In addition, the incidence of newly diagnosed head and neck cancer cases among the elderly is expected to increase by more than 60% by the year 2030.[7]

In the realm of head and neck cancer, squamous cell carcinoma of the head and neck (SCCHN) is the most prevalent and challenging malignancy to treat and is thus the focus of discussion. The treatment for SCCHN has become quite complex, necessitating multidisciplinary teams and multimodality therapy. Historically, tumors of the head and neck have been treated primarily with open surgery–alone approaches. The use of postoperative adjuvant radiation therapy (RT) became common in the 1970s, although its introduction in SCCHN began several decades earlier. Mounting data subsequently followed demonstrating that adjuvant treatment with RT improved locoregional control rates, thus improving overall survival. Further investigations have also led to the use of RT alone for the primary treatment of certain early-stage SCCHN with excellent outcomes. Along with surgery and RT, a third efficacious modality to treat SCCHN is chemotherapy. Investigated most thoroughly in the last decades of the 20th century, chemotherapeutic regimens, as a neoadjuvant therapy or in combination with RT in the postoperative setting, have shown great promise as an adjunct therapy in further improving oncological outcomes. In the mid to late-1990s, concomitant chemoradiation therapy (CRT) became a viable primary treatment option for certain patients with advanced-stage SCCHN. Yet, despite the continued advances in the therapeutic options available for SCCHN patients over the past 20 or more years, overall survival (OS), disease-free survival (DFS), functional outcomes, and toxicity profiles from therapy have remained relatively poor.[8] To date, patients with SCCHN continue to have some of the lowest survival rates of all major cancer types.

In the era of multimodality therapy, treatment paradigms for older patients with head and neck cancer are not well defined. The majority of patients with head and neck cancer will present with advanced (stage III and IV) disease requiring multimodality therapy.[9] Combined surgery, radiation, and chemotherapy cause significant acute toxicity and long-term morbidity, thus reducing compliance to therapy and decreasing quality of life as well as life expectancy. These morbidities can be profound in older patients, secondary to comorbid medical conditions and impaired functional status. As a result, older patients are often considered poor candidates for multimodality treatment and are therefore less likely to receive standard of care therapy compared with younger patients.[10,11] This bias against optimal treatment in the elderly may jeopardize their chance of cure. A retrospective series from Ortholan et al noted deviation from institutional protocol for head and neck cancer treatment in greater than half of older patients.[12] Although standardized treatment plans should be based on clinical stage and prognosis, age-related comorbidities and frailty need to be taken into account. Healthy older patients should be treated as aggressively as younger patients,[13] and treatment plans should be adapted in higher-risk frail elderly patients to balance the goal of curative treatment with an increased risk of treatment-related morbidity and mortality.[12]

In addition, older patients are often ineligible for the large prospective, randomized trials[14] on which treatment paradigms are based (**Table 21.1**). For example, in a recent meta-analysis of 93 clinical trials, only 692 of 17,346 patients (4%) were ≥ 70 years of age.[15] Thus the outcomes of these studies may not be applicable to older patients. Despite recommendations not to include age limits in large prospective trials, many ongoing trials continue to have upper age limits in their inclusion criteria.

Limited data suggest that selected older patients have survival outcomes similar to younger patients when treated primarily with surgery. In particular, several retrospective studies have matched older patients to a younger cohort and have shown no difference in survival outcome.[16–18] One study matched 115 patients who were ≥ 70 years of age by tumor type and stage to 115 patients < 70 years of age and found no difference in 5-year survival rate.[16] In addition, multiple nonmatched retrospective studies have shown similar results.[19,20]

An integral component of treatment planning is access to a Head and Neck Tumor Board Conference. Once a cancer diagnosis is confirmed, optimal treatment strategies are designed and individualized during a multidisciplinary tumor board. A multidisciplinary approach to patients has been shown to alter diagnosis, stage, and treatment modalities in head and neck cancer patients in nearly a third of patients.[21] Change in treatment was significantly more common in cases of malignancy, occurring in 24% of patients versus 6% of benign tumors. Significant changes in treatment were also noted to be largely escalations in management by incorporating multimodality therapy.[21] Furthermore, discussion at a multidisciplinary head and neck tumor conference may serve as a forum to mitigate bias that continues to surface in the literature regarding the elderly patient population with respect to treatment stratification.

Quality of Life Assessment and Comorbidities

The challenge in identifying surgical candidacy in the elderly population begins with preoperative quality of life assessment. Quality of life is a multidimensional concept that includes evaluation of positive and negative aspects of life.[22] Quality of life refers to "a patient's appraisal of and satisfaction with their current level of functioning compared with what they perceive to be possible or ideal."[23] There is limited quality of life data available in older head and neck cancer patients. The reason for this is unclear; however, subjective evaluation using validated quality of life questionnaires may be especially challenging in older patients. Treating physicians quite often believe that older patients have more side effects and toxicities from treatment and have more difficulty adjusting to their cancer diagnosis, thus overestimating the problems faced by their older patients with cancers and potentially affecting the aggressiveness of care.[24]

Although preconceived notions regarding the disproportionate impact of surgical therapy in the elderly persist, several studies have demonstrated no differences in posttreatment quality of life between older and younger head and neck cancer patients. A prospective assessment of surgically treated patients with head and neck cancer studied quality of life at 3 months postoperatively and observed no age-based differences.[25] An institutional database analysis of quality of life in 289 patients with head and neck cancer stratified by sex and age determined that, although global quality of life assessments are predicted by age, head and neck–specific metrics are not.[26] This is supported by a similar analysis using head and neck–specific quality of life instruments.[27] These findings were further confirmed in a long-term prospective observational study demonstrating that age did not impact on the quality of life for up to 6 years after diagnosis.[28]

Interestingly, younger patients may report worse quality of life outcomes after treatment for head and neck cancer. In a prospective study comparing quality of life, 78 older patients and 105 younger patients with head and neck cancer undergoing surgery were stratified based on baseline changes in physical function.[27] Although older patients had worse

Table 21.1 Median age in important multimodality randomized trials on head and neck cancer

Trial (see page 245)	Randomization	Results	No. of patients	Median age, years (range)
Larynx preservation studies				
Department of Veterans Affairs (VA)[1]	Definitive sequential chemotherapy + radiation vs. surgery + postoperative radiation	OS: no difference; larynx preserved in 64%	322	62 (24–79)
Radiation Therapy Oncology Group (RTOG) 91–11[2]	Sequential chemotherapy + radiation vs. concurrent chemoradiation vs. radiation alone	Larynx preservation; LC: better with concurrent chemoradiotherapy	547	59 (26–79)
European Organization for Research and Treatment of Cancer (EORTC) 24954[3]	Sequential chemotherapy + radiation vs. alternating chemotherapy and radiation	No differences	450	55 (35–76)
Definitive chemoradiation with standard fractionation studies				
Groupe Oncologie Radiotherapie Tete Et Cou. (GORTEC)[4]	Radiotherapy with concurrent chemotherapy (carboplatin + 5-FU) vs. radiotherapy alone	OS, DF, and LC were all improved with chemotherapy	226	55 (32–74)[a]
Intergroup trial[5]	Radiation alone vs. radiation with bolus cisplatin vs. split course RT with bolus cisplatin and infusional 5-FU	Did not meet accrual; OS was improved with RT and bolus cisplatin	295	57 (25–80)[a]
RTOG 97–03[6]	RT with daily cisplatin and 5-FU vs. RT with daily hydroxyurea with 5-FU vs. RT with weekly cisplatin and paclitaxel	Phase 2: All three regimens feasible	241	56 (21–83)
Hellenic Cooperative Oncology Group (COG)[7]	RT alone vs. RT with cisplatin vs. RT with carboplatin	OS improved with concurrent chemotherapy; cisplatin with best median OS and TTP	128	57 (31–78)
United Kingdom Head and Neck Trialists Group 1 (UKHAN1) Trial (nonsurgery arms)[8]	RT alone vs. RT with concurrent chemotherapy (VBMF or M alone) vs. RT with adjuvant chemo vs. RT with concurrent and adjuvant chemotherapy	Improvement in EFS with RT + concurrent chemotherapy	713	60 (17–84)
Bonner trial[9]	RT + concurrent cetuximab vs. RT alone	LC and OS improved with cetuximab	424	57 (34–83)
Definitive chemoradiation with hyperfractionation studies				
Brizel trial[10]	Hyperfractionated RT alone vs. hyperfractionated RT + cisplatin and 5-FU	Improvement in LC with chemotherapy and trend in OS, RFS	122	59[a]
Jeremic trial[11]	Hyperfractionated RT alone vs. hyperfractionated RT + daily cisplatin	OS, LRPDFS, and DMFS improvement with concurrent chemotherapy	130	61 (39–70)
German trial[12]	Hyperfractionated RT alone vs. hyperfractionated RT + carboplatin and 5-FU	1-year survival with local control benefit for concurrent chemotherapy	263	57 (28–73)

(Continued on page 234)

Table 21.1 *(Continued)* Median age in important multimodality randomized trials on head and neck cancer

Trial (see page 245)	Randomization	Results	No. of patients	Median age, years (range)
Swiss trial[13]	Hyperfractionated RT alone vs. hyperfractionated + cisplatin	LC and DFS improved with cisplatin; no difference in OS or time to failure	224	~ 55 (33–74)
GORTEC 99–02[14]	Standard fractionated RT + concurrent carboplatin and 5-FU vs. accelerated hyperfractionated RT + concurrent carboplatin and 5-FU vs. very accelerated hyperfractionated RT alone	Most favorable outcomes in conventional chemoradiotherapy arm	840	56.6 (34–75)[a]
Postoperative chemoradiation studies				
RTOG 9501[15]	RT alone vs. RT with concurrent cisplatin	LC and DFS benefit with chemotherapy	459	~ 56 (24–80)[b]
EORTC 22931[16]	RT alone vs. RT with concurrent cisplatin	LC, PFS, and OS improved with chemotherapy	167	54
French trial[17]	RT alone vs. RT with concurrent carboplatin	No difference	144	55.5[a]
UKHAN1 trial (surgery arms)[8]	RT alone vs. RT with concurrent VBMF	No difference	253	~ 58 (32–81)

Abbreviations: DMFS, distant metastases-free survival; ECOG, Eastern Cooperative Oncology Group; EFS, event-free survival; FU, fluorouracil; LC, local control; LRPFS, local recurrence progression-free survival; M, methotrexate; OS, overall survival; PFS, progression-free survival; RFS, recurrence-free survival; RT, radiation therapy; TTP, time to progression; VBMF, vincristine, bleomycin, methotrexate, and fluorouracil.

Used with permission from VanderWalde NA, Fleming M, Weiss J, Chera BS. Treatment of older patients with head and neck cancer: a review. Oncologist 2013;18(5):568–578.

[a]Mean age.

[b]Total of 25 patients who were > 70 years old (5%).

physical functioning prior to treatment, the difference remained constant throughout treatment, indicating that the older patients did not have a higher relative decrease in physical functioning compared with younger patients.[27] In addition, younger patients reported more pain at 6 months than older patients.[27] This difference is not limited to physical performance only, given that one retrospective study of 638 patients demonstrated that patients older than 65 had better long-term physical and emotional functioning than younger patients following surgery.[29] These findings may suggest that older patients experience fewer quality-of-life difficulties than their younger peers. Alternatively, they may suggest that older patients are less likely to report changes in quality of life due to differences in perceived expectations. Although the current data suggest that older patients do not have worse quality of life following treatment, the subjective nature of quality-of-life end points makes it difficult for clinicians to interpret these data for their individual older patients.

Another important preoperative assessment in the elderly is a careful evaluation of medical comorbidities. One case-control study did not identify significant differences in postoperative complications, mortality, or recurrence in a diverse population of patients with head and neck cancer stratified by the age of 70 who were treated surgically.[16] Despite data suggesting that age itself does not influence outcomes in head and neck cancer,[30] it stands to reason that patients with medical comorbidities and poorer functional reserve (common issues in older patients with SCCHN) would experience more and/or worse treatment-related toxicity.

The literature on head and neck cancer surgical outcomes stratified by medical comorbidities reveals mixed and conflicting conclusions. In one retrospective evaluation, medical comorbidities, independent of age, did independently predict postoperative complications.[31] Another demonstrated an increase in 30 day postoperative mortality in older patients (3.5% mortality) as compared with that in a younger cohort (0.8%).[32]

However, the authors here concluded that, given the relatively low rate of perioperative mortality, age alone should not be a contraindication to aggressive surgery. In a large retrospective analysis of 310 patients over age 70 with mucosal and salivary head and neck cancers, the authors determined that medical comorbidities (measured on the Adult Comorbidity Evaluation-27 index, see Appendix) and performance status (using the Karnofsky performance scale [**Table 21.2**]), as well as age > 80, all independently predict survival.[33] Finally, another study limited to patients > 80 years of age indicated that age did not impact on survival in early-stage disease but was a strong predictor of poor overall survival (median, 8 months) in patients with advanced-stage cancer.[34]

A new paradigm to emerge in the evaluation of candidacy for treatment may be defined not by age but by frailty. In a population study of 61,740 elderly patients,[35] *frail elderly* is defined as 66 years of age or older with comorbidity scores of 2 or higher and was examined as an independent variable in an analysis that included the previously described independent variables as well as acute medical complications, surgical complications, dysphagia, and weight loss as dependent variables.[17] Frail elderly status was additionally examined as an independent variable in analyses of short-term mortality, surgical complications, acute medical complications, length of stay, and costs that included an interaction term between frail elderly status and weight loss. The median age in this study was 73 years (range, 66–104 years) and did not differ significantly between groups based on comorbidity status; however, patients 80 years of age or older were more likely to have advanced comorbidity. Cardiovascular diseases and chronic pulmonary disease were the most frequent comorbidities and had an increased prevalence in patients with advanced comorbidity scores.[35]

Multinomial regression analysis was performed to identify variables associated with frail elderly patients, identifying a cohort that was significantly more likely to be 75 years of age or older, required urgent admission, and had significantly increased risks of acute medical complications (**Table 21.3**). Multiple logistic regression analyses of independent variables associated with the risk of in-hospital death and complications are shown in **Table 21.4**. After controlling for the effects of all variables, statistically significant independent predictors associated with the risk of in-hospital death were urgent or emergent admission, age 75 years or older, hypopharyngeal primary site disease, procedure, pedicled or free flap reconstruction, weight loss, and frail elderly

Table 21.2 Karnofsky performance scale status definitions rating (%) criteria

Able to carry on normal activity and to work; no special care needed	100	Normal to no complaints; no evidence of disease
	90	Able to carry on normal activity; minor signs or symptoms of disease.
	80	Normal activity with efforts; some signs or symptoms of disease
Unable to work; able to live at home and care for most personal needs; varying amount of assistance needed.	70	Cares for self; unable to carry on normal activity or to do active work
	60	Requires occasional assistance but is able to care for most of personal needs
	50	Requires considerable assistance and frequent medical care
Unable to care for self; requires equivalent of institutional or hospital care; diseases may be progressing rapidly	40	Disabled; requires special care and assistance
	30	Severely disabled; hospital admission is indicated although death not imminent
	20	Very sick; hospital admission necessary; active supportive treatment necessary
	10	Moribund; fatal processes progressing rapidly
	0	Dead

Used with permission from Oxford Textbook of Palliative Medicine, Oxford University Press; 1993:109.

Table 21.3 Multivariate logistic regression analysis of variables associated with frail elderly status

Variables	Relative risk ratio	95% CI	*p*-value
Age 75–79 years	1.29	1.14–1.45	< 0.001
Age ≥ 80 years	1.23	1.08–1.40	0.001
Female sex	0.84	0.75–0.95	0.004
Urgent/emergent admission	1.21	1.06–1.38	0.005
Laryngeal primary tumor	1.47	1.31–1.65	< 0.001
Oropharyngeal primary tumor	1.47	1.31–1.65	< 0.001
Acute cardiac event	4.52	4.00–5.09	< 0.001
Acute pulmonary edema/failure	2.41	1.95–2.98	< 0.001
Acute renal failure	3.39	2.55–4.50	< 0.001
Acute cerebrovascular event	10.49	5.32–20.68	< 0.001
Sepsis	1.95	1.35–2.80	< 0.001
Pneumonia	2.05	1.75–2.42	< 0.001
Urinary tract infection	1.52	1.19–1.95	0.001
Weight loss	1.60	1.31–1.94	< 0.001
Short-term hospital stay	3.68	2.38–5.68	< 0.001
Other facility	2.60	2.24–3.02	< 0.001
Home health care	1.53	1.35–1.73	< 0.001

Abbreviation: CI, confidence interval

Used with permission from Genther DJ, Gourin CG. Effect of comorbidity on short-term outcomes and cost of care after head and neck cancer surgery in the elderly. Head Neck 2014.

Note: Procedures were categorized by severity as **minor** (excision/destruction of lesion, tonsillectomy, and partial glossectomy, with or without neck dissection; and neck dissection alone when performed as the index admission procedure) and **major** (partial or total laryngectomy, esophagectomy, total glossectomy, pharyngectomy, mandibulectomy, and maxillectomy, with or without neck dissection).

status. Postoperative surgical complications were significantly associated with urgent or emergent admission, major procedure, pedicled or free flap reconstruction, and weight loss, but not frail elderly status. Finally, acute medical complications were significantly associated with frail elderly status, age 75 years or older, urgent or emergent admission, major procedure, flap reconstruction, and weight loss.[35] Although the data presenting are conflicting, the evidence favors a comprehensive treatment approach in patients with head and neck cancer, with appropriate modifications in those with multiple comorbidities, which may assist surgical planning and help take preventive measures to minimize potential complications.

Factors to Consider in Surgical Procedures for Elderly

Preoperative Nutrition

Nutrition in the elderly is often impaired without the acute or chronic impacts that the presence of a head and neck cancer would create. Alterations in the senses of smell and taste as well as social isolation often create a relative anorexia with diminished caloric intake. This combined with decreased activity leads to a loss of lean body mass. In the setting of SCCHN, the presence of malnutrition plays a vital role in wound healing.

Table 21.4 Multivariate logistic regression analysis of variables associated with risk of in-hospital death and postoperative complications

Variable	Odds ratio	95% CI	*p*-value
In-hospital death			
Urgent/emergent admission	1.82	1.19–2.79	0.005
Age 75–79 years	1.60	1.01–2.54	0.04
Age ≥ 80 years	2.60	1.79–3.76	< 0.001
Hypopharynx primary site	2.41	1.31–4.44	0.005
Major procedure	1.63	1.03–2.61	0.04
Pedicled or free flap reconstruction	4.26	2.43–7.46	< 0.001
Weight loss	1.64	1.00–2.69	0.047
Frail elderly	3.55	2.57–4.90	< 0.001
Postoperative surgical complications			
Urgent/emergent admission	1.30	1.06–1.60	0.01
Major procedure	2.49	2.01–3.08	< 0.001
Pedicled or flap reconstruction	7.32	5.49–9.82	< 0.001
Weight loss	2.00	1.63–2.46	< 0.001
Acute medical complications			
Urgent/emergent admission	1.49	1.30–1.70	< 0.001
Age 75–80 years	1.38	1.24–1.55	< 0.001
Age ≥ 80 years	1.76	1.57–1.98	< 0.001
Female sex	0.84	0.75–0.93	0.001
Medicaid	1.85	1.19–2.87	0.006
Major procedure	1.28	1.14–1.43	< 0.001
Pedicled or flap reconstruction	2.09	1.74–2.51	< 0.001
Weight loss	2.92	2.42–3.53	< 0.001
Frail elderly	3.71	3.32–4.14	< 0.001

Abbreviation: CI, confidence interval.

Used with permission from Genther DJ, Gourin CG. Effect of comorbidity on short-term outcomes and cost of care after head and neck cancer surgery in the elderly. Head Neck 2014.

Note: Procedures were categorized by severity as **minor** (excision/destruction of lesion, tonsillectomy, and partial glossectomy, with or without neck dissection; and neck dissection alone when performed as the index admission procedure) and major (partial or total laryngectomy, esophagectomy, total glossectomy, pharyngectomy, mandibulectomy, and maxillectomy, with or without neck dissection).

Preoperative consideration of how to deliver adequate nutrition must be addressed given that one of the three phases of swallowing will be affected after surgical intervention. A study evaluating nutrition impact symptoms, defined as key determinants of reduced dietary intake, weight loss, and reduced functional capacity of patients with head and neck cancer before treatment, suggests that symptoms before treatment may adversely affect nutritional intake, weight/body mass index (BMI), and the functional capacity of patients with head and neck cancer.[36] Diagnosis, management, and treatment of symptoms were essential in preventing weight loss. To do this, patients must be assessed for nutrition impact symptoms (NISs), such as dysphagia, mouth sores, xerostomia, dental problems, and difficulty chewing. The extent of dysphagia is graded from 0 to 4, from no dysphagia (grade 0) up to dysphagia for all kinds of oral intake including liquids (grade 4).

A patient-generated subjective global assessment tool (PG-SGA)[37] was used to systematically collect information on the NISs of the patients, and linked to dietary intake and weight loss. The PG-SGA is a validated nutritional screening technique for patients with cancer, which includes NIS, dietary intake, height, weight, weight loss history, and functional capacity. A PG-SGA score ≥ 9 indicates a higher nutritional risk, and in this report 31% of patients fell into this category.[36] This study prospectively assessed 341 patients from the Canadian health care system and found that the presence of anorexia, dysphagia, and mouth sores among others were predictors of significant weight loss from reduced dietary intake.[36] A BMI of < 18.5% was associated with a decrease in survival (p-value = 0.001). Patients with T1 and T2 tumors had fewer NISs than those with T3/T4 tumors.[36]

Patients in this series in the study by Kubrak and colleagues[36] were of mean and median age of 62 with 40% of the patients over the age of 65. The most profoundly affected group were those with oral and pharyngeal cancers. Of the patients with BMI < 18.5, who accounted for 5% of the study population, a greater proportion were older than 65 and most likely to have oral and pharyngeal cancers. Indeed, the patients with these cancers had the most weight loss. The survival of patients was worse in univariate analysis for PG-SGA > 9. The strongest impact on survival was BMI ≤ 18.5 and a reduced functional capacity. For example, patients with a BMI of ≤ 18.5 had a survival average of 519 days versus 1,263 days for a BMI of > 18.5 ($p < 0.0001$) (**Table 21.5**). The assessment and management of NISs is not systematized or even considered prior to treatment.[38,39] A standardized nutrition instrument may provide an opportunity to optimize outcomes in the geriatric patient population and optimize functional status during and after treatment.

The study highlights the value of PG-SGA screening because it allows assessment of weight loss and causes in light of potential upcoming treatments. Second, it frames involuntary weight loss in the context of current dietary habits/intake and swallowing function. Last, it makes it possible to treat causes of NISs, especially pain. This consideration weighs in on treatment decision making in our group and likely others.

For this reason, another study attempted to generate a prediction model for percutaneous endoscopic gastrostomy (PEG) placement in head and neck cancer patients.[40] A cohort of 152 patients were analyzed, taking into consideration the following parameters: age, gender, BMI, staging, size and localization of the tumor, or need for a neck dissection. Decisive predictive parameters for needing a PEG included size and localization of the tumor in the oral cavity, resection of the root of the tongue or the oropharynx region, and performance of a neck dissection.[40] Specifically, T3 and T4 oral cavity tumors necessitate preoperative PEG placement. Tumor location in the posterior floor of the mouth, root of the tongue, and oropharynx are predictive of preoperative PEG placement irrespective of T stage. This study cohort was taken from 2005 through 2010, prior to Food and Drug Administration (FDA) clearance of transoral robotic surgery (TORS). TORS data for oropharyngeal SCCHN demonstrate that PEG may not be necessary in this group. Studies in patients undergoing TORS reported 2% and 0% of patients being gastrostomy tube dependent at 1 year (in the setting of adjuvant therapy).[41,42] Studies from three other institutions reported a cumulative gastrostomy tube rate of 1.4% (2/139) at the time of surgery and 30% (32/107) placed expectantly at the time of adjuvant therapy.[43–45] Negative margin surgery in the setting of TORS can lead to deintensification of the use of radiation and potentially negate the need for chemotherapy. At the University of Pennsylvania Cancer Center, some patients, especially those with lower risk pharyngeal cancers, are treated with postoperative radiation to the neck only to mitigate the need for PEG during adjuvant therapy.

Neck Dissection

General considerations in surgical approaches for head and neck cancer invariably involve manipulation of the neck. This includes the cervical spine and great vessels, in particular the carotid. Although there are no practice guidelines for monitoring the cervical spine, if, during the workup of an elderly head and neck cancer patient, the radiologist has expressed concern for stenosis according to the neck computed tomographic (CT) scan, a dedicated cervical spine study is ordered in our practice. In addition,

Table 21.5 Univariate and multivariate survival analysis of patient and nutrition characteristics derived from the Patient-Generated Subjective Global Assessment (PG-SGA) for patients with head and neck cancer at presentation

	Univariate analysis		Multivariate analysis	
Variables[a]	p **value**	**Hazard ratio (CI 95%)**	p **value**	**Hazard ration (CI 95%)**
Sex				
Male	0.23	1.3 (0.8–2)		N/S
Age				
≥ 65 years old	0.001	1.8 (1.2–2.7)	0.008	1.7 (1.1–2.5)
Tumor classification (T1/T2)				
T3/T4	≤ 0.001	2.6 (1.8–3.9)	0.001	2 (1.3–3.2)
Treatment category (no treatment)				
RT/RT surgery	0.001	0.3 (0.1–0.6)	≤ 0.001	0.2 (0.1–0.5)
ChemoRT/surgerychemoRT	0.01	0.4 (0.2–0.8)	0.005	0.3 (0.1–0.7)
Palliative treatment	0.05	2.2 (0.9–4.3)	0.60	1.2 (0.5–2.8)
Tumor localization (oral cavity)				
Salivary gland	0.51	0.6 (0.2–2.1)		N/S
Paranasal sinuses	0.21	2.1 (0.5–8.8)		N/S
Pharynx	0.27	1.8 (1–2.2)		N/S
Larynx	0.14	0.5 (0.2–1.1)		
N/SMI category (> 18.5–24.9)				
≤ 18.5	≤ 0.001	4.1 (2.1–8)	0.001	3.1 (1.6–6.1)
≥ 25–29.9	≤ 0.001	0.1 (0.07–0.3)	0.10	0.6 (0.4–1)
≥ 30	≤ 0.001	0.8 (0.01–0.3)	0.07	0.6 (0.3–1)
PG-SGA (< 9 Score)				
≥ 9 Score	≤ 0.001	2.1 (1.4–3.1)		N/S
PG-SGA components (an/ssence)				
Grade 1 weight loss	0.007	1.6 (1.1–2.4)		N/S
Reduced dietary intake	≤ 0.001	2.3 (1.5–3.7)		N/S
Nutrition impact systems				
Anorexia	0.02	1.7 (1–2.7)		N/S
Nausea	0.94	1 (0.3–2.8)		N/S
Constipation	0.15	1.4 (0.8–2.5)		N/S
Mouth sores	0.003	1.9 (1.2–2.9)		N/S
Dysgeusia	0.71	1.1 (0.6–2.0)		N/S

(Continued on page 240)

Table 21.5 *(Continued)* Univariate and multivariate survival analysis of patient and nutrition characteristics derived from the Patient-Generated Subjective Global Assessment (PG-SGA) for patients with head and neck cancer at presentation

Dysphagia	0.001	1.9 (1.3–2.8)		N/S
Feeling full	0.031	1.8 (1–3.2)		N/S
Pain	0.049	1.4 (1–2.1)		N/S
Dental pron/slems	0.14	1.4 (0.8–2.2)		N/S
Xerostomia	0.80	1 (0.6–1.8)		N/S
Other	0.594	1.1 (0.6–1.8)		N/S
Reduced functional capacity	≤ 0.001	2.4 (1.6–3.5)	0.001	

Abbreviations: RT, radiotherapy; chemo, chemotherapy; BMI, body mass index; N/S; not significant; PG-SGA, patient generated subjective global assessment.

Used with permission from Kubrak C, Olson K, Jha N, Jensen L, McCargar L, Seikaly H, Baracos V. Nutrition impact symptoms: key determinants of reduced dietary intake, weight loss, and reduced functional capacity of patients with head and neck cancer before treatment. Head Neck 2010;32(3):290–300.

[a]Reference category in the parentheses.

intraoperative sensory evoked potentials (SEPs) are monitored, particularly when positioning the neck in extension. The patients for whom we use this type of monitoring note symptoms with extensions during assessment at the preoperative history and physical appointment.

In general, retrospective data suggest that the risk of postoperative stroke after neck dissection varies from < 1% to 4.8%.[46,47] Theoretically, this risk is higher in patients with preexisting carotid stenosis or atherosclerosis, which is more prevalent in elderly patients.[48] Moreover, the management of high-grade carotid stenosis is complicated by prior oncological treatment. Carotid ultrasonography has been advocated as a screening mechanism for patients scheduled for neck dissection, although no studies have confirmed its role, nor has it become accepted routine practice.[49] Nevertheless, in some cases, elderly patients with head and neck cancer may benefit from either imaging or subspecialist consultation or both before either neck dissection or radiation to plan appropriately.[50] Indeed, surgeons operating on elderly patients should be mindful and cautious when positioning the neck and manipulating the carotid sheath.

Supracricoid Partial Laryngectomy

Supracricoid partial laryngectomies (SCPLs) result in complete and bilateral resection of the paraglottic space, including, when required, one arytenoid cartilage on the tumor-bearing side. When compared with the conventional vertical partial and supraglottic laryngectomies, SCPLs appear to be the conservative laryngeal procedures that most disturb the sphincteric function of the larynx. Aging impairs oropharyngeal motor command and laryngopharyngeal sensitivity,[51–53] as well as esophageal motility.[54] Modifications of the pulmonary physiology related to aging also greatly increase the risk of atelectasis and pneumonia in the postoperative period in this group of patients.[54]

In the setting of potential dysphagia and aspiration, head and neck surgeons must give special consideration to the functional results encountered in assessing elderly patients presenting with endolaryngeal carcinoma, which is oncologically amenable to SCPL. Currently, there is no consensus on the parameters defining the ideal elderly patient for SCPL. In one series, several variables, including gender, age, medical history, tobacco consumption, associated neck dissection, arytenoid cartilage resection, type of reconstruction performed, and laryngeal RT were examined, and none were found to statistically increase the risk for aspiration after SCPL.[19] On the other hand, univariate analysis revealed that postoperative aspiration was less likely if repositioning of the pyriform sinus and inferior constrictor muscles was performed (p = 0.01).[19] This maneuver allows for repositioning of the pyriform sinuses laterally to the reconstructed neoglottis. Such repositioning may result in better propulsion of the bolus at the time of swallowing, therefore reducing the risk for postoperative aspiration.

Although current evidence suggests that age by itself should not be considered as a deterrent to SCPL, aspiration remains a risk. Severe aspiration (grade 3) was noted in 21.7% of patients in this same study but was temporary, given that permanent gastrostomy for liquid intake and completion total laryngectomy were required in only one patient.[19] Another study described three elderly patients managed with SCPL-CHP and found that one patient developed bronchopneumonia from aspiration and another required completion total laryngectomy.[55] This experience prompted the authors to state that SCPL-CHP was not advisable in patients over the age of 65.[55] Late aspiration has been documented in one patient that died of aspiration-related complications 3 years after SCPL-CHP with arytenoid cartilage disarticulation,[19] therefore suggesting that long-term functional follow-up is necessary when SCPLs are performed in elderly patients.

Total Laryngectomy

Total laryngectomy, defined by complete removal of the laryngeal framework to create a tracheostoma, has proven oncological results for the treatment of late-stage SCCHN. However, communication after total laryngectomy is a critical component of quality of life and therefore an important consideration in terms of patient selection. Postlaryngectomy communication is undertaken using a team approach that relies on a preoperative assessment by a speech-language pathologist and a comprehensive discussion of available communication options.

There are essentially two types of artificial larynx. The pneumatic larynx is activated by respiratory air from the tracheostoma via a connection to a tracheal cannula. This voice device has the advantage of not requiring a battery, and the fact that the pitch varies with breath pressure results in fundamental frequencies that are more gender-appropriate. Despite this they have not won widespread acceptance, probably because patients regard them as cumbersome and do not like the plastic or metal tube that serves to transmit the sound from the vibrator at the stoma to the mouth. The second type of artificial larynx is the electrolarynx, a handheld battery-driven device that uses a diaphragm, acted on by an electromechanical vibrator. When the diaphragm is held tightly against the neck, vibrations are transmitted through the soft tissue and emerge from the vocal tract, where the user modulates them with the mouth to create speech.[56]

Effective postlaryngectomy communication can also be restored by surgically creating a tracheoesophageal puncture (TEP), or a fistula through the tracheoesophageal party wall. This may be performed either primarily during laryngectomy or secondarily when the tracheostoma is fully healed. Once the fistula has been created, a prosthetic tube (~ 4 mm in diameter), containing a one-way valve, is inserted. When the tracheostoma is finger-occluded, this device diverts exhaled air through a one-way valve into the neopharynx and mouth, creating a gurgling sound, which is then modulated into words. With this technique, aspiration is generally not a risk, and more air is available to produce a more fluent and sustained sound. A further advantage is that, when the surgical procedure for the insertion of the voice prosthesis is performed at the time of the laryngectomy, the patient can be trained to speak within a few days, with psychological benefits.[57] Disadvantages are that, in most cases, a thumb is required to occlude the stoma during speech, and the voice prosthesis allows air to flow from the trachea to the esophagus. Frail and elderly patients or those with neurological disorders such as Parkinson disease do not have the proprioceptive capabilities to care for their valve, which needs daily cleaning, or to occlude the stoma to speak. In both these groups, such a device is not appropriate, and an alternative means of communication should be sought.

Free Tissue Transfer

As microsurgical techniques have advanced, free tissue transfer has evolved to become the preferred modality of reconstruction after head and neck cancer ablation.[58,59] Previous studies have suggested that free tissue transfer can be performed in selected patients that are 65 years of age or older.[60–65] However, most studies focus exclusively on the flap survival, flap-related complications, or comparable results to those of younger patients (often < 65 and ≥ 65 or < 70 and ≥ 70) and demonstrate that there is no difference between comorbidity and complications in both young and elderly head and neck cancer patients, suggesting difficulty in predicting the postoperative morbidity and mortality in the elderly subgroup.[60,63,66]

It is of paramount importance that we understand the safety and feasibility of complex microsurgical reconstruction in this patient population. In elderly patients undergoing head and neck surgery, potential perioperative complications appear to be related to the preoperative comorbidity status.[66] The American Society of Anesthesiologists (ASA) physical status classification (**Table 21.6**) on the one hand can be used for individual estimation for the peri- and postoperative risk factors, and on the other hand it might correlate with the in-hospital mortality of the patients.[67] One study focused on free tissue transfer outcomes and found that an elderly cohort of over 70 years of age had a significantly higher ASA score than a younger group (age 65–70), which correlated with an overall more eventful postoperative course for those in the older group that included arrhythmias,

Table 21.6 American Society of Anesthesiologists (ASA) Physical Status Classification System

ASA Physical Status 1	A normal healthy patient
ASA Physical Status 2	A patient with mild systemic disease
ASA Physical Status 3	A patient with severe systemic disease
ASA Physical Status 4	A patient with severe systemic disease that is a constant threat to life
ASA Physical Status 5	A moribund patient who is not expected to survive without the operation
ASA Physical Status 6	A declared brain-dead patient whose organs are being removed for donor purposes

Courtesy of American Society of Anesthesiologists website: https://www.asahq.org/clinical/physicalstatus.htm.

bronchopulmonary pneumonia, gastroparesis, and delirium.[68] In evaluating 13 octogenarians undergoing free flap reconstruction of the head and neck, medical complications were fourfold higher when compared with a younger cohort (62% vs. 15%).[69] The authors determined that free flaps were dependable in this age group; however, they cautioned against their use.[69] Complication rates in this cohort were then controlled for a higher ASA class in octogenarians, and despite this there remained a statistically higher complication rate in elderly patients (67% vs. 29%).[69] When comparing the two elderly subpopulations, patients aged 70 to 79 years versus those 80 years and older, the overall complication rate (35% vs. 59%), medical complication rate (12% vs. 41%), and perioperative mortality (8% vs. 18%) were significantly higher in the over-80 subset.[65] Nevertheless, flap success rates remained near identical at 96% for those aged 70 to 79 years and 100% for patients 80 years and older.[65] The authors concluded that free flap surgery can be performed successfully in well-selected elderly patients, but with increased medical complications. In fact, flap success in patients 90 years and older has been reported for 10 cases.[70] Four medical complications occurred that included one case of pneumonia and three cases of arrhythmia. There were no mortalities after 8 months of follow-up. Two recipient-site complications occurred (one infection and one fistula), and the flap failure rate was 0%. One late complication developed 7 months postoperatively involving infection and nonunion of the mandibular reconstruction. The authors conclude that medical and flap-related complications in patients 90 years and older are consistent with rates previously reported in elderly patients and note that this population can tolerate free flap reconstruction with favorable long-term outcomes.[70] This relatively low mortality rate highlights the efficacy and importance of careful preoperative evaluation and optimization in the elderly patient population.

In major head and neck surgery necessitating reconstruction, substantial blood loss is possible. The extent of blood loss and the subsequent need for transfusion depend on the patient's condition, disease stage, tumor size, and complexity of operative procedures.[71,72] Preoperative evaluation includes hemoglobin levels, which were found to be within normal ranges in both the older (age > 70) and the younger (age 65–70) groups.[68] On average, however, lower levels were seen in the older group. Despite no significant difference in intraoperative blood loss between these two groups, the need for intraoperative blood transfusion of at least 2 units was significantly higher in the older group.[68] Interestingly, blood loss of > 220 mL is a significant predictor for postoperative medical complications; thus the surgeon should aim to achieve minimal blood loss.

Because free flap reconstruction is an integral component of oral cavity, oropharyngeal, and total laryngectomy defects, particular understanding of potential wound complications is paramount. The incidence of wound infection in head and neck cancer surgery remains controversial, with reported rates ranging from 11 to 47%.[73,74] Wound infection rates were 40% and 19% for the older (age > 70) and younger (age 65–70) groups, respectively ($p = 0.003$). The rate of flap loss (< 1 week postoperatively), including partial and total flap loss, was low at 4.1% (4/73) for the younger group and 10.6% (10/94) for the older group, with no significant difference between these two groups.[68] The high flap success rate of both groups is consistent with those of large series from major microsurgical centers, where studies of flap success rates ranged from 91 to 99%.[75,76] Compared with the previously published literature, in which 5 to 25% of transferred flaps require reexploration within the first week postoperatively due to circulatory compromise or neck hematoma, the reexploration rate is 5.5% in the younger group and 10.7% in the older group.[77] As a matter of fact, there is no clinical evidence demonstrating a higher incidence of flap loss or vessel thrombosis in the elderly patients, even for those over the age of 70. Therefore patients with cancers that would benefit from microvascular reconstruction should be offered this modality. The use of synchronous two-team surgery should lead to compressed surgical times.

Summary

In summary, the teams treating elderly (aged) patients with head and neck squamous cell cancers should offer these patients and their families the state of the art in treatments. The use of preoperative assessment tools for nutrition, functional status, and comorbidities will help identify patients at higher risk. These individuals can then be offered therapy to optimize the outcomes of the standard treatment, or be presented with customized management options that account for comorbidities and individual circumstances. The team is critical to the successful care of elderly patients. The incorporation of geriatric specialists or teams will likely be beneficial and more common. There is no doubt that with the current boom of healthy aging and virally related malignancy, the number of patients needing treatment will increase. As the aging population increases, and in parallel the number of patients with head and neck malignancies, the geriatric multidisciplinary team will assume a greater role in assuring optimal care and outcomes in this very special subset.

References

1. Parker SL, Tong T, Bolden S, Wingo PA. Cancer statistics, 1997. CA Cancer J Clin 1997;47(1):5–27
2. Pallis AG, Fortpied C, Wedding U, et al. EORTC elderly task force position paper: approach to the older cancer patient. Eur J Cancer 2010;46(9):1502–1513
3. Siegel R, Ma J, Zou Z, Jemal A. Cancer statistics, 2014. CA Cancer J Clin 2014;64(1):9–29
4. Patel SC, Carpenter WR, Tyree S, et al. Increasing incidence of oral tongue squamous cell carcinoma in young white women, age 18 to 44 years. J Clin Oncol 2011;29(11):1488–1494
5. Gillison ML, Broutian T, Pickard RK, et al. Prevalence of oral HPV infection in the United States, 2009-2010. JAMA 2012;307(7):693–703
6. National Cancer Institute. Surveillance, Epidemiology, and End Results Program. http://www.seer.cancer.gov
7. Smith BD, Smith GL, Hurria A, Hortobagyi GN, Buchholz TA. Future of cancer incidence in the United States: burdens upon an aging, changing nation. J Clin Oncol 2009;27(17): 2758–2765
8. Carvalho AL, Nishimoto IN, Califano JA, Kowalski LP. Trends in incidence and prognosis for head and neck cancer in the United States: a site-specific analysis of the SEER database. Int J Cancer 2005;114(5):806–816
9. Argiris A, Eng C. Epidemiology, staging, and screening of head and neck cancer. Cancer Treat Res 2003;114:15–60
10. de Rijke JM, Schouten LJ, Schouten HC, Jager JJ, Koppejan AG, van den Brandt PA. Age-specific differences in the diagnostics and treatment of cancer patients aged 50 years and older in the province of Limburg, The Netherlands. Ann Oncol 1996;7(7):677–685
11. Fentiman IS, Tirelli U, Monfardini S, et al. Cancer in the elderly: why so badly treated? Lancet 1990;335(8696): 1020–1022
12. Ortholan C, Benezery K, Dassonville O, et al. A specific approach for elderly patients with head and neck cancer. Anticancer Drugs 2011;22(7):647–655
13. Grénman R, Chevalier D, Gregoire V, Myers E, Rogers S. Treatment of head and neck cancer in the elderly: European Consensus (panel 6) at the EUFOS Congress in Vienna 2007. Eur Arch Otorhinolaryngol 2010;267(10):1619–1621
14. VanderWalde NA, Fleming M, Weiss J, Chera BS. Treatment of older patients with head and neck cancer: a review. Oncologist 2013;18(5):568–578
15. Pignon JP, le Maître A, Maillard E, Bourhis J; MACH-NC Collaborative Group. Meta-analysis of chemotherapy in head and neck cancer (MACH-NC): an update on 93 randomised trials and 17,346 patients. Radiother Oncol 2009;92(1):4–14
16. Kowalski LP, Alcantara PS, Magrin J, Parise Júnior O. A case-control study on complications and survival in elderly patients undergoing major head and neck surgery. Am J Surg 1994;168(5):485–490
17. Clayman GL, Eicher SA, Sicard MW, Razmpa E, Goepfert H. Surgical outcomes in head and neck cancer patients 80 years of age and older. Head Neck 1998;20(3):216–223
18. McGuirt WF, Davis SP III. Demographic portrayal and outcome analysis of head and neck cancer surgery in the elderly. Arch Otolaryngol Head Neck Surg 1995;121(2):150–154
19. Laccourreye O, Brasnu D, Périé S, Muscatello L, Ménard M, Weinstein G. Supracricoid partial laryngectomies in the elderly: mortality, complications, and functional outcome. Laryngoscope 1998;108(2):237–242
20. Barzan L, Veronesi A, Caruso G, et al. Head and neck cancer and ageing: a retrospective study in 438 patients. J Laryngol Otol 1990;104(8):634–640
21. Wheless SA, McKinney KA, Zanation AM. A prospective study of the clinical impact of a multidisciplinary head and neck tumor board. Otolaryngol Head Neck Surg 2010;143(5): 650–654
22. The World Health Organization Quality of Life Assessment (WHOQOL): development and general psychometric properties. Soc Sci Med 1998;46(12):1569–1585
23. Cella DF, Cherin EA. Quality of life during and after cancer treatment. Compr Ther 1988;14(5):69–75
24. Kahn SB, Houts PS, Harding SP. Quality of life and patients with cancer: a comparative study of patient versus physician perceptions and its implications for cancer education. J Cancer Educ 1992;7(3):241–249
25. Derks W, De Leeuw JR, Hordijk GJ, Winnubst JA. Elderly patients with head and neck cancer: short-term effects of surgical treatment on quality of life. Clin Otolaryngol Allied Sci 2003;28(5):399–405
26. Silveira AP, Gonçalves J, Sequeira T, et al. Geriatric oncology: comparing health related quality of life in head and neck cancer patients. Head Neck Oncol 2011;3:3
27. Derks W, de Leeuw RJ, Hordijk GJ, Winnubst JA. Quality of life in elderly patients with head and neck cancer one year after diagnosis. Head Neck 2004;26(12):1045–1052

28. van der Schroeff MP, Derks W, Hordijk GJ, de Leeuw RJ. The effect of age on survival and quality of life in elderly head and neck cancer patients: a long-term prospective study. Eur Arch Otorhinolaryngol 2007;264(4):415–422
29. Laraway DC, Lakshmiah R, Lowe D, Roe B, Rogers SN. Quality of life in older people with oral cancer. Br J Oral Maxillofac Surg 2012;50(8):715–720
30. Sarini J, Fournier C, Lefebvre JL, Bonafos G, Van JT, Coche-Dequéant B. Head and neck squamous cell carcinoma in elderly patients: a long-term retrospective review of 273 cases. Arch Otolaryngol Head Neck Surg 2001;127(9):1089–1092
31. Boruk M, Chernobilsky B, Rosenfeld RM, Har-El G. Age as a prognostic factor for complications of major head and neck surgery. Arch Otolaryngol Head Neck Surg 2005;131(7): 605–609
32. Morgan RF, Hirata RM, Jaques DA, Hoopes JE. Head and neck surgery in the aged. Am J Surg 1982;144(4):449–451
33. Sanabria A, Carvalho AL, Vartanian JG, Magrin J, Ikeda MK, Kowalski LP. Comorbidity is a prognostic factor in elderly patients with head and neck cancer. Ann Surg Oncol 2007;14(4):1449–1457
34. Italiano A, Ortholan C, Dassonville O, et al. Head and neck squamous cell carcinoma in patients aged > or = 80 years: patterns of care and survival. Cancer 2008;113(11):3160–3168
35. Genther DJ, Gourin CG. Effect of comorbidity on short-term outcomes and cost of care after head and neck cancer surgery in the elderly. Head Neck 2014. doi: 10.1002/hed.23651. [Epub ahead of print]
36. Kubrak C, Olson K, Jha N, et al. Nutrition impact symptoms: key determinants of reduced dietary intake, weight loss, and reduced functional capacity of patients with head and neck cancer before treatment. Head Neck 2010;32(3):290–300
37. Ottery FD. Rethinking nutritional support of the cancer patient: the new field of nutritional oncology. Semin Oncol 1994;21(6):770–778
38. Lees J. Incidence of weight loss in head and neck cancer patients on commencing radiotherapy treatment at a regional oncology centre. Eur J Cancer Care (Engl) 1999;8(3):133–136
39. Jager-Wittenaar H, Dijkstra PU, Vissink A, van der Laan BF, van Oort RP, Roodenburg JL. Critical weight loss in head and neck cancer—prevalence and risk factors at diagnosis: an explorative study. Support Care Cancer 2007;15(9):1045–1050
40. Wermker K, Jung S, Hüppmeier L, Joos U, Kleinheinz J. Prediction model for early percutaneous endoscopic gastrostomy (PEG) in head and neck cancer treatment. Oral Oncol 2012;48(4):355–360
41. Weinstein GS, Quon H, O'Malley BW Jr, Kim GG, Cohen MA. Selective neck dissection and deintensified postoperative radiation and chemotherapy for oropharyngeal cancer: a subset analysis of the University of Pennsylvania transoral robotic surgery trial. Laryngoscope 2010;120(9):1749–1755
42. Weinstein GS, Quon H, Newman HJ, et al. Transoral robotic surgery alone for oropharyngeal cancer: an analysis of local control. Arch Otolaryngol Head Neck Surg 2012;138(7): 628–634
43. Genden EM, Park R, Smith C, Kotz T. The role of reconstruction for transoral robotic pharyngectomy and concomitant neck dissection. Arch Otolaryngol Head Neck Surg 2011;137(2):151–156
44. Moore EJ, Olsen SM, Laborde RR, et al. Long-term functional and oncologic results of transoral robotic surgery for oropharyngeal squamous cell carcinoma. Mayo Clin Proc 2012;87(3):219–225
45. Sinclair CF, McColloch NL, Carroll WR, Rosenthal EL, Desmond RA, Magnuson JS. Patient-perceived and objective functional outcomes following transoral robotic surgery for early oropharyngeal carcinoma. Arch Otolaryngol Head Neck Surg 2011;137(11):1112–1116
46. Thompson SK, Southern DA, McKinnon JG, Dort JC, Ghali WA. Incidence of perioperative stroke after neck dissection for head and neck cancer: a regional outcome analysis. Ann Surg 2004;239(3):428–431
47. Selim M. Perioperative stroke. N Engl J Med 2007;356(7): 706–713
48. Nosan DK, Gomez CR, Maves MD. Perioperative stroke in patients undergoing head and neck surgery. Ann Otol Rhinol Laryngol 1993;102(9):717–723
49. Atik MA, Ates M, Akkus NI, Altundag O, Altundag K. Preoperative Doppler sonography for prevention of perioperative stroke in head and neck cancer patients undergoing neck dissection: is it beneficial? J Clin Ultrasound 2007;35(1):38–39
50. Rechtweg J, Wax MK, Shah R, Granke K, Jarmuz T. Neck dissection with simultaneous carotid endarterectomy. Laryngoscope 1998;108(8 Pt 1):1150–1153
51. Mortelliti AJ, Malmgren LT, Gacek RR. Ultrastructural changes with age in the human superior laryngeal nerve. Arch Otolaryngol Head Neck Surg 1990;116(9):1062–1069
52. Aviv JE, Martin JH, Jones ME, et al. Age-related changes in pharyngeal and supraglottic sensation. Ann Otol Rhinol Laryngol 1994;103(10):749–752
53. Calhoun KH, Gibson B, Hartley L, Minton J, Hokanson JA. Age-related changes in oral sensation. Laryngoscope 1992; 102(2):109–116
54. Evers BM, Townsend CM Jr, Thompson JC. Organ physiology of aging. Surg Clin North Am 1994;74(1):23–39
55. Alajmo E, Fini-Storchi O, Agostini V, Polli G. Conservation surgery for cancer of the larynx in the elderly. Laryngoscope 1985;95(2):203–205
56. Norton RL, Bernstein RS. Improved LAboratory Prototype ELectrolarynx (LAPEL): using inverse filtering of the frequency response function of the human throat. Ann Biomed Eng 1993;21(2):163–174
57. Mathieson CM, Stam HJ, Scott JP. Psychosocial adjustment after laryngectomy: a review of the literature. J Otolaryngol 1990;19(5):331–336
58. Wei FC, Celik N, Chen HC, Cheng MH, Huang WC. Combined anterolateral thigh flap and vascularized fibula osteoseptocutaneous flap in reconstruction of extensive composite mandibular defects. Plast Reconstr Surg 2002;109(1):45–52
59. Serletti JM, Higgins JP, Moran S, Orlando GS. Factors affecting outcome in free-tissue transfer in the elderly. Plast Reconstr Surg 2000;106(1):66–70
60. Shestak KC, Jones NF, Wu W, Johnson JT, Myers EN. Effect of advanced age and medical disease on the outcome of microvascular reconstruction for head and neck defects. Head Neck 1992;14(1):14–18
61. Coskunfirat OK, Chen HC, Spanio S, Tang YB. The safety of microvascular free tissue transfer in the elderly population. Plast Reconstr Surg 2005;115(3):771–775
62. Ozkan O, Ozgentas HE, Islamoglu K, Boztug N, Bigat Z, Dikici MB. Experiences with microsurgical tissue transfers in elderly patients. Microsurgery 2005;25(5):390–395
63. Beausang ES, Ang EE, Lipa JE, et al. Microvascular free tissue transfer in elderly patients: the Toronto experience. Head Neck 2003;25(7):549–553
64. Furnas H, Canales F, Lineaweaver W, Buncke GM, Alpert BS, Buncke HJ. Microsurgical tissue transfer in patients more than 70 years of age. Ann Plast Surg 1991;26(2):133–139
65. Howard MA, Cordeiro PG, Disa J, et al. Free tissue transfer in the elderly: incidence of perioperative complications following microsurgical reconstruction of 197 septuagenarians and octogenarians. Plast Reconstr Surg 2005;116(6):1659–1668, discussion 1669–1671
66. Kao HK, Chang KP, Ching WC, Tsao CK, Cheng MH, Wei FC. Postoperative morbidity and mortality of head and neck can-

cers in patients with liver cirrhosis undergoing surgical resection followed by microsurgical free tissue transfer. Ann Surg Oncol 2010;17(2):536–543

67. Hightower CE, Riedel BJ, Feig BW, et al. A pilot study evaluating predictors of postoperative outcomes after major abdominal surgery: Physiological capacity compared with the ASA physical status classification system. Br J Anaesth 2010;104(4): 465–471
68. Tsai CH, Chang KP, Hung SY, Chen WF, Cheng MH, Kao HK. Postoperative morbidity in head and neck cancer ablative surgery followed by microsurgical free tissue transfer in the elderly. Oral Oncol 2012;48(9):811–816
69. Blackwell KE, Azizzadeh B, Ayala C, Rawnsley JD. Octogenarian free flap reconstruction: complications and cost of therapy. Otolaryngol Head Neck Surg 2002;126(3):301–306
70. Wester JL, Lindau RH, Wax MK. Efficacy of free flap reconstruction of the head and neck in patients 90 years and older. JAMA Otolaryngol Head Neck Surg 2013;139(1):49–53
71. Taniguchi Y, Okura M. Prognostic significance of perioperative blood transfusion in oral cavity squamous cell carcinoma. Head Neck 2003;25(11):931–936
72. Szakmany T, Dodd M, Dempsey GA, et al. The influence of allogenic blood transfusion in patients having free-flap primary surgery for oral and oropharyngeal squamous cell carcinoma. Br J Cancer 2006;94(5):647–653
73. Barry B, Lucet JC, Kosmann MJ, Gehanno P. Risk factors for surgical wound infections in patients undergoing head and neck oncologic surgery. Acta Otorhinolaryngol Belg 1999; 53(3):241–244
74. Penel N, Lefebvre D, Fournier C, Sarini J, Kara A, Lefebvre JL. Risk factors for wound infection in head and neck cancer surgery: a prospective study. Head Neck 2001;23(6):447–455
75. Wei FC, Jain V, Celik N, Chen HC, Chuang DC, Lin CH. Have we found an ideal soft-tissue flap? An experience with 672 anterolateral thigh flaps. Plast Reconstr Surg 2002;109(7): 2219–2226, discussion 2227–2230
76. Kao HK, Chang KP, Ching WC, Tsao CK, Cheng MH, Wei FC. The impacts of liver cirrhosis on head and neck cancer patients undergoing microsurgical free tissue transfer: an evaluation of flap outcome and flap-related complications. Oral Oncol 2009;45(12):1058–1062
77. Chen KT, Mardini S, Chuang DC, et al. Timing of presentation of the first signs of vascular compromise dictates the salvage outcome of free flap transfers. Plast Reconstr Surg 2007; 120(1):187–195

Trial References for Table 21.1

1. The Department of Veterans Affairs Laryngeal Cancer Study Group. Induction chemotherapy plus radiation compared with surgery plus radiation in patients with advanced laryngeal cancer. N Engl J Med 1991;324(24):1685–1690
2. Forastiere AA, Goepfert H, Maor M, et al. Concurrent chemotherapy and radiotherapy for organ preservation in advanced laryngeal cancer. N Engl J Med 2003;349(22):2091–2098
3. Lefebvre JL, Rolland F, Tesselaar M, et al; EORTC Head and Neck Cancer Cooperative Group; EORTC Radiation Oncology Group. Phase 3 randomized trial on larynx preservation comparing sequential vs alternating chemotherapy and radiotherapy. J Natl Cancer Inst 2009;101(3):142–152
4. Calais G, Alfonsi M, Bardet E, et al. Randomized trial of radiation therapy versus concomitant chemotherapy and radiation therapy for advanced-stage oropharynx carcinoma. J Natl Cancer Inst 1999;91(24):2081–2086
5. Adelstein DJ, Li Y, Adams GL, et al. An intergroup phase III comparison of standard radiation therapy and two schedules of concurrent chemoradiotherapy in patients with unresectable squamous cell head and neck cancer. J Clin Oncol 2003;21(1):92–98
6. Garden AS, Harris J, Vokes EE, et al. Preliminary results of Radiation Therapy Oncology Group 97-03: a randomized phase ii trial of concurrent radiation and chemotherapy for advanced squamous cell carcinomas of the head and neck. J Clin Oncol 2004;22(14):2856–2864
7. Fountzilas G, Ciuleanu E, Dafni U, et al. Concomitant radiochemotherapy vs radiotherapy alone in patients with head and neck cancer: a Hellenic Cooperative Oncology Group Phase III Study. Med Oncol 2004;21(2):95–107
8. Tobias JS, Monson K, Gupta N, et al; UK Head and Neck Cancer Trialists' Group. Chemoradiotherapy for locally advanced head and neck cancer: 10-year follow-up of the UK Head and Neck (UKHAN1) trial. Lancet Oncol 2010;11(1):66–74
9. Bonner JA, Harari PM, Giralt J, et al. Radiotherapy plus cetuximab for squamous-cell carcinoma of the head and neck. N Engl J Med 2006;354(6):567–578
10. Brizel DM, Albers ME, Fisher SR, et al. Hyperfractionated irradiation with or without concurrent chemotherapy for locally advanced head and neck cancer. N Engl J Med 1998; 338(25):1798–1804
11. Jeremic B, Shibamoto Y, Milicic B, et al. Hyperfractionated radiation therapy with or without concurrent low-dose daily cisplatin in locally advanced squamous cell carcinoma of the head and neck: a prospective randomized trial. J Clin Oncol 2000;18(7):1458–1464
12. Staar S, Rudat V, Stuetzer H, et al. Intensified hyperfractionated accelerated radiotherapy limits the additional benefit of simultaneous chemotherapy—results of a multicentric randomized German trial in advanced head-and-neck cancer. Int J Radiat Oncol Biol Phys 2001;50(5):1161–1171
13. Huguenin P, Beer KT, Allal A, et al. Concomitant cisplatin significantly improves locoregional control in advanced head and neck cancers treated with hyperfractionated radiotherapy. J Clin Oncol 2004;22(23):4665–4673
14. Bourhis J, Sire C, Graff P, et al. Concomitant chemoradiotherapy versus acceleration of radiotherapy with or without concomitant chemotherapy in locally advanced head and neck carcinoma (GORTEC 99-02): an open-label phase 3 randomised trial. Lancet Oncol 2012;13(2):145–153
15. Cooper JS, Pajak TF, Forastiere AA, et al; Radiation Therapy Oncology Group 9501/Intergroup. Postoperative concurrent radiotherapy and chemotherapy for high-risk squamous-cell carcinoma of the head and neck. N Engl J Med 2004; 350(19):1937–1944
16. Bernier J, Domenge C, Ozsahin M, et al; European Organization for Research and Treatment of Cancer Trial 22931. Postoperative irradiation with or without concomitant chemotherapy for locally advanced head and neck cancer. N Engl J Med 2004;350(19):1945–1952
17. Racadot S, Mercier M, Dussart S, et al. Randomized clinical trial of post-operative radiotherapy versus concomitant carboplatin and radiotherapy for head and neck cancers with lymph node involvement. Radiother Oncol 2008;87(2):164–172

Appendix [Courtesy of the Washington University School of Medicine; all rights reserved]

IF YOU HAVE QUESTIONS, PLEASE CALL 314-362-7394 AND ASK FOR ASSISTANCE.

Adult Comorbidity Evaluation-27

Identify the important medical comorbidities and grade severity using the index.
Overall Comorbidity Score is defined according to the highest ranked single ailment, except in the case where two or more Grade 2 ailments occur in different organ systems. In this situation, the overall comorbidity score should be designated Grade 3.

Cogent comorbid ailment	Grade 3 Severe Decompensation	Grade 2 Moderate Decompensation	Grade 1 Mild Decompensation
Cardiovascular System			
Myocardial Infarct	☐ MI ≤ 6 months	☐ MI > 6 months ago	☐ MI by ECG only, age undetermined
Angina / Coronary Artery Disease	☐ Unstable angina	☐ Chronic exertional angina ☐ Recent (≤ 6 months) Coronary Artery Bypass Graft (CABG) or Percutaneous Transluminal Coronary Angioplasty (PTCA) ☐ Recent (≤ 6 months) coronary stent	☐ ECG or stress test evidence or catheterization evidence of coronary disease without symptoms ☐ Angina pectoris not requiring hospitalization ☐ CABG or PTCA (>6 mos.) ☐ Coronary stent (>6 mos.)
Congestive Heart Failure (CHF)	☐ Hospitalized for CHF within past 6 months ☐ Ejection fraction < 20%	☐ Hospitalized for CHF >6 months prior ☐ CHF with dyspnea which limits activities	☐ CHF with dyspnea which has responded to treatment ☐ Exertional dyspnea ☐ Paroxysmal Nocturnal Dyspnea (PND)
Arrhythmias	☐ Ventricular arrhythmia ≤ 6 months	☐ Ventricular arrhythmia > 6 months ☐ Chronic atrial fibrillation or flutter ☐ Pacemaker	☐ Sick Sinus Syndrome ☐ Supraventricular tachycardia
Hypertension	☐ DBP≥130 mm Hg ☐ Severe malignant papilledema or other eye changes ☐ Encephalopathy	☐ DBP 115-129 mm Hg ☐ DBP 90-114 mm Hg while taking antihypertensive medications ☐ Secondary cardiovascular symptoms: vertigo, epistaxis, headaches	☐ DBP 90-114 mm Hg while not taking antihypertensive medications ☐ DBP <90 mm Hg while taking antihypertensive medications ☐ Hypertension, not otherwise specified
Venous Disease	☐ Recent PE (≤ 6 mos.) ☐ Use of venous filter for PE's	☐ DVT controlled with Coumadin or heparin ☐ Old PE > 6 months	☐ Old DVT no longer treated with Coumadin or Heparin
Peripheral Arterial Disease	☐ Bypass or amputation for gangrene or arterial insufficiency < 6 months ago ☐ Untreated thoracic or abdominal aneurysm (≥6 cm)	☐ Bypass or amputation for gangrene or arterial insufficiency > 6 months ago ☐ Chronic insufficiency	☐ Intermittent claudication ☐ Untreated thoracic or abdominal aneurysm (< 6 cm) ☐ s/p abdominal or thoracic aortic aneurysm repair
Respiratory System			
	☐ Marked pulmonary insufficiency ☐ Restrictive Lung Disease or COPD with dyspnea at rest despite treatment ☐ Chronic supplemental O_2 ☐ CO_2 retention (pCO_2 > 50 torr) ☐ Baseline pO_2 < 50 torr ☐ FEV1 (< 50%)	☐ Restrictive Lung Disease or COPD (chronic bronchitis, emphysema, or asthma) with dyspnea which limits activities ☐ FEV1 (51%-65%)	☐ Restrictive Lung Disease or COPD (chronic bronchitis, emphysema, or asthma) with dyspnea which has responded to treatment ☐ FEV1 (66%-80%)
Gastrointestinal System			
Hepatic	☐ Portal hypertension and/or esophageal bleeding ≤ 6 mos. (Encephalopathy, Ascites, Jaundice with Total Bilirubin > 2)	☐ Chronic hepatitis, cirrhosis, portal hypertension with moderate symptoms "compensated hepatic failure"	☐ Chronic hepatitis or cirrhosis without portal hypertension ☐ Acute hepatitis without cirrhosis ☐ Chronic liver disease manifested on biopsy or persistently elevated bilirubin (>3 mg/dl)
Stomach / Intestine	☐ Recent ulcers(≤ 6 months ago) requiring blood transfusion	☐ Ulcers requiring surgery or transfusion > 6 months ago	☐ Diagnosis of ulcers treated with meds ☐ Chronic malabsorption syndrome ☐ Inflammatory bowel disease (IBD) on meds or h/o with complications and/or surgery
Pancreas	☐ Acute or chronic pancreatitis with major complications (phlegmon, abscess, or pseudocyst)	☐ Uncomplicated acute pancreatitis ☐ Chronic pancreatitis with minor complications (malabsorption, impaired glucose tolerance, or GI bleeding)	☐ Chronic pancreatitis w/o complications

Cogent comorbid ailment	Grade 3 Severe Decompensation	Grade 2 Moderate Decompensation	Grade 1 Mild Decompensation
Renal System			
End-stage renal disease	☐ Creatinine > 3 mg% with multi-organ failure, shock, or sepsis ☐ Acute dialysis	☐ Chronic Renal Insufficiency with creatinine >3 mg% ☐ Chronic dialysis	☐ Chronic Renal Insufficiency with creatinine 2-3 mg%.
Endocrine System	**(Code the comorbid ailments with the (*) in both the Endocrine system and other organ systems if applicable)**		
Diabetes Mellitus	☐ Hospitalization ≤ 6 months for DKA ☐ Diabetes causing end-organ failure ☐ retinopathy ☐ neuropathy ☐ nephropathy* ☐ coronary disease* ☐ peripheral arterial disease*	☐ IDDM without complications ☐ Poorly controlled AODM with oral agents	☐ AODM controlled by oral agents only
Neurological System			
Stroke	☐ Acute stroke with significant neurologic deficit	☐ Old stroke with neurologic residual	☐ Stroke with no residual ☐ Past or recent TIA
Dementia	☐ Severe dementia requiring full support for activities of daily living	☐ Moderate dementia (not completely self-sufficient, needs supervising)	☐ Mild dementia (can take care of self)
Paralysis	☐ Paraplegia or hemiplegia requiring full support for activities of daily living	☐ Paraplegia or hemiplegia requiring wheelchair, able to do some self care	☐ Paraplegia or hemiplegia, ambulatory and providing most of self care
Neuromuscular	☐ MS, Parkinson's, Myasthenia Gravis, or other chronic neuromuscular disorder and requiring full support for activities of daily living	☐ MS, Parkinson's, Myasthenia Gravis, or other chronic neuromuscular disorder, but able to do some self care	☐ MS, Parkinson's, Myasthenia Gravis, or other chronic neuromuscular disorder, but ambulatory and providing most of self care
Psychiatric			
	☐ Recent suicidal attempt ☐ Active schizophrenia	☐ Depression or bipolar disorder uncontrolled ☐ Schizophrenia controlled w/ meds	☐ Depression or bipolar disorder controlled w/ medication
Rheumatologic	**(Incl. Rheumatoid Arthritis, Systemic Lupus, Mixed Connective Tissue Disorder, Polymyositis, Rheumatic Polymyositis)**		
	☐ Connective Tissue Disorder with secondary end-organ failure (renal, cardiac, CNS)	☐ Connective Tissue Disorder on steroids or immunosuppressant medications	☐ Connective Tissue Disorder on NSAIDS or no treatment
Immunological System	**(AIDS should not be considered a comorbidity for Kaposi's Sarcoma or Non-Hodgkin's Lymphoma)**		
AIDS	☐ Fulminant AIDS w/KS, MAI, PCP (AIDS defining illness)	☐ HIV+ with h/o defining illness. $CD4^{+} < 200/\mu L$	☐ Asymptomatic HIV+ patient. ☐ HIV^{+} w/o h/o AIDS defining illness. $CD4^{+} > 200/\mu L$
Malignancy	**(Excluding Cutaneous Basal Cell Ca., Cutaneous SCCA, Carcinoma in-situ, and Intraepithelial Neoplasm)**		
Solid Tumor including melanoma	☐ Uncontrolled cancer ☐ Newly diagnosed but not yet treated ☐ Metastatic solid tumor	☐ Any controlled solid tumor without documented metastases, but initially diagnosed and treated within the last 5 years	☐ Any controlled solid tumor without documented metastases, but initially diagnosed and treated > 5 years ago
Leukemia and Myeloma	☐ Relapse ☐ Disease out of control	☐ 1st remission or new dx <1yr ☐ Chronic suppressive therapy	☐ H/o leukemia or myeloma with last Rx > 1 yr prior
Lymphoma	☐ Relapse	☐ 1st remission or new dx <1yr ☐ Chronic suppressive therapy	☐ H/o lymphoma w/ last Rx >1 yr prior
Substance Abuse	**(Must be accompanied by social, behavioral, or medical complications)**		
Alcohol	☐ Delirium tremens	☐ Active alcohol abuse with social, behavioral, or medical complications	☐ H/o alcohol abuse but not presently drinking
Illicit Drugs	☐ Acute Withdrawal Syndrome	☐ Active substance abuse with social, behavioral, or medical complications	☐ H/o substance abuse but not presently using
Body Weight			
Obesity		☐ Morbid (i.e., BMI ≥ 38)	

OVERALL COMORBIDITY SCORE (Circle one.)

0	1	2	3	9
None	Mild	Moderate	Severe	Unknown

22 The Role of Neuropsychology in the Evaluation and Treatment of Geriatric Patients

Thomas Swirsky-Sacchetti and Caterina B. Mosti

■ Introduction

What Is Neuropsychological Assessment?

Neuropsychology is the science of brain–behavior relationships. Neuropsychological assessment is the objective measure of brain functioning in which a person's performance is compared with individuals in that person's normative group (i.e., similar age and educational backgrounds). Although brief and/or computerized batteries are now available, a comprehensive battery measures all major domains of neurocognitive functioning, including overall intelligence, learning and memory, expressive and receptive language, sensory and motor function, and complex problem solving/executive function. A good neuropsychological evaluation should also include a measure of personality/emotional functioning. Fixed batteries (e.g., the Halstead–Reitan neuropsychological battery) are becoming less popular in the wake of flexible batteries, in which the test composition is dictated by the particular needs of the patient and the specific referral question. A full comprehensive battery can sometimes require up to 6 hours of testing, but most batteries developed for the geriatric population are of necessity briefer but with every attempt made to evaluate all of the aforementioned cognitive domains to some extent. Although briefer computerized batteries such as ImPACT (ImPACT Applications, Inc., Pittsburgh, PA) have gained popularity in the assessment of sports-related concussions, many of these batteries have limited use with the elderly due to inadequate norms, the inherent discomfort many elderly have with computerized assessment, and the limited ability of the clinician to clearly understand and adequately diagnose the patient's problems with only 20 to 30 minutes' worth of data. Even one of the most widely used neurological screens in clinical practice, the Mini-Mental State Examination (MMSE), has been shown to have limited utility in a white matter dementia,[1] underscoring its limited utility with common forms of dementia, such as vascular dementia, which predominantly affects white matter.

Abbreviated batteries have their utility in a screening capacity, but referral questions are often complicated in the elderly and require "pattern analysis" (i.e., an inspection of the individual's strengths and weaknesses across the aforementioned modalities). These strengths and weaknesses are identified within a context of the patient's overall intelligence and educational/occupational background. For example, one would have higher expectations for someone of superior intelligence, such that even a technically average or low average score on a memory task might have implications for the onset of an incipient dementia. Given the prevalence of depression and other emotional issues in the elderly, the neuropsychologist must also factor in the contribution of emotional variables. This is also done by pattern analysis, wherein various subtypes of dementia present with differing patterns, each of which differ from normal aging changes in the brain and/or a primary emotional etiology. To do pattern analysis, a more comprehensive evaluation covering intelligence, learning and memory, receptive and expressive speech, sensory/motor functions, and executive functions is required.

Neuropsychological Functioning in the Elderly

There are a host of well-documented changes in brain functioning as a result of normal aging. The brain slows in information processing speed and is less adept at "fluid" measures of cognition, which require quick adaptation and adjustment to unfamiliar tasks. In contrast, "crystallized" intelligence, such as one's long-term knowledge base for occupationally related material, vocabulary, or the rules of grammar, may continue to increase with age, depending on one's intellectual curiosity. There is a wide range of normal variation in the cognitive aspects of aging, similar to physical aging, which is why norms based on age and education are crucial in interpretation of testing results.

Mild cognitive impairment (MCI) is defined as the diminution of one domain of cognitive functioning with other domains remaining intact. Subtypes of MCI have been identified, with the amnestic subtype (i.e., predominant memory impairment) being the one subtype more likely to convert to dementia. Petersen et al reported that the prevalence of MCI in a nondemented population of older adults ages 70 to 89 is ~ 16%.[2] Considering that many of these individuals will convert to dementia, the importance of the potential contribution of cognitive issues in the elderly cannot be underestimated. Given increased longevity and better medical treatment, the prevalence of various forms of dementia is increasing.

Dementia is an umbrella term under which many subtypes of cognitive decline may fall. Rates of dementia in those ages 71 and older are at ~ 13.5%. Incidence of dementia among adults ages 71 to 79 falls at ~ 5% but jumps to 37% in adults ages 90 and over.[3] Although Alzheimer disease is perhaps the most widely discussed dementia, there are several other dementia subtypes, including multi-infarct (vascular) dementia, frontotemporal dementia, and subcortical dementias. Alzheimer disease is characterized by progressive and diffuse cognitive decline with prominent memory decline, often without a clearcut onset. Vascular dementia presents with more isolated domains of cognitive impairment, and is usually characterized by deficits in executive functioning with relatively intact aspects of memory. Frontotemporal dementia is characterized by atrophy of the frontal and/or temporal lobes of the brain responsible for planning and judgment and understanding and production of speech, respectively. Hallmark symptoms of frontotemporal dementia can include increasingly erratic or impulsive behavior, which may be the first signs of a problem, as well as changes in language. Subcortical dementias, such as those associated with Parkinson and Huntington diseases, tend to result in slower speed of processing or inability to initiate activities and are in contrast to the forgetfulness or language difficulties associated with cortical dementias (e.g., Alzheimer disease).

The most common form of dementia is Alzheimer disease. Most agree that histopathologically confirmed Alzheimer disease constitutes around 45% of the dementia population, with vascular dementia, representing roughly another 25%. Of course, these two forms are not mutually exclusive and can co-occur in roughly another 20%. Frontotemporal dementia, with an estimated prevalence rate between 2 and 15%,[4] and Parkinson dementia, estimated to affect less than 1% of adults ages 65 and older,[5] are some of the more common "rare" dementias.

Neuropsychological assessment is useful in helping to differentially diagnose normal aging and the dementias, documenting response to treatment, helping the patient/family with decisions regarding needed level of care, and setting up appropriate expectations for the patient (i.e., determining if the patient is capable of managing finances or driving an automobile).

Cognitive Rehabilitation with the Elderly

Cognitive rehabilitation refers to any activity designed to improve cognitive functioning. Li et al[6] and Reijnders et al[7] provide excellent reviews on cognitive interventions in older adults, those with MCI, and even those with mild dementia. The use of computerized brain training programs and video games to stimulate brain functioning in the elderly is becoming more popular, although more research is needed to objectively measure any beneficial effects. There is increasing research support for using various cognitive interventions in the elderly population,[8] with more success obviously realized in those with MCI or mild dementia as opposed to moderate–severe dementia groups. Rehearsal-based techniques for memory enhancement have demonstrated efficacy. Compensatory techniques take two forms (i.e., external and internal). External compensatory techniques simply change or rearrange the environment with the use of external crutches, so that the same function (e.g., remembering tomorrow's appointment), is done with the use of a crutch (e.g., a calendar notebook or smart phone). Internal compensatory strategies involve rehearsal based strategies or to using different physiological pathways to accomplish the same task in an effort to avoid or to minimize reliance on dysfunctional areas. Multimodal imprinting is the technique of using more than one sensory modality for memory encoding (e.g., a list of shopping items can be encoded by auditory verbal rehearsal or by forming a mental picture of those items on the checkout counter) thereby using vastly different brain regions.

Neuropsychology and Presbycusis

One illustrative example of the intersection between neuropsychology and geriatric otolaryngology is presbycusis, which will be treated in more detail because there is a growing body of evidence supporting the association between presbycusis and cognitive decline in the elderly.[9,10] In evaluating the potential contributing factors of brain involvement in presbycusis, it is not just the assessment of receptive (and expressive) language that is more germane to central presbycusis, but also the assessment of other brain functions such as memory, executive functions, and processing speed, which are increasingly seen to be not only relevant, but of crucial importance in diagnosis and treatment.

It is increasingly clear that the comprehensive evaluation and treatment of older adults with presbycusis is based on a model in which several levels of etiology, such as peripheral functioning, central auditory processing, and cognitive functioning, are included.[11] Some prefer a simplified classification system of peripheral versus central etiologies. Central presbycusis has been defined by Humes et al as "age related changes in the auditory portions of the central nervous system negatively impacting auditory perception, speech-communication performance, or both."[9] Humes et al studied older and young adults, the vast majority (90%) of whom had not worn hearing aids.[9] They administered 6 cognitive measures, 17 psychophysiological measures, and 9 different measures of speech understanding. Of the 12 measures in which older adults performed significantly worse than younger adults, 6 were cognitive measures. This further underscores the importance of considering cognitive functioning in working with the elderly with presbycusis. Pichora-Fuller and Singh noted two conceptual models for describing the relationship between cognitive and central auditory processing components with peripheral etiologies, and argue for an integration of these models.[12] The "site of lesion" approach holds that distinct anatomical sites are organized hierarchically from the bottom up (i.e., peripheral, central auditory processing, and cognitive processes, respectively). This system has proven useful for differential diagnosis of conductive, sensorineural, retrocochlear, or central hearing loss. However, Pichora-Fuller and Singh argue that this schema doesn't account for overlapping systems, which are guided by afferent encoding as well as efferent feedback. The other model described is a "processing view" model, in which a bidirectional influence and the interaction of lower-level sensory and higher-level cognitive processes is the schema for understanding the functions of hearing, listening, comprehension, and communication. The processing view model necessitates the involvement of cognitive functions of attention and memory as well as language. The authors argue that understanding how sensory and cognitive domains interact is an important precursor to remediation. Pichora-Fuller and Singh also include the role of social-emotional factors because both perceptual stressors (noise) and cognitive stressors (memory loss) can affect the social well-being.[13] Cox et al also highlight the importance of the emotional functioning of the older individual, which can have a reverberating effect on the perceived success of treatment.[14]

Cognitive Domains of Importance in Presbycusis

Whereas one can argue that all domains of cognitive and emotional functioning are relevant to the evaluation and treatment of presbycusis, the areas of attention, memory, and executive function have thus far been most researched.

The role of attention takes on more salience as one moves from the relatively artificial context of listening to one stimulus source in a quiet background to the more realistic, everyday-life. Inunctional hearing required in noisy environments with more than one source of speech or other competing demands, the listener has to focus not only on the "what" of speech but also on the "where" and sometimes the "when."[12] Selective attention refers to focusing on one source of stimuli and inhibiting others. Alain and Woods demonstrated that older adults' difficulty hearing in a noisy context may reflect a decline in the ability to inhibit irrelevant stimuli.[15] Divided attention refers to the allocation of attentional resources to more than one stimuli simultaneously, a common demand of daily life (e.g., listening to a phone message and writing down salient notes as a reminder). When hearing-impaired listeners were required to perform two tasks simultaneously, Rakerd et al found that listening to speech was especially effortful.[16] The brain regions subserved by attention depend somewhat on the type of sensory stimulation that is involved, although most would agree that the bilateral frontal lobes play a major role in the regulation of attention and the inhibition of distracting factors. Neuropsychological testing of attention includes both visual and auditory attention, as well as tasks with varying demands (e.g., divided attention, alternating attention, sustained attention, and attention with simultaneous competing demands).

Memory is perhaps the most researched of all cognitive domains. Comprehension of lengthy speech passages is aided and abetted by recall on the initial portions of the passage. There are many schemata for organizing this complex brain function. A temporal dimension of immediate recall, delayed recall, and remote recall can be used to characterize a memory task. Another aspect of memory depends on whether something is consciously or unconsciously learned. Explicit memory refers to recall of material that you consciously intend to remember (e.g., information from this chapter or tomorrow's appointments). Implicit memory refers to unconsciously learned memory or learning of skills and habits, although one may not be able to recall the exact time and place of acquiring a particular skill (e.g., how to use a hammer). The memory task can also be conceptualized according to whether the individual has to produce the stimuli or simply to recognize them from among confederates. Recognition memory may be significantly better in someone who is encoding the memory but has difficulty with retrieval or recall. Cued recall (e.g., providing the first sound of the word to be remembered), is another way to differentiate between encoding and retrieval problems. Memory, especially explicit memory, relies heavily on the hippocampal regions of the mesial temporal lobes. However, as the complexity of the task increases (e.g., learning a long list of words), frontal lobe resources are also used.[17] The assessment of memory is often the most time-consuming portion of a neuropsychological battery and is especially important in differential diagnosis of normal aging, mild cognitive impairment, and various dementing conditions. Memory of material presented aurally, visually, and through the tactile modality is tested for immediate recall and delayed recall, with a variety of cueing and recognition trials clarifying the distinction between encoding versus retrieval problems. Gates et al aimed to measure central auditory processing across three groups of older adults—those without memory impairment, those with mild memory impairment, and those diagnosed with dementia.[18] They found that central auditory processing worsened across memory impairment groups, even after controlling for age and peripheral hearing loss. These findings suggest that memory may adversely impact central auditory processing in the elderly independent of sensorineural hearing loss.[18]

Working memory refers to holding information in a temporary store long enough to perform some action with it, such as writing down a confirmation number or transferring an appointment date to a calendar. It is considered by most to be one type of executive function. Discourse processing has been studied using the working memory model posited by Baddeley.[19] Information initially heard is held in a temporary store long enough for it to be processed on a deeper level, and this is done quickly enough for the next cluster of information to be heard. When information is presented too quickly, the working memory demands of the elderly may be overloaded due to normal aging changes in processing speed. Similarly, when sensory information is presented in a degraded form due to peripheral issues, the working memory system may be overstressed and may break down. Erb and Obleser examined neural speech processing in a group of older adults with varying levels of sensorineural hearing loss as well as younger adults.[20] Their findings indicated that both young and older adults had similar levels of behavioral adaptation to degraded speech stimuli. However, older adults with increased levels of hearing loss demonstrated greater activation of the anterior cingulate cortex as well as the middle frontal gyrus for speech comprehension.[20] Recently, researchers aimed to investigate the relationship between executive function and hearing loss in a nationally representative sample of older adults. A subset ($n = 605$) of older adults ages 60 to 69 from the National Health and National Examination Health Survey was administered the Digit Symbol Substitution Test (DSST)—a subtest from the Wechsler Adult Intelligence Scale (WAIS-IV) used to measure executive function and psychomotor speed—in addition to standardized audiometric testing.[21] Results of this study indicated a significant negative association between hearing loss and cognitive function among older adults, even after controlling for several demographic and cardiovascular factors (diabetes, smoking, hypertension, stroke).[21] The magnitude of the reduction in cognitive performance was associated with a 25 dB hearing loss and an age equivalent of 7 years. Importantly, hearing aid use was associated with higher DSST scores. However, future studies should aim to replicate this finding, because only 13 hearing aid participants were included in this group.[21] Lin et al extended these findings by analyzing the relationship between a more comprehensive neurocognitive battery and audiometric testing in another nationally representative sample of adults over the age of 55.[22] Participants were administered tests of mental state (MMSE), memory (Free and Cued Selective Remind Test [FCSRT]), executive function/attention (Trail Making Test B, Stroop Mixed), psychomotor and processing speed (Trail Making Test A, Stroop Color and Word Naming), and verbal ability (Category and Letter Fluency, American Version of the Nelson Adult Reading Test [AMNART]). After adjusting for age, sex, education, diabetes, smoking, and hypertension, hearing loss was significantly associated with lower scores on the MMSE, memory free recall, and Stroop mixed. Associations between Trails A and B approached statistical significance. Thus the associations between hearing loss and memory and executive function were stronger than those between hearing loss and measures of verbal ability or processing speed.[22]

Similar findings have been reported, even in mixed samples of older adults with and without memory loss and dementia. Gates et al administered an extended audiological battery and executive function testing to a mixed sample of both healthy and memory-impaired older adults ($n = 313$).[23] The audiological battery consisted of several tests, including (1) peripheral audition, (2) auditory-evoked potentials, and (3) central auditory tests including Synthetic Sentence Identification with Ipsilateral Competing Message, Dichotic Sentence Identification, and Dichotic Digits. Executive functioning testing consisted of the Trail Making Test, Clock Drawing, Stroop Color and Word Naming, and subtests from the Cognitive Abilities Screening instrument to measure mental concentration.[23] Importantly, an executive functioning composite score was significantly associated with all three measures of central auditory processing but not with primary auditory pathway measures. The Trail Making Test Part B, aimed to measure mental set shifting and mental flexibility, was most strongly associated with auditory outcomes.[23]

Neuroanatomical Support of Central Presbycusis

Neuropsychological research has increasingly used structural and other imaging measures in addition to traditional paper-and-pencil tests. With the increased use of functional magnetic resonance imaging (fMRI), diffusion tensor imaging (DTI), and other advanced brain imaging techniques, there is a growing body of literature suggesting neuroanatomical changes associated with hearing loss. Although imaging research has traditionally focused on deficits in the primary auditory cortex located within the temporal lobe of the brain in regard to presbycusis, newer research suggests that changes in brain morphology associated with hearing loss may be more widespread than previously hypothesized.

Hwang et al compared fMRI findings of 12 healthy elderly and 12 young adults.[24] Their findings included reported lower activation of the auditory cortex, particularly in the anterior and posterior regions of the superior temporal gyrus (STG), in older adults while listening to speech sounds. These effects were amplified when older adults were required to listen to speech in noise. Of note, there was a marked decrease in activation of the posterior region of the STG, suggesting that functional changes associated with central presbycusis may start in this region.[24] Eckert et al employed factor analysis to divide hearing metrics into high- and low-frequency sounds among a sample of 49 older adults.[25] High-frequency hearing loss, generally found among those advanced in age, was associated with decreased gray matter in the auditory cortex and increased cerebrospinal fluid. These findings suggest atrophy of the auditory cortex with increased hearing loss. Eckert et al indicate that further research is needed to investigate whether there are specific subtypes of hearing loss (e.g., low frequency vs. high frequency) that may be more strongly associated with central presbycusis.

In addition to morphological changes within the temporal lobe, recent research suggests that presbycusis may be associated with changes in several regions of the brain. Boyen et al used voxel-based morphometry (VBM) to investigate morphological differences between those with hearing loss and those with hearing loss and tinnitus.[26] Compared with the hearing loss group, the tinnitus group had greater gray matter in the superior and medial temporal lobes. Interestingly, hearing loss as well as tinnitus was associated with decreased volume in the frontal and occipital lobes.[26] Similarly, Wong et al's study reported that larger and thicker prefrontal cortex volume was associated with better speech perception in older adults, but not in younger adults.[27] The authors concluded that better prefrontal cortex functioning may facilitate speech perception in the elderly and supports the "decline-compensation" hypothesis, which posits that decline in sensory processing abilities due to aging can be accompanied by use of more general cognitive areas as a method of compensation.

Unlike the Wong et al study, Profant et al were unable to replicate findings suggesting involvement of the frontal lobe in presbycusis.[28] Their study included comparison groups of young adults and two groups of older adults with expressed and mild presbycusis. Overall, older adults had less gray matter than young adults. Those with *all* levels of presbycusis had decreased volume of the Heschl gyrus and decreased thickness of the planum temporale. Interestingly, research indicates no abnormal auditory cortex morphology in young adults with congenital deafness,[29] suggesting a neuroanatomical component to presbycusis in the elderly. Increased white matter in the temporal lobe and increased radial vectors under the Heschl gyrus—both associated with neural degradation—were also found among the presbycusis groups, indicating a role of the central auditory processing cortex in central hearing loss.

The practical implications of integrating neuropsychological assessment into geriatric otolaryngology are widespread and extend beyond routine auditory testing. Clinicians need to take cognitive factors into account when working with this population and understand that impairments may extend beyond obvious sensory deficits.

The Evaluation of Surgical Patients

Another important role for the neuropsychologist is in the evaluation of surgical patients. The American College of Surgeons in collaboration with the American Geriatric Society recently issued best practice guidelines for working with geriatric patients.[30] Among the 13 important areas cited by the authors as requiring preoperative assessment in geriatric patients were cognitive impairment/dementia and decision-making capacity. The authors recommended that, even for patients without a known history of cognitive impairment or dementia, a detailed history and cognitive assessment be strongly recommended. This is particularly important because a patient and/or family caregiver may not realize the presence of cognitive impairment and may simply attribute it to normal aging. The patient and/or family may also be in denial of fairly serious cognitive issues for a variety of reasons. The presence of cognitive impairments may interfere with the patient's ability to understand the purpose of and the likely outcomes of the planned surgical procedure, and may clearly interfere with the capacity to make informed decisions. Neuropsychological testing can also be helpful in determining these capacities in patients with a clearly established diagnosis of mild cognitive impairment or dementia. It is important to remember that, given varying levels of dementia severity, even a diagnosis of dementia does not automatically preclude the patient's ability to understand the purpose of a planned surgery and the likely outcomes. The best practice guidelines also note the importance of documenting preoperative cognitive status because postoperative cognitive dysfunction is common but difficult to evaluate objectively without the record of baseline cognitive status.

Depression should also be assessed preoperatively according to the best practice guidelines. As noted earlier, depression can often masquerade as an organic cognitive issue (i.e., pseudodementia). The role of depression in predicting surgical outcome has been well established in several medical specialties. Rosenberger et al found in a meta-analysis that depression and other psychosocial factors (e.g., social support) played a significant role in recovery and were predictive of surgical outcome even after accounting for relevant clinical variables.[31] Smith et al reported that depression was one of the strongest predictors of poor outcome following endoscopic sinus surgery for chronic rhinosinusitis.[32] A comprehensive neuropsychological evaluation will assess for depression in the elderly patient, and contextualize findings on objective measures suitable for use in this population. Some popular depression measures that include common somatic symptoms of depression may overinflate a normal older patient's depression score. Contextualization is of vital importance in understanding depression and what to do about it. An older patient may have a "reactive" depression in the context of just having lost a spouse or loss of independence/function. In this case, supportive psychotherapy might be the best treatment recommendation, whereas medication may be more appropriate for someone with a long-standing history of depression without clearcut precipitating factors.

Concussion and Mild Head Injury

Elderly patients are more at risk for falls due to a variety of medical issues, which places them at greater risk for concussion and closed head injury. Among the most common physical symptoms of concussion are dizziness and tinnitus, and the elderly are more vulnerable to persistent symptoms in these areas, as well as in cognitive areas,[33] perhaps due to lack of "cognitive reserve." Research indicates that anywhere from 23 to 81% of concussion patients report dizziness within the first few days of head injury; however, the literature also suggests that symptoms of dizziness can persist several years postinjury.[34] Dizziness may be due to peripheral vestibular injuries or to structural damage within the brain, including diffuse axonal injury or contusion to the brainstem and/or cerebellum.[35] Likewise, postconcussive symptoms such as migraines or anxiety may contribute to or exacerbate symptoms of dizziness in postconcussive patients.[35] Elderly patients presenting with dizziness or tinnitus should be carefully screened for a history of fall(s) even if not accompanied by a direct blow to the head or loss of consciousness. Referral for neuropsychological testing can help in determining the nature and extent of any persistent concussion-related cognitive deficits and how these are distinguished from normal aging or dementia. These deficits may coexist with dizziness, tinnitus, or other physical postconcussion symptoms and may certainly complicate treatment of the latter. Treatment for any concussion-related emotional changes (e.g., depression, irritability, anger management issues) as well as cognitive rehabilitation for the cognitive issues will have a beneficial effect on the patient's ability to understand and follow through with a treatment protocol.

Clinical Implications

Neuropsychological assessment of elderly patients is increasingly vital to accurate diagnosis and treatment of a variety of ear, nose, and throat patients. There exist several easily accessible cognitive measures aimed to assess gross cognitive function in patients at little to no cost to the clinician that would be appropriate for use as gross screening measures. Likewise, they are simple to administer and interpret and thus are appropriate for all levels of familiarity with neuropsychological impairment. For example, one study found that administration of a simple letter–number sequencing task aided clinicians in detecting speech recognition deficits.[36] However, if frank cognitive deficits are apparent or if patients have difficulty with a screening measure, clinicians should refer patients for a more thorough neuropsychological examination. Emotional functioning is equally an important consideration because this has been shown to affect how older individuals adjust to, comply with, and rate satisfaction with treatment. The clinician who senses that depression and anxiety or issues of social isolation are at play should make referrals to a mental health professional for further evaluation and treatment.

Importantly, there exist several compensatory strategies aimed to reduce cognitive impairments among the elderly. These methods, including rehearsal-based strategies to improve memory and reliance on external aids such as memory notebooks or calendars, have been shown to be of use in memory-impaired older adults. Such interventions may also be useful in treating older adults presenting to the ear, nose, and throat specialist who exhibit some cognitive deficits. In particular, those with central auditory processing disorders may benefit from computer-based training programs or other newer cognitive rehabilitation efforts[37]; however, future research is needed to establish their utility in this population.

References

1. Swirsky-Sacchetti T, Field HL, Mitchell DR, et al. The sensitivity of the Mini-Mental State Exam in the white matter dementia of multiple sclerosis. J Clin Psychol 1992;48(6):779–786
2. Petersen RC, Roberts RO, Knopman DS, et al; The Mayo Clinic Study of Aging. Prevalence of mild cognitive impairment is higher in men. Neurology 2010;75(10):889–897
3. Plassman BL, Langa KM, Fisher GG, et al. Prevalence of dementia in the United States: the aging, demographics, and memory study. Neuroepidemiology 2007;29(1-2):125–132
4. Onyike CU, Diehl-Schmid J. The epidemiology of frontotemporal dementia. Int Rev Psychiatry 2013;25(2):130–137
5. Aarsland D, Zaccai J, Brayne C. A systematic review of prevalence studies of dementia in Parkinson's disease. Mov Disord 2005;20(10):1255–1263
6. Li H, Li J, Li N, Li B, Wang P, Zhou T. Cognitive intervention for persons with mild cognitive impairment: A meta-analysis. Ageing Res Rev 2011;10(2):285–296
7. Reijnders J, van Heugten C, van Boxtel M. Cognitive interventions in healthy older adults and people with mild cognitive impairment: a systematic review. Ageing Res Rev 2013; 12(1):263–275
8. Hampstead BM, Mosti CB, Swirsky-Sacchetti T, Cognitively-based methods of enhancing and maintaining functioning in those at risk for Alzheimer's disease. J Alzheimers Dis 2014 Aug 11. [Epub ahead of print]
9. Humes LE, Dubno JR, Gordon-Salant S, et al. Central presbycusis: a review and evaluation of the evidence. J Am Acad Audiol 2012;23(8):635–666
10. Parham K, Lin FR, Coelho DH, Sataloff RT, Gates GA. Comprehensive management of presbycusis: central and peripheral. Otolaryngol Head Neck Surg 2013;148(4):537–539
11. Committee on Hearing, Bioacoustics, and Biomechanics (CHABA). Speech understanding and aging. J Acoust Soc Am 1988;83:859–895
12. Pichora-Fuller MK, Singh G. Effects of age on auditory and cognitive processing: implications for hearing aid fitting and audiologic rehabilitation. Trends Amplif 2006;10(1):29–59
13. Pichora-Fuller MK. Cognitive aging and auditory information processing. Int J Audiol 2003;42(Suppl 2):S26–S32
14. Cox RM, Alexander GC, Gray G. Personality and the subjective assessment of hearing aids. J Am Acad Audiol 1999;10(1): 1–13
15. Alain C, Woods DL. Age-related changes in processing auditory stimuli during visual attention: evidence for deficits in inhibitory control and sensory memory. Psychol Aging 1999; 14(3):507–519
16. Rakerd B, Seitz PF, Whearty M. Assessing the cognitive demands of speech listening for people with hearing losses. Ear Hear 1996;17(2):97–106
17. Swirsky-Sacchetti T, Mitchell DR, Seward J, et al. Neuropsychological and structural brain lesions in multiple sclerosis: a regional analysis. Neurology 1992;42(7):1291–1295
18. Gates GA, Anderson ML, Feeney MP, McCurry SM, Larson EB. Central auditory dysfunction in older persons with memory impairment or Alzheimer dementia. Arch Otolaryngol Head Neck Surg 2008;134(7):771–777
19. Baddeley A. The episodic buffer: a new component of working memory? Trends Cogn Sci 2000;4(11):417–423
20. Erb J, Obleser J. Upregulation of cognitive control networks in older adults' speech comprehension. Front Syst Neurosci 2013;7:116
21. Lin FR. Hearing loss and cognition among older adults in the United States. J Gerontol A Biol Sci Med Sci 2011;66(10): 1131–1136
22. Lin FR, Ferrucci L, Metter EJ, An Y, Zonderman AB, Resnick SM. Hearing loss and cognition in the Baltimore Longitudinal Study of Aging. Neuropsychology 2011;25(6):763–770
23. Gates GA, Gibbons LE, McCurry SM, Crane PK, Feeney MP, Larson EB. Executive dysfunction and presbycusis in older persons with and without memory loss and dementia [published correction available in Cogn Behav Neurol. 2011;24(1):39. Note: McCusrry, Susan M corrected to McCurry, Susan M]. Cogn Behav Neurol 2010;23(4):218–223
24. Hwang JH, Li CW, Wu CW, Chen JH, Liu TC. Aging effects on the activation of the auditory cortex during binaural speech listening in white noise: an fMRI study. Audiol Neurootol 2007;12(5):285–294
25. Eckert MA, Cute SL, Vaden KI Jr, Kuchinsky SE, Dubno JR. Auditory cortex signs of age-related hearing loss. J Assoc Res Otolaryngol 2012;13(5):703–713
26. Boyen K, Langers DRM, de Kleine E, van Dijk P. Gray matter in the brain: differences associated with tinnitus and hearing loss. Hear Res 2013;295:67–78
27. Wong PCM, Ettlinger M, Sheppard JP, Gunasekera GM, Dhar S. Neuroanatomical characteristics and speech perception in noise in older adults. Ear Hear 2010;31(4):471–479
28. Profant O, Škoch A, Balogová Z, Tintěra J, Hlinka J, Syka J. Diffusion tensor imaging and MR morphometry of the central auditory pathway and auditory cortex in aging. Neuroscience 2014;260:87–97
29. Penhune VB, Cismaru R, Dorsaint-Pierre R, Petitto LA, Zatorre RJ. The morphometry of auditory cortex in the congenitally deaf measured using MRI. Neuroimage 2003;20(2): 1215–1225
30. Chow W, Rosenthal RA, Merkow RP, Ko CY, Esnaola NF; American College of Surgeons National Surgical Quality Improvement Program; American Geriatrics Society. Optimal preoperative assessment of the geriatric surgical patient: a best practices

guideline from the American College of Surgeons National Surgical Quality Improvement Program and the American Geriatrics Society. J Am Coll Surg 2012;215(4):453–466

31. Rosenberger PH, Jokl P, Ickovics J. Psychosocial factors and surgical outcomes: an evidence-based literature review. J Am Acad Orthop Surg 2006;14(7):397–405
32. Smith TL, Mendolia-Loffredo S, Loehrl TA, Sparapani R, Laud PW, Nattinger AB. Predictive factors and outcomes in endoscopic sinus surgery for chronic rhinosinusitis. Laryngoscope 2005;115(12):2199–2205
33. Shapiro S, Swirsky-Sacchetti T. Neuropsychological deficits in minor head injury. In: Mandel S, Sataloff R, Shapiro S, eds. Minor Head Trauma. New York, NY: Springer; 1993:86–106
34. Alsalaheen BA, Mucha A, Morris LO, et al. Vestibular rehabilitation for dizziness and balance disorders after concussion. J Neurol Phys Ther 2010;34(2):87–93
35. Fife TD, Giza C. Posttraumatic vertigo and dizziness. Semin Neurol 2013;33(3):238–243
36. Vaughan N, Storzbach D, Furukawa I. Investigation of potential cognitive tests for use with older adults in audiology clinics. J Am Acad Audiol 2008;19(7):533–541, quiz 579–580
37. Gates GA. Central presbycusis: an emerging view. Otolaryngol Head Neck Surg 2012;147(1):1–2

Index

Note: Page numbers followed by f or t indicate figures or tables, respectively.

T

U

V

W

X

Z